W9-AEO-614

Dedication

The Phoenix rises out of the ashes of all those who have died in the name of human rights and particularly all those millions of unknown saints and martyrs who have suffered torture, pain, brutal imprisonment and who now lie quiet beneath the earth.

Let them now rise with one voice and cry to the hearts of living men and women that they too may make the right of self-determination and freedom of mind and body into a flaming torch of the human spirit.

This book is dedicated to those who will carry this torch of the spirit through the generations of a coming higher evolution. To them I give the name of genius. Whether president or peasant, whether mother or son, they are the real heroes of life.

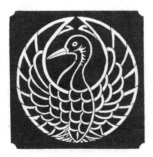

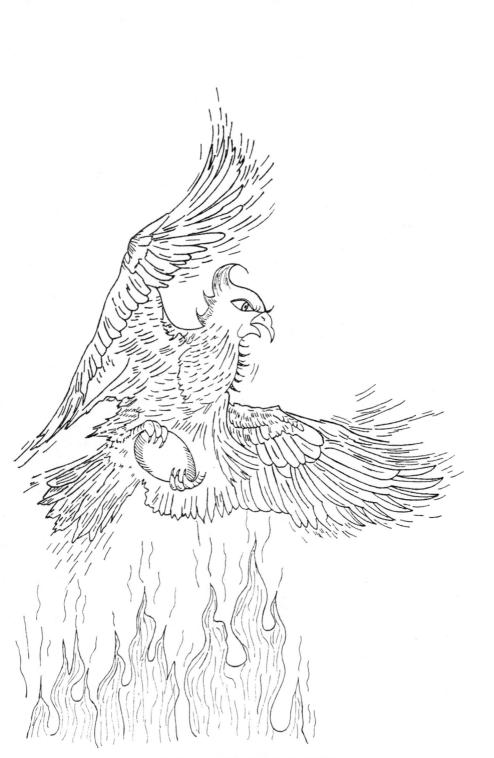

THE PHOENIX

THE PHOENIX

The Phoenix is a very mythical bird and I doubt if anyone in history has ever seen one. As a symbol it represents that soaring of the human spirit which at certain times in history signifies the dying of an old order and the birth of a New Age. The ancient Chinese described the bird to be like an eagle with a brilliant scarlet and gold plumage. They said that the dying Phoenix flies to the city of the sun and immolates itself on the altar in the temple of the sun. Out of the ashes of its own funeral pyre springs the new Phoenix from the flames. Taking its father's ashes and embalming them in an egg of aromatic frankincense and myrrh, the Phoenix rises once again on its long journey across the world to the temple of the sun. Its coloring of scarlet and gold, its miraculous rebirth and its connection with the primordial fire of the sun was meant to be a symbol of the birth of the universe itself. As a symbol of eternal birth and rebirth the Phoenix stands for immortality and life after death in the early Christian cultures, but in ancient Egypt, Arabia and India, in Japan, Greece, Mexico and in China, this universally-acclaimed bird symbolized not only life after life but the eternal passing of the old age into the new.

The Phoenix is always associated with the worship of light in all the world's cultures. Its age varies from the Egyptian estimate of 1,461 years to the Hindu 97,200 years. As a symbol of eternal life it spread to Rome so that the Phoenix appears on the coinage of the Holy Roman Empire as a symbol of the eternal city. The Christian church fathers adopted the Phoenix as an illustration of the resurrection of Christ. The eagle was adopted by the founders of the United States as a national symbol of freedom with upswept wings because the eagle is said to resemble the Phoenix in size. The German eagle, representing mastery and empire of earth, is seated with its wings down by its side symbolizing the earthbound power of the solid germanic character and was chosen to represent the glorious birth of a master race.

And what of our supersensitive modern age? With our sensors stretching to the outermost edge of the mysterious universe, what will the modern Phoenix see with its eagle eye as it rises from the ashes of a world destroyed by its own egocentric drives for power and selfish ambition? The Phoenix lives and dies and rises in everyone and its vision of the world to come is our own vision of the limits of the universe. The Phoenix flies off the outermost edge of the universe along the rays of our radiotelescopes and dies only to return back into our eyes as consciousness. The Phoenix lives long and patiently in the human prison which limits our vision until it flies off to return like an echo of some long distant memory.

Perhaps the Phoenix is calling us with a sweet melodious voice but does anyone hear its music? There are many who crave to hear that melody that is heard only with the inner ear. This book is written for those who have not lost the ability to listen, who still have the vision of the Phoenix and can look directly from its eyelids at the unfolding world mirrored in our own consciousness. And what if we cannot see? The beauty of the immortal world can only be real if we can see through the ugliness of the world. If we can fly with the Phoenix into the heart of the sun we will see nothing but the dazzling beauty of its light. But how many want to fly into the sun? Only the ONE—the Phoenix—the rising Self.

THE GREAT SEAL OF THE UNITED STATES

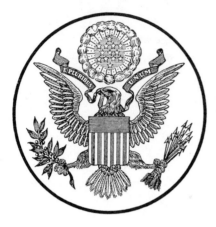 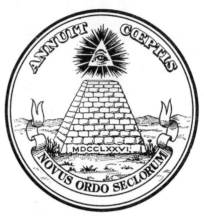

From Hunt's *History of the Seal of the United States.*

The bald eagle, emblem of America found on every dollar on one side of the Great Seal of the United States, has its wings in upward mode of flight, "on wing and rising" instead of "displayed", representing the Phoenix soaring towards the stars and the sun. The bald eagle was not named for a bald head, which it does not have, but the name comes from its pure white head and neck feathers which contrast with its brown body. Symbolizing the effortless mastery of the air (spirit) and the majesty of its stately flight and keen vision (perception), it was picked after the founding fathers in 1776 had already chosen the Phoenix. But because the seal was several years in preparation and went through three committees of Congress until 1782 and several cuttings of dies until 1904, the final form was an adaption to the American eagle. The founding fathers, who were Freemasons, placed an olive branch in its right talon and a bunch of arrows in its left. This symbol of the rising Phoenix grasping in its claws both the olive branch of peace and the arrows of power, flies upwards with a trailing ribbon in its beak on which we find the words, "Out of many one people".

The first Great Seal of the United States (1782) was designed by William Barton with a different bird's head altogether, representing a Phoenix. The neck was much larger and there was a tuft of feathers at the back of the head quite different from the eagle which appears on the Great Seal of 1904. The founders were eager for it to be a Phoenix. Its body was much larger and thinner and the beak did not resemble that of an eagle. Benjamin Franklin declared the eagle was an unworthy bird to be chosen as the emblem because it did not have a good moral character. Its later adaption upon the second design of the Great Seal is really as a conventionalized Phoenix, symbolizing the regeneration of creative energy. The unfinished pyramid on the reverse side shows the eye of God as the capstone representing the light of consciousness. The words

GOD FAVORS OUR UNDERTAKING,

A NEW ORDER OF THE AGES

are obvious references to the rising of a New Age of consciousness as the primary reality. The symbol represents the coming together of consciousness and concrete matter. This reality of science and spirit means the discovery not only of the sensory phenomena experienced by the brain and body but also the process of observation and understanding of consciousness.

THE SYMBOL OF NUCLEAR EVOLUTION

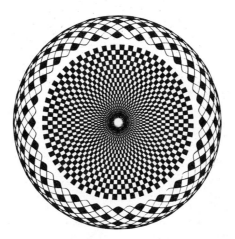

THE GREAT SEAL OF THE COSMOS !

The Creative Spirit of the almighty ONE abides at rest in silence in the void at the Center. It proceeds in expression by moving in three ways simultaneously:

★ Inwards from periphery to point (creating involution)—*Gravity*

★ Outwards from point to periphery (creating evolution)—*Light*

★ Spirally (creating growth)—
  Synthesis

Ultimately it returns to a state of rest, or equilibrium, at the Center, enriched by experience through contrast between Light and darkness.

The concentric circles in this symbol represent both the peripheral radiations of potential moving inwards, so that they create a boundless space within the center and the outward-moving waves of radial energy emanating from the center. The resultant pattern gives a visual representation of the movement, or Life, of the Creative Spirit and the spiral motion inherent in it.

The inner concentric circles represent the spheres of consciousness of the inner life, and the outer concentric circles represent the spheres of consciousness of the outer life. The boundary where they meet represents the surface, or limit, separating the inner from the outer life of each individual, which is the seat of consciousness and the region of creative activity. The white spot in the center represents the Light of the inner spark of life that resides within the core of every being, the white hole that is each individual's link with the Absolute.

When all gaps in consciousness are filled, and all these spheres of consciousness are fully developed and integrated into a unity, full enlightenment is attained, and Cosmic Consciousness is achieved.

The circular surround symbolizes the network of creative thought arising from the meditations of all integrated groups and individuals throughout the world, interwoven into one universal network of unity. The intersections of these waves of thought embrace the whole world in a cobweb of linked thought. If this is full of good will it becomes a cobweb of light, a magic framework of united creative will-to-good, from which all can draw strength and inspiration.

ACKNOWLEDGEMENTS

Twenty-five loving people have helped me to manifest this book in all its many stages. They have labored as if it were their own book and so it has become theirs as much as mine. Or let us say that it belongs to everyone who reads it and has no particular author other than love and devotion.

I feel grateful to have had such selfless co-workers, particularly the editors who shaped the words for others to receive them. I thank Robert Massy for his good work on layout and illustration, and I thank Pamela Osborn, Ary King and Susan Welker for their long hours typesetting. Thank you Sibyl Greene and Julie Fritz for mock-up. Thanks to Bruce Cryer for organizing proof-reading and technical editing and for compiling the Index. And thank you to twenty of my students for jumping in so willingly to proof and reproof the book. My blessings.

I appreciate the artists who gave their skill and meticulous care to their illustrations, namely Stephanie Herzog, Susan Belanger and Joanne Jonas. For responding to typing and printing needs I thank Wendy Rickert, Sonia Beasley and Roger Smith. For picture research my thanks go to Michael Hammer. For the cover painting I thank Liisa Rahkonen and for cover design and photography I thank my son John. I also thank many unnamed artists whose God-given talents have made this work more than what it would have been without them. Credit has been given wherever I knew the origin.

An important part of creativity is to be kept free of disturbance and correspondence and I owe this gift of peace to my wife Norah who protected me from many responsibilities.

I acknowledge with gratitude those unmentioned scientists, thinkers, and gurus as well as historical personages such as Krishna, Christ, Buddha, Lao Tzu, Socrates and Einstein who have inspired and triggered much of this work and who have provided the ladder by which I could look over their shoulders at the world to come.

Finally I acknowledge all those humans, both incarnate and discarnate, who have contributed invisibly and osmotically to the contents of this book. I hope that I have said what was in their hearts and minds. Foremost among these would be my father and mother who both had so many thoughts they could never express. I honor them both for nourishing the vehicle of expression and for loving me in spite of my apparent lack of appreciation.

May all these wonderful people find fulfillment from their giving.

Christopher Hills
February, 1979

CONTENTS

PART ONE
INTO THE FIRE

PART TWO
VEHICLE OF. TRANSFORMATION: THE HUMAN BRAIN

PART THREE
TUNING TO
THE COSMIC PROGRAM

PART FOUR
MANIFESTING THE VISION

EDITOR'S NOTE: For those wishing to do deeper study, we have footnoted many of the author's other works to encourage more detailed research of the subjects discussed in this book.

PART ONE

INTO THE FIRE

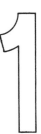

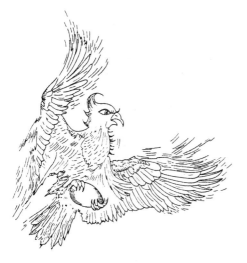

THE
ULTIMATE
ORGANISM

At some point in your evolution you have perhaps begun to reach outside the narrow parameters of self-interest and to feel concern for the plight of others. The pictures in magazines of the starving children of Biafra or the refugees in Viet Nam have brought a sudden remembering that somehow you are connected with these sad-eyed foreign children whom you never met. Feeling guilty that you can't do more, perhaps you send some money or organize a program at the level of local government. A few, whose scope is broader, will try at a national or international level to accomplish some worthwhile task. Acting in this spirit of concern, in 1964 I began working together with Professor Hiroshi Nakamura of Tokyo, Japan. Later I secured a grant for a pilot project in 1968 from US president Lyndon Johnson's administration to develop an inexpensive way of feeding the starving people of the world. The knowledge was available already—a process for growing unique

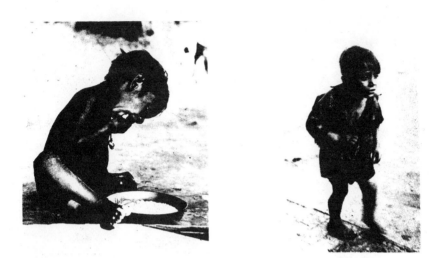

foods in the ocean by modern scientific techniques of aquaculture—but the project needed financial backing. The grant was abruptly cancelled by the incoming President Richard Nixon's administration. Today, nearly fifteen years later, there are thirty-nine factories producing this same chlorella algae in Japan commercially, because they discovered a special growth factor and a cancer-reducing agent in it. It is so much in demand in Japan that it is priced almost weight-for-weight with gold. Yet the US government has still done nothing to produce it on a large scale as we had planned all those years ago. Even though there are thirty-nine factories in Japan and Okinawa, the officials still say it can't be true. "If it is true, why hasn't it been done?" they say. But they will not buy a plane ticket to Japan to go and look for themselves.

Feeding the world's hungry children would be a feasible and practical service to mankind, but compared to the major task of bringing permanent peace between warring and competing nations of the world, it is nothing. To feed the world's millions is possible *now;* it only depends on the will to do it. But the other mammoth task of bringing peace or even researching the causes of war, does not depend on human conscious will. Everyone says that peace is what we want; everyone agrees that weapons should be beaten into plough shares; but because peace depends on the quality of man's evolution and the levels of his consciousness, it cannot be willed, legislated, commanded, coerced, policed or wished into existence.

The only person who can evolve the quality of your consciousness is you. You live in a world which is in danger of obliteration by nuclear warfare and to send a check to the hunger fund cannot stave it off for even one moment.

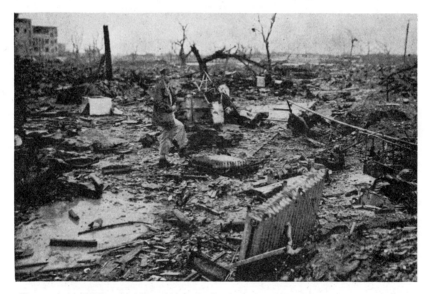

The atomic bomb left nothing but rubble and twisted metal to show that people had once lived in this section of Hiroshima, Japan. Sixty percent of the city was totally destroyed. The terrific force of the blast was felt for miles. Note the radiator in the foreground.

We all live with this dread event hanging over us, but we put it out of our minds because we are only a housewife, a businessman, a student, only one tiny individual in a vast network of political forces.

"I'd like to help, you say, "but what can one person do?" My answer to you is:

YOU HAVE THE POWER IN YOUR HANDS IN EVERY MOMENT TO MAKE WORLD PEACE A LIVE POSSIBILITY FOR THE FIRST TIME IN HUMAN HISTORY!

During the Kennedy-Nixon debates of 1958, John F. Kennedy won the hearts of American youth by his spirit of positive action: "Don't ask 'What can my country do for me?' Ask 'What can I do for my country?' "

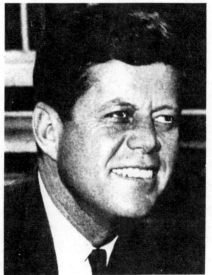

J.F. Kennedy

The Peace Corps proved that the willingness was there. People *did* want to be involved in their nation, but they had no avenue until the President created one. It is my purpose in this book to create for you an avenue not only into the nation but into the world and into the whole of creation. If you choose to walk this pathway, it will cost you self-sacrifice and hard work, but you will have the chance to make a deep and lasting change in the fabric of the world which cannot be

made by any other means than this self-transformation which I call
NUCLEAR EVOLUTION*.

The so-called "peace researchers" study past wars, make sophisticated computer studies of the apparent causes of war, of revolutions
and their build-up, of economic poverty, of the manufacture of weapons,
and so on, readily attributing the causes of war to anything from
industrial strife to political philosophy. If we read this "peace research" we find most of it supported by foundations who seem
interested in producing erudite abstract theory which will never be read
or used by pragmatic politicians who live by the dictum of what is
possible. We should not condemn this paper work nor should we
despise the naive efforts of idealistic revolutionaries to bring peace by
force and violence. But if we look with full unemotional clarity, we can
see that none of this "peace research" or "revolution" really gets to
the root cause of war, namely that nations fight for the exact same
reasons that two people fight.

Wars are not caused by external forces but by the shadows, fears,
aggressions, delusions, confusions and desires within groups of people.
The tensions which exist as psychological forces within individuals
build up into the aggregate tensions between nations.

Academicians who investigate the herd instinct and the behavior
of crowds know that the mass of people can be roused by skillful
manipulators to commit acts contrary to their better natures. When the
German people awoke from the Nazi dream in 1945, they asked
themselves, "What made me go along with it? Am I so bad as they
say?" But even this herd behavior comes back to the same cause in the
end. If the German people had looked at the quality of their consciousness, they would have known their capacity (hidden deep inside the
minds of busy housewives and good-natured burghers) to acquiesce in

---

* I have set forth the vision of this evolutionary process in *Nuclear Evolution:
Discovery of the Rainbow Body* (1977), which clearly shows what enormous potential
lies within your grasp and how it can effect deep change in the nucleus of your being. It
deals with such matters as those described in these Chapter headings: *How Humans
Transmute Light... The Experience of Time... Kundalini... The Influence of Color and
Light on Personality... Science and Spirituality.*

the murder of six and a half million Jews in the name of a private ideal: the Reich, the Fatherland, the Aryan supremacy. How many did not believe in this seductive ideal?

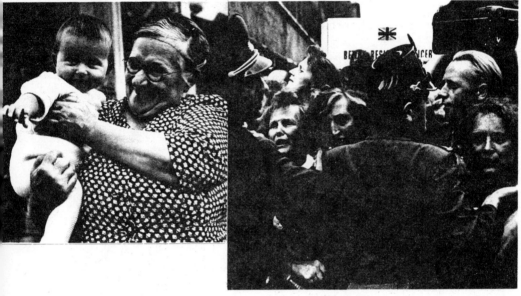

Germany. Mildred Grossman

How could the German people have come to know the workings of their consciousness and been more clear-seeing when the signs first appeared in that movement which would later bring them to world-wide disgrace? How can each of us come to know ourselves beyond the boundary of the self-image, the national image and the cultural programming in our memories and mind-computers? In this book I will talk about the World Peace Center and invite you to become part of it. Miscommunication, conflict, and pain in your relationships with others will perhaps mirror back to you that you are not a center of peace in yourself, much less in the world. Yet there are concrete and practical techniques by which you can become that sort of person who creates peace wherever he goes, just by the vibration he emanates, regardless of the ideals he holds or the words that he speaks. Nuclear

Evolution is not an evolving of the intellect into higher and higher ideals but is a growth in the deepest stratum of one's being. And the World Peace Center is not necessarily a geographical location but a space in your heart. Anything which is in the human heart can be given to any place on earth. First Nuclear Evolution must find its people, then the place of peace will manifest irrespective of any social or political philosophies.

For this reason you will find this book very different from those writings which set about solving socio-political problems in socio-political terms from inside the socio-political framework of concepts. This book is intended to be unfittable into the present concepts of a society which is unqualified to pass judgement upon anything it has not already tried. Society regulates and rules out what it calls "bad", whereas Nature is big enough to include all degrees and levels of her evolution at once and is constantly bringing forth to our awareness the richness and novelty of the universe around us. Consequently, this book does not shirk the work of looking at the planetary manure heaps and shoveling some of the cosmic dirt of man's five million year history. The theme of this book is that, in spite of all that was wrong and that still is wrong, if we really look at how it got so wrong, we can then invent something new and exciting and try it out. This is the evolutionary spirit: discarding that which does not work, embracing that which makes life full and fit to be lived.

Nature is exciting and it has invented everything which excites man most, from sex to real love. The next million year leap is concerned with a spiritual orgasm that ends in the birth of the ultimate organism. There is something common to all life which we can call a natural principle, or the constitution of nature, or the laws of being, or whatever. The name does not matter as long as we discover what it is. Although there is enough in this book for every pessimist to delight in, the whole emphasis is that these negative events are steps in evolution, merely transitory stages toward the ultimate optimism. To discover the stimulus which triggers the emergence of the evolutionary program in mankind after five million years of darkness is the social goal of this book. It employs the actual processes of all living systems by viewing the worst environment in history as the best environment for a fundamental change. Christ said, "I came not to call the righteous but the sinners to repentance." Out of the foulest manure grows the most beautiful flower. Human beings are flowers grown from human seeds planted in the soil of consciousness. We must not be afraid to look at the state of our garden and assess the work to be done.

Usually a picture like this one will make us close a book and turn away. It is sickening. It hurts. We can feel what the little boys must

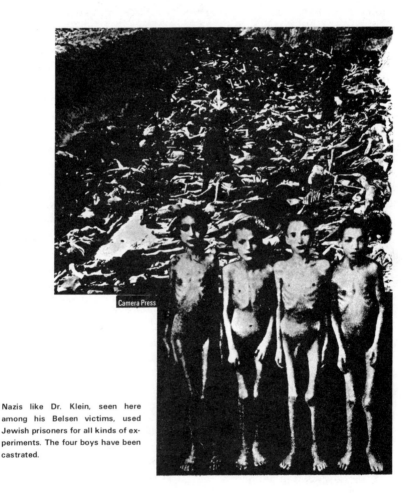

Camera Press

Nazis like Dr. Klein, seen here among his Belsen victims, used Jewish prisoners for all kinds of experiments. The four boys have been castrated.

have been feeling. We try to get inside the minds of the experimenter who would do such a thing to another human being, but that hurts even more. We can see that he must not be able to feel the feelings of the boys or to see that they are like himself and that it is his own self he is butchering. How did he come to have so little capacity for empathy? Is he some freak of Nature that he is unable to feel for another person? And yet, we ourselves find it necessary to cut off our awareness at a certain point. Someone says to us, "Stalin murdered forty thousand people per month." And in our minds we say "So what! There are so many terrible things in the world; one cannot afford to think about them." We are inundated in the newspapers with violence, and on the television fictitious violence is added to the already towering heap. Genocide, rape, murder, vandalism, war. So what!

In order for the manure of life to nourish a flower, one has to have enough humility to root oneself firmly in the humble earth and to see that earthy quality for what it is. One has to see that indifference is a kindred spirit to murder, rape, and butchery, and that even though it hurts to open up our caring and begin to do something about the state of the world, we cannot shirk it any longer and still feel good with ourselves. Once we see how we shut off awareness and pretend there is nothing we can do, once we see ourselves turn away and go on about our business, leaving the world stewing in its mess, we cannot claim innocence any longer. Every housewife turns to her partner at the bridge table with a look of innocence that says "I'm okay. It is okay for me to be playing cards. Surely you can't expect me to get involved in all that political mess!" And her partner, because she wants to use the same excuse, returns her look with unspoken sympathetic absolution. Together they go to church on Sunday and in all sincerity pray for the world, after first praying for all their loved ones. And on Sunday, perhaps they will catch a very tiny glimpse of that total creation of which they are a part. But on Monday, they dare not look into the pit. Life goes on in the same safe careful ruts year after year, and if all goes well, nothing changes.

If we could once realize that all the pain and fear and depressions which darken our inner peace grow out of a willingness to separate from the rest of mankind and from nature and from the entirety of creation, then we would see how our decision to look after only our own happiness and our own security is really the pathway to *in*security and insures that we will never quite be truly happy. Life is a mirror of what we are. If we make ourselves small, small joy must be our reward. Let any man or woman test this out. Expand your world to include someone you did not wish to include; do something for the whole that means sacrifice at the level of your private wishes. Change an attitude. See how swiftly the universe will mirror back to you good fortune. I do not mean that you will be rewarded by feeling you did the right thing or that you'll feel some pious "good" feeling if you do a good deed. I am talking about something far beyond good deeds and trying to feel like you are a good person. I am talking about the deep inner change that is necessary in order for a human being to become attuned to the whole and begin to let go of his private separated existence. The cosmic mirror will reflect or give back to such a person his heart's deepest wish, because he has been willing to give it up or set it aside for something higher.

The ultimate organism is you. And you are part of the ultimate organism of the enlightened state which Christ called the "Kingdom of Heaven". This kingdom is already here and you don't have to go traveling anywhere or escape this beautiful planet to enter into it. It is common to all nature which breathes, eats, and grows. All living organisms move, breathe, digest food, assimilate nutrition, excrete wastes, grow, reproduce and respond to stimuli. The ultimate organism understands every one of these steps but particularly evolves itself in the step called "growth". To understand growth is to understand change; to understand change we must first understand the process of excretion. As you read this book and eat its ideas as mental nourishment, you may find the food unacceptable to your present gut. Don't worry about digesting this food; the portions you excrete may be the richest manure for your growth.

How large is your body? How far can it grow? What is the extent of your awareness? Does it reach two feet outside your physical body or six blocks away or three hundred miles or does it extend to the other side of the world? If it does, then everything and everyone it encompasses is part of you, just as every cell of your body is you. Even at the purely physical level, the body has its politics, just as the mind has its locks and doors. Every organism in your body competes for nourishment from the whole you. Can you supply all your cells (including the cells of your larger Self—the whole of humanity and the entire cosmos) with fair treatment and equality for all? Can you do justice to all and do justice to yourself at the same time? The ultimate organism uses this blend of selfless selfishness which is common to all nature. What's good for your cells is good for you. So we have no option but to be an altruistic organism for we cannot be happy and fulfilled until we have made *social awareness* as exciting and evolutionary as the dance of life itself. The ultimate organism, like all other organisms, is sensitive to stimuli, but most of all it is supersensitive to the whole, and responds to love.

I CAN'T WAIT

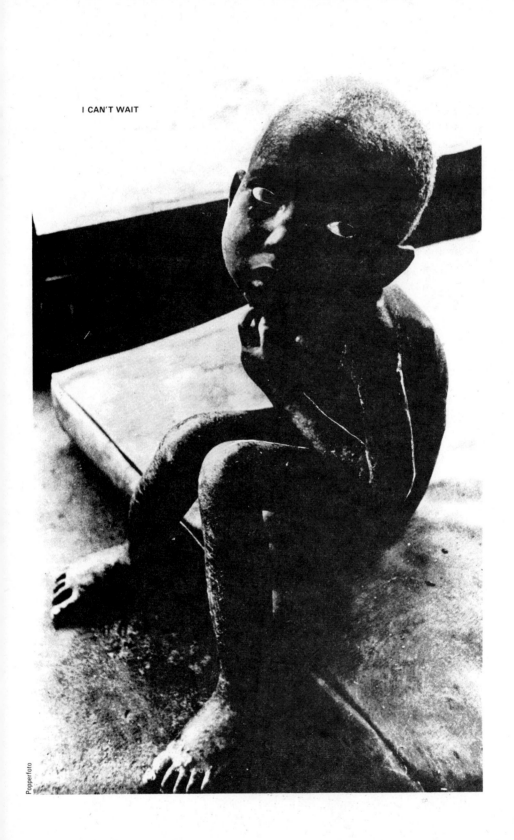

Popperfoto

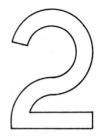

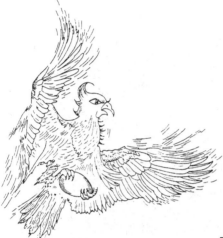

THE IMPOSSIBLE DREAM

As I write I feel conscious of the negativity of the world which weighs heavily upon the actions of human beings like a wet blanket. Even as a small boy I felt this sense of tremendous work to do in society, and the minds around me seemed dull and unquestioning. People seemed accustomed to exploitation, war, poverty and a whole host of abstract evils whose concrete realities were perhaps too terrible to face or to feel. But children are more open to direct perception and I knew that these awesome responsibilities were somehow mine. From that first realization (in me or in you) that an ordinary person, through his own growth and rebirth, can bring forth a new world—from this first glimpse to the actual manifesting of the dream is a distance whose miles, fathoms, heights, years, and intensities are measured in human consciousness. Each person who can catch the dream becomes a seed which brings its fruit to bear in others, and so it spreads.

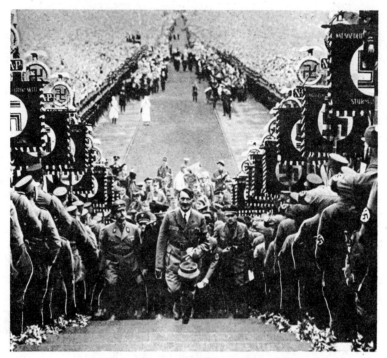

It is characteristic of man that he exalts the evil and crucifies the good.

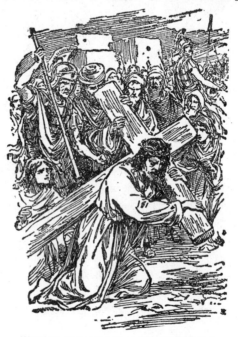

Would the world recognize a living Christ today?

It has always struck me as strange that weeds and bacteria spread and multiply so fast while the good agricultural seeds and flowers take so much human effort. Our thoughts are like this. If we do not discourage the negative strains of our mind-stuff, then doubts and fears and uncaring spread like an epidemic not only through our own inner world but from person to person. In order to get a higher quality seed, we have to breed a higher level of consciousness by cultivating the medium in which our thoughts appear to "happen". But the world is heavy with apathy and blindness and the dream often seems impossible.

I began to see why the ancient prophets were so given to ranting and vituperation as my own caring grew and deepened amid the mass indifference of mankind. All that most people seemed to want was to be left alone to pursue their own lives, earning money to spend on their desires, so how could they want a new method of government badly enough to create one? I looked at the world's people—not at the small cliques of power-seeking individuals who do not understand their own unconscious drives for domination and rule, but at every man and woman—and I thought to myself, "Will they ever try something new with enough enthusiasm to make it work? How can people have any sense of conviction about a theory which hinges upon a major change in their own consciousness without any guarantee that it will work?"

If, like Hitler, one proposed the Third Reich and appealed (in a cloak of idealism) to each person's drive for power and supremacy, then a dynamic energy would spring to manifestation. But if, like Christ, one is stuck with the unpopular message that "he that would gain his life must lose it," then the bands do not play nor the armies march, and only a few will find the strength to lift up the wet blanket and emerge into the light. It is a fact of the human situation that the many will be sucked into seductive movements which cannot deliver what they promise, movements which beguile the majority because most people, including many intelligent persons, cannot foresee the future outcome.

Those of us who do want the light feel some sympathy with the idealism of revolutionaries who are now at this moment fighting to bring social change about by violence because they too are frustrated by the dead weight of these attitudes. Yet can we trust these violent idealists to bring us a manifestation any greater than their own limitations of thought or to give us anything but the hard work of endless naive schemes which come to nought? History is full of idealistic revolutions which have come to nought, and yet mankind is the same—unchanged and unenlightened.

If not with guns and rockets, how can we combat this monumental uncaring in the human race which instinctively says, "it can't work" or "I will try when I see it is already working," or "why should I think of becoming a cosmic being when I can't even handle my *own* problems?" "What is the use of all this theory about self-government to someone whose belly is crying out for the next meal?" "How real is this dream of peace when three quarters of the human race are focussed entirely on immediate survival?" The answer to these age-old arguments is becoming increasingly clear. Whether we are a peasant ploughing up the pasture and sowing crops or a computer expert making plans, we really have no option because our survival does not depend any longer on bread alone. Survival now depends on care and the evolution of love. Even those who have plenty to eat find it hard to care. If we are only caring about our *own* stomachs while other stomachs are empty, then can we ever be fulfilled and will we ever be filled full? Or will we keep on trying to stop that gnawing sensation deep inside us which we never can satisfy with things and pleasures and power and status and food and fame? It only grows more bottomless the more we gratify it.

What would you do right now if someone told you about a group of joyful people who had found an ideal way of living and whose faces shone with the radiance of fulfillment? You immediately become suspicious of a place too good to be true. "Another one of those utopias," you think. Yet a friend confirms it is a place where enduring bonds of love are built and tested in the fires of open conflict, a community where each person is free to express himself or herself without fear and where everyone's views count and are heard because the responsibility is their own and their behavior is not controlled by any government or structure. In this community, the members change their governing institutions the moment they become boring, stultified and bureaucratic, because their own understanding of consciousness is the self-regulating mechanism which brings order in society. A common purpose binds all the members together and enables them to resolve all conflicts creatively. If you really believed that there was this place on earth where fulfillment and peace of mind could be found, where the right conditions for external peace and justice for all permeated the way of life, would you sell everything and go?

Idealistically people believe that they would respond, but in practice we would first think of all the difficulties in moving. Doubts would creep in and all the attachments to our present life would reassert themselves. However, if someone came along and said, "We are forming a group of people to work out the conditions for an *expected* state of peace to be achieved in some future evolutionary advance and we want to put you on a committee along with a lot of famous names," what human being would not step forward and offer himself? The fact is that it is easier to involve people in something that is *going* to happen, *might* happen or in something that we can *talk* about, than it is to get people to put energy into something which already exists. There is just some peculiar ego blindness, some love of glamor, which prevents many a person from working on something already in existence, especially if it is in the vanguard of society at the edge of the future with the wilderness yet to be tamed and the holy grail yet to be won. People would rather be heroes in imagination or on letterheads only. They would rather identify with the hero in the TV films vicariously than awaken the hero in their own lives.

If that state "so devoutly to be wished" has actually been achieved by some people already without our help, then what is so new becomes a threat instead of an inspiration. We cannot understand how society or science got a jump ahead of us and it makes us feel uncomfortable. So instead of finding out where that place is and whether the reports are true, we repress the good news and go our own way. The fact is that those long lists of people, those organizations and committees and letterheads with promotion campaigns behind them, never do achieve the results aimed at, nor do they ever change mankind. What is the reason? The reason is that all those names who give their contribution or have their reputation on the masthead are all doing such important famous things already that only a minimal amount of their time, their being, their resources is ever committed. All they have invested in the new scheme is their name.

When I first began to work toward world peace, I gathered together, in an organization for Research into the Creative Faculties of Man, experts from all over the world. I traveled from country to country talking to people like Prime Minister Nehru, Adlai Stevenson, Prime Minister David Ben Gurion, Prime Minister Michel Debré and many others. But in the end we made no great contribution to the world and so I began again, this time with a small collection of very ordinary people whose most extraordinary trait was just a willingness to give their time, energy, and love to a project that required hard work and self-sacrifice for as long as it might take, their only reward—the priceless luxury of having a high purpose in their lives. So I know by experience that names on paper do not bring peace. Words do not bring peace. Actions unless purely motivated and free of ego invest-ment do not bring peace either but more often bring conflict.

Let me give an example from real life. As I said in Chapter 1, about fifteen years ago I thought the only way to solve the world food problem was to grow algae in the oceans and lakes to get protein for the starving people of the world. I gathered together the experts who had already grown algae or had already designed plans for algae aquaculture farms and with a colleague set up an office in Japan, the home of aquaculture, where millions of pounds of seaweed are grown every year on farms which extend as much as fifteen miles across the Japanese coastal waters. The Vice President in charge of our office was a famous microbiologist who had been asked by Emperor Hirohito (also a university trained microbiologist) to solve the problem of the Japanese food crisis during World War II. An experimental factory was created at a cost of $3 million and was put into commercial production after the war. Professor Nakamura, the Vice President, was consultant to the Russian space program and many other commercial companies who use algae, including the Japanese pearl king who had hired Nakamura to produce an algae food for oysters and was so pleased that he gave him a monthly stipend for life. Professor Nakamura's father was the chancellor of a Tokyo university during the war and so he came from an impeccable Japanese academic background.

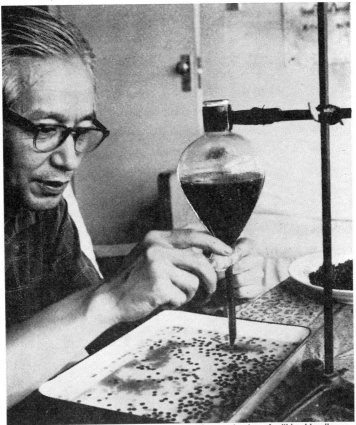

Dr. Hiroshi Nakamura is shown demonstrating production of edible chlorella peas and chlorella spaghetti by a patented method of coagulating the algal suspension.

However, when the plan was presented in 1968 to the United States government agencies, no one could believe that the answer could already be in existence. No one would actually fly out to Tokyo to see an aquaculture pond for themselves, but all the officials had their own ideas as to what would save the world's millions from starvation. One of these alternatives was for making protein by growing yeasts on cheap petroleum which has since gone up from $2.50 per barrel to $14.00 as a result of the Arab oil embargo. Another was making protein biscuits from fishmeal residues. Naturally all these plans were being lobbied for and the push was on for government finance by powerful oil companies or fishmeal companies. Fishmeal since then has become an important fertilizer and there is no surplus today.

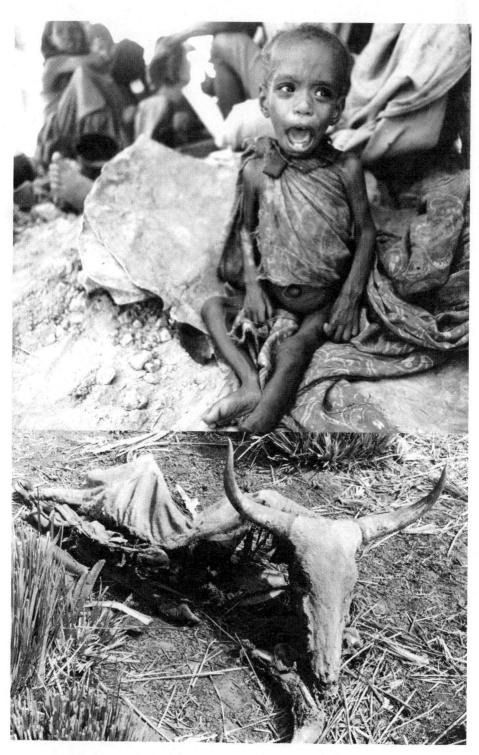

SHORTAGE OF FOOD, A WORLD PROBLEM   United Nations, J. Frank, C. Purcell

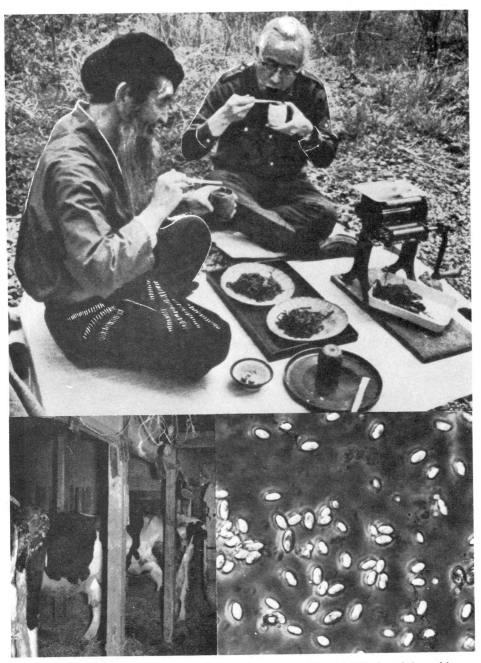

Cattle feeding on algae.

Scenedesmus obliquus (x600). One of the useful strains for cattle feed.

ALGAE, FOOD FROM SUNLIGHT*, A WORLD SOLUTION

* "Food From Sunlight" by Christopher Hills and Hiroshi Nakamura, publ. University of the Trees Press.

The officials of the United States government AID program decided that there must be a test pilot program to decide if my claims were true. They granted $1 million after a great effort of organizing all the factors to establish a plant in Bangalore, with the University there contracted to test the reliability of this protein food in a cattle feeding program. All this notwithstanding the fact that the algae program was *already* being worked and researched in animal husbandry and that the results had been published in detail and in the public domain.* A flight to Japan costing a few hundred dollars would have convinced anyone. Nevertheless we went along and did a lot of work for over two years. The project was given top priority status by the Indian government from the Prime Minister down the chain of command. Then a new American president was elected and his first act, just as we were about to start, was to cut back foreign aid twenty-five percent on all existing projects and to cancel all grants for projects like ours which were not yet paid out. This was done across the board, regardless of the value of the projects. Those projects which were to be continued would have to be resubmitted to the new administration and renegotiated. The paper-work was voluminous and required expensive expert legal counsel. We did not have the time and resources to spend another year with cap in hand, waiting for a dole out to be given to us so that we could feed the world.

But the interesting part of this tale came ten years later when we contacted the National Science Foundation and spoke to an official who had already given a small NSF grant to a sewage engineer to grow chlorella algae. The NSF man had never heard about our world-wide project. He could not believe it. The only ponds in the USA according to him were the experimental ones in Berkeley which the NSF was financing. Although I told him there were other successful ponds in Kansas which were actually feeding cattle commercially, he could not listen and said we would have to apply for funds by going through the small experiment in Berkeley because the whole field was unproved, new, speculative, and he had heard that there were difficulties in harvesting. We assured him that harvesting difficulties had been solved

---

* Original material now available in *Food From Sunlight,* by Christopher Hills and Hiroshi Nakamura. 384 pages, University of the Trees Press.

in the ten years since our AID grant was withdrawn, and several more commercial Chlorella factories had sprung up in Okinawa, Taiwan and Japan and that an air ticket to Japan would save repeating all the experimentation in the very unsuitable location in Berkeley.

After visiting the Berkeley engineer, our staff informed the NSF man that the engineer who was undertaking the project was almost totally ignorant of our algae growing methods, knew nothing of former efforts in other parts of the world in different species of algae such as Spirulina, and believed himself to be the only one pioneering the field! We suggested, as there were now thirty-nine commercial factories operating, that it would be stupid to do years and years of research again since in Japan and Taiwan the factories were all automated. Plus every Japanese knew about the particular species of Chlorella and Spirulina algae since they had now become fashionable food additives. He insisted that the government had no funds for any other projects in this area until the two acre ponds at Berkeley had proved or disproved whether it was feasible. We reiterated that it must be feasible with thirty-nine factories already in existence.

That was two years ago and the situation is the same today with our great American nation, whose technology could feed the world and greatly improve on the Japanese concepts. People continue to starve. Officials continue to draw their big salaries. Lobbyists continue to prevent funds from leaving their pet projects which don't work. And the world continues to think that we must keep on researching to find a new way to feed the world.

When the Army and Navy inquiry boards probed into the details of the surprise attack on Pearl Harbor that found America so unprepared, they found confusion and lack of co-ordination between the armed services. But the very next day President Truman asserted that the whole country was as much to blame as its military leaders for the lack of preparedness that brought America defeat in the first blow of World War II. One could say the same for fifteen years of American neglect which enables the very same nation, Japan, to be several years ahead in the fight to feed the world.

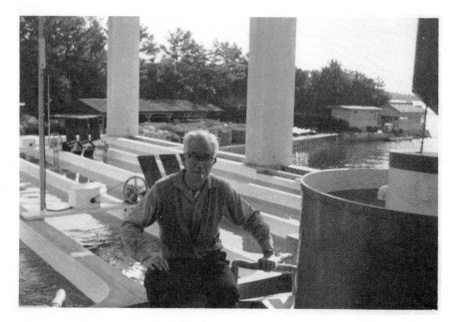

Professor Nakamura at his algae tanks in Japan.

If people concerned will not fly to Japan to see for themselves an actual algae utopia in existence, accomplished already and commercially profitable, what would people do if they heard that there was a place on earth that had solved the problem of peace? The algae problem of feeding the world is a minor one compared to the communication problem between myself and this Doctor of Science at the National Science Foundation, because the world food problem is only an effect of that ego-blindness which blocks real communication. The fact is that famine, war and most other human problems are born out of this same blind unwillingness to see the obvious. If someone says that there is a place where the problem of peace and war has been solved creatively, what will humans in positions of power go out and do? They will feel terribly threatened that it happened already in spite of them and without their knowledge. The same thing happens in science, in medicine and in government departments every day. How could it be true, the ego thinks, that I was so ill informed that something is actually happening in my own field that I do not even know about? Intolerable thought! Go away, repress the information, disregard it, do not test it out for it might be true and if it is, then I will have to re-evaluate everything, including myself. Therefore ignore it, like a human ostrich with its head in the sand, until it becomes overwhelmingly impossible to avoid.

The same blindness exists toward a parallel experiment in conscious evolution of society which has actually been going on for over ten years in several stages. This book covers some of those stages in a process of natural growth called "Nuclear Evolution" which is only just now coming to the notice of the general public. However, there have been many so-called experts in various political and social movements who have known about it and have turned a blind eye to it in favor of various expensive schemes of promotion for future projects. Because they are so obsessed with these promotional methods they can never have time to stop and think or develop an inclination to try out the techniques and methods which already exist. Instead they romanti-cally chase after the will-o'-the-wisp in their imaginations. Why is this? The answer need be no further than your own self.

Ask yourself again: what would you feel right now if someone you trusted told you that he actually knew of a group of people who had discovered a political system for making conflict creative, turning painful emotions into growth experience, transmuting anger and frustra-tion into emotional steam for enlightenment? Ask yourself not just as a fantasy or a "what if" but as a live practical option which actually presents itself in your life. Would you say, "so what?" or would you sell everything and go there? This book is written solely for those who would pack their bags, sell their house and business and be willing to start all over, bringing nothing but themselves. It is not written for fence-sitters whose "wait and see" consciousness excludes them from flying to Japan or risking a penny worth of ego. It is written for those who want to live life without phoniness and to transcend the fabric of lies which permeates everyday existence. It is mostly written for those who have stopped deceiving themselves that the world will get any better until mankind gets to know itself better. In fact, the book is written for the few, not the many, hoping that the many will think they are the few.

To begin to care, to *decide* to care, in a world where very few others are caring, is to discover the hero in yourself—that quality you felt as a child but had almost forgotten was there, that part of you which could see the truth when everyone else seemed satisfied with compromise, the part that would have aimed higher if even one parent or teacher had asked for it, the part that felt some thrill inside whenever it saw goodness or love in another. The impossible dream of Nuclear Evolution is to touch this deep core of being inside you, where the hero still wants to give everything he's got for something really worthwhile. This nuclear center has within it the seed of our evolution and our destiny. All it needs is a drop of water and a little ray of light to bring it into life.

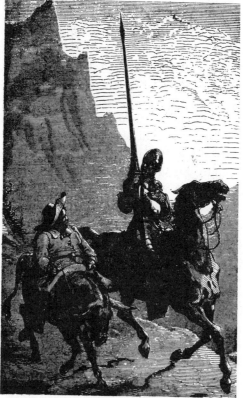

Culver Pictures

The delusion that you are getting along okay is the ostrich-like consciousness which prevents such a radical change. That quality in you which opts for stability at the expense of growth, prevents you from risking what might bring the ultimate reward. Perhaps this portrait of a typical young man I know can be a mirror for you. After college he volunteered to join the Marines and went to Viet Nam in a spirit of adventure. He was resisting marriage to his fiancee because to him it meant adopting the whole boring materialist life with babies and washing machines and being tied to a mundane job. The hero in him longed for more excitement from life than to repeat the same drama his parents had lived and their parents before them. But he did marry and got a job and began to accumulate things and invest in property. More and more each year he is shaped and molded by the life he has chosen.

"As soon as I get enough money," he says, "I'm going to quit and live a different way." He believes he can get to the right end by employing the wrong means. But means and ends are the same in the long run of evolution; there is no separation between them. If you eventually reach the right ends by the wrong means you will never enjoy the results. Thus our young Marine fools himself. He rationalizes in this way, so that he will not see himself nourishing one side of himself while neglecting another deeper part that wants to be free of all the social expectations and cultural brainwash he was programmed with in childhood. He longs with a passion he is no longer in touch with, to find out who *he* is, not just be what the world expects him to be. But he has not the courage to risk; and each year as he acquires wealth and comforts it becomes less and less likely that he ever will risk his possessions for a new life. Like the rich young ruler, when Christ said, "Sell all that thou hast and give to the poor and follow me," he turns sorrowfully away.

Inside each of us is this uniqueness crying to be born, yet sold for a bit of security or a scrap of approval. This unrisking, unalive part of us is the wet blanket of apathy which cannot bring itself to see the Truth and cast our lot with it. Most of the people who make up society are feeling this shaky uncertain stability, this "I'm really okay", and yet if you probe more deeply, they are not really fulfilled. Ask yourself. Is your happiness really whole or is it just a surface over deeper unmet needs and unheard longings?

We do not know, until we unlock the doors of the brain, what vast potentials are inside us all, for the brain is the instrument of evolution and the doorway to infinite realms of spiritual discovery. There are many who feel that "spiritual" is a synonym for "weak", "soft", "naive" and "stupid"—especially in the realm of politics, which prides itself on survival in the ruthless competition of the strong and the cunning. In America the kind of spirituality that has guided politicians has had a vaguely sentimental quality and did in fact weaken the foreign policy, the diplomatic communication and the public image of this country. The Russian dissident Solzhenitsyn who was expelled from his own country and was given hospitality in America, recently caused a storm by exposing this very weakness. He complains that instead of standing up for Truth and risking all for it, the American society hinges upon legalistic and moralistic platitudes. If we reject this mirror of ourselves because Solzhenitsyn is too unflattering, then we will miss an opportunity to survey where we are at. If we look at ourselves objectively perhaps we will see how naive it is to think that going to church is spiritual or to think that "doing good" will make us popular. It is naive to feel that by sending money overseas we are sharing ourselves. The spiritual life is not living a sentimental idealistic version of a book saint. Spirituality means looking at what is actually happening. And this is what Solzhenitsyn asks of us, that we face the reality that America, just to earn a few dollars, is supplying the technology with which the Russian dictators will attempt to defeat the freedom of America. We are building Russian truck factories, selling advanced computers, oil technology, building chemical plants and selling wheat to make the very anti-God succeed. How can this be spiritual? Real spirituality is to stand up against the forces of human oppression, not to listen to words and naive arguments about detente, not to believe that our own words will mean anything at all unless we back them up with character and integrity. People all over the world believe that Americans are suckers for any demand for money because they feel guilty about their affluence. Americans also have a compulsion to be liked, so they don't come on strong. This brand of American spirituality was born out of innocence and nurtured in the cradle of material abundance. But there is another kind of spiritual fiber that is tough and which grows like the weeds and bacteria in conditions where nothing else can flourish. How do we come to this lean and hard kind of spiritual consciousness which is centered in Truth and which sees so clearly the nature of Reality that courage and total integrity are the natural fruit of its flowering? There are many in this era who have tried to arrive there by reading books or by following certain teachers, forming communities, or doing good deeds for fellowman. Others have tried to climb to that consciousness through drugs. In a frantic quest for "something" the youth of this era have plunged into the experience of hope and disillusionment and, although they have not arrived at the kingdom of heaven, yet it has brought forth that condition in which the true seed may fall on fertile ground and begin to grow. There are weaknesses yet to be confronted but at least the soil has been tilled, and people feel in the air that a New Age is about to dawn. How have we come to this exciting threshold of a dream that once seemed impossible?

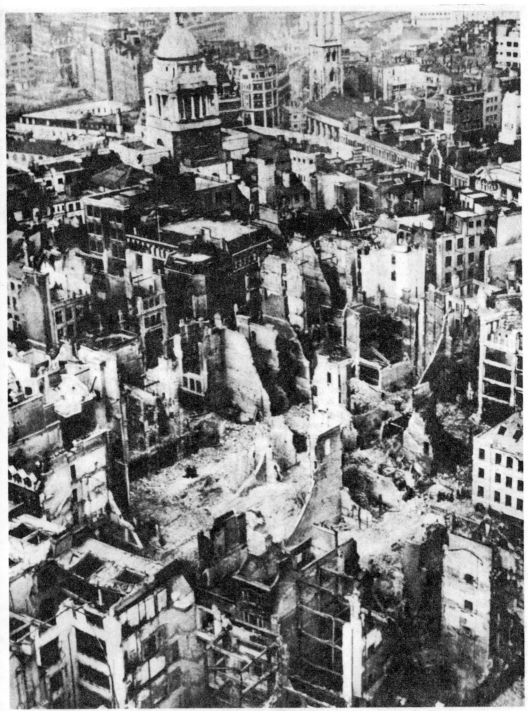

United Press International

War-torn London in 1941.

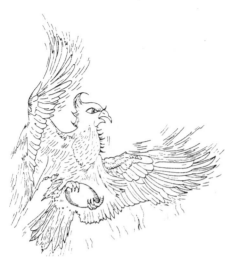

HOW THE
SPIRITUAL
COUNTER-
CULTURE
WAS BORN

The world had seen the ravages of violence on a gigantic scale and in its most beastly form when the whole world was raging at war—Germany, Japan and Italy against the British, the Americans and the Russians. After that, one began to wonder if hatred and killing were plunging the world into a darkness greater than that of the Dark Ages. The Vietnam war went on for years after the world war, sapping the life blood and flesh not only of living people but also the vitality of the great economy of the United States. Was there an inscrutable design behind all this killing, maiming and brutality? Krushchev, the Russian Premier, made an announcement in 1960 to the Kremlin presidium that they now had the means to destroy all life. Was it a secret weapon of psychotronic

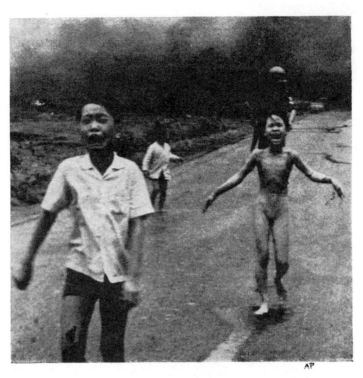

Americans were shocked by the atrocities of the Vietnam War.

power which could explode in the psychic hyperspace and derange
the minds of the enemy? We still do not know.

We now live in the post-Vietnam period which covered a decade of
violence. At this time of writing (1978) it seems incredible that there is
no major war going on in the planet. The thirty years of almost
constant war between Israel and the Arab Nations is at this moment
climaxed by peace talks in Cairo between Israel and the Egyptian
president Sadat, who broke the deadlock by going to his enemy's camp,
Jerusalem. Sadat is pleading for a peaceful solution. But his allies,
Syria and Libya, have rejected him openly as a traitor. The world
vainly hopes that the prospect of another war is over, but fighting with
Syria and Libya is inevitable if they maintain their present attitudes,
because seemingly they do not believe that anything but war can solve

the problem of creating an independent Palestinian state. Various guerilla wars are going on in Africa at this time, mainly in Ethiopia, Somalia, Angola, Rhodesia and Uganda with little promise of wider escalations, but the prospects of a world conflagration are all around us. The Arab nations, using as a potential weapon the embargo of oil which is vital to the operation of the US and European economies, have increased the price five hundred percent and another cut off of supplies would threaten the present fragile stability of world economy. All this will have changed in the shifting patterns of the world scene when this book is read five, ten or twenty-five years from now, but one thing will remain. We will not solve our problem of creating a model for participating self-government by the year two thousand unless some grass-roots movement for a radical change for self-rule sweeps the countries of the old world with their deeply grooved patterns of culture. The tinder box is dry. Anything can happen socially and economically, and everyone can feel the electricity and uncertainty in the air. These are the conditions in which the flames of a dying age consume the Phoenix and bring forth something new.

THE FIRST SPARK

The reaction against violence came in the years of the sixties from adults with sensitive feelings and from youth. But even then, in recoil from the napalm bombs, the urgency of the cosmic message was not being seen—namely that

MAN HAS TO LEARN TO LOVE SOON OR HE WILL NOT SURVIVE THE PRODUCTS OF HIS SCIENTIFIC INGENUITY!

During the sixties the idealism on the university campuses of America and Europe was marked by an international interchange between members of the SDS—Students for a Democratic Society. Eventually their movement was infiltrated by radicals and leftists and the moderates went back to their studies, but in the early days, the movement began with an insight into the world's most pressing need:

"Our work is guided by the sense that we may be the last generation in the experiment with living. But we are a minority—the vast majority of our people regard the

temporary equilibrium of our society and world as eternally
functional parts. In this is perhaps the outstanding paradox:
we ourselves are imbued with urgency, yet the message of
our society is that there is no viable alternative to the
present...

Loneliness, estrangement, isolation describe the vast distance between man and man today... We would replace
power rooted in possession, privilege, or circumstance by
power and uniqueness rooted in love, reflectiveness, reason,
and creativity. As a social system we seek the establishment
of a democracy of individual participation, governed by two
central aims: that the individual share in those social decisions determining the quality and direction of his life; that
society be organized to encourage independence in men and
provide the media for their common participation.*"

Unfortunately, no one in the student movement evolved this working
alternative system. However naive the claim may seem to cynics, this
book aims to provide such an alternative. Its essence was already
available during the student revolution at the time of the above
statement. I published the plan first as the *New Book of Changes*
(1963), and six hundred copies were sent to major universities. It was
reprinted again in 1968 as *Christ–Yoga of Peace* with an introduction
written by the pacifist philosopher Bertrand Russell. Eighty-five hundred
copies sold by word of mouth, but its time had not yet come.
Distribution in England on a national scale was almost non-existent
because no major publisher would accept it as a viable commercial
proposition. So it was published by the Centre Community Association,
Centre House in London, which was committed to testing out an
experimental community and using it to validate the theory of Nuclear
Evolution in a real life situation.

---

* From Students for a Democratic Society, The Port Huron Statement, June 1962.

Perhaps a short review of the turbulent background since the 1960s will show whether the time is coming at last for the method whose cornerstone is the growth of individual participants in a self-governing community. We can easily see as we look at the movements for change in the 1960s, that this growth was missing.

CAMPUS REVOLT

American and European campuses erupted in political tensions between generations. The activity seemed to grow into doctrinaire forms such as the motto "You can't trust anyone over thirty." The causes of this conflict were different according to who was speaking. Marshall McLuhan insisted that its potent force arose out of the media revolution represented by the children born into an electronic society which demanded rapidity of results. Some observers felt that the new generation were the children of the affluent society. Not having to work for economic subsistence like their parents, and liberated from economic pressures by grants and parental lavishness, they were free to indulge in extravagant or arrogant thinking and to follow their ideals. Many thought the student revolt was a total rebellion against the materialist culture which cast the students in what they saw to be artificial and phony roles as prospective fodder for the giant corporations. Any large organization became a social enemy which had prostituted its power and deprived youth of choice, in order to "process" society for meaningless 9:00 to 5:00 rat race work schedules. The young people saw adult society wallowing in hypocrisy and therefore adopted the politics of personal openness and integrity.

The university was the nearest large organization available to the young revolutionaries so it became the prime target of their anger against the authoritarian organizational structures. They rebelled against the assembly line production of Ph.D.s in higher education and rightly demanded more relevant classes. An articulate minority swayed the moods of estrangement and hostility and orchestrated the techniques of confrontation so that activism dominated the university life of the decade.

TRAGEDY AT KENT STATE

The extent of student unrest and antiwar feeling was dramatized by the confrontation of Kent State University students and Ohio national guardsmen. The guardsmen fired (right), in what they later claimed was self-defense, at the crowd of 1,000 students who had rallied to protest US involvement in Cambodia. Below, a girl screams as she realizes that a student, Jeffrey Glenn Miller, is dead. The tragic results—four students killed and nine injured—set off a nationwide reaction and led to further disorders and violence across the country.

RIGHT, JOHN A. DARNELL/LIFE: BELOW, JOHN P. FILO/VALLEY DAILY NEWS

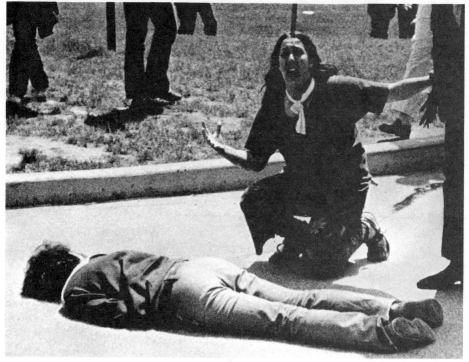

A worldwide wave of student protest swept through universities everywhere, stimulating sit-ins and angry take-overs of campus buildings, mass arrests ending in the shooting of four students by American National Guardsmen at Kent State University in 1970. By this time the SDS had become a militant organization and their leaders were

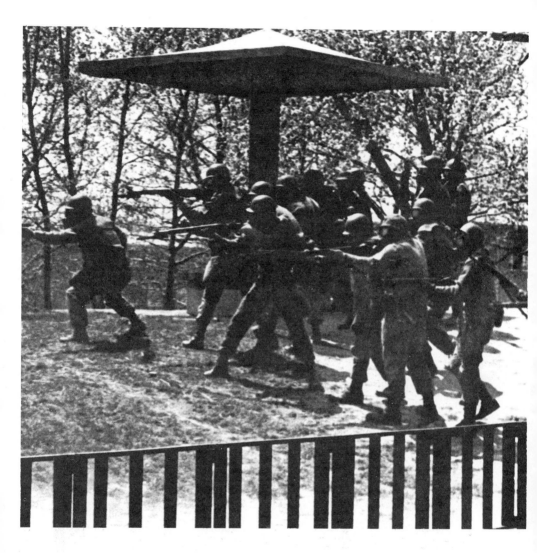

rigid ideologues advocating Trotsky policies and simplistic use of taxpayers' money. Avoiding any leadership or centralization, shunning any plans, and shouting against any intellectual elitism, they espoused decentralization, self-determination over their affairs, and voluntary small communities. While one section of the movement shouted generalizations like "Make love, not war!" another faction of radicals became the "New Left".

I attended a conference in the Round House in London in 1967 at which leading figures of the student revolution railed at the forces which prevented the transformation of society. I remember going up to the microphone after Herbert Marcuse and asking him what he meant by the word "imagination" which he had used several times during his speech, since he related his total philosophy to the use of that human quality. I asked him point blank to say what research he had done into the quality of imagination and also whether other philosophers had said what it was. I myself had done several years research on the important role of our imagination in the evolution of the species and I thought if he could say what it was that philosophers had never said about it, his words would then have more relevance. I was thinking about the primordial power that created the universe and is inherent in all men as the transforming dynamic of all true vision. The danger of would-be world changers is that they invariably "jump the gun" into idealistic, even sentimentalized action without taking into account this cataclysmic agency of the imagination behind every effective evolutionary change that has ever been made by mankind. The air was electric as I spoke because I was criticizing the current guru of world change in 1966, whose Marxist writings had largely been responsible for the campus disturbances. Marcuse was considered the one person in academia who was "telling it like it is", rather than going along with the system for grant money. I was rocking the boat of the one who had rocked the boat, and howls of repressed student anger went up from his admirers. This was the technique at the time, to start a chant of group voices going. They began to chant "we want action, we want action" and I was shouted down by people who did not know what I was talking about.

What *was* I talking about? That very thing! The senseless demand for action, before we had got our imagination clear and straight! I was talking about going into action half-baked, without preparation. I tried to say that I was for action too, but action which had researched its motives and was based on empirical knowledge, not on some outlandish Marcusian theory. It was no good. The students wanted action at any price. Even violence was good, they said, if it brought change. But I could see clearly that they had nothing new to offer, no alternative society nor anything original except resistance to what they felt was definitely wrong. The calls for action grew louder. "We don't want to discuss imagination," called out one. And another shouted, "Let Marcuse speak." So I shrugged my shoulders and stepped down from the microphone. Marcuse came back to reply. "It is true," he said, "I have hung the whole of my theory on the idea that the value of action is determined by the imaginations of people and the prevailing images in society, but I cannot tell you what imagination is; I only know we have to change our imaginations to change the future." Afterwards we talked on the stage and he confessed he had done no research into imagination and that research would have to be done by people like me. I walked away disappointed that people were so blind that they listened to rhetoric and clever ideas that had no real visionary transforming power. How long could any change last or even succeed in the first place unless we tapped primordial images of how things could be, should be and will be?* It is not enough to criticize the bad, without ourselves seeing clearly what is the good.

As the war in Vietnam began to escalate, the New Left emerged as the new wave. Protests against the war grew until angry students attacked institutions of learning for their scientific collaboration with the military-industrial complex. Companies manufacturing weapons, chemical defoliants, napalm, or research grants supplied by the military or CIA, all became targets for the growing numbers of disaffected students who were becoming liable for draft into the army. Undergraduates and some radical professors increased their defiance of authority. Sit-ins, riots, vandalism of computers and science buildings caused the universities to bring in the local police. Thousands of students were arrested. During 1968-69, as a result of public violence, student radicalization became more politicized and out of control. Student leaders who took over the SDS were now actively organizing sedition and recruiting an urban guerilla force. The New Left ideology tried to explain why it rejected American society and why it needed to use violent methods. Its radical extremists spurned the values at the core of American democracy and saw America as hopelessly corrupt and oppressive. Freedom of speech, tolerance of others' ideas and

* For a deeper study of the primal imagination in the universe see *Nuclear Evolution* pages 77-105, the chapter called "Penetrating the Imagination Barrier".

differences, change through discussion and consent rather than by decree, all were regarded by the radical New Left as bourgeois qualities. No one knew whether or not the SDS was being financed by the communists to foment rebellion. The organizers always seemed to have money, yet they did not work. The key recruiting people of the student protest spent their time circulating leaflets, neglecting classes, promoting their radical meetings daily and taking over all decision-making organs in the student body.

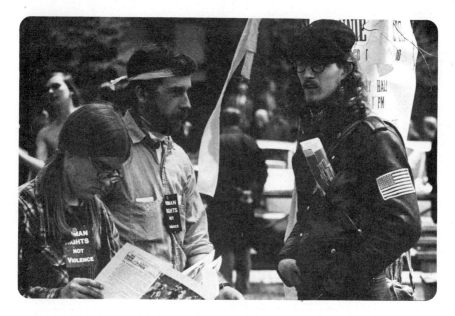

Many students who were originally sympathetic to the SDS did not go along with the violence. Their aim was to stop the systematic destruction of human beings on all levels of society, in the ghettos, on the battlefields, and destruction of the environment.

MARCUSE

Many Americans were shocked and believed the revolt of the young was the result of a communist plot to subvert the US constitutional process and take over "the system". Liberals, who believed there were two sides to every argument and insisted on working to improve society from within the system, became the target of ridicule and condemnation by the New Left. Herbert Marcuse, the chief ideologist of the New Left blended Marx and Freud (two outmoded thinkers) to advance the idea that the industrial-military complex, on which the affluent society depended for full-time employment, had developed a non-terrorist totalitarian hold over society and that the large welfare budgets of USA, England and other countries had corrupted the working classes. The workers, he said, had been lured by affluent consumerism into capitalism and thereby disqualified themselves as an agent of revolution. Therefore any revolutionary change and hope for social transformation could now only come from the exploited classes, the persecuted and resentful and the revolutionary pressures from outsiders. Marcuse argued that it was right to forcibly repress the capitalist exploiters of society and indeed anyone in the free social system who held anti-social ideas. He also insisted that the students who were the *new* agents of revolution had the natural right of armed resistance as all oppressed minorities had if legal methods of change proved impractical. He said of these minorities, "They use violence not to start a new chain of violence but to break an established one. No third person, least of all the educator and intellectual, has the right to preach to the oppressed about abstention from violence."

Perhaps we could have asked him by what right did he, an educator and an intellectual, preach violence? He seemed to have totally forgotten how he came by this right by emigrating from Munich to a free democratic society where all rights are guaranteed. Today, fifteen years later, Herbert Marcuse admits that there are grave errors in Marxist thinking and that Marx was wrong in certain supposedly scientific predictions, namely the demise of capitalism which was inevitably to be overturned by the agents of revolution in the form of the proletariat. However, he still maintains that Marxism is valid as a philosophy because of several other important predictions. These predictions sound like common sense to every businessman and ordinary person but Marcuse advances them as important proofs of Marxian wisdom—the prediction, for instance, that capitalist companies would eventually swallow up the small businessman and become huge corporations which would dominate world trade and thereby become even greater exploiters of the working class. Marcuse sees this prediction coming true in the growth of the great multinational corporations whose bigness, however, does not exploit the working class which has disappeared, but exploits everybody.

Marx could, in 1867 when he wrote *Das Kapital,* afford to be self-righteous in his predictions, but modern Marxists are faced with a very different set of circumstances. Marcuse maintains that the workers in Western economies have become capitalists by their ownership of industrial shares and that now capitalism not only exploits people everywhere, but rapes entire national economies which have been converted to the production of war machines and wasteful weaponry. He mentions nothing about the conversion of over thirteen percent of the entire gross national product of the Russian Marxists to weaponry nor the publicly aggressive and hostile attitudes of communists generally, nor the deliberate policy of all communist nations to undermine democratic rights and institutions. In a world starved of love and integrity, he mentions nothing of the official communist attempts to encourage espionage and irrational conflicts among races within the Western democracies, nor the orchestration of destructive and divisive forces among labor unions.

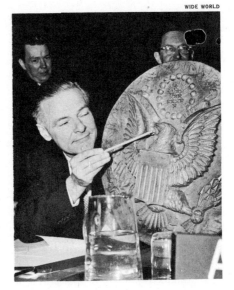

WIDE WORLD

Henry Cabot Lodge, the U.S. Ambassador to the United Nations, shows a Soviet spying device: a hidden microphone in a carved wooden gift to the U.S. Ambassador in Moscow, during a meeting of the security council in May, 1960.

He ignores the Marxist cell technique of infiltration, particularly in England where the subtle control of key positions in the labor unions has brought the British economy to its lowest ebb. Continuous strikes and disregard of all labor contracts have caused rampant inflation in Britain, thereby robbing the population of its former high standard of living. At first the people felt the love and fairness of the new socialist ideals, but now the British public feels terribly exploited by the strike weapon, and of course the government can do nothing because it is itself a socialist labor government. Marcuse sees this as the fulfillment of the Marxist prediction that capitalist expansion would cause the exploited working classes to rebel against the ruling class. The fact that in Britain the labor rebellion is against the state-owned post office, the state-owned coal mines, the socialist state-owned motor company and the state-owned electric utilities seems to have missed his attention.

A person without any political acumen whatsoever could have predicted that big efficient organizations would swallow up small ones, especially in capital intensive industries where large resources are required to finance heavy industrial equipment in oil exploration, steel, cement, computers, etc. The inevitable price of this big ruthless efficiency is that prices will go up once small competition is eliminated. To validate Marxism as a scientific discipline with such predictions when they have been obvious truths for centuries, even to capitalists themselves, is politically academic and unreal. More interesting are the predictions Marx *failed* to make. Since Marx, the joint stock corporation has emerged, something which Marx did not foresee. If he had foreseen it, he would have realized that there was not just one inevitable outcome for capitalism but many directions that it could go. Perhaps he could even have realized the potential of the joint stock company as an evolutionary tool of society, as in the concept of Common Ownership outlined in the economics section of this book. If Marx or anyone else had glimpsed this possibility, then we might have seen a different type of organism developing in the joint stock company, less parasitic, less exploitive and more geared to love and cooperation.

THE INEVITABILITY OF LOVE

Love is no longer a sentiment which is inappropriate to the tough,

practical world of business but now becomes essential for survival of
the human species. We have no choice. Without love and tolerance,
the joint stock company which abuses its freedom in the market place
will eventually be destroyed by its own rapacious greed. The voice of
the people and the lives of dolphins and whales and the pollution of our
precious rivers from industrial poisons can no longer be ignored. The
large companies must cultivate love and become caring for the world or
perish. In short they must become beautiful; they must become instruments of charity and wealth, which distribute some of their excessive
profits to humane ends.

It becomes increasingly obvious that love is now no longer a luxury
nor an added jewel in the living of a good life, but a dire necessity for
the survival of mankind. Could we explode love in the hyperspace?
Could the ingenuity of man in fact create machines, TV screens or
vehicles of radiance which could take the vibrancy of human love,
experienced in one place in the heart, and radiate its cosmic frequency
pattern out on the same powerful radars used for antiballistic missile
destruction? And what of beauty? Could that also be thought of as no
luxury but a dire need for the survival of the entire human race? Our
sensitivity to beauty is not separable from our sensitivity to each other
and to the invisible spiritual dimensions of our own being. The ugliness
of our physical environment testifies to the poor quality of the consciousness that created it, just as our physical eyes also make visible

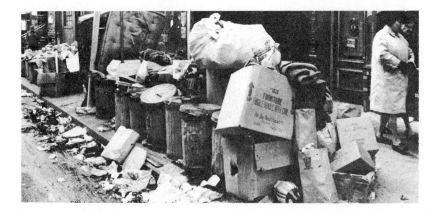

the kind of spirit that dwells behind them. Your spirit and mine relate to one another with a crude or a refined vibration that is directly connected to our capacity to respond to beauty. If we searched out beauty with the same intensity we pour into the search for power, what kinds of love and beauty might we discover?

It is the vision of this author in this book that human society and human relationships can be made into an instrument of beauty so dynamic and powerful, so overwhelmingly truthful and revealing of love, that hatred and conflict will be eventually seen as a bad waking dream. We have been given everything we need to make the world work, except love. This must come from within us, from our heart, from the center of our being, and then our efforts will receive a response from life because we are in tune with the universe. Love is the only contribution we really have to make. All else has been given. Consciousness, power, wealth and supreme intelligence have all been given by an all-wise Creator, but love must come from us. It is the price we pay for heaven, the effort we must put forth to make the world work more abundantly. Man thinks that he must gain power and wealth by his own efforts, but these have already been woven into the nature of man. All he must do is unblock them in himself. To unblock them he must learn to love; this is the key to the flowering of all other powers. All powers, whether of money, artistry or social achievement, if they cannot be administered with love, are vanity and come to naught. What pulls the insects and animals into reproduction of their species if it is not love? What will be needed to pull man into survival of his species if it is not love? Hate has had a long fling. In the years which prepared the way for the counterculture, only hatred and division and destruction of the system were preached by the Marxists. After fifty years of absolute power, all the communists had to offer was the Russian revolution that failed to make its ideal happen and created a country that was riddled with coercion and political malevolence. In the 1960s, all over the world, in China and in emerging countries, love was out and the power of the gun was in fashion. To speak of love and peace was to invite ridicule in a world where only violence supposedly got results.

THE BEAST IN NEW DISGUISE

The movement called "the New Left" originally arose as a reaction and rejected violence and instead called for active civil disobedience against the self-perpetuating power structures which were leading the world to nuclear suicide. Had they offered some positive solution along with negative protests, perhaps they might have accomplished more. Even Bertrand Russell, who could have been a potent force for creating an entirely new social order in the West, was too busy at this time organizing sit-down strikes and disarmament protests to think up an answer to the problem of social order with freedom, even though he had confessed to me that it had been his main interest all his life. The time was not yet right. The rejection of violence by the New Left did not last long before the new leaders of the "Weathermen" faction of the SDS saw American society as totally corrupted and beyond all salvation. They decided that the only way to deal with an unconscious destructive society was to destroy it. Bombings claimed by Weathermen are still going off in cities and universities all around the world as this book is written. The fanatic element believes that the violence of their ideology succeeds in unmasking the "establishment" by provoking it to retaliate and thereby radicalize more people. When these bombings killed innocent bystanders and did little more than cause expense for replacement of the bombed facilities, the militant left then claimed that the establishment system had disarmed the dissent by absorbing it. The Attorney General cracked down on the New Left, and the "Weathermen" were driven underground.

At this time of writing (1978) these violent revolutionaries have little standing among the serious students of the country. These activists are still admired by a fringe of alienated leftists who believe, like Marx and Mao Tse Tung, that the only way to social change is through the barrel of a gun. But the majority can see that even if these fanatics managed to destroy the entire system, they have never issued any plan for an alternative society. Nor do they have anything to say about who will be eligible to run it. One thing is absolutely clear: the American people would not want any of *them* to run it, because ruthless killers who believe they have a right to dictate how others run their lives, even at the cost of the lives of others, only appear as supreme egotists, totally blind to their own inadequate beings. If they could do some work on themselves and the corruption of their own values, then the public might give them some respect as idealists, but to kill and destroy because you yourself cannot create anything is, in the eyes of most Americans, a psychological sickness, at best a mind corrupted by its own passions.

THE HIPPIES

Political activism did not excite everyone, and there were an equal number of students in the sixties who felt society was finished as a high technology system, since it robbed people of freedom to flow, to be, to do what the spirit felt good with in the moment. Rather than changing society, there was a move towards dropping out of it and creating an alternative scene. Originating with the "beatniks" of the fifties, the hippies of the sixties were less verbal, much younger and were eventually joined by all classes as a movement to change "lifestyles". The beatniks were a literary movement which wrote about what the hippies lived out. Disdaining suits, ties and "square" clothes, the hippies grew long hair, wore bright and unusual clothes, and attempted to find identity in being "original". The adult world was labeled "uptight" and "plastic", and the young hippies congregated all over the European world at beautiful places where they could just be themselves. They called themselves "flower children" and they celebrated, away from the "sit-ins" and activist confrontations, at "be-ins", and "love-ins", and their slogan was "flower power" because of their custom to give flowers to uptight people.

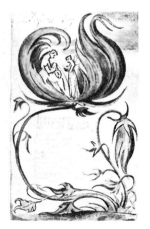

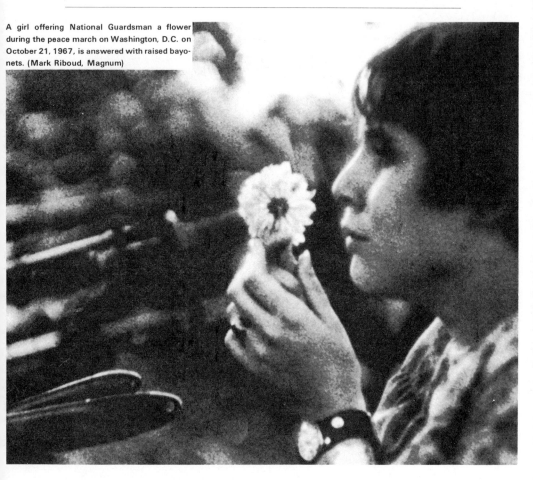

A girl offering National Guardsman a flower during the peace march on Washington, D.C. on October 21, 1967, is answered with raised bayonets. (Mark Riboud, Magnum)

However, they could easily help themselves to *your* flowers that you spent three months growing and tending every day, with the nonchalant comment "All flowers belong to God."

A spontaneous gentleness characterized the movement. I remember a busload of hippies organized by Simon Vinkenoog arriving at our center in London from Amsterdam to attend the annual Stonehenge festival of the Druids. The Chief Druid, a doctor who lectured weekly on herbs, homeopathy and Druid knowledge at our London community, invited me to preside over the summer solstice at Stonehenge and be crowned with the traditional laurels. The hippies turned up with a professional camera crew and thousands of feet of colored film, plus the "King of the Hippies" from a community living in caves in the Greek islands. They were all nice people and obviously some had money. Somehow I felt the marriage of money with enthusiasm for the quaint traditions and ceremony was another fetish, a desperate search for roots and meaning in a bygone age. All were dressed in expensive flowered gowns and velvet pants in vivid colors, reminiscent of the actors in a Medieval play. "What was motivating them?" I thought. Something was driving them, inside their beings, some identity was restlessly searching for something they knew had been lost, but they did not know what it was and so they too were lost, like children lost on a strange planet. I felt with them the yearning of a whole generation for the missing love in the world. They were impatient to find it, trying this drug and that ritual.

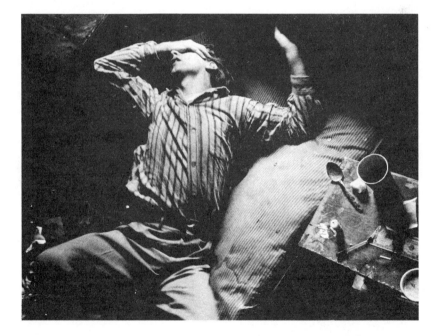

Today it was Druidic magic, tomorrow perhaps a busload to Lourdes, a perfumed garden in Persia, a certain beach in Goa. I could feel the thing that was eluding them. I knew that nothing but a dilettante manifestation of their movie would ever materialize. Ten years later I met the "King of the Hippies" in a California fleamarket. "Whatever happened to all that film?" I asked. "It's still all there," he said, "we never got around to editing it." Five years after that I met him again in the street outside my own front door. "How's the Greek Islands?" I asked. He said, "Never went back there since Stonehenge." I asked, "What happened to all that expensive color film footage you shot?" He answered, "You know that young director, he's got it and never did anymore with it." In my mind's eye I flashed back to all those starry-eyed children of the sixties, thinking they had found the love ethic that was transforming the world. They were going to live life as it was meant to be, without hassle or struggle. Drugs, marijuana and free love and all our wish-fulfillments were now magically possible in the affluence of the computer age. Work was only for old fogeys and taxpayers.

I have mentioned this incident because it was typical of the *laissez faire* everywhere I went in the sixties. On the village green with flowers, weddings just by mutual agreement, babies brought into the world to be shared with everyone because they too were like God's flowers, even though their earthly father was unknown. Sex was a communion like drugs were a sacrament; money was the universal oil on the wheels of life, like food was grown by God in the field. Love flourished and youth established an international grapevine through Tolkien's images of Middle Earth. Soon hippies joined together in communes wherever they could find a beautiful place. A forest in the mountains, a papaya farm in Hawaii, everywhere I went I found a commune movement reminiscent of the nineteenth century religious communes. Buildings were taken over in London, Amsterdam and San Francisco, some by squatters in squalid conditions, others by richer scions of wealthy families who liked the freedom and the good loving vibes of a new wave. A building in a metropolis would become overcrowded. A group would split and go off into the country and establish communes in the most beautiful wooded areas of the rural world. I decided to visit some of them scattered around the USA in New Mexico, Arizona, Colorado and California. I wanted to know if they really had found their answer to the riddle of life. Did they find the missing love in the idyllic settings of the communes? I wanted to know how the communes were run and who made decisions. Who controlled the land and who controlled the money? I wanted to know if the authorities they had escaped in the governments and bureaucracies of the national systems had reemerged in the disguise of the pied-pipers of folk gurus. Furthermore, was it real? Having given many years' thought to the community problem of organization, I met and visited with many who were searching for the ideal way of life. I discovered none with an answer to the real question in my mind: how to grow selfless without acting out some dreamlike fantasy which could only last until the reality of group life penetrated the ego structure. And what is the reality of group life? It is living so closely with people that all the hang-ups, negatives, quirks and unawareness have to be dealt with, including our own. I found sharing in the places that I visited, and I found caring, but nowhere could I find the answer to world survival. They were not independent persons but were offshoots of the affluence. They would die on the vine unless they could face internal conflict as well as handle and resolve the conflict in the world outside. Yet by 1970 several hundred communes had spread like wildfire across the country. A worldwide network of several thousand people would be moving from one commune to the other, and an amazing grapevine system developed so that one could know whenever a "happening" was going to take place. An incredible number of customs, diets, creeds and

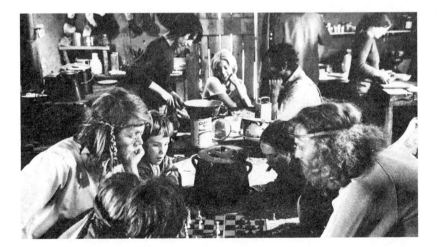

Communities were formed with a vast variety of creeds and lifestyles.

attitudes existed, from the totally selfish to some very unselfish ideas of collective property, group sex, free love and children, but usually with little responsibility for the consequences. Life in the communes was at survival level unless you had a secret stash of money. The motto, "Do your own thing", "turn on and drop out" was the philosophy of the hippie phenomenon. Drugs, mainly LSD and marijuana which had become the stable sacraments of the movement, then moved on with a rapidity beyond the detection of parents, to the "experience seekers" in colleges and high schools. Students at all levels from all classes were trying to blow their minds and expand their consciousness. The model was Aldous Huxley's ingestion of mescaline given him by Dr. Humphrey Osmond who coined the expression "psychedelic" to describe the psycho-mimetic effects which Huxley described in his book *The Doors of Perception,* published ten years before the hippie revolution.

Following on the psychedelic visions and the attempt to find oneself through drugs, and interwoven with a dozen dazzling fashions in clothes, came the craze over Tolkien's characters who symbolized for youth the mysterious powers which were trying to take over the darkening planet. Again I wondered was it real, and would the energy of transformation be able to work through myths and symbols or did it need to reach us not vicariously but touch us directly in our own lives? All over the world Tolkien's Gandalf, the white magic wizard who was out to save the world from the machinations of Mordor, became the new hero. For a long time a member of our London community was talking about starting a magazine for youth, using Tolkien's mythology as a vehicle. I challenged him to go ahead and do it instead of talking about it. Thus the magazine "Gandalf's Garden" became a popular expression of the freedom of the counterculture across the schools of England. Later it led to the foundation of a hippie pad place in a cheaper part of the city but again the same problem caught up with it and the personalities involved parted in disillusion and bitterness. The ego conflicts, desires and wish fulfillments, those shoals upon which all the great schemes are wrecked, were not considered beforehand. Like the commune movement, Gandalf's Garden faded from the scene like a fond memory of the idyllic tropic island.

As the hippies came to the fore so did the age of rock music, bursting upon the scene with its ear-piercing amplification of the rock beat. Music played an extremely important role in the gathering together of the cultural forces of youth. The Beatles from England and later the Rolling Stones subtly became the cultural mouthpiece of the young. Bob Dylan was the bard of the new culture. Hollywood, looking for new heroes and for new markets, made films and records which sold by the millions. Every youth's ideal was to become a superstar and cut a disk which would hit gold or platinum (sell a million or more) and to become rich, influential, effective and potent.

The height of the new movement towards sound communication in the mass came during a period of huge music festivals beginning in 1969 at Woodstock with four hundred thousand young people sympathetic to the lost hippie scene. Holy men from India, a big string of big name bands and crowds summoned to communion through the network

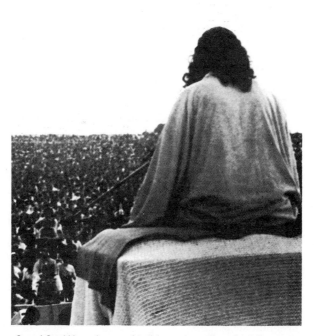

Swami Satchidananda, one of India's greater yogis and a colleague at the World Conference on Scientific Yoga, was involved in the Woodstock Festival.

made up the formula for success. Along with Swami Satchidananda, Yogi Bajan and Swami Vishnudevananda I was sent a ticket to appear at the Atlanta festival shortly after Woodstock. I wondered what I was doing there all the way from London amongst the clouds of marijuana smoke, watching the thousands of young people sitting passively on the ground turning on, stoned with drugs, listening to the deafening beat of where it was all supposed to be at. What was missing? Love of a kind was there. Everyone was smiling and kind. Enthusiasm ran high. New Age business in tie-dies, leather bags and incense flourished. Then on the second day the tough motor bikers came in, smashed the barricades and opened up the gates and the crowd swamped the ticket office and rushed past the gate uncontrolled. Thousands got in free while many paid heavily for their advance tickets. But the hippies were too mellow to let it bother them. The promoter lost money and a collection of several thousand dollars was made to help him but no one knew what happened to the money when the promoter did not get it. Thus another behind the scenes drama was branded a success! My thought was, "What does all this have to do with the world of reality, the world of inner growth and outer peace?" This two day feast of sound when everyone was loving could not be kept up for a week, let alone for a lifetime. The intensity of experience in real life is not a festival, but a continuous program. I decided that this movement upon the face of the waters of modern life was not the way to go and nothing would ever come of it. Later that year at another rock festival held at Livermore Speedway in California, the whole event was broken up by violence and invaded by the Hell's Angels motorcycle group, resulting in four deaths. This event led hippies everywhere to wonder where the love-ins and flower power had gone. The movement degenerated into shouts of "kill the pigs", meaning the police. Said one hippie, "We failed to confront the pig in ourselves, the childish egotistical selfish irresponsibility." Nevertheless the flower generation went through some beautiful experiences and they learned eventually that to share everything indiscriminately was an invitation to those selfish ones posing as hippies to rip off the generous ones, to take their mates, their food, their energy and money and give nothing in return. The movement ended in the political activists' attempt to use violence and confrontation in the context of the hippie ethos, and the Youth International Party or Yippies was formed.

YIPPIES

The Yippie tactics were to create confusion and to make a rhetorical mockery of the courts and even of revolution itself. The leaders' contribution to society is summed up in their statements, "Revolution for the Hell of it", "Confusion is mightier than the sword", "When in doubt, burn", "Fire is the revolutionary's God", "Burn the flag", "Burn the churches", "Burn, burn, burn". This did not impress the world but it made sensational headlines. It successfully killed any remnant of respect for hippie or yippie from the people who supported the country with their taxes. Nor could the young people respect this brand of idealism even though they rejoiced that someone had the nerve to "cock their snooks" at the solemnity of the established ritual of law.

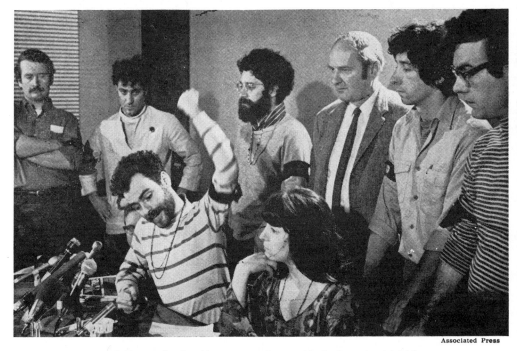

Associated Press

Jerry Rubin, pounding the table, at press conference with other 'conspiracy' defendants.

BY THEIR FRUITS YE SHALL KNOW THEM

Between the ceremony of the law, with its frightening dignity, and the reality of life as it is lived spontaneously beyond the form-filling for government bureaucrats, exists something real and untaxable, and the young were in touch with it. It was the *psychic income* that made life a celebration rather than let it become an endless slavery to officialdom and government requirements. The complexity of any organized activity, the number of forms and the control by government through the information required to feed the voracious appetite of society's computers had become too much. The revolt of the personal against the impersonal government machine was total. But this youthful revolt could only happen in the free democracies of the world! In any socialist country the revolt of youth would have been put down with tanks, guns and jailers. The full weight of regimentation would have been felt. As it was, the hippie revolution ended in a whimper.

The following account was told to me by an American student of that generation who was perhaps deeper than some in her desire to transform society, yet her experience was typical of many:

"I was in Czechoslovakia in the summer of 1968 when the Russians invaded and I was slightly leftist, sort of into the SDS. I felt great concern for the world situation and had gone to Europe not as a tourist but to live among the people to get to know their hearts and how they viewed life. The atmosphere in Prague at the time was very exciting. There was a burst of creativity in the arts and sciences and a pregnant feeling of liberation was in the air. The intellectual climate was very open and progressive. At least that was the vibration I sensed in the people I was talking to. When Russia invaded it was a rude blow that quenched the liberal, humanitarian feeling with one fell swoop. An aura of fear soon replaced the feeling of expectation. My friend and I were quickly ushered out of the country but happened to get on the wrong train car to Vienna and ended up going through Hungary without a visa. We were stopped about sixty miles inside Hungary when the police came through to check our visas and forcefully yanked us off the train into a little country railroad station where we were interrogated. I was frightened. All my socialist idealism was now being confronted with the rude facts and the reality of the communist army.

It wouldn't have been so bad if they hadn't mishandled us. They grabbed me by the shoulder and pushed me wherever they wanted me to go, from this room to that, as if I wouldn't be willing to walk by myself. Finally they must have realized we were harmless and we were left in a waiting room until another train came and we were directed to go back to Czechoslovakia.

But again we were pushed with unnecessary force into what turned out to be a cattle car, and we were sandwiched like sardines practically nose to nose with many other people. My imagination flashed to the movies I'd seen of Nazi Germany. Like the Nazis, the Hungarian communist army and police had no feelings; they were insensitive. It was a particularly dangerous situation because we were in Hungary at the moment when Czechoslovakia was being taken over by Russia, just as Hungary had been invaded by Russia years before. The atmosphere in Hungary was cold and uptight and everyone knew what was happening in Czechoslovakia.

It was hot in the cattle car. We had to stand all the way, nowhere to sit down. People sweating. Nobody smiling. I looked at the Hungarian women with their heavily lined faces and dark, drab clothes. They looked just like the unflattering books on communist countries had said. I was nervous because I wasn't going to Vienna but only back to Czechoslovakia, which was still a dangerous place to be. But soon we were on the train from Czechoslovakia to Vienna and then to Yugoslavia.

Yugoslavia had a friendly light atmosphere similar to what

we had experienced in Prague when we first arrived, though
not quite so free.

Still somewhere in the pit of my stomach I had a longing to
be on the safe shores of America. This was unusual for me,
because for the past five years I had scoffed a bit at the
liberties of America, looking only at the injustices. We went
back to London for a few days but even there, I didn't feel
totally at peace. When I finally landed in Chicago, I felt
that I could relax securely and I realized that somehow (I
am not a sentimentalist and I don't want this to sound
sentimental, but) somehow all that old stuff you learn in
school about the American constitution and the Bill of
Rights and the founding fathers and the great stability of our
nation and the right to the pursuit of happiness and all that
stuff suddenly meant a lot more to me."

THE COUNTERCULTURE

The vision of Marx ended in violence. The SDS ideal of civil
disobedience was swallowed up in the violence of the "Weathermen".
The hippie movement for love and harmonious living somehow gave
birth to the yippie movement with its wanton burning of property just
for the hell of it. Clearly the overthrow of the beast, flourishing through
the centuries like a virulent virus, will take more than drugs and flower
power. It will require us to determine the cause of our callousness, the
reason for our blind dependence on government, our docility toward its
evils, which we can never do if we are blaming the system or escaping
responsibility for it. This unwillingness to look *in*side, rather than
*out*side is why the movement of the sixties failed in its purpose and
brought the sad feeling of a lost vision, the resignation to encroaching
social forces of the dull unchanging status quo which dampens every
fashion and spreads over the planet like a wet blanket to shatter the
ever-wondering child, killing "enthusiasm" (the Greek word for the

God within). Studies of this generation ten years after the student revolution show its leaders and spokesmen now securely nestled in administrative business jobs all across the country. When asked why they have adapted to the system they once fought with such conviction, they only laugh, as if to say, "That was just kid stuff."

Out of all these mixed movements, the hippies and the political radicals and the varieties of revolt, from left wing activism to the rock concert and the drug trips, emerged the present day counterculture which rejected a society geared to achievement, professionalism, and "authorities". It was a counterculture unified by moods rather than ideas. The unspoken purpose was to create a change in consciousness along artistic and spiritual lines. Beginning around 1972-73 the straight society began to find some excitement in the rock and roll beat and to smoke marijuana to relieve their tensions, while trying to make it to the top or to make their marriages work or just to be able to listen and cut out the clamor of the TV or shut the world outside off. Was the whole hippie movement to end in nothing more than this minor variation of the same mediocrity we had before? Had the generation of the student revolutions made no dent in society at all? Now that the fervor had died down, nothing was happening. After President Nixon pulled American troops out of Viet Nam, that was it. Poof! It was gone. What was there to turn to? What answers had been distilled from the new communities and the student reactions—the love-ins and the be-ins, the soul searching, the sincere draft resisters who spent years in prison? Where did the idealism go? One college student expressed the feeling poignantly:

> "In the fall of '67 I went on the famous anti-Viet Nam march to Washington, thinking I was part of some big beautiful movement that was really going to change the world. But when I got to Washington I found that most of the students there were ranting young adults who had a lot of disappointment with their parents, with teachers, and with the system and needed to vent their feelings. They had no deep penetrating insight into society and no real way to change the world or even themselves. They didn't even look at themselves and their egocentricity.

I felt a great sense of loss. I felt displaced. We spent the night at the Pentagon with planes swooping low over us and eerie sirens filling the air, tear gas grenades going off, and I had a deep feeling that there was no place for me. I was there because of my urgent feeling about people being killed in Viet Nam in a senseless war. But our society, represented by the Pentagon and the government and the planes, had no feeling for what we were trying to do. Their one thought was, "Let's get these hippies out of the way." And yet I didn't feel like a hippie or like a revolutionary either. They seemed like a bunch of disturbed kids throwing tantrums to me. I walked away from the whole scene, from the Pentagon, from the crowd, in tears, totally disillusioned. My romanticism had entirely died. I had gone with the fervor and devotion of a righteous cause, but I found only emptiness. I had already ditched the prospect of a dull American dream with a house in suburbia and kids. Now I had to ditch the peace movement as well. I was looking for an ideal and an identity, but there wasn't anything. A few others seemed to be coming to the same realization when we got back to college from the march. Some turned to drugs. But I was looking for meaning and purpose, not an escape."

Into the vacuum and meaninglessness of it all sprang the Eastern teachings of consciousness, which had been absorbed by thousands of young people who had traveled to seek their souls in India, in the Eastern countries of Persia and Turkey, and in Europe where the new fashionable political movements had taken on spiritual overtones.

I had been moved by the Eastern teachings some years before the fashion and went to India in search of spiritual enlightenment. While all this ferment was going on in the worlds of politics and academia and the drug scene, I returned from India to England in 1965 and founded a center to group together all those working for a New Age consciousness. During 1965 I had been giving lectures at Caxton Hall, and various groups had indicated that London had no center at which to carry out all the new growth techniques. So we started London's first growth center. We began with monthly meetings between the leaders of the different movements which were emerging at that time in England and we called these meetings the "Round Table". In the ecumenical spirit, we welcomed all exponents of spiritual life, all those engaged in real self-transformation. Many other social movements sprang into being around the same time. Our Centre Community in London held nightly classes in Sanskrit for three years 1967-70 with Dr. Rammurti Mishra and held lectures on other nights by well-known

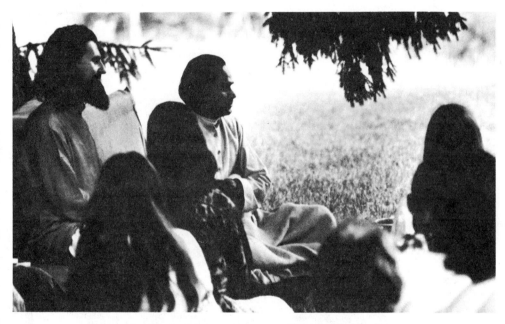

Dr. Rammurti Mishra and Christopher Hills at Ananda Ashram.

spiritual teachers such as J. G. Bennett, Ven Sangharashita, who founded the Western Buddhist order from our Centre after returning from twelve years in India, Count Keyserling, Thomas Maughan, Paul Twitchell, Sant Keshavadas, Swami Muktananda, Swami Satchidananda, John Coats, head of the Theosophical Society, Dr. Heydenriech of the Steiner Society, etc.

Many new age groups used the lower three floors of our seven story building as headquarters for their budding movements. We organized pilgrimages and conferences in India, registered the World Yoga Society in Lucknow in the capital city of Uttar Pradesh and sent out thousands of Centre Newsletters, BUT THE EXPECTED REVOLUTION IN CONSCIOUSNESS DID NOT COME. Alan Watts, a popular writer on Zen, Buckminster Fuller, an originator of the geodesic dome, psychologist Ronald Laing and scientist Andrija Puharich all said the New Age was already here, that it was happening, that the messianic movement had come. I looked around the scene and saw that the nuclear transformation of the human ego-structure and public knowledge of the levels of consciousness which could transform society was still a long way off. Fashion and glamor and enthusiasm could not be mistaken for solid achievement in the transforming work on ourselves.

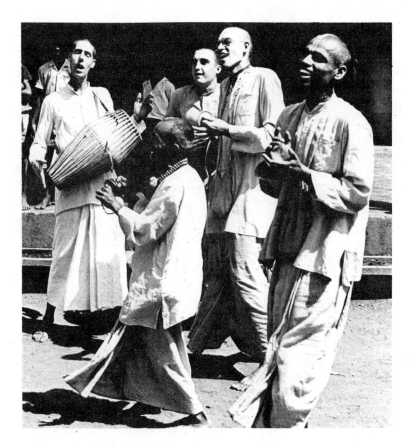

The same year that I returned to London to found the Centre Community Association, the Ven. Chogyam Trungpa left Oxford University to found a Tibetan Buddhist meditation center in Scotland. But these early centers were just the forerunners of a movement that did not really begin to come into its own until the seventies. About 1970 Trungpa visited the USA and founded the Naropa Institute and a group of meditation centers to teach the Buddhist tradition to an ever-growing group of seekers. Trungpa's book *Cutting Through Spiritual Materialism* (1973) was better than the usual spiritual books. He talked like one who had done the hard work of dismantling the ego structure, but had he really done it? I don't know. But I know that the Naropa Institute had a very intellectual vibration and one could feel the long line of scholarly Buddhist monks transmitting the Buddhist tradition down through the centuries, in infinite detail and complexity talking *about* the spiritual life instead of actually living it.

Tibetans are the most egoless people I know. But they are not yet egoless enough to transcend their deeply rooted culture of quaint stories, personalities, hierarchies of lamas, etc. They want to get Buddhism across, even though the spiritual trip is nothing but a long mountainous difficult journey if you go by the traditions in *any* culture. If instead they could have found the links between Buddha, Christ and Krishna, this simple "essence knowledge" would have said to the world: "Hey, we can forget that Buddha was a prince before he was a buddha or that Jesus was a carpenter before he was a messiah. We can forget that Naropa was a chancellor or that Buddha fasted fifty different ways or that Milarepa turned green through eating nettles. All we need to know is that the egg (the nucleus of our being) is just like the yolk of a chicken's egg which is just a mass of yellow—very simple." That is the trouble with truth. It is too simple. How do you recognize that what you've got, twirling around in your own head is the cosmic egg, the yellow mush all jumbled together, the chemical gene structure all mixed together in the DNA prior to cell division. The feathers of the Phoenix are hidden there in the yolk. The flower's blossoms are written in the bulb. Our destiny is written in the simple nuclear stuff of consciousness waiting for us to discover it. All this was waiting, deep inside the people who *externally* were going through the motions of creating a New Age of the human spirit. Including myself.

Life was a ceremony but was it real?

THE WORLD CONFERENCE
ON SCIENTIFIC YOGA

In 1970 the Centre House Community in London organized the
World Conference on Scientific Yoga and I traveled the United States
to interest scientists in the effects of the yogic disciplines on altered
states of consciousness. A six month tour yielded fifty Western
scientists who committed themselves to coming to New Delhi if I
would get the yogis to come together. Having founded the Institute for
Psychic and Spiritual Science in 1962 in New Delhi, it was not
difficult for me to organize a large steering committee consisting of
ministers of government (Health Minister, Railways Minister, Deputy
Leader of Congress) and various Indian political figures who could
attract the yogis out of their traditional isolation in ashrams. I asked
my eldest son to visit a long list of ashrams and personally invite the
swamis. We hired the largest government building in New Delhi and
opened the conference to a full house of several thousand people at the
Vigyan Bhavan. Eight hundred yogis and fifty Western scientists
attended the seven streamed conferences running side by side. The
organizers for J. Krishnamurti asked if they could put up their own tent
alongside our demonstration tent, and I agreed as I felt the integrity of
Krishnamurti was a necessary antidote to the traditional Indian guru
who enslaved disciples by making them dependent, instead of teaching
them to think for themselves. This was 1970. From about this time
onwards the spiritual counterculture was underway. About thirty former
hippies from Katmandu, some with doctorates in Sanskrit, some just
drop-outs from American colleges, helped me run the conference along
with three of my own students from Centre House. We kept to an
American space-age time schedule, an unheard of thing in India. It was
really seven conferences at once, all running parallel.

The book *The Greening of America* by Charles Reich seemed to
reflect briefly what I was striving for in beginning the London Centre
and in organizing the World Conference on Yoga. Reich referred to it
as Consciousness III. But actually I was aiming at more than a new
fashion, more than a transcending of the culture of the nineteenth

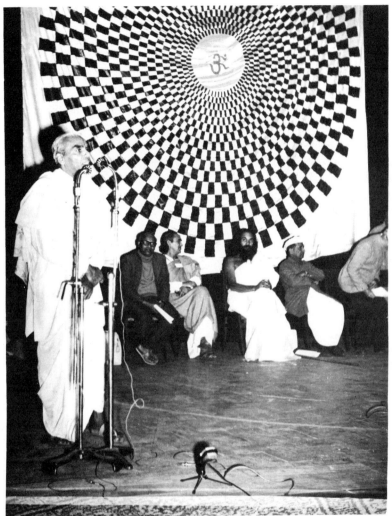

B.K.S. Iyengar, India's most well-known Hatha Yogi, chairman of one of the committees at the World Conference on Scientific Yoga. Other chairmen from left to right, Dr. M.C. Modi (Bangalore), Swami Rama (USA), Swami Dhirendra Bramachari (New Delhi), Dr. B.L. Atreya (Varanasi).

century capitalist society and its subsequent managerial revolutions. I was aiming at nothing less than the complete transformation at the nucleus of being, the transformation of the reality of the self into all other selves. Of course that was optimistic, even messianic, for the time has not come even yet as I write.

Through all the violence and rhetoric of the student revolution, through the years of the hippies, the rock music concerts, the fashion for Eastern teachings, exotic trips to Katmandu and the drug culture, I kept asking myself, "Is this it?" I had experienced the feeling of "Now is the time" once before when I gave up business and became a researcher of the nucleus of man's lost being. And now I was waiting for that feeling to come again, the feeling of some momentous turning point. I would see people enthralled in one spiritual fashion or another, people who obviously thought inside themselves, "This is it! It's really happening!" But I could see clearly the phases of my own path being re-enacted in their lives.

When I was into politics, I helped found a new political party and became Vice President of it. When I was into religion, theology and Christian ethics, I felt like becoming a priest and getting a parish. When I was into Indian philosophy and had studied the *Vedas* and the *Gita*, I wanted to become a wandering Sadhu, free as a bird and without possessions. When I was into psychic research and divining, I wanted to use the "powers" for the benefit of the human race. And when I started my own Centre and community in London, I traveled to other communities in America to see "what was real" about them and to ask myself would they last or was this all just the transition towards some gigantic, fantastic, bizarre and inconceivable step in evolution. At each place I had the feeling, "The time is not yet." I arrived at Pondicherry to meet with a friend who had known Sri Aurobindo for many years and was head of the World Union Movement there and who wanted me to meet the Mother of the ashram. Deep inside I felt this might be it, the contact with an Indian yogi who had seen the vision of man's evolutionary spiral and would somehow be a link with all my years of research. Just before we were about to meet for the first time, I received a small card from the Mother, given to my friend who had just been telling her about my work. I opened it and on it was

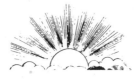

written briefly, "Not yet." I began to wonder, "Am I missing the flood tide that is happening or is there something missing in all this which I cannot see?" Everyone was saying the New Age was here, that this guru and that guru had the answer. In 1961, Maharishi had arrived unknown in London and I was having lunch with Lady Cripps at my London hotel. Sir Stafford Cripps had been one of the key people involved in giving India its independence. She pushed toward me the leaflet announcing Maharishi's first arrival and told me he had hired the Royal Albert Hall to give initiations in meditation techniques and said I should do the same. Something inside me said, "This role is not for you. The Maharishi may be able to help many people with these basic techniques of Hindu meditation but for you, there is another way that does not involve platforms, entertainment hall speeches and Madison Avenue promotion." Something said, "If God is really with you, what do you need all these human methods of promotion for in order to get across the obvious?" All these teachers flooding into the counterculture were filling some deep need in people for identity, for comradeship, for community of experience at the spiritual level, and yet something was saying, "Not yet." I wondered if it would all pass by as a fashion in the excitement of the times.

There was a great desire in the churches to put the teachings of Christ into one ecumenical movement where Christ's spirit, rather than his words, would bring back that magic into Christianity which would sweep people off their feet into the new world of life more abundant. Yet the more I looked for essence, the more I saw that the needs and the spiritual hunger were being satisfied by the husk. The kernel was missing. I wanted to feel the whole big movement happening every-where, not just in England or America or among the fashionable cults of Eastern teachings, or the encounter groups, the hippies and the radicals, but something I could feel was affecting the whole of society. Even the most popular gurus were reaching less than one percent of the population and I thought, "That is not what I'm looking for. I'm looking for a WAVE!" I knew that deep in the Christian religion there was the essence of yoga, that what Christ had taught to his disciples was the union of self with the whole. But the parents and society did

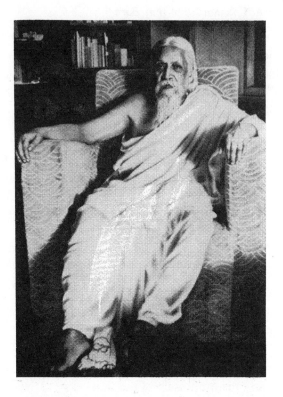

Two of India's last great yogis who were effective in world change gave the world an idea of the ancient works from which the more recent yogis have been living.

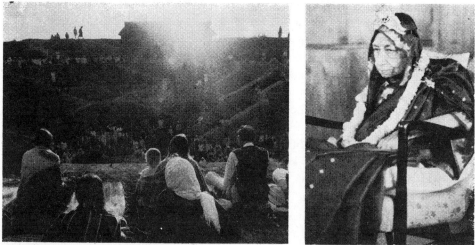

Dominique Darr—Gamma

Aurobindo disciples at the crater in Auroville and 'the Mother'. From Hindu mysticism, a plan for social reconstruction and world unity.

not flow with the counterculture. Many people took the drugs, the psychedelic fashions, the new colors, the old outward forms of the new Eastern religions but they were like the Revivalists of England a hundred years before, intoxicated with religion and yet fundamentally unable to see that they were missing the main thing.

What was the main thing? Some dynamic overview which saw all the parts of the counterculture fitting together like a hologram as it emerged from the different sections of society. It was that feeling as if one were living in a time when history was definitely being made. People would tell me excitedly when we first went to the moon, "This is it! Man's entry into space. Man will never be the same. He has seen a picture of planet earth from afar, taken from the moon. His consciousness will be changed forever." I looked at them and wondered what they knew about human nature. To me, no one was changed by going physically to the moon. I thought, "Maybe there is something wrong with me. Maybe I am too skeptical. Perhaps it takes more facts, more research to get me off the ground." Nothing short of the penetration of the nucleus of being, the direct fertilization of the cosmic egg would convince me that Nature had made all things ready. Salvation for man could only come about in God's way in God's good time.

Month after month, year after year the time flowed on and I traveled asking myself, "Is the time near for the coming of the push? Has the time come when all will hear and all will respond? It was 1972 and my friends and colleagues, Swami Satchidananda and Dr. Rammurti Mishra and I decided to start a World Yoga University in America and prepare a funding brochure. I came to live in America and to look for a place to begin the work, but again I got the message, "Not yet. The time is not ripe." I sent out the beautiful printed brochure but the response came back to me—the time is not yet.

It seemed as if the whole world were turning toward the East. But I had been East and seen the sorry state of society which had emerged from the great teachings and laws of three thousand years of philosophy. I had lived in that society in which religion and philosophical thought were united in one, yet the flowering of that thought in the real world had yet to come. Then someone said, "Don't you realize that all your

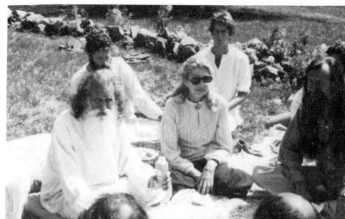

Christopher Hills and Swami Satchidananda meeting in California.

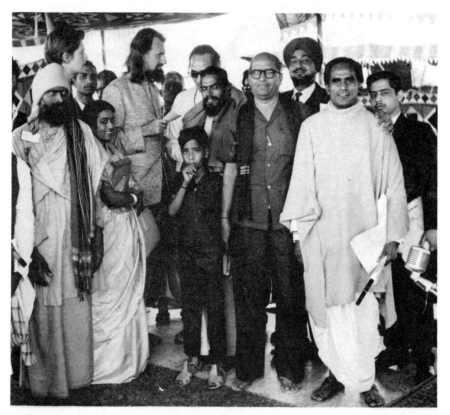

Christopher Hills with Rammurti Mishra (second from right) and participants in the 1970 World Yoga Conference.

Eastern meditation and philosophy affects only a tiny portion of the American population?" I saw that the response to all these new Oriental waves was coming from a deep need for spiritual experience in tens of thousands of Americans who were learning the old contemplative traditions, but not more than a handful would really get into these new waves and even if they did, they would be no better at the practice of these disciplines than they were at their own Christian practice of prayer and contemplation. Spiritual exercises in the religious life of the West had also, just like the East, been mainly for those few who took up the monastic or religious direction or for those like myself who had begun rethinking the biblical tradition and Christian spirituality. For the millions who daily toil and are caught in the net of their own thoughts, there could be no liberating exaltation, no vibrant contact with the beauty of the world and the perfection of the cosmos, while communication and sharing with each other was yet so superficial. To listen to a lecture, to meditate and pray together on a Sunday, to read books of spiritual stories of those who lived long ago (Marpa, Milarepa, Mary and Joseph, Radha and Krishna) seemed to repress originality and turn people into imitative cardboard puppets acting out life. What I wanted for the earth was the feeling of being in *love* with life, in love with God and intoxicated with the sound of everything vibrating just as it is! I wanted to get beyond words, quotations, concepts and scriptures to the real stuff.

My worst fears—that this new era in which Americans were turning to the Eastern philosophy and beginning to practice the art of meditation would be misused and would unconsciously strengthen the ego trips of those who wanted some ostentatious recognition—were confirmed. The tendency to wear beads and bracelets and meditation pants and to regurgitate half-digested concepts about Krishna, Buddha, Shiva and so on, made me feel that the West was failing in the actual manifestation of the Eastern teachings. In some way they were romanticizing the idea of reaching the egoless state in exactly the same way that the Christian pacifists, the communists, many scientists, and most religious fanatics romanticize unity but totally ignore the reality of the oneness of spirit and matter, even though it is all around us. There are just as many enlightened people in the West as there are in the East. It is just that in the West they are less visible and harder to find, because they live in a skeptical culture where truth is ever changing, whereas the East lives off its truths of three thousand years ago. To transplant these truths into the West could not, in itself, work a spiritual transformation. Several million Westerners may have been practicing some form of Eastern discipline or have heard of the I Ching or taken Karate back to its underlying Buddhist pacifist origins. I had myself turned Eastward, been a sadhu, known the religions and sacred Eastern chants, yet for me the same thing was missing from Eastern practice that was missing in our own Christian practice, namely *the world-changing, world-shattering, world-transforming penetration of our ego structure with the all-consuming love of the whole.* It was this missing dynamic contact that motivated Westerners to turn, unsatisfied, to try other practices. We were all looking for the same thing that works, the messianic feeling of "Now is the time" of the last days when the world will be transformed from top to bottom, from East to West. I knew it was not to be found in any particular tradition. A new insight was needed and it must have a scientific base, not a *religious* base but a *spiritual* one that made our different ideals, thoughts and scriptures mere commentaries on our own direct experience of God. We must enter the holy temple of the cosmic egg and find the flame of the original nucleus, the sacred fire which makes us come alive again and write *new* scriptures and write new stories and sing new songs and chants to God! Yet to those imprisoned within narrow minds these were sacrilegious words amounting to supreme arrogance. Such exuberance could be mistaken for religious fanaticism. What was needed was a method of slowly unfolding the nuclear self which didn't need to live in the past, study the past, dote on the events and personalities of the past but a method which looked to the bright future and turned to the unfolding evolutionary intelligence in all our social relationships so that our very house and village became a temple of the Divine. A contemporary form of scientific reality and spirituality is needed in the West, one that is able to incorporate the ever-changing truth of science into a never-changing framework of cosmic consciousness. We need the penetration of the primordial nucleus not in some abstract concept but as a realization that our own consciousness *is* that nucleus, and that we can never know it directly until we know what consciousness is beyond its mental, conceptual, idealistic thought structures which are only bubbles floating on its surface.

Nuclear Evolution is such a penetration of the structure of our experience of consciousness and it is therefore the key to the ONE Reality which Christ and Krishna, Buddha and Moses, Lao Tzu and all great sages clothed in their own different cultural garbs. They were all really saying the same thing but in the concepts and cultural idiom of their times. Nuclear Evolution is for our times and contains the simple essence of all these spiritual teachers in its insight into the nature of creation and the evolving consciousness which experiences it. This was the missing element in all this traditional "looking back" which did not energize our consciousness to look forward to the dazzling nature of consciousness itself—how to take hold of the raw stuff of our minds and shape its worth into something which can be communicated, shared and loved.

What *is* this shaping of worth? What *is* the true essence of the spiritual life that is so liberating to human consciousness and yet has constantly frightened people away in every era of history? One of my students at the University of the Trees says it perhaps better than I can:

> "When the teachings of spiritual yoga first came to me I thought it was a lot of hogwash, this business of men lying on nails and sitting all day apparently doing absolutely nothing. The miracles that were claimed seemed impossible outcomes of such practices. But then I met some people who had practiced meditation and spiritual disciplines, and I was very moved by their radiance. The kindness they showed to each other, the respect and sensitivity toward each other's inner worlds was a revelation to me, and I wanted to be part of them more than anything in the world.
>
> I began to meditate with them and began to experience a part of myself that I never knew I had. Deep feelings of love, care for nature, unity with others' hearts made me feel that I had found the key to life. I plunged headlong into Eastern teachings and felt that the sensitivity they brought and the refined consciousness they unveiled was the answer to the world's problem, certainly the answer for the youth

that had rejected Western materialism.

But after the initial entrancement with the Eastern teachings, my friends and I were confronted with the hard facts of dealing with our material needs. Several of my friends had children and soon were sucked right back again into traditional social roles and responsibilities. A lot of time, energy and consciousness was given to what was called "getting it together on the physical plane". Most of the people got bogged down and were not able to mesh their ideals with the practical reality of everyday life. So our group split apart and I was left feeling that there was something that hadn't been answered by the Eastern teachings.

My group had a cut-off point at the place where they didn't know themselves any deeper. If they got involved with nitty gritty relationship problems with their mates, no one had any answers. When they would work together on an enterprise and certain money problems would come up, they didn't know how to deal with the egos rising in each other. The soul love never wavered, but everyone ended up doing their own thing.

I decided that the only way the Eastern teachings could be lived to the full was to escape into a monastery, because that is the only place you could sustain the higher consciousness and not be bombarded with the intense challenges of present day material existence and communication. My friends and I were missing several levels of communication, not because we didn't want them but we hadn't the foggiest idea where to look. And neither do most of the Eastern teachers. They tell you to give it to God and transmute the problem in an idealistic devotional way. Not until I began to study Nuclear Evolution did I find any tools at all for dealing with life as it is.

Creative Conflict gave me the means to probe unconscious motivations and to find in myself and others the depth of communication that was missing on other levels in all the movements I had been through—liberal politics, the hippie culture, encounter and transpersonal psychology, even devotional yoga. I discovered that Creative Conflict does not talk about ego but deals with it in living situations, and this ego penetration, in my experience, is the only thing that releases pure unconditional love and truly fills that hole inside that people are always trying to fill.

THE FUTURE

Groundwork for the basic spiritual training of ego confrontation is now being laid by countless spiritual movements of every variety from Hindu to Sufi, from Christian to Transpersonal Psychology—all focusing on the one most important factor in changing anything whatsoever about our external world: the development of the individual self. For until an individual has lived through an experience, he cannot help another through it or even perceive that another is *going* through it, because he doesn't know what "it" is, or he knows only abstractly. If you have ever had the experience of being "helped" by someone whose advice did not come from actual living experience and personal growth, you will know that a person cannot change the world by preaching or telling others how to do it before he has done it himself. This is why ego confrontation, through Creative Conflict or other techniques, is so imperative to creating the New Age. The only problem that the world has or has ever had is personal and group selfishness, and every individual must study and master that enemy in his own psyche before he or she will know what to do about it in the world. This means working on oneself in real life situations, not just reading spiritual books or having discussion groups or doing affirmations or repeating mantrams. How can we know truth direct instead of reading it second hand?

Already the public has begun to realize that the answer they are seeking is well beyond the analysis and rationality of academia. More and more people are turning to yoga and meditation practice as the way into the peace that is beyond all the structural and institutional solutions. And because the fusing power of meditation is so tremendously powerful, in time it will bring to us a direct experience of the ideal of "community" as a total feeling of togetherness. Therefore a nuclear relationship in society is about to begin on a wider scale, a relationship that will eventually result in the "ultimate organism" cooperating with a set of laws shared with and evolved by the whole participating membership of society in the final quest for wisdom. Even socialism and capitalism will emerge from the dialectic with a completely new system which will unite the warring halves of this earth in the triumph of love as the ingredient of survival.

Does this sound like an extravagant claim, an impossibility? How will such a union ever come about? The answer is very simple. It will originate with individuals as the participants emerge out of the counterculture to change the political structure—strong, centered individuals who know themselves and know how to work together with others and have worked on their own unconscious motivations enough to set aside ego and become the willing agent of evolution, an instrument of the cosmic intelligence and a direct channel for the only One who really has the power to change the world. This long sought dream will come about not by anyone making messianic claims to special teachings from entities on high, not by giving false spiritual expectations to gullible but sincere people, not by asking people to give up their critical judgement. The New Age will come by training people to think for themselves. But first the world of human consciousness must be charted and its oceans and reefs mapped. We must plumb the depths of the heart, for only in the heart are people open to that penetrating force of total love which binds us—even to our enemies. At present people cannot communicate their real depths even in close relationships because they do not yet understand that genuine deep communication takes place only in the nucleus of being and that social evolution can therefore only happen at the level of the heart.

The transformation of the nuclear center of being of each person cannot be resisted nor controlled by political force; neither can it be regimented by political legislation. The heart is totally defenseless against real love and caring. Hence many have repeatedly mistaken the promises of those who came with an appeal to the heart but who abused the trust of the people. Lenin promised the oppressed millions of Russia a freer and better life, but in his own heart another motive was paramount but unspoken: he intended to *use* them as the energy and power which he needed in order to make the revolution happen. The elitism which shaped his concept of the "vanguard" of the revolution later came to fruition in the rigid hierarchy of the communist party, and the masses were left with an even worse domination than before.

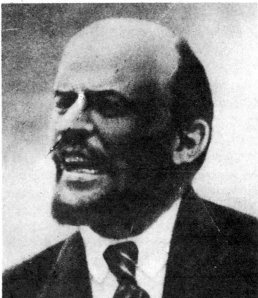

Lenin expounding the ideal of unity with the masses.

If the West can show that it really cares for the rights of our Russian repressed brothers and sisters while still rejecting their system of a repressive society, the two opposing systems will eventually respond to a non-violent solution of the existing hostility. This caring for human rights is the most important thing we can do to change the world vibration from negative to positive, for it is not material concessions or hand-outs of money, technology, food and aid that will give us any survival from destructive thoughts and actions. These material supports only bolster a false system in its errors. In any case, material help in technology or agriculture is only viewed by the communist peoples as the typical capitalist tendency to sell to the highest bidder in order to feather its own nest. This is what is taught officially in the schools of Moscow. But what the Russians want is what they have never had from their own people or from others: that is the understanding of the deep Russian heart which has through centuries of time allowed repeated exploitation by power cliques. We must all now see that violence and coercion by the State cannot bring communion in spirit. Nor can any group of idealists ever hope to bring world change by speaking even the highest truth or the wisest of prophecies. The cosmic fire must penetrate to the heart beneath all the words and beyond all ideals. This is why the group "nucleus" at the University of the Trees is not offering some merely intellectual ideas picked out of the sky but are actually creating right now an evolutionary system taken direct from Nature and from human nature in the daily operation of a specific constitutional instrument. This decision-making instrument is still evolving and will always be evolving as long as people understand that it is no more than a crystallization of their own evolving consciousness.

Programmed into the theory of Nuclear Evolution is the freedom which will not allow any theorist or idealist ever to take over again, without first proving empirically that his schemes can work with ordinary human beings. We have had in America since 1973, located at the University of the Trees, an empirical Nuclear Evolution community focussed on self-rule which brings growth for each individual participant and gives freedom of self-government in tune with the laws of nature. When the experiment reaches the right ripeness, it will begin its work of turning on the rest of the world, beginning with those who are ready and who now form the body of the counterculture.

Out of this background and parallel to the development of the present counterculture this system of nuclear government has been slowly evolving. While the youth movement was looking externally for "experience" rather than "self-knowledge", the way of Nuclear Evolution could not emerge. To negate the external culture that we live in is not as necessary as to feel the birth pangs of the New Age inside one's own self. Now self-knowledge and Nuclear Evolution must be tested in the wider experiment of growth reflected in those mirrors of our own egos—our fellowman.

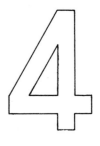

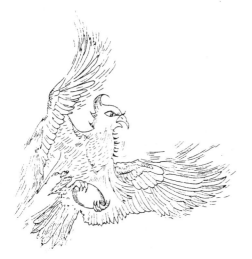

THE
WORLD
MIRROR

When life goes wrong, the natural human tendency is to blame someone near to us or blame the government or blame God, but the evolutionary energy is triggered only when we are strong enough to look for the cause within our own consciousness. With this kind of receptivity, communication is transformed. And when an entire group of people is committed to this kind of self-inquiry and self-honesty, the group vibration is lifted to a level of refinement that is found nowhere in the world that I have ever seen. Even in monasteries and spiritual ashrams, where the vibration is said to be very high, this holy energy of total transformation which comes from the evolutionary spirit working dynamically in an intensified and concentrated way, is not to be found. To create this energy or group consciousness was my purpose in founding the University of the Trees in Boulder Creek, California. The people gathered at the University of the Trees have committed themselves to Nuclear Evolution through the techniques of Creative Conflict. In other words, they have made a commitment to own their negativity and to receive feedback from one another as a "soul mirror" and to work on themselves until their consciousness is free of all limits which their personal history has placed upon it.

In the mythological story of the *Bhagavaad Gita* the field of action is the consciousness of man's mind and the heroes and villains are symbols of the different parts of human beings which must be conquered in order to preserve the world against its own self-destruction through ignorance. If we apply the analogy to the political field we find polarization of political forces symbolized in the powers of good and evil lined up in battle for men's souls. Right and wrong images of life compete for survival on the battlefield of Kurukshetra—the field of karma, governed by the laws of action. Everyman's battle between the selfish and selfless images of his mind is the history of his incarnation in this world. In the *Bhagavaad Gita*, the hero Arjuna, forced to do battle with his own kinsmen, is symbolic of every man in battle with his own lesser self. What an unthinkable thought that we should fight the very feelings and attitudes which we identify with as "me". As Arjuna says, "If I kill these desires, how can I ever enjoy my wealth, or any other pleasure?" Once the self-sense is gone, how can we enjoy life? This is the deep fear of every human being which keeps each person locked inside his ego, lest life lose its luster and excitement. "If we kill them," says Arjuna, "none of us will wish to live.": The evil king, Dhritarashtra, kinsman of Arjuna and Krishna, is the selfish ego inside us all with whom we must do battle in the name of righteousness or right action. This ego, with its desires, attachments, needs and ambitions, is the identity we treasure and yet is the source of all our pain and all our conflict; it darkens our life and leaves us feeling empty and unfulfilled. The ego is our enemy and yet it is also our most beloved self. We know this self-righteousness of the ego in others when we say, "He is his own worst enemy," and we know we are talking about the mental blindness of the person who does not see that the cause of his difficult situation is himself. It is not without accident that the evil king in the story of the *Gita* is blind and has to watch the battle through the eyes of another.

The World Peace Center works its constitution through Creative Conflict in order to fight our natural human tendency to separate ourselves from the whole and thereby place the responsibility for inner conflict on someone else or on some external field of action we call *society*. To fight this battle between outside and inside, good and evil, right and wrong action, is the purpose of yoga and it is also the purpose of the social yoga of the World Peace Center constitution-making process. The new politics is, then, a spiritual discipline and Creative Conflict is a Western form of yoga which need not be done in ashrams but can be practiced in society at large. It is a device of the enlightened consciousness that sees with clear perception that years spent developing the spiritual self with gurus isolated in ashrams away from the battlefield of society, leads not to action but to the supreme narcissism which must always be reflected in the mirror of the world state. If the state of the world is in dire conflict and ready to destroy itself, where are those supreme powers of yogis who have been prepared in the ashrams of the world? Where are the sages from the caves of the Himalayas? Are they now in our midst in the heat of the battle like Krishna and Arjuna?

The internal battle and the external battle are one and the same. Those military arms and weapons, in which the ignorant place their faith, reflect their deep distrust of the evil in another, because in themselves the Evil One (selfishness) holds sway, and the ego sits upon the throne of consciousness. This fearful, mistrusting, insecure and yet powerful king and kinsman is the one thing we must conquer and triumph over in the social union of a planetary consciousness. The foe is within, yet the battlefield is the world. Enlightenment cannot be merely the self-centered enlightenment of one individual, achieved in some remote cave or by merely looking at one's own face reflected in some far off lake in a Himalayan valley. It must be right here and now in the sweat and blood of the spiritual battle for men's souls. Are the retreats and hermitages of the world an escape from facing the violent birth of a new universe? Did God shrink from violence in the mad crucible of the first few seconds of the creation of all the atoms? How did Brahman* achieve the dynamic peace to be found in the expansion of the atoms of the cosmic egg?

---

* Brahman is the Sanskrit word for Universal Being or Pure Consciousness.

Our modern heroes have shrunk away from the ruthless task of rooting out the continuous violence which crowds our TV sets. We have tacitly agreed to the training of our children as the future killers of the world and we create in them those believers in the ultimate finality of death. Have the heroes fainted at the thought of telling mighty Mammon to stop exploiting the environment of the planet and to clean up his act?

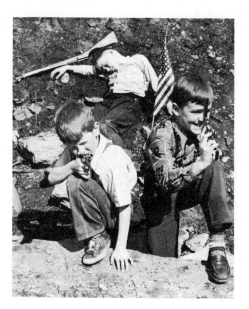

The Phoenix is eternally born to bring to us the message of the *Gita,* of life's eternal battle in our consciousness, coming down from the steep mountain paths and caves of the Himalayas to the homes of our future voters and idealistic makers of political dreams. For we must have crystal clarity on this fact: we are now poisoning our own nest with the false, naive and immature thought that to watch violence and competition for survival on the screen of the world scene is but a catharsis of human aggression. The conflict and aggression of the world is not on the screens, but in us. Only there is the war of our own consciousness fought and only there can selfishness and violence be ruthlessly exterminated. This is the true yoga of Creative Conflict with its promise that we may give birth to a new age of spiritual politics and save the world from itself.

The method of decision-making in the constitution of the World Peace Center is modeled on this concept of the entire earth divided in battle, in a life and death struggle for the ego, with all its worshippers of might and power on the one hand and on the other hand the selfless lovers of man, who rule through love. It would seem that love and power are arrayed upon the battlefield of life, with mighty rockets and tanks and guns on one side and the puny single individual heart yearning for peace on the other side. But the struggle is more subtle and not a simplistic either/or, to fight or not to fight, to love or to die. The point is, we *must* fight, whether we like it or not. The choice is only in the *way* we fight and in the skills we use to disarm the usurper that is sitting on the seat of power. Most people cannot understand that guns cannot be silenced by guns but only by changing the minds which pull the triggers. To do that we will first have to experience and understand the way our own minds gain power to preserve the ego. Only our heart works with love. How many of us are actually in touch with our heart's deep longing to be united with the one Self in all? Whatever pain and suffering we may have in our lives, it cannot compare with this deep unconscious pain in the heart that is longing to give itself away. Most of us spend all our lives seeking to *be* loved, not realizing that even when we are finally able to get it, the love is not enough and we are left still searching. Only when we give love are we fulfilled.

What does the tension feel like inside a person when he or she is pulled by two different drives at the same time: on the one hand the egocentric personal drive to gratify basic longings for acceptance, respect, security, and on the other hand that more subtle drive, deep at the heart's core, prompting us to our destiny, urging us to grow toward awareness of our larger Self, our connectedness with others, and our responsibility for that wholeness which we have turned our backs on, not just once or twice but at every moment? One young woman experienced it this way:

"I was a very introverted person and loved to sit in my
study reading and writing, feeding my mind and soul with
higher and higher and higher ideals. In my life, however, I
was avoiding contact with people almost entirely. I was
hiding even from friends, much less taking responsibility for
the whole world. I did not let myself compare the lofty
ideals with my own manifestation, because I felt trapped in
my antisocial nature and thought I could not overcome it.

As far as I knew, I was happy. But now, looking back upon
those years, I realize that the self-obsessed quality of my
search for Truth was intensely painful to me and although I
was happy, I never experienced fulfillment. The more
desperately I sought for the inner-peace that was my goal,
the more I found that until I could relate with others and
find external peace in situations which tested me and touched
my emotions, I would never have peace within.

When I moved to the University of the Trees, I was
answering a need to be part of life and to give of myself—a
need much deeper and far more imperative than the need to
"get" anything, even love. Having opened to this kind of
testing, I felt the pain of living, loving and feeling come as a
tremendous shock, after all those years of safety. Yet I find
that even when my emotions are unhappy, I am fulfilled.
Sometimes when my emotions are churning and my personal
life seems hopelessly tangled, I can feel my spirit singing,
and I see that it is content."

The powerful personal longings that we feel inside all come from
the mechanism of the ego and its way of separating our consciousness
from the situation we are in. Life presents us with opportunities every
day to learn of our selfishness and egocentricity, and the few who listen
to life, find her simple message—the knowledge of the Self—enthroned
only in the heart. All human beings have inborn drives and impulses to
control, and they incarnate on this earth to learn about them. The
entire present and future of our world depends on our learning more
about the vast regions of superspace between each atom of our being.

Where can we get this knowledge? This secret knowledge is available only to those who search for satisfaction and fulfillment in service to the world. The goal of Nuclear Evolution is nothing less than a way for the whole of mankind to become the vanguard of a new race of space beings. We don't need to go out into space to become a space being. The joke is that we already are space beings whether we like it or know it or not.

Habits of thought die hard, and the greatest of all wet blankets upon the human spirit is the feeling that we are no more than what most of our parents told us we were. The journey into the core of Self or Being, the exploration of the unconscious and discovery of the capabilities still harnessed within the brain—these contain the greatest answers for world and individual peace. There is no separation between these two kinds of peace. There is no way to undo our interconnectedness with the rest of the world. To seek only for our own personal betterment is the illusion of the separative ego which cannot see that the world and "other people" are only a mirror reflection of itself. The world seems many but is really only One, and it is not Nature's way to evolve only one part of her creation. Evolution is happening to the whole, whether we choose to flow with it or not. Therefore, any real transformation of society will require some stretching of the individuals who make up that society. This is the fundamental premise of the World Peace Center.

COMMUNICATION: OUR MOST REVEALING MIRROR

The World Peace Center is the name I have given to the activity of thousands of small groups who one day will come together as one great movement of overlapping circles. This plan is predicated on the realization that without better people, better systems cannot work. So far the individual has lagged behind the more sophisticated methods of group decision-making which have evolved through systems such as computers, parliaments, democracies, companies, and the system of dictatorships set up by the Soviets. To transform or replace these systems of large human decision-making organisms we must embark on a worldwide search at the small group or family level for better

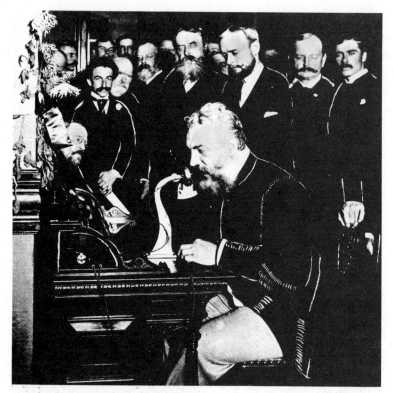

Alexander Graham Bell: he made iron talk.

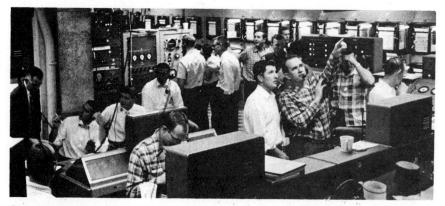

Communication and control

ADVANCED TECHNOLOGY DOES NOTHING TO IMPROVE THE QUALITY OF COMMUNICATION.

systems which at the same time produce better people. There must be a better way. To believe that the system, however idealistic, is somehow more safe or better than the people who run it, has been the naive belief of mankind up to now. We tend to feel an awe for scientific method that is somehow greater than our faith in dry cerebral scientists. We feel respect for the government, though we know the politicians are corrupt. We have a reverence for Christianity despite centuries of mediocre Christian preachers and teachers who could not in their own personal evolution back up the true message of Christ. We must now come to know that no instrument is better than its player, no tool is better than its user, and even the artificial intelligence in a computer is no better than its programmer. The problem is that we ourselves are also people who cannot always back up with our being what we preach with our mouths. We talk to one another, yet somehow we do not communicate.

People get used to poor communication and accept it as part of life. Children soon learn that they cannot speak their real feelings with their parents, and the parents are frustrated too. They feel they must mold and guide their children but often cannot get through to them. We try new systems, new machines, we build rockets to the moon, and yet there is something unfulfilled, some contact with others not made. A wife and husband love each other yet they drift apart, and neither mentions that they are mostly relating in superficial ways and that something is missing. A man is growing old. To whom can he talk and say that he is afraid of death? A child hears he is loved, yet can't quite feel it is true. He is insecure and feels alone. A woman's friends will not invite her when they gather to be sociable. She does not know why. They smile but say nothing. In our lives we have these gaps in communication, gaps in our lives, and we are so accustomed to them that we hardly notice. Our brother is a bit ruthless and in small ways he wrongs us. But he is a loved one. For the sake of family harmony we say nothing. Twenty years later, he is twenty times more ruthless than before. These are the ways of human life. Technology cannot alter our drives and motives nor improve our relationships. What *does* determine the quality of our love, hate, anger, greed, fear, generosity or gentleness? What kind or quality of consciousness does it take to even raise such a question? We are told that the fault lies with the system. What utter nonsense! We are talking in this chapter about changing society by working on *ourselves* and we have to realize that this work begins and ends with communication. Most human problems spring from this one common source.

NOT UNTIL OUR COMMUNICATION IS RIGHT WILL WE BEGIN TO SEE THAT WE ARE ONE

If you think how simple is this truth, you will be amazed that we could be so unaware of how important communication really is.

It is a fundamental point of this book that quality of communication (not speed or ease or quantity but *quality*) can only be improved if we improve both the consciousness which is communicating and the consciousness which is listening. But listening is very rare. Real listening is getting your own responses and reactions out of the way long enough to hear not only the words of another person but the message between the lines, the vibration of his being. Any political system which ignores this fundamental fact will eventually peter out of the evolutionary spiral. The evolutionary intelligence moves over vast periods of time, so it becomes imperceptible, but it eventually roots out all irrelevance from existence as surely as it roots itself into the fabric of life. Therefore the cornerstone of Creative Conflict is receptivity and its goal is genuine being-to-being communication. One cannot listen if one's ego is in the way.

This morning, two years after our last attempt with the National Science Foundation (NSF), we tried again to communicate with the government about the algae project and again met with closed minds. "We have to have papers to show to the president," they said. "We are getting our papers ready to show him now." When we spoke of the previous rival Republican administration which cancelled our project, we met with receptivity, but when we spoke of feeding the world, we were told that the project now being prepared to show to President Carter was based on wheat. Wheat costs much, much more to produce than algae costs, but the budget plan has allotted two billion dollars and there are certain interest groups who would like to supply the wheat. To get past this network of priorities (among which the feeding of the world's starving people is pretty far down the list) we had to actually shout down the telephone line! Such is the state of most human communication.

PROGRESS IS NOTHING NEW

Recently there have been a number of ideas for instantaneous citizen participation in voting procedures, such as electronic ways of registering the will of the people by telephone or computers which instantly record the number of people for or against a particular issue and communicate it to representatives at the seat of government. There have also been a number of world constitutions offered to Americans by members of the World Federalist Union over the past thirty years which aroused little general interest. All of these efforts have centered on the present federal system and have concentrated on improving methods of voting. They had nothing revolutionary to offer apart from faster ways of communicating our will. The issues which affect modern man are not those which need more speed in voting or ease of voting. The speed of decision can have no effect; in fact the voters need to take more not less time and care to decide things rightly, rather than swiftly. Speed may be a modern obsession, but in fathoming the depths of human actions "slow but sure" is faster.

This fascination with speed and cleverness leads to the illusion that mankind is somehow progressing, that the quality of our decisions is improved by our tools. But a man is no more intelligent about *why* he does something with a computer instead of with his head or *why* he drives a car to a destination instead of a horse and buggy. In fact, if a journey would take a week instead of a day, the thinking process on the way might even realize that many of our journeys, trips and motions are totally unnecessary. Some people look back to the positive pioneering spirit that built the haven of American freedom, the dynamic motivation which made America so affluent, and they feel that the only hope for us today is to begin again in the same way, to escape off this crowded planet into space colonies. But we shall only take our negativity with us into the colonization of outer space so that the same problems will arise again. Technology cannot save us from ourselves. If we cannot create a loving group here on earth, is it not a delusion to

92

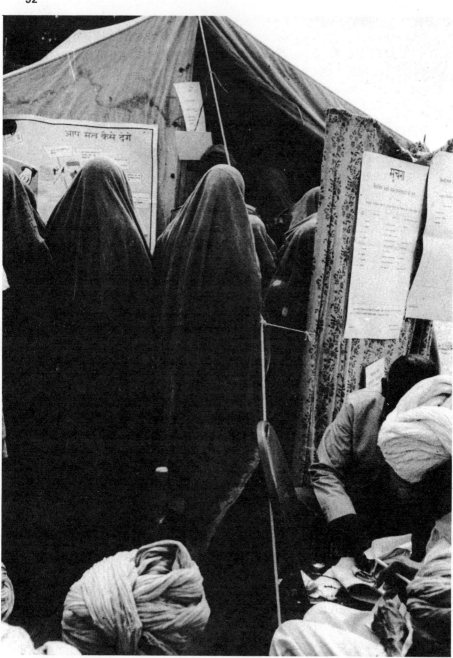

A group of women voters outside a polling tent in the sandy wilderness of western Rajasthan.

think that we can do it on a space station? When we witnessed the landings on the moon we were there with a TV camera in our consciousness seeing the first astronauts walk on the surface. Yet in spite of our sophistication not one new word was said over that tremendously complex system. It was like telephoning your mother in Australia and saying nothing but "Hello Mother."

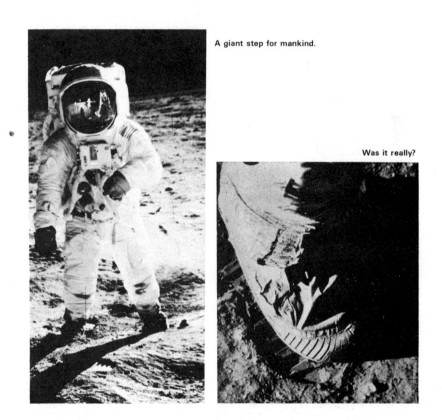

A giant step for mankind.

Was it really?

It is the improved *quality* of our communication which is necessary, not the speed of it nor the amount. The slowest letter written by a genius will always be far more important than a telegram from a moron.

Believing in our communications technology we have said, "Let us bring education, TV, telephones and electricity to the poverty-stricken areas of the globe." Yet those very societies who have "instant communication" have not evolved as individuals any more than those who lack telephone and TV. We know that communication face to face is more efficient than such devices, because we cannot say we "know" someone merely by seeing them on television or speaking to them on the telephone. And even when we *are* face to face, do we communicate? Do those sincere missionaries who devote their love and their lives face to face with the poverty-stricken peoples of the world, actually bring any more than an ideal personality cult into the lives of the masses, which many later reject? Why should they expect blacks to take up the essence of Christ's teaching any more than their white brothers have done in practice? Do not the African countries, the people of Asia and the third world end up resenting the invasion of Christian teachings of non-violence and instead espouse the violent guerilla warfare teachings of Mao Tse Tung?

If there is any way to lift even a corner of the wet blanket and let in a ray of light to people who walk in darkness, it is clear that neither science nor religion has found it. And a new way has to be found. To say this to people committed to Christ seems like blasphemy, but Christ himself said the same thing, much to the displeasure of his fellow Jews to whom the scriptures were more holy than life. Christ put life itself before the scriptures and therefore his way was and still is a new way. It is the quality of what we do and what we are, not what we say that speaks to the soul in every person.

WHAT IS IT LIKE
TO HAVE REAL INTEGRITY?

Now the time has come again when we must re-discover the "way", using both religion and science to tap a wisdom which is very old. This is the way of Nuclear Evolution. This very ancient new idea is simply this: that unless we can grow enough so that we embody and actualize and become a living example of whatever ideal or system we preach, we cannot communicate. Our *being* must communicate what words can never fully say. Several University of the Trees students went to a symposium at a small private school some months ago and shared the platform with two authors of famous books on the Physics of Consciousness. At first these students were a bit intimidated because these acute intellectual minds were insisting that the University of the Trees had not done proper scientific research. They claimed that it had not done experiments that could be reduplicated and validated by others.* But later, as the arguments grew more and more heated, the University students became more and more centered. Their training in Creative Conflict would stand them in good stead and they knew it. Even the audience began to realize that the famous physicists, so knowledgeable in their fields of specialization, knew almost nothing at all about their own emotions. The meeting came to a climax as Sue, the youngest member of the University of the Trees, age 22, turned to one of the physicists, whose emotions were by this time entirely out of control, and insisted that he mirror back the moderator's last communication. When he refused, the audience went up in arms and forced him to repeat her communication to show that he had heard and understood. His arrogance became very obvious to everyone in the audience.

When the students returned home to the University they reported to the rest of us that the scientists had demanded proper experiments. One student summed up the whole difficulty in a simple phrase: "They didn't realize *we* were the experiment." But the audience, feeling the communication of each student's *being*, perceived the truth instinctively and in their hearts were moved to stand up for what they knew. The audience began as a collection of separate individuals but ended as a unified whole, made *one* in feeling by the impact of a few young people who had done some work on themselves. Our bond as a society is a living thing, a thing sensitive to vibrations. The intellectual presentation of the two physicists maintained the traditional division between authority and audience (government and the silent masses) but these "passive" listeners were ALIVE. They needed only the right spark in order to rise up and say where they stood. When such people

---

* It turned out that these "experts" themselves had not done any experiments in the subject they were talking about, whereas I have done reams of research, all scientifically validated, which I can prove to anyone who asks me, though I do not dwell upon that aspect when I write.

are banded together as a World Peace Center, their government will be
alive because *they* are alive. Mere academic knowledge will never be
enough to draw respect and obedience. It will have to be backed up
and balanced by awareness of man as a *whole* being, with a heart as
well as a head.

A NEW IDENTITY

To reform society by technology or to improve our methods of
voting is only patching up an antiquated system. The real evolutionary
step will not come by a better way of voting but only by a better way of
solving the conflict within and between the individuals who will cast
the votes. What we need is something really new, something so vital
and all-engrossing that people become greatly changed and evolved by
the practice of decision-making: a system which works in such a way
as to create a group conscious entity, with each of us conscious of
every other living entity as an integral part of ourself. In the World
Peace Center, the constitution is a direct manifestation of the consciousness of the individuals who create it, day by day. It is a living
expression of their values and their aims and their understanding. So it
is not just a chore and a responsibility for the world "out there" but a
venture inward. As the individuals grow, the living constitution also
grows. It is not a document written by some consciousness hundreds of
years ago, reaching out of the past to govern us in the now.

It is true that even in the most utopian community a constitution is
still a set of *external* rules which say how we shall be governed. And
those people who abhor all rules in favor of self-discipline are quite
correct: there would or should be no need for governments if human
beings *could* discipline themselves. However, I have noted that all
those who object to even a minimum number of rules are those whose
behavior is most lacking in the minimum amount of self-discipline.
Actually rules are only *ways of doing* things. All rituals are ways of
going about certain cultural occupations and they save us having to
repeat instructions every time we pray, get married, crown the king, or
deck the town mayor. Similarly the law courts are rituals of human
behavior which have enshrined the rules of a complex society into the
legal system. Any constitution merely describes the intellectual tools

by which the traditional methods and concepts of government are formed into an operating system. But when these rules take on a life of their own and begin to reflect a legalistic totalitarianism rather than self-government, then each one of the individuals in the group must learn to determine clearly where the bottom line must be drawn between themselves and the larger group.

We are so used to big government that we adjust to its encroachments almost without noticing, but once you get into a small self-governing group or a business or a club, particularly if it requires your time, money or energy, you soon become acutely aware of this line, and you begin to feel the group encroaching upon your personal freedom. Gaining a real control over this subtle line is the answer to the human riddle of individual freedom in the free society versus the "totalitarian self" of communist society. This riddle of life presently splits the planet into two separate warring halves, and the survival of each depends on their ability to synthesize the individual freedom of democratic society with the social responsibility for the *total*itarian whole. A synthesis must take place between the **thesis** of self-centered freedom and the **antithesis** of external totalitarian discipline. And the creative tension between the two becomes the life-force for both individual and social growth. Herein rests the dynamism that is missing in most people's lives. True democracy means self-government not in name only (being counted) but a taking hold, a shaping of our worth. In relation to the group, we define who we are in the delicate balance between freedom and responsibility.

Governments and their rules need not be arbitrary collections of institutions, committees, and councils acting separately from the people who produce them. Governments *can* be, if we know how to make them be, living arrangements of complex activities. But they can make this living growth ONLY if the participating individuals themselves are willing to change and grow. The constitution must not be some ideal which is far out ahead of what we are as a people. The ideal must be an expression of what we *are* and what we can embody. The Marxist ideal of sovereignty for all is a bright flag of freedom flying above the grey walls of oppression in every communist country. Only the few dissidents have dared openly to confront the discrepancy between the

ideal and the actual way of life imposed on the people. In America the
Bill of Rights, that sounds so lofty and inspiring, may seem a mockery
to the victims of racial slights and intimidation and discrimination in
courts of law.

To regard a constitution as sacrosanct, an awesome piece of paper,
difficult to amend and change, is stifling to growth. Many people cling
to the stability of their "holy cow", however antiquated, because to
consider change makes them feel insecure. As individuals we deal with
our feelings of insecurity by building self-confidence and seeking ego
food. Often the most confident-seeming person—the one who lets
everyone know his good points and makes others aware of their weak
points—is the most unsure inside himself. His strength is not real and
solid but is a false confidence built on faulty foundations and misinforma-
tion about others. To get to a real and solid security, he must be strong
enough to let go of his inflated self-image and be someone more
ordinary and yet more real. Similarly, as a nation, our feeling of
security, rooted in a strongly written constitution, is also fake security.
For an individual or for a nation there is only one way to grow and
evolve and that is to bring our manifestation more into line with our
self-image or with our written documents. Our security is not in
legalistic phrases of a constitution but in our creation of a *living*
constitution through responsible involvement with other people. Once
we do get involved, the constitution ceases to be a "Thou shalt"
document and becomes an interaction with real human beings. Then
love enters in and a new sense of righteousness is born—not *self-*
righteousness ("I know what is best for you") but the ability to take
"right action" because you care enough about others to know what
they are feeling. If a constitution is only a set of rules with which you
comply, there is no call to expand your heart. But if you look on the
constitution as guidelines for living with fellowman, then inevitably
your heart is involved and your love is called forth. If this love is
missing, the constitution is a legal farce.

A SPIRITUAL NECESSITY

We can escape our responsibility for righteousness and leave these
problems for the politicians to handle, but most politicians are more

interested in their own careers than in you or me. Who shall look out for your freedom, your growth, your future if not yourself? We cannot afford to abdicate this responsibility for the conditions of life right now by becoming mentally caught up in the excitement of a purely idealistic or utopian future. Even if it is not our cup of tea, we must be willing to participate in the everyday political scene in order to guide social life toward the future. Most people feel that they do not know what to do or how to do it. It is not just a matter of joining your local political party. It is a matter of taking responsibility for what happens to you. This awakening to the world as an extension of our own vibration, through caring, is the real meaning of the word "spiritual", because our individual spiritual growth cannot be divorced from the constant re-creation of the ultimate social organism. One is the outgrowth of the other. Some people plant flowers in their own back yard. Others do their best to make a garden of the world. Those who believe themselves to be spiritual seekers and yet are not motivated to involve themselves in social governing, belie the very essence of spirit, which is expansion. People are willing to passively let society affect their lives because they do not see that spirit is radiation *outwards* in action, vitality, caring, and creativity.

This passivity appears in its most exaggerated form in Marxism, which says that our spiritual nature is passively acted upon and formed entirely by our social system. On the contrary, it is obvious that

ANY SOCIAL SYSTEM IS FORMED OUT OF OUR SPIRITUAL INTELLIGENCE OR THE LACK OF IT

We need only look at life as it is actually lived under the communist regimes now established in several parts of the world. Those who extoll it without actually living there and "knowing" first-hand should go there. On their return they will make better dedicated workers for the real synthesis. The fact is, the Marxian hypothesis about the human spirit is 180 degrees out of phase with the laws of the universe, and the communist manifestation proves it. Yet our Western manifestation is not that much better. We are not radiating either but are living the same life of contraction. Just as billions of Christians have lived out the letter of the law and entirely missed the spirit of Christ's teachings, so too both communists and capitalists the world over are living out the opposite of their own ideals. Therefore a true synthesis of these two systems of government lies in the union of the individual with the whole, so that the world becomes a mirror of each person's energy and love, and this caring is reflected back to each of us in deep fulfillment.

NARROW IS THE WAY

The members of the World Peace Center are committed not just to ideals for the future but to individual growth in the here and now. This is the rub. Who actually *wants* to change? No one. This is why Christ said, "Straight is the gate and narrow is the way which leadeth unto life and few there be that find it." At the University of the Trees, people laughingly admit to one another, "Even the people who *want* to change don't want to." A commitment to self-change is a very rare thing in the world. One member of our center had a realization of this basic fact of human nature and expressed it as follows:

> "I went home to visit my family in hopes of rest from the intense pace of life at the University of the Trees, but I met with the same human conflicts that we deal with in our Creative Conflict meetings. After a long and frustrating argument with my sister-in-law which lasted until three o'clock in the morning, she turned to me and said "I'm not *ready* to change." I was stunned. I had become so accustomed to living with people committed to listening and to growth that I had spent hours trying to communicate with her and never once stopped to ask if she had any intention of changing anything at all about herself. Like most people, she was eager that *I* should change but was unwilling even to meet me half-way."

The secret of commitment to the Creative Conflict technique is that people care enough to change. Then they can begin to live in harmony together and, once they do, they reach a threshold of evolution that is like the birth of a new organism. The incredible power in even a small commitment is like the power sleeping inside the atom which is released by nuclear fission. It is that "holy energy" I spoke about before, that evolutionary dynamism which can re-create the world. The new organism which will be created is not *based* upon the constitution, as though one precedes the other, but is one with it. Therefore the constitution of the World Peace Center is not a legalistic description of an institutional approach ("The System") but can be seen as the track record of the way a group has functioned together as a living whole.

GROUP CONSCIOUSNESS

When molecules become cells and individual cells become organs and the organs become a human body, the organism called man begins to have a history. The brain then records this history in time through memory which ties the whole organism together conceptually with its environment. However, the concept of *the whole* is not really formed by the environment but by each single person, by his or her own power of consciousness. By recognition and identification with the "whole" rather than with our ego as a separate part, the union with the totality takes place from within. The union can never result from any external or totalitarian pressure or coercion, but is completely self-programmed. A kind of *divine marriage* takes place when the individuals of society, like the individual brain cells, begin to function together to create a higher level of organization and accomplishment. The written form of the constitution can be likened to the conceptual memory. But the nature of "group consciousness" and the "union" process, by which the individual members become fused as one, is the embodiment of the real constitution. The word *union* in Sanskrit is spelled "yoga" and therefore the process can be described as "social yoga".

To map out this new step in evolution and to achieve a gradual social synthesis of separate egos is the purpose of this book. This is the something new that Nuclear Evolution has to offer to society and to the individuals which make it up. The idea of fusing men into one brotherhood may sound a bit familiar, since politicians and philosophers have used the same language for centuries to talk about society and its ideals. However, most of us have long since stopped believing that people could *really* be fused into one organism with the same love that binds our cells together in a living body. For centuries, the monasteries and ashrams have looked upon yoga and discipline as the perfection of the individual soul in the cloistering of the few rather than the many. Yet even in these small, dedicated groups, a genuine "group consciousness" has never manifested because the filial religious love is still only love of one ego for another person. What is the something new that can make us believe, even for a moment, that total union and "group consciousness" is possible? What is the something new that can make us want this union enough to pay the price it will cost us to change? Did not much of the world embrace Christianity and throw out the Christ for precisely this reason: that the cost was too high? And is it not all the more discouraging when we see what a heavy and lumbering thing a normal group can be? To think of a group ever producing a work of art or a concerto by Beethoven or a theory like Einstein's is an unthinkable thought. In fact, it has been proved over and over again in certain fields of creative human endeavor that groups in general produce less quality, less action and more talk, less good and more evil than any individual that ever lived.

Many a time, in the years of trying to build a group-conscious assortment of individuals, my heart has fallen to its greatest depths when the group has spent hours, weeks, months deciding to do what I myself could do in one afternoon all by myself with one hand tied behind my back. Many times I have reminded myself that the patience of God and the long span of evolution had to be my model. If I went out and did the job myself, the group would not grow, nor would the individuals that comprise it ever understand the wider dynamic and potential of the individual *self* versus the *group.* I've often thought to myself, "Let somebody else do the work on group consciousness. Why does it have to be me? All I want to do is sit in the sun and write. And after I'm done, I can point to a pile of books and say, 'See, that's what I've accomplished.' But if I foolishly invest my life in working with a bunch of people, then I have nothing to show for it but their growth, and most of them don't even realize it." These negative thoughts haunted me in the back of my mind during years of travel, forming groups which repeatedly failed to match my expectation. The doubts only went away when I realized that the results of my efforts didn't really matter, because my own attitude and motivation were the real source of my fulfillment. There didn't seem to be anyone else to do the work, and I could see it had to be done. I knew that I had to be responsible for the group (for the world) because I am the group. As long as we are imprisoned in our ego we cannot truthfully say that we are the group or realize it and least of all experience it. What does it feel like to get this insight so that we do see it as something new and not just some concept in a book? What brings it alive and makes it a living experience of love? What does it mean when we say, "I am the group"? It means nothing less than "God consciousness", not as an ego thinking we are God but not seeing any difference which separates us from God. The first time I confided this realization to another human being was on a mountaineering trip with a close friend whom I loved very much. I lost a friend. He completely projected his own egotism onto me and virtually accused me of saying I *was* God. I tried to point out the subtle difference between the loss of ego which sees no differences between itself and the whole, and the kind of ego he was talking about. But it was no use. He kept insisting that I was claiming to be God, which I was not. I did not want to be God and was quite happy being an inseparable part of the whole. But I experienced no separation from God and I was foolish enough to say so. Years later I experienced this sense of oneness even more deeply. I was standing in a bedroom looking at my own face in the mirror when suddenly I realized that the eyes looking back at me from the mirror were not mine but were the eyes of my teacher, whom I loved very much. It is hard to express in words the deep love for all creatures that springs from such an experience of oneness. It is an incredible kind of love, and it is locked inside every heart.

I knew that once people could come to this same realization they would make that fantastic evolutionary leap in which cells become organs and organs become bodies and bodies beget brains and memories and then something becomes possible in the world that was not possible before. The difference between the level of consciousness in the atoms of your body and the much more widely ranging consciousness in the complex workings of your thought processes as a total person—your memories, hopes, dreams, disappointments, inventions, plans, feelings, intuitions—is vast. And yet the only difference is that the atoms and molecules have formed "group consciousness" in your cells. They work as a harmonious whole. Your other levels in ordinary consciousness as yet do not. Once people see that they *are* the world (in the same way that your hand must realize it is *you* and not some separate member) then individual people become organic wholes and a new threshold in consciousness is reached. This is not just an idea or a feeling that we *should* have. It is a deep, transforming experience that we can and will have because it is our potential to do so, just as our cells had the potential to become organs. The same vast leap to group consciousness is possible to us now in whatever degree we can realize a new identity with the whole of mankind.

The human race, acting as one, can accomplish goals like going to the moon, which no genius, however enlightened he may be, can accomplish on his own. The fantastic thing about going to the moon is not the trip itself but the fact that human cooperation can achieve anything that it imagines. It only remains now to apply an even greater spirit of cooperation in mind and heart, not to a trip away from the earth but to the challenge of staying here and finding our real place on earth. For this reason, even if you are one of those who is bored by politics and cherishes a challenging self-image of the rugged individualist, then group consciousness is calling you from a higher level of your own potential to open to a new idea NOW. Can you be big enough in your individuality to lose yourself in the whole group without losing your uniqueness or your power to act on the authority of your own soul? Such a statement may appear paradoxical and illogical to some who are bound to egocentric ways of looking, but if we reflect on those who have followed nature's patterns we see clearly that all truly great people have thought in that selfless, non-egocentric way.

KURUKSHETRA:
FACE TO FACE WITH THE NEGATIVE

Group consciousness is Nature's own way, and it is Nature which has formed the group in Boulder Creek, California, with whom I am now working. One by one they were drawn to the area, without the means of any communications media or lavish advertising, without any particular promotional effort on my part to draw them. They just came. And despite the rigor of self-discipline required by the life here and the work on themselves, most of them who commit themselves to self-growth stay. What drew them? And what keeps them here? The way of life here goes against the very selfish core of human nature that tells us to work for ourselves, to look out for number one, to survive. And yet they stay, and their light draws others. The new ones don't want to come. They are afraid of facing their own negatives. But they see a light and they cannot stay away.

It is true that some who come to do this work on themselves do not stay to see it through. One young woman who has been with us just a few months has just this week decided to leave. At one of the University of the Trees dinner groups, she complains that certain people are sending her a bad vibration. The other eleven people, however, experience just the reverse. They say that this young woman is sending out a vibration so hostile and belligerent that it is difficult not to respond to it in kind. So in actual fact, the newcomer is herself *creating* the bad vibe that is coming back to her. Physical violence has followed her all the way through childhood, college and through two marriages. And everywhere she goes throughout the rest of her life, unless she makes a radical change in her being, people will continue to send her a hostile vibration. Why? Because

THE OUTSIDE WORLD IS ONLY A MIRROR

and it cannot send us anything other than what we ourselves are putting out.

This situation is difficult because the woman in question is so reactive and defensive that communication with her is almost impossible. She replies to all comments as if she were conducting a press conference and does not let anyone get through to her heart or touch her emotions. "I'm not ready to be this selfless," she says, "I intend to keep working on myself, but I want to be selfless somewhere else than here." Someone replies, "You know, what you are really doing is running away from facing yourself. It is okay if you are not ready to be selfless, but at least don't kid yourself about it." The words do not get through because this person is seeking a "cause" which will feed her own ego's needs. Already she has two socially respectable causes that offer an outlet for her natural belligerence. She will not accept a cause that requires her to look *into* this inner violence rather than simply to express it. Why not? Because this negativity is her very self, her identity, the lifeblood of her ego which intends to survive, no matter what.

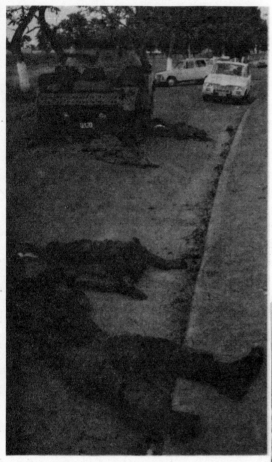

Civil war in Lebanon, not between nations but between religions, makes a mockery of the Arab Moslem and the Christian ways shown in this photo.

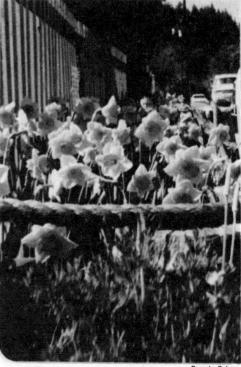

Pamela Osborn

When human beings can grow like flowers and take themselves and their consciousness as a garden for composting and weeding they can create beauty like this street at University of the Trees.

I am not suggesting that anyone repress the negative energies within them but only that they be willing to look within and to work with whatever is real, even if it is unpleasant. This is the timeless battle of mankind that Arjuna fought in the *Bhagavaad Gita,* coming face to face with the negative part of his own self. Since the negative is Nature's way of teaching us to become positive, our negativity need not be rejected as worthless but is the good manure in which our finer selves may flower. To own and get into our negativity in a positive way and to see it as an opportunity to duplicate Nature's way is to understand that even excreta is the fuel for plant organisms that trap the light. We need only remember that the light of the universe itself (the excreta of stars) is our life. What is absorbed and re-radiated out of our beings, our eyes, our minds and in the words of our mouths is our own psychic excreta that the universe somehow turns back into light.

How can human beings use the negative picture and expose it like a photograph and see its positive image? Through the technology of Creative Conflict we can obtain so many positive prints from the one negative condition of human consciousness, that we see how light does actually turn the negative into positive. This exciting prospect for man is outlined in my book *Nuclear Evolution.* How we can clear the excreta of our minds and turn the constipation of centuries of self-delusion into light is the purpose of Nuclear Evolution. It requires no more than the will (the heart) to test its proofs: to open ourselves to the mirror which comes to us through our life situations or through the honest feedback of a group committed to openness.

The difficulty of the task need not throw us into a pit of negativity. We must make up our minds once and for all that the hero's task is to clean out the Aegean stables, with their accumulated excreta of centuries of living. To do the impossible we need the insight of the hero, Hercules, who found himself eternally condemned to shovelling the manure of ages and decided instead to divert a river to wash the muck away. This is the crucial point. How do we get together as a group and find a way, through using the stream of consciousness? The mighty river of consciousness is the only power which can wash away from man's mind those limitations put there by human consciousness through suggestion and self-hypnosis over the centuries. Only conscious-ness can remove what consciousness has created. This is the nuclear secret of our incarnation on this planet if we can face it: that no matter how big the world seems and no matter how powerless we feel to change it from its present course, we do have the power to change our *own* course and in so doing become that hero who can also change the world. The real hero is not me or you but that limitless love and limitless power of consciousness which pours through any man or woman whose heart is big enough to let it in. To whatever extent we are able to do this, the instantaneous change in our world (however large or small that world may be) will mirror back to us the tremendous power of our freedom and the awesome size of our responsibility.

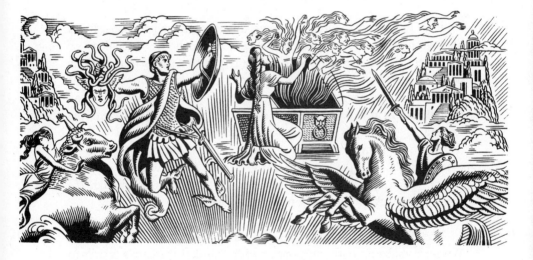

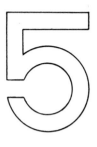

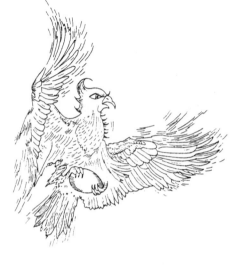

THE
NEW AGE
LEADER

The New Age leader is not only committed to serving others but also risks everything in that service, meaning that his* own fulfillment will only come when he is totally giving of himself and not holding something back. So one of the qualities of the nuclear leadership that must be present is SELFLESSNESS. Leadership in the ordinary world is full of selfishness, achieving fame and power for oneself and bestowing it on others in order to make henchmen and followers. A selfless person, however, does not seek advantage over another nor does he rise on the backs of others nor does he attempt to gain anything for himself, but merely leaves it to the group or to the cosmos to reward him with a sense of satisfaction. And he does not believe in

---

* I am using the pronoun "he" for convenience, but of course the true leader may be either male or female since the prime criterion is selflessness.

failure, because failure to do something really big and important and difficult is not really a failure. If someone is frightened of failing and allows that fear to take him over, then he won't tackle very much. He'll be content to risk very little of himself. So a New Age leader and one who is going to practice Nuclear Consciousness must be prepared to risk a lot, in fact to risk everything, since, if he lost everything and failed, this itself would teach him more than if he risked very little and succeeded. So the whole attitude of a nuclear leadership is almost 180 degrees opposite to that which you find in regular politics. Instead of trying to gather wealth and power and fame and reputation, one is doing the opposite, getting rid of power, getting rid of wealth, as it were, and building up the social wealth, the common wealth.

If one is going to become a leader because there are certain privileges involved, then we can never have a nuclear leadership, we can never have a leader who can think of everyone as part of himself. And what kind of example would it show if a spiritual leader became great merely because everyone else worked their butts off and he used that love and energy and sent everyone else out to work, so that he could sit on a gilded throne being adored by his followers? Is this a trap? Is there anything New Age in that, or is it just disguised spiritual materialism? Is our investment going to be in setting the guru on a throne or will we invest our consciousness in cleaning up our act? Is not sitting on a guru's throne the same thing as becoming president or leader of some political party or of some movement but with a spiritual veneer on top? Is it not just the need of people to have some focus— father figure, guru, call it what you like—who obligingly sits on a golden throne and dresses up in fine robes so that he can be adored and thereby fill the need of people who are really looking for an escape instead of thinking for themselves? They expect a guru to think for them, do everything for them, and they trust him to decide their life and everything in it and they throw themselves, as it were, in surrender at the feet of someone who is supposed to know better. Is this really New Age? Or will that person force everyone to look at themselves and think for themselves and achieve self-mastery like *he* has done?

If we are going to become leaders then we have to look inside and ask ourself, "Are we eligible to pass through this test?" The ancient myths used to tell of a hero who had to pass through certain tests that were set by the cosmos, not by man, since human tests could always be fixed, but tests set by the cosmos were always impossible ones for ordinary people. So Nuclear Evolution* is a bit like that, finding the Golden Fleece. It sets an impossible task so that whoever should get it will become a hero, the hero merely being the one who dedicates himself to the goddess Hera, the female side of Zeus who was the most powerful god and who could fix up any problem in the universe. But his wife, Hera, had one power that was equal to that of Zeus. She could bestow her favor or grace on any man or woman she should choose and that grace, if a man could acquire it, would enable him to do the impossible and become as one of the gods. This Greek idea was symbolized in the journey of the hero, the becoming of the archetypal leader who sets an example, so that human beings become capable of doing the impossible, since the possible is rather boring. What is interesting in life about doing things that are possible? Isn't that being consigned to an eternal Bingo game or everlasting politics? What is the challenge and what is the growth in repeating and repeating the possible?

Nuclear Evolution, then, is asking us how can we become a hero and recover that lost part of ourselves that at some point in our lives died? At various ages in different people the heroine or the hero dies, and we begin to accept everything rigidly when people or society says "That's how it is." Up to a certain age there is a hero alive that does not accept other people's reality but says "No, I'm going to think for myself. I'm going to be someone who matters, someone who leaves an impression or mark on this life, not one who just passes through it without leaving any trace." And in every young person up to a certain age, that hero or heroine is still alive. Then comes that moment of

---

* Nuclear Evolution is that process by which we grow and unfold our full potential, just as a beautiful flower grows to perfection from its tiny seed or nucleus. My book, *Nuclear Evolution: Discovery of the Rainbow Body,* (University of the Trees Press, 1977) lays the groundwork for *The Rise of the Phoenix* which describes Nuclear Evolution at the social level. The process of growth that unfolds the perfection of world peace springs from such a tiny ordinary seed that anyone and everyone can begin to create it here and now in the rich soil of his own consciousness.

deadness when the one who strives to do something extraordinary suddenly accepts the ordinary as the reality, and that is when life becomes boring, stultified and life's magic has gone out of it and the child is imprisoned in the adult world: the same boring repetition and parroting of truths which are just like pedantic words being spun with no one really living them out, no one really listening. We all know these truths. Everyone knows the truth, but do they live what they know? They settle for something second best. But the leader of a nuclear community or a nuclear center is someone in whom the hero has never died or the heroine is still alive, or it is someone in whom it has been reawakened and reborn. That quality is the quality on which Hera smiles and bestows her grace. Whatever it is in the universe that gives grace or makes a person feel spontaneous and bubbling with energy and drawing from sources that are non-human, that "something", whatever it is, (we call it grace) is the sole objective of Nuclear Evolution, that attunement to the universe that sets us on the most important journey of all, the journey of the soul into those worlds of light in which the impossible can take place.

Life is a miracle. The impossible is always possible with God. If we truly believe in the power of consciousness as God, not as some abstract quality or being "out there" running the show, but that same stuff that is singing its note inside our own head, thinking all the thoughts, running the cells and recreating them every second, if we think of consciousness as God then we realize that anything is possible with consciousness. And what greater thing can there be in the whole universe than realizing that that consciousness in everything that one sees and experiences is a reflection of the ultimate glory of that purified consciousness which is deep in the heart of the nucleus that gave birth to the entire total universe? That spirit which can do the impossible when consciousness is eligible is the sole objective of Nuclear Evolution and the sole power that can raise up men and women from their present low ordinary state of existence. The true leader is that one who holds to that vision and is guided by that vision, surrenders himself or herself to that supreme power of consciousness sitting at the heart of every nucleus, that one who is the most attuned wherever it may be, in whatever part of the world, that one is a true leader of the human race, whether he is known or unknown. The most evolved person on the planet will be the one who is most attuned to that grace and that power to achieve the impossible. Such was the dynamic that lived in the mind of Christ and lives in the minds of all great men and women who carry the torch of the Eternal One through time. They are not single entities but the end of a long chain of torch-bearers, heroes from the Greek times and before, who carry the torch of the human spirit through great periods of darkness and through certain moments of history emerge to hold aloft that torch so that others may see the way and have faith in the consciousness that enables them to be themselves. That is the essence of true leadership, knowing that we ourself are one of those torchbearers who carry that awareness in our own heart.

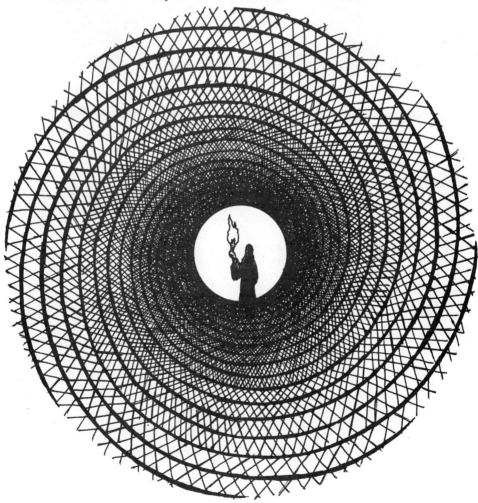

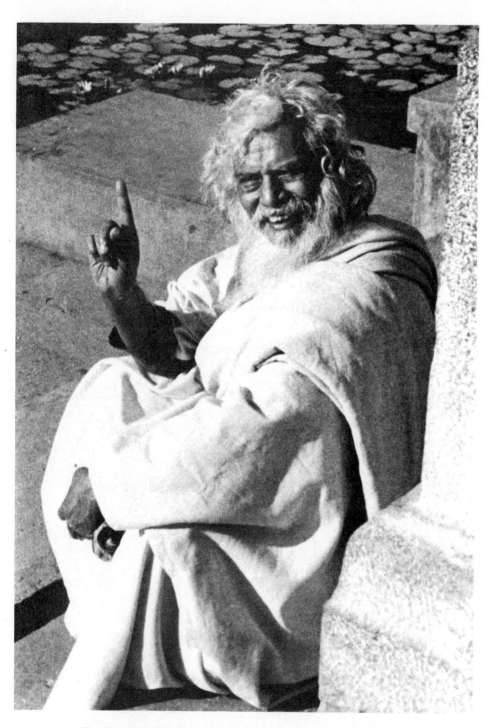

This man embodied the One quietly without allowing a cult to grow up around him.

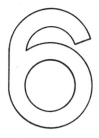

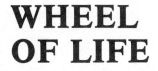

WHEEL
OF LIFE

The leaders of violent revolutions always claim to be saviors of the poor, the downtrodden and the exploited, but what is their true motive beneath all the words? If we consider the full scope of the world's history we would need a thick volume to give all the examples of the inner worlds of revolutionaries and leaders. The sheer complexity of the different views of the protagonists, the opinions prevailing and the inner motive which spawned the revolutionary ideas would all make an intellectual feast for any scholar and give the reader something to identify with. But it is just this identification process which is the real problem in all revolutions and idealism.

The merits of capitalism and communism as political systems were not the real issue in the communist revolution, despite what its leaders wrote and preached. By looking at the French Revolution or the repression of the Christians during the first 400 years after Christ or by getting into the fanatical world of the Puritan soldiers under Cromwell we can see that the real issue in any revolution is people's inner conflict, insecurity, apathy, gullibility, aggression, envy and idealism.

In order to make this real we must give examples which are relevant to our present world. Here again we have an identification problem; the world does not wish to identify with man's suffering, genocide, violence or disturbance. It wants to blot it out, close its eyes if at all possible and hope the conflict will go away. How can we make the subject of violence attractive? How can we make conflict something we research and go into rather than escape? Surely only the aggressive ones will respond to examples of pain and stupidity, of continuing blood baths and human bestiality. Those of a gentle passive nature will be turned off and gravitate to words of peace, inspiration and beauty. Because of this human willingness to turn away from pain and ugliness and seek the pleasant, we find that people soon ignore and even forget

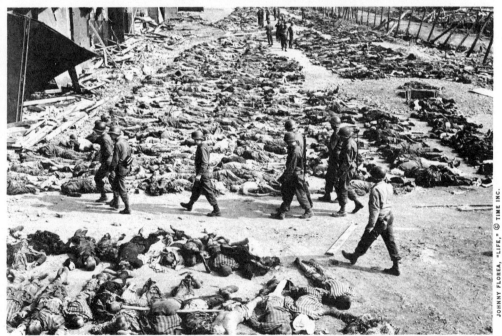

Corpses of Nazi victims at concentration camp near Nordhausen, Germany, Spring 1945. While this genocide is notoriously racist, millions more are quietly eliminated throughout the world in slave camps and prisons, under dictatorships and totalitarian governments without our knowing.

the world's plight. Only when we are the ones with our souls beaten to pulp with torture, only when we can identify with the horror of a political jail as if we were the victim, can we be motivated to work for the release of prisoners. When these events are far away in Chile or Cambodia, Siberia or the French Revolution, we feel grateful that our own freedom is not affected and that we can ignore them. But is

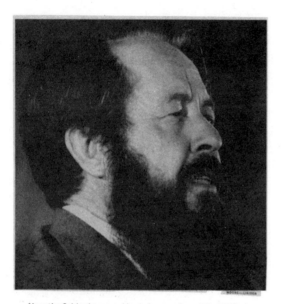

"Freedom is indivisible... One must take a moral attitude toward it."

Alexander Solzhenitsyn speaking before members of the US Senate.

freedom indivisible? Is not our own freedom, our own happiness, our own conscience bound up somewhere deep down with the consciousness of others? Is blame, guilt, or ignorance of the situation as a whole, with us? There are certain people who self-righteously point the finger at the evil in others, the lack of spiritual wisdom, the political immaturity and conceit of others, and these feelings motivate them to fight, bomb, kill and annihilate anyone who disagrees. Even innocent bystanders are drawn into events. How innocent are we of all this blind arrogance?

Just as in the time of the French Revolution, modern revolutionary fervor throughout the world revolves mainly around the idealistic question of who will wield power—certain groups of the wealthy few or the impoverished many? But when the masses fight for the power and win it, they install leaders who then become a new upper class basking in wealth and power, and the common man again becomes the under-dog. Mild reforms have occurred, but the real change has not. And so the wheel turns, perpetuating the division between powerful rulers and the weak who are ruled. In capitalist countries, such as the USA, where democracy is supposed to put power in the hands of "the people", we find that the wealthy are still in control through powerful lobbying for congressional favors and the distribution of public monies, and through mass advertising which persuades the public to buy their reality. In communist countries, which are supposed to be a haven for the masses, the Party has created a new class system where the masses dare not even question a party decision without fear of reprisal.

Is it possible to get off this wheel of life and find the still center where distinctions between ruler and ruled which keep the wheel turning, disappear? If we can look at world politics as a wheel with different ideologies and isms as the spokes, we can see that communism and capitalism are diametrically opposite to each other, and all other isms lie somewhere in between the two. By looking at the evils in both

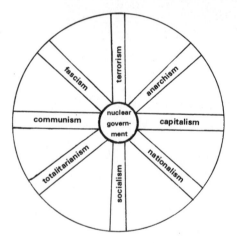

systems and the good in both systems, we gain insight into the fundamental problems of human nature that are manifested outwardly in our world political life. By looking at the root of the fundamental problems common to both and synthesizing the best of both systems we arrive at the hub of the wheel, and at nuclear government.

But the problem is difficult and on a vast scale. Utopias and small communities have been attempted like the Quakers, the Oneida community, Walden Two, Kibbutzim, etc., and all have failed to bring about a mass movement towards fundamental change. The views have either been too narrow or the excitement of life in the wider society has caused the children to leave the small community in search of stimulation.

How can we organize a nuclear government and a community which is going to solve the world's problems and offer all the intensity of the dynamic attractions of the larger society? We ask ourself the important question: how can a mere handful of people begin a small community and solve the world's problems without seeming absurd in the worldwide context? Does it depend upon numbers? Is it the potency of the thought or is it dependent on the number of people who try to play political games against the huge backdrop of the "real world" political scene? We are reminded that communism did not begin with more than one man with one disciple. Marx and Engels certainly did not believe their political theory was absurd just because only two men at that time believed in it! Then again, Christianity, involving huge political areas of the world and empires based in Rome, began with one man! Yet we must ask ourselves: can twenty people* setting out with all the good will in the world fix it all? What the Presidium of the Supreme Soviet and the collective brains of great governments cannot do, can the small community, fired with an evolutionary Truth accomplish and so overshadow revolutionary power? Such a utopian experiment seems unreal, as remote as the tortures of Siberia, as far away as the crucifixion of Christ.

An examination of the motivations of an evolutionary revolutionary

---

* Twenty people doubling their membership for seven years totals a community of 1280 people, the maximum number considered optimum for deep communication for all.

like Christ, Darwin or Einstein, whose revolutions were self-propagating through knowledge, or the drives dominating the frustrations of a revolutionary like Marx, Lenin or Mao Tse-tung, whose self-righteous fervor required the murder of millions, can lead us to real understanding of the causes of violence. But can twenty people with stars in their eyes start a community, write a constitution, work out their own salvation in juxtaposition with all this heavy world stuff we hear about every day on the news? The answer is that if you have twelve people and a Christ or fifty people and a Mao Tse-tung or one hundred people who even read *Das Kapital*, you have enough. The personality is merely a focus for the right ideal at the right time. The purposes, goals and failures of small communities generally must be discussed against the ripeness of the times and not in terms of members or resources. Who could have foreseen that Christ who had no money bags would one day own millions of churches whose bells ring out from the hilltops of small villages everywhere on Sunday all over the planet? Or that Marx who died in abject poverty would one day have the resources of the entire Soviet Union to point rockets for the total destruction of capitalism that he prophesied? Christ's methods took hundreds of years to become politi-cized in Rome and the Soviets took fifty years to become a dominant world power. What strange turns of history are coming in the future to make our skepticism, our knowledge of political realities, our present values and arguments and reasons of no account? What new insight into Nature could turn our reality upside down?

Nature's model of government is from the nucleus of the cell outward. The message of life is coded into the DNA located in the nucleus and shared with the entire cell by the RNA messengers. Yet the nucleus without the cell is helpless. All parts of the cell work together for the harmonious functioning of the whole. So although the nucleus informs the cell body, it is not more important than the rest of the cell. In theory, communism believes that it is based on Nature's model, that the Party is no more important than the masses; but in practice, Party members receive much greater privileges, depriving the masses and creating strife and divisiveness on the subterranean unconscious levels in the cell of communist life. In Nuclear Evolutionary terms, following Nature's model of government means that union between the nucleus, the DNA, RNA and the cell body, must take place *within each*

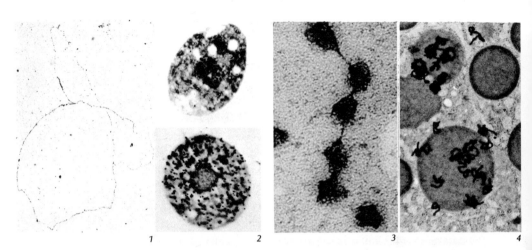

The above picture shows the stages of communication as the nucleus of an intestinal bacteria is synthesized into cell proteins. Figure 1 shows the DNA replicating. Figure 2 shows RNA forming in the nucleus at top and later in the cell fluids. Figure 3 shows a strand of messenger RNA linking a nucleic acid in the sequence of translating the message of the DNA language. Figure 4 shows the final sequence of the production of a cell. The nucleic acid here has been treated with radioactive tritium in order to see it. Individual people are like DNA molecules which hold the complex memory of cosmic happenings. To communicate their knowledge to each other there must be replication. Communication is replicating of information in another person through the biological vehicle of cells, nerves, brain and the messenger chemicals (emotions) which transmit the cosmic knowledge in the nucleus (consciousness).

individual. Together we stand at the center and selflessly serve all the parts who are each other, and together we take responsibility for the whole, serving different roles as need be, but not confined or limited to a role—free to be both the whole and the part. For as long as we are content to be only a part, to govern or allow ourselves to be governed, we will never be fully alive, fully responsible for ourself, fully in tune with Nature's message which is to master our own Self-realization. Nuclear government is Self-government with our "Self" being our Cosmic Body of which all persons are part. The hub is the heart pulsing through the whole; it is there that the World Peace Center lies.

THE REAL DIALECTIC

The greatest good in capitalist theory is the thesis of the freedom of Spirit. But this freedom has been abused to exploit the poor and deny others that same expression of freedom. As a result there has been a swing of the pendulum. Communism arose as a backlash, an antithesis against this capitalist freedom of the few at the expense of the many.* Communism's theoretical purpose is to return freedom to the common man. The greatest good in theoretical communism is its vision of the potential of the many, its group consciousness and cooperative sharing. But in practice communism denies this freedom of the spirit in order to force a group consciousness. Its theoretically-conceived cooperative society has become a coerced society. To eradicate the ills of capitalism, the baby (Spirit) was thrown out, by communism, with the bathwater (exploitation). The thesis of God was replaced by the antithesis of matter, and all that had to do with religious feeling was condemned as evil—the cause of apathy and the perpetuation of oppression. God was rooted out in favor of the hard, cold reality of economics. The dualistic nature of humanity is nowhere more vividly portrayed than in this dialectic between God and man, Spirit and matter, capitalism and communism which is now waging war on many levels in all humans throughout the planet. Nuclear government is not an ism. It sees from a different perspective and is a synthesis of the best in all isms—the freedom of Spirit in capitalism and the group consciousness of man in communism—and thus it is the union of Spirit and matter. The resolving of the age-old duality of Spirit and matter is before the planet now as the polarization between the one force and the other reaches its greatest extreme in individuals and nations.

How can the nuclear government of the World Peace Center be achieved in the heart of every man, woman and child? To the reader of this book 100 years from now, what will the poised juxtaposition of communism and capitalism, of rockets and nuclear warheads of opposing systems mean? As remote as the French Revolution is to us now, it is hard to be concerned and identified with the suffering and insecurity of the people at that time, or the gullibility of idealists who are always taken in, century after century by those who arouse our self-righteous anger. Do we have the foresight to predict the shape of the new society 100 years from now when the great revolutionaries themselves have

* The Bureau of Census shows five percent of the people own eighty-three percent of the stock in American businesses.

prophesied and seen the trends all wrong? What is our responsibility for creating the new vision, creating the images which motivate, the examples to illustrate the impasse between revolutionary idealism and apathy, between change and conservative stability? In the chapters to follow we will look at some real examples from our present world situation which do not take a genius or a prophet to predict the outcome. In order to get a fresh view, a different perspective, we will look at these all too familiar situations from inside-out, not as a commentator and an opinionated onlooker without any power to influence events, but as a participant who knows that history will actually be written by us and not by some safe spectator 100 years hence.

By discussing small communities and big theories and real political power over life and death and by looking at the subtle power of the human spirit at work behind the well-known personalities who act as a focus for human thoughts, drives and emotions, we will see how to grasp the nettle by the hand and take the big plunge into the nuclear center, by the total commitment of our own consciousness. This commitment at the back of all great movements for human evolution is the only real power there is that will automatically and effectively change the world outside. The only real power that any of us has at this very moment is to change ourself. If we believe naively that we have the power to change others, we will eventually face the truth that all such change is superficial and idealistic. Those others too are the only ones who can deeply change themselves. To yearn for this power to control others is a mark of our own inability to know ourself. This ignorance will be a vital factor in our need to change ourself. It will determine whether or not we overcome the self-perpetuating power complex and create a nuclear government.

Whether you have been politically involved in social demonstrations and rallies or taken sides in the socialist revolution against capitalism, the fact is the same: you alone, not the laws nor the philosophy in your head, will change your consciousness. Laws, systems, ideas, intellectual structures, are merely the pegs to hang our particular thoughts upon. These thoughts, flitting constantly through our minds, are bound tightly into habitual patterns of doctrine and dogma. They are only the excreta of our state of being, our level of evolution, our confusions and inner conflicts. Only consciousness can change them from within. To believe that they can be imposed on the world or upon others by force, by coercion or by teaching or propaganda, is the twentieth century delusion. Direct experiential knowledge of the Nuclear Self is more potent than any nuclear bomb, more transforming of our own purpose and aims than any particular philosophy of life. Human slaves of political systems are no more important against the background of evolutionary time than a scarecrow's head full of straw. One person with nuclear consciousness can change the world, and twenty people embarking with group consciousness along the evolutionary revolutionary course can penetrate the shadows of a million blind slaves in a matter of years. When a person sees how blind he is, how stupid and gullible he has been, no one kicks him harder than his own foot. This is the beginning of wisdom, the beginning of the power that overturns the world, the beginning of the new Phoenix!

Thus we need not worry about the smallness of the numbers who will start the nuclear communities of the World Peace Center. The global villages of today's youth and the razzle dazzle electronic capability of instant communication are only waiting for something important to be said. They are the infrastructure through which the Phoenix sends out its sweet song—the song that transcends the blood and killing and torture and the mendacity of man, and the song whose wistful longing tones are born out of the pity of those ashes. For man does not see without pain, and he does not become peaceful without conflict.

The community that can acknowledge and resolve conflict without aggressiveness and without violence, the group that can understand the nature of frustration, the individual who becomes free of disturbing thoughts, has the answer to the world problem. In such a man or woman is the seed of all successful world change for he or she becomes an instrument of evolution, the archetype and the megatype who carries within, the solution to human conflict. How can such a grandiose evolutionary scheme be effected through the puny efforts of human beings? How can ordinary people aspire to act on a stage of worldwide proportions?

Only in small groups and together can we get off the spinning wheel of life and stand in the still center where all dualities become one. The World Peace Center is made of individuals in small communities who practice nuclear government in their own lives, in their businesses and in their immediate society. Every member becomes an instrument of peace, embodying peace in their own being and thus carrying the center with them wherever they go. Only with this love, action and commitment to each other can the World Peace Center be established and spread.

What kind of people would choose to join the World Peace Center? "Am I that kind of person?" we ask. From many walks of life some have already caught the vision and determined to become the vision. Let us march down our own spoke of the wheel with them as we read through this book and resolve our own inner dualities that together we may march towards the center. Can we reach the hub to capture the vision beyond our ego self and rise like the Phoenix into the synthesis of our greater Self?

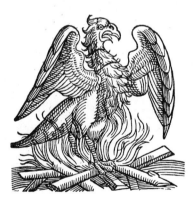

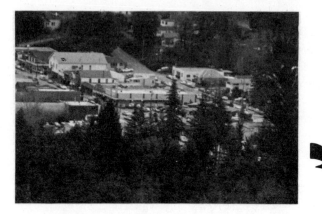

The University of the Trees perfects itself as a pure seed for a
new system of government.

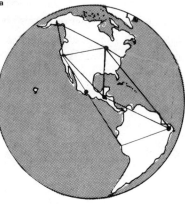

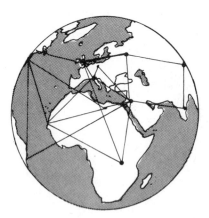

Seed communities grow inside existing political
structures in a peaceful non-destructive manner
as world peace centers.

APPENDIX TO CHAPTER

EDITORS' NOTE

MARCHING TOWARD THE CENTER

One day at an editorial meeting the editors, Ann and Debbie, suggested that having some personal statements of how people came to be at the University of the Trees would illustrate better what we mean by marching toward the center of the wheel of life. So Debbie set out to interview various members of the group. The following are excerpts from the interviews, statements about the lives of people now at the University of the Trees made by the people themselves. Seven excerpts out of many were chosen by the editors that reflected widely different backgrounds. They are being included here as an appendix to this chapter to separate it from the work of the author, Christopher Hills. The purpose in including these is to show that anyone can begin a real live nucleus which probes the nature of individual and group consciousness together with people from all walks of life provided it is based on love. The interviews were spontaneous and informal, in response to Debbie's questions. The simple, conversational style has been preserved in the transcriptions. The basic questions asked were, "How did you come to be here at the University of the Trees?" and, "Can you trace the events in your life that brought you to wanting to investigate your real Self?" The interviewer's questions were deleted from the transcript to create one continuous flow from the speaker.

Roger

Before I came here I was feeling a real sense of lack. All the things I was trying weren't satisfying, so I'd go around and try different things to see which one would resonate. At one point I thought that the thing I wanted to do was become a working class hero kind of person, so I went out and I got a job doing hard manual labor, lifting bags of cement and things like that, but the people I was interacting with didn't have the ideals about what we were doing that I did. To them it was drinking beer, chasing after girls, just this whole frame of mind that didn't want to get into the deeper questions, so that if I started talking with somebody about those deeper questions there would be kind of uncomfortable silences, and that didn't feel fulfilling. Then I wanted to try for something a little more lucrative, figuring that if I got my material trip together then I'd be in a better situation to do something. I tried being a salesman but the same thing happened . . . it was always deep down underneath, the motivations that were driving the people weren't really for truth or for any kind of higher purposes. It was more of a, "Well, I just do the best I can and survive" kind of thing. I got involved with the United Farm Workers, thinking, "Well, this is a crusade to better the working conditions," and so forth. And that was fine, except all I was doing was feeding my ego. "Oh, here I am helping undertrodden masses lift themselves up by their own bootstraps a little bit." But still the thing inside me that wanted to be answered was there. So I went back to school and there I met some teachers with nice ideas but still, even if they said they had a good idea and the words sounded fine, their being and the way they manifested it was ringing false. And there were ego trips going on in me, a lot of judgements, a lot of games. And then I happened to meet Debbie and she turned me on to what was going on here at University of the Trees. Something clicked that felt real, because it seemed to synthesize the spiritual and the religious questioning that was in me with the kind of hard-nosed practicality I was looking for.

When I met Christopher he was talking about colors and some far-out ideas. I liked that, but it wasn't what he said as much as the conviction, self-conviction that he had that really drew me to find out what on earth was making him so self-assured. Then gradually I found out that that certainty was based on a kind of integrity in a lot of different areas, whereas in the past I'd find that the people that I'd put up on the pedestal would have flaws and then I'd start to chip away at their image and eventually I'd want to move on to something else. Christopher's integrity makes me feel that I don't need confirmation from other people to know that there's something real, that I can follow the truth because it feels right for me. When he sees a gap in someone's consciousness he points it out and there's no ego involved. It's sort of like, well, that's just the way it is. Whereas when I see a flaw and I make some comment about it, there's ego in it. I can feel it. So the fact that I'm seeing the flaw and can make a remark somehow I use as ego food. Then it always backfires. So I'm learning this other way to give feedback and check out my own ego too.

In all my college studies the stress was on empiricism and it had to be something that could be put in an experimental duplicator so that other people could duplicate it and everybody in the world universally could experience it through their senses, etc. But yet there were insights that were more in touch with the emotions and more intuitive kinds of things that I thought were just as real, just as valid, yet science can't explain all those things. But Christopher was able to put them into a context in a way that you could account for that, in a way that didn't make them seem spaced-out cousins to physical facts. It meshed so much with what I was intuitively seeking for. I'd say the main thing that I've gotten as a result of being involved here is to be able to go inside myself to verify and find out what's true instead of always searching out there for somebody else's definitions which never quite fit. There's some deeper kind of reality that encompasses and brings together all these perspectives. Instead of something static, or some one truth, it's something constantly alive, changing and evolving.

Before I came here I was always modifying my perceptions to fit with what other people thought, especially people from whom I wanted approval, thinking we had to agree in ideas in order to have some resonance. And what I've learned is that the only way that the union that I want can happen is for me to really come out with where I'm at and then there will be something to work with, and that's been a real change in confidence. Of course you have to begin with people who can hear you, who are doing the same thing. Then you can go into a wider world and be real too. People like it. What keeps me here is the love, or the kind of nitty-gritty confrontation of the soul that doesn't beat around the bush and go through a lot of compensations. Also, the vision that what we're doing here is something that's going to have some kind of lasting effect, the start of something that's going to go on. And more than anything else, it's that feeling inside that there's a connectedness and that it's going to get deeper, that the community thing is just going to get deeper and deeper.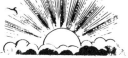

Phil

Just before I came to University of the Trees I was searching for some way to serve. I'd been through different trips and seen what other people were doing with their lives and decided that I wanted to serve in some capacity. I wasn't into the money trip. I was somewhat into adventure, wanting to be into something exciting and fulfilling and challenging, something that would challenge me to become more than I was. My values were sort of a cross section of what I thought was the best of all the different religions, and I was trying to get some kind of an overall perspective of what life was about and what were common cross-cultural values. I was trying to get into that and trying to see what bound people together and what boundaries they created—like national boundaries, or racial or whatever. I had been turned off of Christianity because of the dogmatism in it. So I'd become an agnostic because I had to admit to myself I didn't know if what they were telling me was true or not. But when I was in Thailand with the Air Force I got into Buddhism and Buddhism gave me the other side and I was able to see the good things in Christianity as a result of seeing a fresh approach to what spirituality was about. I was attracted to Buddhism by the way people lived in Thailand. They lived what they believed day by day and their lives were integrated with their spirituality. It wasn't just go to church on Sunday; it was like every day they were cooperating. There was a happy sharing spirit. If people didn't have enough, there was more of a help-him-out attitude. They seemed to be more cohesive as a society because of what they believed in together and they practiced an equality I felt lacking in Western society. Then when I got back to the US I felt like I'd stepped off the planet into another dimension of reality and I was able to get a fresh look at Thailand. I wanted to go back. I had sort of a mini-enlightenment experience there and it convinced me that enlightenment is a real thing and is possible to achieve, so I wanted to have it and it made me goal-oriented, to get enlightened.

I tried to get back to Thailand in every way. I tried the Peace Corps and that didn't work. I tried to get a job there teaching English and that didn't work. So I went back to school to get a Master's degree to go into the foreign service so I could get there. You need to have a job so that you can stay there. But I came upon University of the Trees. It appealed to me in that it was speaking the same truth, but was a less structured, less authoritarian, less conventional way to enlightenment. I could see that I was chasing an ideal image of what spiritual life is in wanting to go to Thailand and become a monk. Somehow the fantasy vanished after I came here. I saw it as an escape in not facing the reality of what I was born into and I think I was born into a situation here in the US to try to understand and be part of and help guide the direction somehow of what's going on. If I went to Thailand I'd be out of the action and I'd be on the sidelines, though I was *thinking* I'd be in the middle of it. I dreamed I'd get enlightened and then come back and be some kind of savior or something, but now I see it's all tied together and you have got to do the work at the same time because you can't make that separation. It's a delusion. You get enlightened by doing and by serving not by removing yourself from it and sitting down in a cave and spacing out.

So I came here when I was working on my Master's thesis. I had some insights into the nature of consciousness. It was the most important area of study for me as I could see how it led to enlightenment. I had been researching everything I could get my hands on in the field of consciousness and I was still searching for some answers. I was at the end of my rope as far as my research went and then everything I found at the University of the Trees filled all the holes. The universal field could be proved and Christopher's insight into the universal field of consciousness brought everything from the spiritual down to the material and linked it all together with some kind of coherent vision of the whole, and that was what had been lacking in all the other research I'd seen. And getting into Nuclear Evolution and the different levels of consciousness . . .well I was able to look at the study of consciousness from all those different levels instead of just going the intellectual route and getting very stuck in one tunnel vision concept of looking at it. Up to that point most of what I'd read about consciousness was pseudo-scientific, some of it was mathematical; it was very theoretical and not too much based on experience. Of course there was the mystical, but it was never tied to anything provable or practical. The thing I like about University of the Trees is its practical down-to-earth stuff that works and is based on experience that you can see in your own life and show others because they can see it in their life.

How did I get into all this? Well I was into security. I'd been convinced when I went into the military that that was a good way to go as a career. You know your life is taken care of, all the benefits and the retirement and all. But then I saw that to get that I had to sell my soul. When I went into the service the Viet Nam War was on and I was going to be drafted and maybe given a gun and sent over there to shoot. So I went into the Air Force which was non-combatant and I went into personnel. I was interested in people and got to see first hand the problems people were having with the military and what it was doing to their lives. It was also an information network and I was in the middle of it so I knew some of the deals that were going on and what people's attitudes were. I saw a lot of good people dedicated to something they believed in but also deep down realizing that there was something wrong. I mean, it's hard to explain; a lot of it was people wanting the security trip like me. Everyone being told what to do, not being required to think for yourself, being given orders and following them without questioning. Then you see people who are giving the orders and you know they don't know what the hell they're doing and you're being forced to take orders that you don't like and passing them on. I refused to do it sometimes. I thought they were immoral, unethical. Like in the middle of a war people were getting rich and having a great time, while other people were getting killed and there were certain rules about getting assignments back to the States and on one occasion the commander of the base pulled strings to reassign someone back to the States when there were other guys ahead of him who wanted to go back and couldn't. I was in a position to say no because what they were doing was against regulations. I was legally right, but I was in a situation where if I did that I would probably have been threatened with a court-martial—you see there was an undercurrent. I started to balk at cutting the orders and I was confronted by my superior, a major. He ordered me, threatened me to do it. So I did it. I mean it wasn't a big thing, no one was getting hurt, but it was the principle of the thing and then being forced to do it. So I decided to leave the service, security or no. The people in the military just felt they were doing their little job. They weren't seeing how they were keeping the whole thing going and had a part in the responsibility. But with this incident I was just completely awakened to what was going on. I had been told all these high-sounding idealistic things about duty, honor, country, service, peace, and I was seeing over and over the exact opposite going on in reality, so I felt like I'd been brainwashed and duped and betrayed.

So here on campus I'm sometimes wary. I'm committed but I sometimes have a conflict between my personal will and the group's will. The authority trip. But I'm seeing more and more how it's okay to go along with the group decisions *as long as I put in my input* so it becomes part of the whole. And the group's decisions are then my decisions and they usually do pan out to be good ones. I see more and more they really are for my own good and the group thing isn't a separation. All decisions are consensus and if they weren't we'd each be doing our own thing or trying to lay trips on each other. But if we're open then the group consensus is powerful and doesn't create mixed feelings in people and still overcomes the little separations. I didn't want to go through life just being a bump on a log, doing a job and going home to TV. I'd been through that trip, almost got married to a lady who was into that trip. It just wasn't fulfilling. I was very self-sufficient, raised on a farm, and I knew I could always take care of myself if I had to. I studied political science in undergraduate school and I always read extensively to keep up with current events. I even thought about going into government service before I entered the military. I figured democracy was the best thing we got, our version of course, and I had some feelings for grass-roots democracy. It wasn't until Thailand and the military that I began to feel brainwashed into believing the American dream. I began to do a lot of serious thinking about politics, government and societies. In fact my Master's degree was to be in this field, international politics, but my research kept taking me deeper into people's motivations and then into consciousness and that's why I'm here.

I began to come here on Friday nights and I could feel the energy. Christopher's personality intimidated me but also thrilled me at the same time. And the love in the group, the group vibration, the group spirit, I knew there was something here beyond any one person, something you couldn't see but you could feel. I'd never experienced anything like that before. It was the oneness. In spite of any surface separations and tensions, there was something holding it together, something very strong and cohesive that would withstand just about anything. There was a strong will, strong determination to make the vision real instead of just talking about it, dreaming it. It woke me up to myself and still is.

Richard
When I think about what brought me here I get a kind of sense of awe. Like I can remember being in Idaho and I can remember standing in a field and looking out over the hills and I remember I was crying. I remember I made a vow to a bush, you know, that I would try and learn to love, and it was kind of a stupid thing. I'd read in a Don Juan book about some guy talking to a bush and I thought I would love to emulate that and I wanted to find a man that knew . . .and it was such a deep yearning. I used to walk up in the hills and mountains all by myself, but there was always this feeling that I wished that I knew a man that I could be with that knew everything there was to know. that I could be close to that guy some way and he would look on me as one of his students. And things didn't go well in Idaho and I remember looking up at a star one night and it was just kinda like this feeling inside that said "Go back West". And my wife Sue and I packed up and went to California and I went to plant some trees for a month up north to get some money. I'd been reading Krishnamurti, the first time I had read some real spiritual work, and it said that you had to see yourself in everything, you had to see how you were

the cause of things, and I really tried looking at that, it got me, you know. And the day before the job ended I got real, real scared! Something in me said you got to go back to Sue, she's out of wood and you gotta get out of here, they're going to get you. I got real paranoid. I was in the best physical shape I've ever been in in my life, running up the side of mountains every day for a month with a hoe-daddy in my hand and a thousand trees in my pouch.

I'd put all my imagination into the books I was reading and I really got screwed up. And as I left with my friend about a mile out of town I suddenly had this flash that I'd done the wrong thing and that I was very prideful, and I caught a flash of that pride and it just killed me. I couldn't believe it, I just panicked, I felt lost, like somehow I'd condemned myself to hell. I got home to Sue and I knew I needed meditation. I never heard of any meditation that I knew of but I knew I needed it. I was getting worse so we went to a doctor and the doctor introduced me to the *Lazy Man's Guide to Enlightenment,* believe it or not. He was a medical doctor, but he intuited that I had had an experience that was spiritual, even though it was messed up. I wasn't into drugs, oh I smoked a little grass, you know, but I didn't know what was happening to me. I committed myself to a mental hospital, and in fifteen days I knew the doctors didn't know, so I got myself together to get out. I thought, this is stupid, this hospital with all these people. And I told all the other inmates there the same. I really yelled at them, beat my fists on the table to try to put some energy into them and the others all reacted of course. But it was really amazing, one of the girls got dressed up for the first time and one of the guys who was almost catatonic showed anger, you know, because I told all the nuts that they got to get out of this. So after I got out I was still dependent on the shrinks and I was still looking for somebody with answers. I saw a sign that said, DO YOU WANT TO BE A PIONEER? And I practically shook to death to think of that, but I *did* want to be a pioneer. And the next thing I knew I was on Christopher's doorstep knocking and Norah answered the door and I told her the basic situation, and she said, "Yeah, I understand." And when I met Christopher I knew I'd found somebody who knew more than anybody else about what had happened to me. And even though I was scared, something inside kept driving me on to find out more. I wanted to be a pioneer, I wanted to be a physical pioneer, find the last frontier, but I never could do it and I never could find out what I was doing wrong. I went to Idaho to get it. I remember looking out my window and there were the trees to the forest and that forest represented the last frontier to me, because I saw society as just creeping over and taking over everything and pretty soon there would be no wild man left, there'd be no free man left. But I wasn't wild and free; I was an economic slave and I was alone and I didn't like it. I tried to farm, but I was no farmer. I thought I wanted to farm because I had an ideal that if you wanted to be a strong free man you should farm, but I didn't want to farm, I didn't want to fight those weeds, I hated weeds.

So I had a consultation with Christopher and he said to me, "You've come this far, you might as well jump off, you know, you can't get much worse; you're in a bad state so you might as well jump off." And I couldn't even believe what I was hearing. It was just like somebody plopped me into a dream, suddenly everything I had imagined was beginning to come true. I felt I'd found the man that I'd looked for or found a reality that was really real. Nobody had ever asked me the kind of questions he did, or made the kinds of statements he made to me. Like knowing you've come that far with your development and knowing that you know what he means, like you've really got to get at it now, you've really got to do something about it. . . you've really got to put your heart and soul into evolving yourself, into getting inside your consciousness and finding out about those realities on an experimental basis; you're the experiment. Of course that's the part I wanted the most and that's the part I ran away from the most. So he was speaking to the part that was scaredest and he always has.

I remember I had images of what a wise man should be. He should be kind, not kill. And there was a bunch of sow bugs sitting on the floor where he had pulled something back, and he sort of methodically stamped every one of them out and I was shocked, you know, "thou shalt not kill." And I was freaked both good and bad that first meeting. Then I did something I've always been glad of. I offered to do work exchange, in exchange for the time that he'd spent with me. I didn't have much at that time and possibly that was a saving grace because that was one quality in me that was still alive—the desire to give. Even though at that time I was so imploded I couldn't get out of myself, I knew that you had to give for what you got or it wouldn't be right. So I made a repair on the shed out back which is still there to this day. But I didn't do it in the way he said I should do it. I felt I was a carpenter, by god, I knew how to do it. But it's proved to be as inefficient as he said it would. Then for my first two years here I had very close feelings to him, but I also reacted to practically everything he did to see whether it fit my image of how he should be. Now I love the teachings here, but then I didn't give a damn for Nuclear Evolution, and I hated Creative Conflict. But I loved him—he saved my life. It was his being I could relate to.

Sue W.

I have skated around on the surface of things a lot in my life. I must have started college—different ones—six times. I kept trying to find which image or which concept would fit myself, and I couldn't. I was one of the marchers in all the Viet Nam protests in San Francisco and at San Jose State. I felt very strongly about politics in college during the '60s and I put some effort into that. I felt a real sense of injustice. In high school I went to presidential conventions and when I was younger to a Republican convention for Goldwater. But in college I switched parties. After college I got involved in trying to make my own life successful and I turned more internal. I had lots of religious feelings as a child but I could never mesh them with what was happening in church. I was a Baptist and when I was immersed I had a rather mystical experience and a few other memories which were deep impressions. But that waned because I could not see an alternative to established religion in high school or college, so I let it drop.

I felt that marriage was the one thing that could possibly bring me fulfillment and there were social expectations to get married. I really loved Richard very much too. I loved his being and his heart, and I had no realistic concept of what marriage was. I say this with hindsight. I just had a very idealistic concept that that's what you did at twenty-two. I sort of bought the whole social idea that that would bring me fulfillment.

After marriage I felt constantly let down by what my expectations were of a relationship and I was totally unprepared even to have one child, which I did do. I did it consciously, thinking it was a good idea. I was all dreams of how lovely it would be to have a baby and have all motherly feelings, which was quite exciting for awhile. But the reality did not live up to what I had anticipated it to be. There was always a gap between my ideal and my reality. I was mostly idealistic. I would get an idea of how things should be and I would try to live up to that. I was always secure. I had a good family that I could trust and rely on. I knew I could always support myself. But if I was too secure I got bored. So I wanted challenges. Before marriage I dumped several boyfriends who were madly in love with me because there was no challenge.

Richard and I mutually decided on a life-style, back to the woods and to the land. But Richard was not whole-hearted about it. I was willing to give it everything, and when I really make up my mind to do something I really do it and I don't have any doubts about it. Like being married. It never occurred to me to leave when the going got rough. I'm too steadfast. So there we were in the woods and one year passed, two years and our savings dwindled and we didn't have our own place yet. I was very frustrated that Richard wouldn't look for our place, our dream. We were only half way and I wanted to fulfill the whole thing to see if it was real. He kept dragging his feet and I became very unhappy. Then Richard got sick. I had so much tension stored up from that whole experience, I tried to help him out but all his strange comments made me feel hysterical. I would laugh at them in a strange way until the doctor told me that I was feeding Richard's trip by doing this. At that time I didn't understand what he meant. I stayed with my folks then. They were really supportive. The doctor made us make a plan for our lives—a, b, c, d—before he'd let Rich out of the hospital. I think Richard wanted some discipline and I wouldn't give it to him. But we rented a cottage and Rich was looking for work as a carpenter. Shauna was a year old when he came home one day and said, "I've had this really interesting talk with this guy in Boulder Creek. He gives a talk on Friday nights and I think I'd like to go." Rich went for a couple of weeks and I didn't think much of it until he asked me to join him. So I said okay. I was suspicious—very suspicious. But he did seem to get something out of it so I went along. You know that first night was one of the most grueling experiences I've ever had. I couldn't sit still for one thing, and I was not into sitting on the floor. I was so uncomfortable. One day Robert came to visit us and he was very nice. I think he showed us a pendulum which was so strange, I couldn't accept that at all. There was something that I liked about Friday night, but it was so painful to come—physically so uncomfortable—and I couldn't control my mind very well. But the man who was giving the talks seemed to look straight at me every five minutes and answer a question in my life as if he was reading my mind. It absolutely freaked me out to the depths of my being and I really could not believe that there was anything like that, that a being in a person could do it. It was incomprehensible, with my Baptist upbringing. I knew that Christ could do those things, but it had not occurred to me that it actually was within the realm of my experience. And so to have someone in such a kind and loving way see something about myself that was a question or a problem to me, and to speak to that part of myself without any vibration of judgement, really turned me on. I was absolutely amazed and blown out by the power of his consciousness. So I had a two-way thing going. There were lots of things that seemed really alien and strange to me, but there was something that kept speaking to me deeper than that so that I wanted to keep coming. And it took me a good year even to be able to sit still for the whole time.

After a while I didn't care whether Richard liked the University of the Trees or not. I felt it was my trip and it didn't have anything to do with him. I was very happy that he was into it so that we could share, but if he had not been I still think I would have come. Now I feel like I have found my stream and there is some resonance that pulls me up that stream. My goal is really the discovery of the rainbow body, and that means to me essentially opening up all the levels of consciousness and I'm finding more and more fulfillment in my life because of that. Richard's and my relationship has improved a hundred-fold since we've been here. I always hung on to this idea of Richard's potential whenever I would get down during those early years. And then he would do something that would really turn me on. So I'd get all my hopes built up again and then he'd do something that would bring me down again. But I always clung to this idea of his potential—maybe at the expense of my own since I've never really felt clear on what my own potential was. But now I'm finding my own center, and Richard is really finding his. Someday I hope we can work as a team, but now we're growing individually together.

Robert
I've always wanted to be very affluent. I must have been very young when I first made that decision because I don't remember making it, I just remember it being there. I remember looking around the neighborhood and seeing that we were one of the poorest houses on the block, and it was a poor neighborhood. So I used to try to get things by the route of talking some of the richer guys out of their toys and things like that. I wanted my share of toys. I never had an electric train set all my life, and the other kids would get electric trains and stuff for Christmas. So at some stage I said, "Okay, I want to prove I'm as good as you, I want a Rolls Royce." Had I stayed in England I'd have had a Rolls Royce by now, no matter what condition, but I would have had one. Then the desire left me for awhile. I was real young, seventeen. I had been going out with Brenda for a few years, and then we broke off. I was very content then to just have a job, earn a nice wage and spend it on buying

things for my mother that she never had, like an electric heater and a washing machine. Then Brenda and I got back together and we got married and the desire started building up again because when you have a wife and a house to support you need money. I started back into the rat race. Before, I'd work and enjoy life. It was nice to have money in my pocket and it was nice to have a reasonable lunch every day and I was just having a nice time. But then Brenda wanted to buy gifts for her mum. Before she married me she hated her mum. When she married me her mum became her best friend. It was real strange, overnight. I quickly changed my job (I was working as a technician in a school) to an industrial job to get more money. But even though my salary went up by one-third, it wasn't enough because she spent all her salary on herself and my salary had to go to the food and rent. I had a problem. I started going to night school five nights a week to colleges all over London. I wanted to have a secure future. I took my third year at one university and at the same time I started taking fourth and fifth year at another university to get it done fast. They didn't know I doubled them up. I got my degree in Physics. In the meantime we had two kids and I needed more money than I could get working in the university. But the companies all wanted to start me off as a recent graduate from college and forget that I had been a technician for five years. The salary I could get was less than my technician's salary before I went to university. The whole English system was upside down. So I wanted to go to the States. I got interested in holography and I heard it was all done in the States. I was turned on to it because I figured in the future we would have holographic films, everything would be holographic.

I couldn't get a job in holography, I tried. It was too new. But I was offered a job as a physicist in Canada. We went to Canada. The job was mechanical—electro-mechanical, developing instrumentation. But Brenda freaked out with a week old baby and being in a new country. She wanted to go back to England. I wanted to come to California. So we agreed to try California and if it didn't work out we'd go back to England. Things were nice for awhile. But we always seemed to be broke. Brenda finally went back to England on a holiday. Then she left for good. I remember crying alot, but I remember feeling let out of prison. She once said, "You never asked me to come back." I never did. I had the kids and that was nice. Soon I became very affluent, without Brenda spending it all. Then Brenda took the kids. I got into a real sex binge, looking for all the things I'd never experienced because I got married so young. Every size, shape, color, that sort of thing. But my back went out. That was hard. Up to then I thought I was Superman. Then I felt like a real old man. I didn't trust myself. . . I can see this in retrospect, of course I didn't see it then. I made money, invested it in real estate and got all my childish wants out of the way. I got a brand new car, an expense account to live on. Anything I wanted I had, so my childhood dreams of being affluent were taken care of. But I realized I didn't trust myself and I wasn't happy. When my back went out again I stayed in bed for a couple of weeks and wondered, "What did I really want to do with my life?" I was real depressed. I flashed on the Bible as what I really wanted and so I read it and felt enthusiastic for about an hour, then got depressed again. I didn't know what I wanted. I moved in with a psychic gal I met at a show in San Francisco where I'd gone to hear about Pyramid Power. She gave me a book to read—Joel Goldsmith. I couldn't understand it. She gave me another and another, but I couldn't understand them. They didn't make much sense to me. Then she gave me *Autobiography of a Yogi* and that I could understand. So I said, "I need a guru." I phoned the fellow who put on the San Francisco show and asked him if he knew any gurus. He'd just met Christopher and gave me his name. I phoned Christopher up and made an appointment to see him.

Christopher asked me what was wrong and I said I was very confused and that three psychics had told me I was Leadbeater reincarnated, and what was I to do. He just said very simply, "If you were Leadbeater, someone would have been waiting for you. Was anyone waiting for you?" I said, "No." Later he said, "Leadbeater was clairvoyant; are you clairvoyant?" I said, "No." So that all dissolved. I signed up for the meditation course and to come to the classes on Friday night. I'd come each week on Friday nights until one Friday night I was sitting at the back, against the wall, and I started wondering what the hell I was doing there because I still couldn't understand all this metaphysical stuff. He used the word "Self", I didn't understand that. And the word "consciousness", I couldn't understand that. He used the word "I", even a simple word like that, but I still didn't know what he was saying, so I wondered what was I doing here. I said to myself, "I don't understand what's going on, so why do I keep coming?" At that moment his eyes met mine and he looked at me and I sort of burst into tears—quietly. I couldn't put words on it, but I realized why I was coming and I just kept coming. I suppose you could say he sent me some love, or I fell in love, I can't put words on it.

Then a place became vacant next door to him and when he asked me if I wanted to rent it I said no because I couldn't visualize myself living in a small town. But within a week I'd moved in. I don't know why, I hadn't consciously remembered the look on Friday night. But it was like when someone once said to me, "My heart is drawn to your heart." It was like that, but not on a conscious level. Since then he's confronted my ego an awful lot. And I would react and even want to leave. So he'd say, "Well, then leave." But I never *really* wanted to. I feel so fortunate to be here, and to be in my life now. I'm a different person. My back stopped going out, hasn't gone out in 4 years, and I can understand things now that I couldn't before. At first when the group started growing I would be jealous of the new people coming in. But now it's such a family. The group consciousness is happening, and I can tune into the Cosmos and talk to the Cosmos and so I can trust myself now because I have the Cosmos behind me. I've put my Physics together with Supersensonics and now that I don't have to be rich anymore I've got everything I've ever wanted.

Michael

I think I must have tried every spiritual trip. I tried everything that came my way. Some were very brief. I was interested in people who made claims about finding the truth, some higher form of wisdom and I wanted to see if this was true. There was a part of me deeply dissatisfied with my life. In high school I had feelings that there were other planes of existence besides just the one I saw. It was a vague feeling at first, then it became stronger and stronger. I was in awe of the coincidence in the way things happened. I used to wonder, if God created the universe, who created God? In college I had many spiritual experiences that blew my mind and I realized that reality was all in my imagination, but I didn't quite understand the part my imagination played in making things what they appeared to be. I could sometimes see an auric/etheric-like structure. It appeared like a whole other universe that operated on another octave of vibration. I would tune into it at various times, it felt like it was existing on a higher frequency of vibration. Sometimes I would feel my body vibrating at a faster pace. Then the physical world would appear like a slow-motion movie. At a certain point the physical movie would disappear and the other world would crystallize. It was like a dream, yet it wasn't. Sometimes I would feel myself at One with everything in the Universe. This was the most wonderful feeling. Drugs did help me have this feeling, but then it was there without drugs too. I stopped taking psychedelics because I wanted to verify what I was experiencing in real life.

I was majoring in architecture at Rhode Island School of Design, but I dropped out the third year and spent that year studying by myself—music and spiritual subjects. I was into Zen and did a lot of reading. I was into astrophysics and how it related to Einstein's Theory of Relativity. I sampled a lot of things. But it was very hard for me to relate to people. I was called "spaced-out" a lot. It was impossible for me to describe what I was feeling and I guess I was sort of not here. That was probably why I sought out spiritual groups and a guru. I had a real nomadic journey. I was initiated into TM, left after four months. None of the instructors could answer my questions. Then I was initiated into Buddhism by a Korean Zen Master and practiced Zen for one year. I wore the robes, used the koans, etc. I left because there was no heart in it. I investigated Guru Maharaji because I was intrigued by the claims made by his initiates. But I didn't feel good about the relationships between the members who lived in the ashram. Finally I went back to college at University of California at Santa Cruz. My roommates were Christian and had frequent meetings in my dorm. I watched baptism rites and saw some people become totally transformed for a few days. Then gradually they would return to their old selves. I tried Eckankar, Summit Lighthouse, Sufi dancing for three months and went to the yoga meetings at the Integral Yoga Institute in Santa Cruz, but I still missed something. I was looking for a deep relationship with people and couldn't find it. I could space out, but I couldn't deal with ordinary human problems and I couldn't find any spiritual group that could help me do that.

Intense feelings of loneliness and separation came to me as I was unable to share myself with others. I decided to visit Sanan, Switzerland and see J. Krishnamurti since I thought he would be able to help me. I was also desperately hoping to meet other people who I could relate to and who had similar problems where we could discuss the negative as well as the positive side of spiritual life. I was very fond of Krishnamurti's books and had read every one. When I got to Sanan and heard Krishnamurti talk I was very disappointed, and there was no real unity among the people as a group. Krishnamurti would speak about what not to do but he would never tell us what to do. There was a rumor about a man who lived in a chalet in the foothills of Sanan who was supposed to be enlightened. It was said that he put down the teachings of Krishnamurti, that he was an old student of his. His name was U. G. Krishnamurti, not related. I went to see him and he asked the small group that was gathered in his chalet why we were there. He said, "That chap is taking you for a ride. Enlightenment is a myth. If you were in that state you would not even know it because that would be the end of you (the self-sense)! So what are you doing here wasting your time trying to get something which you will never know? What you are seeking is so unnatural. You don't want this because this is going to burn the structure of the 'you'. 'You' want to continue, probably on a different dimension, but you want to continue somehow. You are only interested in continuity, continuity of the thing you know and experience—you!" Most people were real offended by U.G.'s very blunt way of pricking the ego and left. But I knew with burning clarity there was a deep wisdom in his words. I had had a taste of something like that before, so I knew it was true. But another part of me felt undermined by the words, "Whatever you do is in the way of That (state)." I left with no direction to go.

It was almost a year later that I met Christopher. He was giving a class on color and the seven chakras in his home. I felt he was in the same state of consciousness as I saw in U.G. and I was elated to find someone with cosmic consciousness only one-half hour from where I lived. I began to go to all the classes and to see him between classes. Everytime I saw him between classes I was completely horrified. He did not act the way a guru ought to. He ate meat and drank alcohol. I was a strict vegetarian and restrained from all intoxicating beverages. I wondered if he was a phoney.

I was very health food conscious and it took me months to reconcile his wisdom with the fact that he ate meat and drank alcohol. He was in super health, so I thought maybe he was one of the few who could transmute all that bad stuff and turn it into nectar. It certainly didn't seem to affect his clarity or his light. I signed up for the three year meditation course and thought I would probably be able to finish it and get enlightened in less than a year since I had already invested a lot of time in the enlightenment trip and felt I was pretty high spiritually. I did the first exercise in Section Zero and nothing happened. I tried and tried but nothing seemed to happen. I thought I was being taken down a blind alley and wondered if J. Krishnamurti wasn't right, that all gurus are useless. Then U.G.'s words echoed in my ears, "Whatever you do is in the way of That." So I was sure I'd fallen into a trap and was going to tell Christopher off. Some of the other people also had difficulty with Section Zero and Christopher was talking about the need for effortless effort. Convinced this was a bunch of twaddle I told him off. Then he started telling me where I was at and saw right through my argument. He even accused me of talking Krishnamurti lingo and I blushed and felt embarrassed. How did he know I had studied Krishnamurti? Then a big iron chandelier hanging over my head broke loose and clotted me over the head, practically knocking me unconscious. Funnily enough, I saw how I was just projecting onto Christopher my own pride and judgement, and that it was unfounded. I felt real remorseful.

My pride and judgements have come out time and time again since I've been at the University of the Trees. The group or Christopher would confront me each time. Sometimes it was hard to see, sometimes I saw. Once I left for six months to join another group, Bubba Free John's, because I felt Christopher had a very big ego he wasn't in touch with. But I came back because there was something that had touched my heart. Something I didn't find anywhere else. Even though Christopher would never build up my ego and made me see how separating and egotistical I was, I wanted to be there. And whenever my pride would rise, life would naturally humiliate me. It's been very hard for me to be open with my feelings and to learn to relate deeply to people. But looking back I can see that the wake I have left behind me and the situations I encountered were all playing on my blind spot, my arrogance that I wasn't in touch with. Here I can't run away from that. I'm cornered. I have to face myself.

Ann

Before I came here I was a housewife. Bob was a good husband. My world was the same as it had been for years and years. I worked on my books, wrote and wrote all day long, did a few chores, went to movies, watched TV. I was working on a book on dreams and before that I'd been working on a book of poetry, and before that I was working on a Ph. D. I was really into the school trip. After I got my Ph. D. I didn't quite know what to do with myself. I got into Bob's trip of fiction writing and teaching. He was an English professor, but I didn't like fiction writing and I hated teaching. Finally my agent said, "Don't write fiction if you don't want to, write non-fiction." It was a big insight to me. That's when I started working in earnest on my dream book. I'd been studying dreams for eight years and that was pretty fulfilling. I was looking for patterns and finding them. I liked Jung and Gestalt. I was also meditating quite a bit everyday. I was always sort of yearning for that something to happen when I meditated, but nothing ever did. I was on a tremendously intellectual spiritual trip and read everything I could get hold of. But they didn't all fit together and I'd practically cry over it. I was real frustrated.

I was totally anti-social, but I had thought that I would reach the world through books. But the world was real far away. And my writing always felt selfish to me. I really worried about it. I didn't want to be famous, I just wanted my work to have some meaning. I didn't need confirmation. I thought people who cared so much about what others thought were real fools. Like other faculty wives, and my best friend, the dean's wife. She worried all the time about her dinners, her looks, what she said. I didn't care at all—I thought. But since I've been here on campus I realize I was probably worse than she was underneath, but I cut off.

I met Christopher through my best friend. She was in London on sabbatical and wrote me that he really was the one. She'd researched it all out, gone to different places. I got sort of a vicarious thrill when she'd describe Centre House and Christopher. I wasn't looking for a guru. I thought that was only for Hindus and Tibetans. It wasn't part of my self-image. But when I heard Christopher was coming to the States on a lecture tour and would give a lecture in Beloit, Wisconsin where we lived and also in nearby Madison, I got real excited. I got to drive to Madison in the car with him and my first impression was that I just *liked* him. His vibe, the gentleness and the twinkle in his eye, the subtlety of his humor and the realness with which he spoke was impressive. You'd ask him a question and there was no phoniness in his answer. I grilled him awhile about all the books I'd read, right down the whole list and he just calmly told me the ones he thought were phonies and the ones he felt were genuine. He didn't say it in a judgemental way. He'd just say, "No, he didn't manifest what he was talking about," or "Yes, he lived that." I could see he cared about light and consciousness and that made *me* care. I was real thrilled.

He said two things about the meditation course that made me want to take it. One was that the second year was about the essence teachings of Christ for you to experience directly, and the other one was that there were techniques you could actually do to stimulate spiritual states, like adoration. I felt, "Wow, I don't have to read about it and wish I were that sort of person. I can learn to feel it. If I'm not there then there's something I can do about it." From that time on I tried to keep in touch. I'd write Norah and order the tapes. The tapes were my lifeline. I was out in the boonies and the vibrations on the tapes got to me. They really touched some deep part and made me feel like I was linked up even though I couldn't be there. I visited the University of the Trees twice, for a week each time. Back in Wisconsin my life continued on as it had done for years, but more and more I felt a regret. I had a feeling that things were really happening at the University of the Trees and I wished I could be a part. I knew I couldn't, but I wanted to. I didn't know what exactly was going on, but it was something important. I wanted to be there. I didn't know how sad I was about not being there, not until this minute. I'm sad now talking about it. I had no idea it was making me that unhappy. I guess I just adjusted to it. And I was happy with Bob. We'd had our life together the same for a long time. We had a happy marriage. We were good friends. But I remember I couldn't share my spiritual life with Bob. He wasn't interested. And he couldn't share his tennis with me. I wasn't interested. So at lunchtime I'd say, "How was your tennis today?" And he'd say, "Six love, six love," or whatever they say. And, "I got the ball into the corner. . . " and I'd give him ten minutes or so. Then I'd sort of stop being interested. Then he'd say, "Well what do you hear from Christopher and Norah?" And I'd have ten minutes. So we could each exchange, but neither of us cared about the other's world. I'd then sort of slip away to do my meditations.

Then I came to visit the University of the Trees for a month and I felt a conflict about going back home. It was just a little inner conflict. I wasn't going to leave Bob or anything. I wanted to be open because everybody was being open and I thought, well, I'll share my little inner conflict. So I did, at tea time one day. And all of a sudden everyone in the whole room started telling me where I could find a job in Santa Cruz. I didn't want a job, I just wanted to share my little inner conflict. I thought, "They don't even *know* Bob and I'm not going on their say-so." But then I threw the *I Ching* and it was quite clear. I must have thrown it a million times to make sure, but I always got a message to join with friends of like mind. So I went back home and was trying to move Bob up to Santa Cruz, because that fit with my ethics. But in my heart I didn't want him to move with me. He was going to move up and be a tennis pro and we'd have to live in some tennis club and I didn't want it. Finally I told Bob, "You know, I don't really want you to come. I want to go alone." And he said, "Go then, don't wait around, do it now." That freaked me out. I packed my bags, and then I'd weaken and he would say, "No, you have to go." This was partly for me and partly because he needed to be free too, only I didn't know that then. And he cried on the way to the airport. I was just devastated by that. It seemed to me I was running out on him.

The month I had been a guest at the University of the Trees I felt such a bond of love in the group. The minute I got here it just included me. I couldn't believe it. I didn't understand it, how it had happened, but I could feel it. Everybody just took me in and it was a circle of love and I felt part of it. It wasn't the studying of the teachings that made me want to stay. I could do that on my own, like I had been doing. I liked Creative Conflict, but I hadn't been through it myself at the time. I was afraid people would find out I wasn't such a sweetheart as I seemed. But I really liked it because I'd always hated to be with people who bugged me and I couldn't say anything to them. When I came here it was like fresh air. The vibe in the group was love but nobody was sweety sweet. They were strong people in a nice way. So I felt resonance with the vibration of the people here. I didn't come just for Christopher by any means. It was 50-50. I felt like these were my people, that I'd finally found them after so many years, people who were like me and I could be myself.

What I found over and over after coming here was that I had a gap between where I was at with my head in my spiritual life and where I was at in my being, and that I really had to start over at Square One. Creative Conflict turned out to be real hard for me. I see that deep down I don't want to lose my ego. I'm afraid of missing out on something in life. So my ego is always giving me pain when things don't go the way I expect with someone or if my love life feels awful. I sometimes wonder, "Where can I run? Back to Bob? I was happy then, and now I'm in pain." But I realize that I wasn't in touch with a heart pain I had before. It was an unconscious pain in the heart. I don't have that kind of pain here. Here I have an ego pain that doesn't want to look at itself. When I stay around Christopher's heart I feel my heart, even though I have to look at my ego. And if I left I'd be turning my back on my heart. Everyone is drawn here by Christopher's heart, by his love. It's not as though it is a person or a personality thing, or just his heart. It's *the* heart; it's *my* heart that I feel in him.

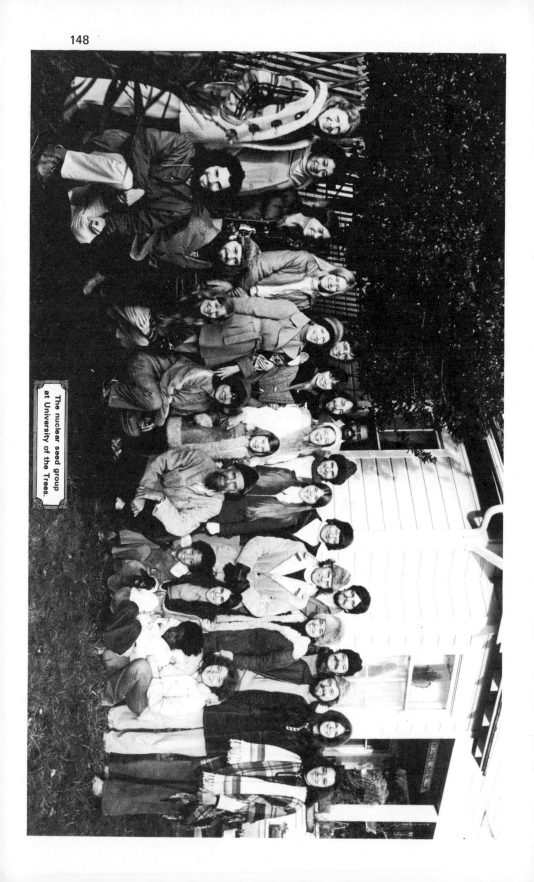

The nuclear seed group at University of the Trees.

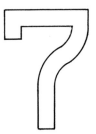

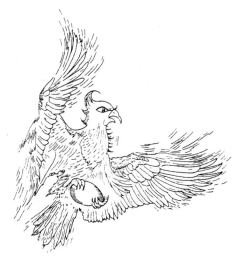

BEYOND THE IDEAL

Political writers who have changed history have done so through the powerful influence of ideals upon human consciousness. Yet ideals are not enough to lift the dead weight of human nature and really change it, because ideals appeal primarily to the conscious mind and leave behind all the drives and images and buried history which we carry with us in that vast storehouse called the unconscious. This unconscious part of us is what takes away our peace. Since it is unconscious, we don't even know it is there, and yet it is who we are. The primary purpose of Creative Conflict as practiced at the University of the Trees is to probe these hidden parts of ourselves. Creative Conflict is a way of life which is based not just upon another ideal but upon an entirely different vision of man. The difference is in its depth of penetration. An ideal can reach the soul and make a radical change in a person or it can be embraced very shallowly in a rush of sentimental feeling leaving the person basically untransformed. Therefore, for every ideal and every impulse toward the light, there must be a cold hard look into the dark. For every feeling of inner peace, there must also be an unsettling of the ego in its self-complacent world, an earthquake of the personality, a shaking of the foundations. This is the only pathway to genuine change and spiritual evolution. All else happens at the level of the conscious mind, which is only the tip of the iceberg, while down below the level of our awareness is the bulk of who we are. The new vision of Nuclear Evolution must include this unconscious but very real level of our being.

In recent brain research, scientists are just discovering the differences between right and left brain functions in our unconscious use of the intuition versus rationalization, but these distinctions have been known to spiritual seekers for many centuries and stand revealed particularly in the ancient Chinese civilization and the I Ching. Today all systems of government are divided into left versus right wing groups or parties and this splitting, too, comes from the conscious mind. The intellect divides reality into polarities of hot and cold, mine and yours, either/or, and in matters of politics especially, sees no middle ground except compromise where a gradient of truth might be found. At this superficial level, we experience a comfortable known reality, neatly ordered by polarized concepts and safely contained by them in clichés. But those who venture to the deeper layers of consciousness discover there an unknown vaster self experiencing the world in an entirely different way with a totally different set of values. Many of our constitutions were written over two hundred years before this psychological and psycho-physical knowledge of man existed in modern scientific form. Even those recently amended like the Russian constitution and the Chinese constitution, do not take into account any of the scientific facts of man's personality but are based purely on idealistic political theories which date back 100 years before the times of the industrial revolution and the antiquated ideas of Karl Marx.

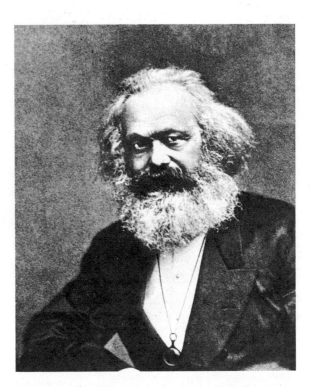

Karl Marx

None of these theories of man or government have been proved correct and in fact the worldwide communist movement has deliberately ignored the results of over fifty years of Soviet testing of the theory. Communists in America and other capitalist countries still believe that the time of revolution is near at hand when they can take over the social capital and wealth generated by the old corrupt system and use it to create the new good system. They are either blind to or silent about the ruthless communist repression in Eastern European countries which are dominated by the quasi-colonialism of the USSR. They refuse to admit that oppression and exploitation of the working classes is the logical result of Marxist-Leninist principles themselves, not merely the Kremlin's version of these. The Marxist dialectic does not solve the question of human freedom nor does it take into account the fact that after sixty years of practice the standard of living in the Russian experiment is several times lower than in the free enterprise system.

Human-Rights

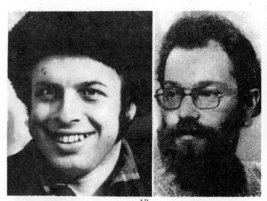

Shcharansky AP Ginzburg

Orlov Ginzburg after incarceration

Orlov, Shcharansky and Ginzburg were leading figures in the small band of Soviet dissidents. They set up a watchdog group that monitored Moscow's compliance with the human-rights provisions of the 1975 Helsinki declaration. Shcharansky, a stocky baldish computer programmer who speaks fluent English, served as liaison between Soviet dissident groups and Western newsmen until he was arrested. Ginzburg a poet and longtime friend of exiled author Aleksandr Solzhenitsyn, administered a fund fed by Solzhenitsyn's royalties to aid the families of Soviet political prisoners.

Ida Milgrom hasn't seen her son, mathematician Anatoly Shcharansky, since last March, when he was jailed for his human-rights activities and told that he faced a potential treason charge—which carries a maximum penalty of death. Petite Irina Orlov has no word about her physicist husband Yuri, who was arrested ten months ago on a charge of slandering the Soviet system. Arina Ginzburg worries about her husband Aleksandr, an editor who was imprisoned last February for alleged anti-Soviet activities. The frail Ginzburg contracted tuberculosis during an earlier term in a labor camp, and she fears that this spell of prison could be tantamount to a death sentence. Each month she travels 110 miles from Moscow to Kaluga prison to deliver a food parcel. Her handwriting on a prison form is the only sign her husband ever gets that she is alive and well.

Under Soviet law, prisoners can be held incommunicado and without legal advice for nine months of investigation. Parliament passed a special decree prolonging the 29-year-old Shcharansky's pretrial captivity for an additional six months, but Ginzburg, 41, and Orlov, 53, are being held without any such legal nicety. The result is lonely, uncertain agony for them and their families. And for the three women who wait at home, arbitrary and petty officials find dozens of ways to make life more uncomfortable.

Hints: Soviet authorities seem to delight in withholding information about the prisoners. When Mrs. Ginzburg asked about her husband's health, investigator Yuri Suchkov replied: "It is not worse than when he was arrested." When arrested, Ginzburg had just spent three weeks in the hospital with pneumonia. Recently another investigator, Viktor Volodin, hinted to Mrs. Milgrom that she may not be allowed to see Shcharansky until after his trial." Does this mean there will be a trial?" she inquired. "I never said that," Volodin responded.

The three women have been stymied trying to hire defense lawyers. Russian attorneys are unwilling to jeopardize their careers by involving themselves with political outcasts, and Mrs. Milgrom has been turned down by twenty of them to date. A number of foreign lawyers have offered to work on the cases—including US attorney Edward Bennett Williams, who was hired by exiled author Aleksandr Solzhenitsyn to defend Ginzburg—but Soviet officials say that no alien attorneys will be granted visas.

House Arrest: Relatives of the prisoners suffer constant harassment. For fear she would make a public protest on United Nations Human Rights Day in December, Irina Orlov was placed under house arrest. While driving to Kaluga with packages for her husband, Arina Ginzburg has been stopped and fined so often for imaginary traffic violations that now she takes the train. "I'd walk to Kaluga if I had to," she shrugs. Mrs. Ginzburg's telephone was cut off more than a year ago without explanation, but she pays for the phone each month anyway to deprive officials of any legal excuse to terminate the service. For Mrs. Milgrom, in contrast, phone calls are a frequent torment. "At all hours of the night, the operator rings to tell me to stand by for a call from, say, America," she reports. "Then after she's woken me up, the operator rings back to say, 'Excuse me, the call will not take place'."

All three families have encountered trouble about jobs. Neither Mrs. Orlov, an artist, nor Mrs. Ginzburg, a language teacher, can find work. "Employers are afraid to hire us," says Arina Ginzburg, who would settle for a position as a maid. Shcharansky's parents live on their pensions, but his older brother Leonid, an engineer, has been called to Communist Party headquarters at his plant and ordered to denounce Anatoly. When Leonid refused, officials left no doubt that he would never again be promoted.

In July 1978, a year later, Shcharansky was sentenced to thirteen years hard labor in the Gulag concentration camp. Ginzburg was sentenced to eight years hard labor, as was Orlov. Since then, Ginzburg has been transferred to two different labor camps. Last August his wife was allowed to visit him She was shocked by the rapid degeneration in his appearance. Ginzburg's wife was even more horrified when she was allowed her first visit. She did not recognize her husband, his physical and mental condition had deteriorated so much. Shcharansky has been moved to three different labor camps and has not been seen for several months.

Fred Coleman—Newsweek;

It ignores the fact that its own origin is not the ideal condition of synthesis which Marx borrowed from Hegelian logic but is merely a total reaction to capitalism, an antithesis to the capitalist thesis but not in any way a synthesis of the best of both. That synthesis is yet to come.

The ideology of communism is written into the Russian constitution—almost a perfect document of human freedom—but the USSR constitution does not reflect where that political system is at in reality. A constitution must evolve not from theory but from a country's actual manifestation. To become the organ of growth for a strong and wholesome society it must be based on the solidity of something real. Just as an individual cannot change until he is willing to see where he is really at, and not where his self-image wishes he were at, so too, society's self-image is seen only in its ideal and usually is not borne out at the level of actual living.

We cannot advance the cause of freedom merely by verbal attacking or by embarking upon the subversion of the systems we do not like. We have to demonstrate an effective evolutionary advance. What attracts the young people of the world to communism? Is it not the thought of a quick end to the world's miserable conditions, an urge for a better way, an ideal, something worth doing with their life which is still before them and not half spent? In affluent countries the young people are jaded with ease. They want to go to the woods and hew houses out of timber, so that there will be some meaning in the house and some meaning in their work.

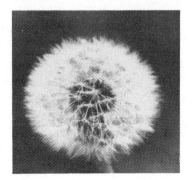

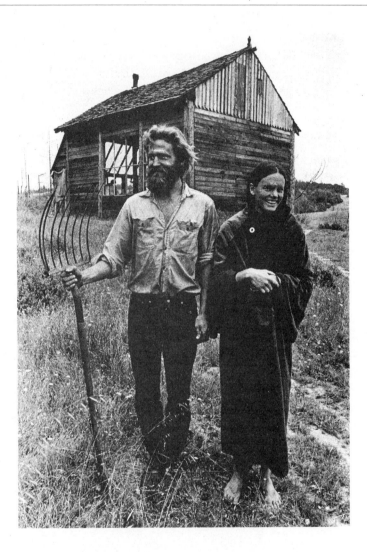

Though American democracy has demonstrated the highest standard of living, the best educated population, and the most libertarian society ever known in human history, it has done little to confront its long list of weaknesses and shortcomings, and this discourages idealists. Worse yet, it lacks the proper rhetoric. It lacks a clear ideal. So the young people of America, because they *need* an ideal, have turned to communism. They have judged communism by its stated ideal while their own country they condemn for its incomplete manifestation. The less experience they have of life, the more they respond to the *ideal* at the verbal level just as they have also done in following after phony gurus and spiritual "masters" without thinking to gauge the manifestation against the words.

The greatest attraction to idealists is that the Marxist-Leninist ideology since its inception has loudly claimed that state ownership of the means of production and the liquidation of the capitalist system will eliminate the causes of war, do away with inhumanity and racial and religious discrimination, and bring about a peaceful world. The actual facts are that communism has divided the world against itself, has exploited international violence whenever it saw the slightest opportunity to conquer or gain influence, and has the largest repressive system in the world. It has created the inhumanity of a totally new class structure with a privileged bureaucracy at the top and about two million state slaves in labor camps at the bottom. How much idealistic fervor can we muster over a cause which is so clearly a divisive force in the world and so little suited to make "a better way of life"? The communist states make war even upon each other. By creating powerful puppet states around it, with the Soviet army in readiness to squash any deviant ideology, the Russian communist system has spawned governments exactly like itself. Therefore conflict between these ruthless and self-seeking powers is inevitable—the Russian invasion of Czechoslovakia in 1968, the military intervention against the Hungarian communists in 1956, the ideological conflict with Peking (escalated by the massing of millions of troops on the Chinese borders, engaging in violent border battles).

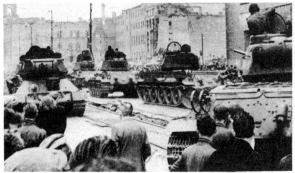

Soviet tanks in Budapest   UNITED PRESS

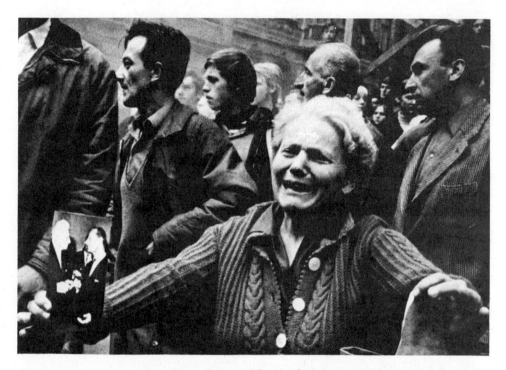

The old lady shows a picture of Prime Minister Dubcek and President Svoboda as the invading Russian tanks roll by in the 1968 takeover of Czechoslovakia whose communist party decided to undertake a different form of socialism. Dubcek's methods were succeeding and the entire country was alive with new freedom. Its success was a threat to Russian failures.

Stalin's attempt to force ideological conformity upon Yugoslavia by threats of violence, political subversion and economic pressures was only resisted by the heroism of Marshal Tito and the determination of the Yugoslav army. The communist ideal—to overthrow the capitalist oppressors—has brought so much more oppression and so much less benefit to people's lives than capitalism has done that its original claims are just a hollow boast. Since its inception, the means used to obtain communist goals of peace have always been violence and force. And this plain fact has stripped international communism of any claims to be a higher level of social organization. For the long awaited unity of the world's peoples we must look in another direction than the activists, revolutionaries and ideologists who are playing political power games with the lifeblood of the earth. If those who lie buried under the soil of the Gulag prisons and Chinese labor camps, the innocent victims of the murderous socialist State, could cry up from the earth, their noise would deafen the living with the hymn of death. And yet the leaders of the socialist State do not feel murderous but on the contrary cast themselves in the role of heroes.

It is difficult to understand this blindness, this clinging to and identifying with the ideal while denying reality, yet it is part of the basic structure of human nature, constantly splitting itself into conscious and unconscious mind in order *not* to see itself as it really is. Every individual, whether communist or no, has this mechanism of self-preservation. So long as our political ideals and constitutions come from the head, from the conscious self-image and its ideals (believed in with all sincerity, so far as we *know* ourselves), then we will not have anything new under the sun, neither in politics nor in life on earth as we know it. Our present structures of society are merely a projection of our consciousness which is ignorant of the nature of human personality, of its drives and how the brain and mind work. The communists make war in the name of an ideal. Their words are lily white while their deeds express the opposite of what they say. So too in our personal lives we are confronted with the same power plays. As long as these actions occur on the individual level, they must also appear on the national level as an effect of human nature. One member of the University of the Trees group told the following personal experience as an illustration of the same basic human nature at work in personal conflicts:

> "I was visiting my mother and overstayed my welcome by several days. My mother wanted me to leave but she did not want to come out and say that she needed to be alone. I think she was afraid that it would sound like she didn't love me, and she may even have been afraid that she really didn't love me. So instead of being straightforward, she began to pick on my appearance so that I would get uncomfortable and leave of my own accord while she would be saying, 'Oh please, stay another week.' She could be the

good generous hospitable person while I was the negative
one who chose to leave. I knew that she maneuvered this
unconsciously and that she did not think of how her remarks
would undermine my confidence in my appearance and
would make me feel much more unloved than if she had just
spoken her real motive."

Such is human nature. How does one person get the upper hand on
another, so that one grows stronger and stronger by making the other
weaker and weaker? In the above example, the daughter put up with
this kind of subtle manipulation for years because she did not want to
risk confronting the mother. Instead she buried her resentment inside
and closed off awareness of the major rift that lay ahead in the future.
Do we not, at the social level, do the very same thing when we live
with situations that are not right? We grumble but say nothing and,
because we take no action, the seeds of a future revolution are sown in
our hearts.

It is the exact same mechanism of human nature by which our
political leaders gain more and more power by capitalizing on our
weakness. How do we become weak while the strong become stronger?
By giving away our strength. Apathy is the natural partner of the
power-seeking drive in human beings and the two energize and feed
each other. In America we don't care enough that we are taxed more
and more every year while the government gains strength in becoming
increasingly bureaucratic so that we eventually find ourselves merely
victims of all the red tape. We look at the size of our government and
feel helpless, but how did it get to *be* that size? The more powerful the
power structure grows, the more hopeless and apathetic one feels,
which only makes the government stronger still. Finally there is
nothing left, either at the individual or the social level but rage,
resentment and revolution and in America, in 1979, as this book goes
to press, a possible taxpayers' revolt.

Why is it that every generation is more apathetic than the last?
Children are born into a world where "the system" is already too big
to fight, before they are even out of diapers. The answer for them is the
same as the answer for any individual who is oppressed by his or her
mother, father, lover, business partner, friend or children. To give up in

despair only makes more oppression, so the only solution is to stand and fight. However there is more than one way to fight. If a bully hits you and you hit him back, then you are fighting on his terms. If a gigantic System steals your freedom and in protest you get a hand-grenade and blow up a building, then you go to jail and the System carries on as usual. In order to beat Goliath, you have to be David. You have to have the universe backing you up. Your cause must be just and your motive pure. Therefore, it is of utmost importance that we do not go off on our own brand of power-trip, criticizing the government, proposing violence, thrashing around with no effect. If the universe is going to back the change we want, then we will have to take a look at how the universe changes things. Nature has ways of making a change. What are they?

For one thing, Nature does not usually change suddenly. She knows that if the thing is to endure it must be built in a slow and steady way. The Marxist way of change is revolution: the overnight transform-ation of society. The Marxists roused the oppressed people of Russia and China to the ideal of freedom, promising that the leadership of the State was only temporary and in time would "wither away," leaving the people free and equal. But the fact is that a self-perpetuating power system will never wither away, particularly if it is enshrined as the very mechanism which provides the means for change. The Marxist way of evolution is to change society by handing down a decree from the Presidium. The Presidium will always be with communism because the philosophers of the socialist State were a product of the belief that the environment shapes mankind rather than mankind shaping the environ-ment. Therefore the most promising material is given the best education to make the best leaders, whose judgement is not to be challenged. The late bloomer or the hidden genius in our society who so often climbs the peaks after adolescence has no room in the Marxist society. To this way of thinking, change comes from outside, not from within. The philosophies of Hegel, Marx and Nietzsche therefore overlooked the subtle force at work in human evolution. They ignored the real structure of human personality and the natural laws of consciousness and instead made reason and logic the new God for the modern state, thereby justifying the use of coercion and punishment for dissident views. First you legislate the change and then you enforce it through violence. But in the hearts of the people, there is no change. First comes the ideal; then society is made to measure up to it. The head imposes "shoulds" upon the heart. Yet the ideal is all theory. Only more Gulag prison camps can be expected as the logical outcome of socialism by force. Even though conditions appear to be improving in Russia—more tolerance, more American radio waves being allowed to broadcast—if the people's spirits ever take a breath of the fresh air of freedom will they not be squelched as they were in Prague when they began to feel liberated? It seems that those whose natures are crude and unrefined are always in a position to persecute the Sakharovs and Solzhenitsyns. How is it that the universe is so designed that those whose consciousness is more evolved are always crucified by those who are locked into false ideals and concepts and, in the name of evolution, lead the world into another 2000 years of darkness?

Any new ideas of social evolution are certain to be crushed by any socialist state. If the communists in France, Italy, Britain or USA ever get their monolithic power machine going in those countries they will immediately crush spontaneity and take away personal freedom as they did in Cambodia, Viet Nam, China, Tibet, Czechoslovakia and every other communist state. For the socialists to see what a mockery of genuine socialism their system really is, they would have to be purged by their own violent system and eradicated by their own methods of silencing the truth.

If these be the fruits of reason and logic, then we cannot trust the mind to save us from ourselves. On the contrary, it leads us nearer and nearer to the complete folly of nuclear suicide. Is there not some higher guiding force that we can follow? If change must come from inside a person and yet no one seems to have any intention of changing, then what can society do to protect itself against ruthlessness and selfishness? The free society and capitalist system has never had an answer to the problem of power-hungry leaders, but at least we can remove them every four or five years under our present system of checks and balances, whereas this same machinery exists under socialism in name alone. The Democratic Union of Socialist Republics is neither a democracy nor a union. The power was given entirely to the State, with no checks or balances built into the system. People thought that they were giving power to themselves because theoretically they *were*

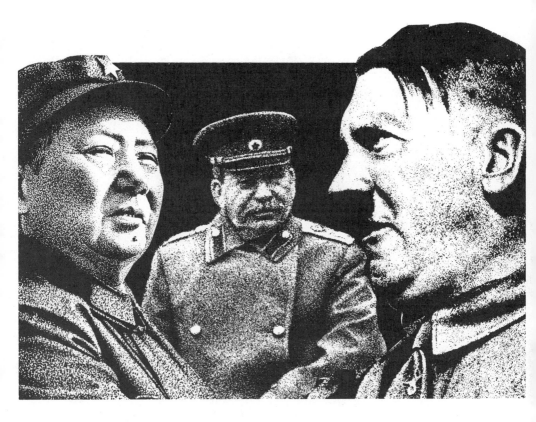

the State, but instead the socialist State became the world's largest exploiting power.

In the West, we have the vast multi-national company without a soul, whose main objective is to make a profit for its investors. It will bribe others, pollute, fix prices, irrespective of basic ethical values. It has shown repeatedly that it will ignore the public weal until forced by communal pressure and laws to clean up its rape of the environment and reduce its exorbitant prices for drugs, consumables, etc. Often the democratic government may force large companies to pay back the consumers, as has happened in American courts.

> **DRUG INDUSTRY. Federal inquiries continue.** Five major drug houses were accused by the Justice Department of conspiring to fix the prices of a broad spectrum of antibiotics—chiefly tetracyclines (Aureomycin, Terramycin)—throughout the 1950's and 1960's. The companies denied guilt but offered to make a cash settlement for "overcharges" to close the matter, allocating $120 million, more than a quarter of which was allotted to individual claims. Legal notices appeared in newspapers explaining how individuals could apply for refunds on tetracyclines purchased on prescriptions. Most of the 50 states agreed to accept this settlement, but a few said that they would take independent legal action.

On the other hand, the communist State has itself taken on the role of the capitalist manufacturers, turning out shoddy goods far below capitalist standards and charging exorbitant prices, paying much lower wages and giving more squalid and primitive conditions along with a regimentation of the human soul far surpassing the financial exploitation of the free economy. The State, being both the employer and the owner of the means of production in the name of the workers, cannot prosecute itself for price fixing nor is there any recourse for the exploited worker who is not free to use the strike weapon to improve conditions.

This domination of the total population by the few is the inevitable result of the philosophy of power as the instrument of change, and the unacknowledged rivers of blood that are seemingly required to establish and maintain these socialist revolutions against the natural will of the people make us ask more urgently: what new system can go beyond this dualism of the exploitative mentality and go beyond the self-righteousness of the master thinkers who believe they can solve the human problem of society through the muzzle of a gun or the power to dictate the course of evolution? The answer comes loud and clear. Those who do not know the purpose of human evolution, who themselves function only on one narrow level of consciousness and cannot see any other level but their own, are not the people we can trust with any power at all. Unless they can first demonstrate their political theories with small groups of like-minded humans, they are merely postulating as Truth their own ignorance of human consciousness.

THIS IS NATURE'S WAY OF CHANGE

She starts small and grows little by little to her full potential. If the

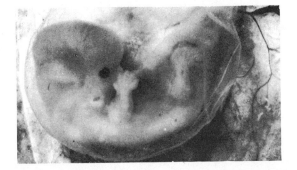

organism has a weakness that makes it unfit to survive, she destroys it and begins again. Her way is slow but her fruits are there for anyone to see. You cannot argue with success! How can we make our own systems as failsafe as the laws of Nature? Only by tuning into ourselves as *part* of Nature.

An acorn does not grow into an oak by external pressure and intimidation; it thrives best when it is allowed to unfold from its own

seed. What is the seed inside a human being that responds to light and grows of its own accord? What guides a human being toward his destiny? Ideals, you may reply. But what inside him *seeks* the ideal, and what responds? What in him chooses the way of justice or turns aside into the love of power? And when he does turn away from the light, what guiding intelligence in life itself brings home to him the error of his choice? It is true that some people take an entire lifetime to learn that the soul cannot be bartered without a very high price to pay, and yet the reckoning does come. After the revolution comes the counter-revolution. After the crime comes justice. If justice seems slow to arrive, perhaps it is because we the victims have an even more difficult lesson to learn from life than that of our oppressors. And we stubbornly refuse to learn it. Until we really look at how we are giving power to those who wish to dominate us, life will continue to mirror back to us our weakness through the painful situations that seem to be "happening" to us. In reality we are "buying" them, though we do not want to pay the price when it comes due. Idealists come with their far-fetched theories of human behavior and expect us to do what they have never achieved themselves. We feel quite virtuous when we become the

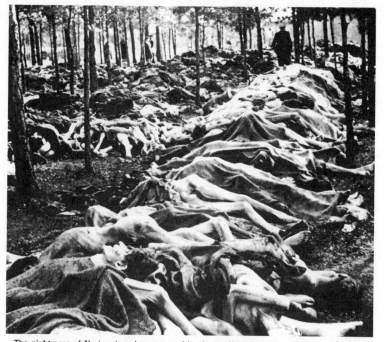

The nightmare of Nazism is only suggested by these piles of bodies at the concentration camp at Belsen, Germany. These victims died of disease and starvation, but millions more —men, women, and children—were deliberately murdered.

devoted follower of this cause or that one, this guru or another, this utopia or its opposite, without a scrap of evidence that any of it is valid. And even when the spiritual teacher who embodies the ideal is a true Christ, what good does it do to create another personality cult and superimpose the ideals upon ourselves from outside, without discovering our own pure consciousness within? The ideals will rebound as we fail to live up to them because of the contents of our unconscious. Ideals alone will never make a perfect society and will never satisfy the real needs of our soul for self-discovery.

Here is the proposal behind this book: let those who respond begin with small experimental communities which offer no threat to the present systems now working in democracies, but may provide models for others who will be turned on when they see something already working. This new method is not concerned with systems which are not working, except to discover solutions to the human dilemma and to put them into practice. About thirty-five people at present are gathered at the University of the Trees to build such a model which will seed the next evolutionary step for human society. There are others quietly working in different places. They live peaceably within the American constitution, yet they are creating their own constitutions as well. The new concepts must obviously allow for the current reality to continue to exist; otherwise a revolution would be needed to overthrow the self-perpetuating power structures. There is no need for revolution. The power of an idea whose time is come will steadily and inevitably replace that which is not working, because the universal law is behind it. It is obvious that neither capitalism nor its reaction, communism, is working. Therefore the time is ripe for anyone to demonstrate a system that does work. And perhaps this time we will not look to reason and logic for our guidance but to the Evolutionary Intelligence itself—that force that can not only set ideals but bring us through the threshing floor of life to embody them. We must have an ideal that is not static and restricting but has the life principle of growth built into it. Such an ideal cannot be dictated by reason but will be based upon what we really are in our hearts and how we actually evolve from the nuclear center of our being. We will learn to "reason by the heart".

To find out the real nature of man it is absurd to focus (as Marx did) only on man's lowest common denominator, his materialism and

166

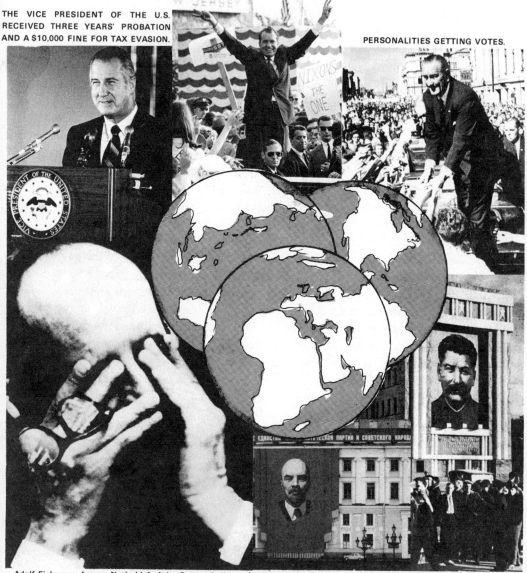

THE PRESIDENT OF THE U.S. STOOPS TO STATING PUBLICLY "I AM NOT A CROOK".

THE VICE PRESIDENT OF THE U.S. RECEIVED THREE YEARS' PROBATION AND A $10,000 FINE FOR TAX EVASION.

PERSONALITIES GETTING VOTES.

Adolf Eichmann, former Nazi chief of the Gestapo's "Jewish Affairs". As chief executor of the Nazi program to wipe out the Jews living in Europe, he sent to death a population almost equal to that of Chicago and Los Angeles combined.

Lenin promised the masses freedom but really wanted their energies to help him form an elite group.

Stalin killed 35 million people at a rate of 40,000 per month by working them to death in labor camps and murder.

**OUR PRESENT SYSTEM
ENCOURAGES THE POWER HUNGRY TO SEEK OFFICE**

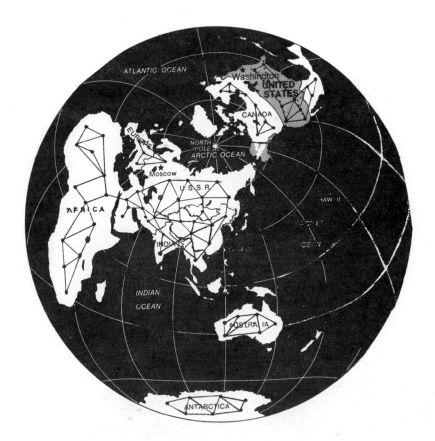

Through interlinking of centers in the natural supersensitive exchange of energy, a planetary grid will be created over the next few years and the concepts of Nuclear Evolution will spread organically over the planet. Those individuals who are even now harnessing the energies of consciousness and of their own volition forming groups to practice new ways of setting up self-governing educational communities, will be given the power of tele-thought.

his basic physical urges. But neither should we settle for those ideal-istic longings which drive us to embrace a concept even when reality contradicts it. Let us instead look to the highest and greatest human beings and see in them the potential of all men. What guided their course? Was it logic? Or was it something infinitely larger and far more wonderful? Socrates was seized with an unshakeable belief that he had been charged with a mission from God to care not only for his own soul's evolution but for the souls of his fellow humans and to teach, via the concrete example of his own life, that too much concern for the body and possessions can ruin the work on the soul. Only if we can risk a look beyond the highest things we know, a look at the really evolved beings of the earth, can we ever find out the secret of the evolutionary process. Only then can any new idea come into the world's awareness and check the headlong course now leading us toward nuclear war.

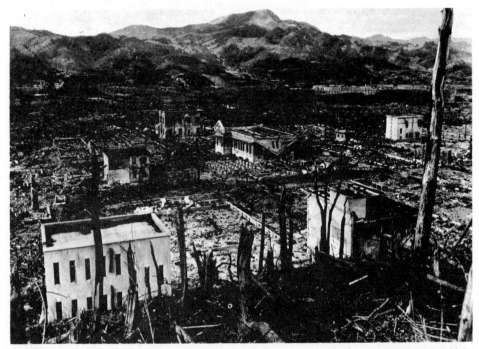

The bombing of Hiroshima on August 6, 1945, followed three days later by the bombing of Nagasaki brought with it a new awareness of man's ability to destroy himself. The fact that only two bombs had killed 114,000 people did not deter nations from developing and stock-piling more sophisticated nuclear weapons.

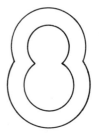

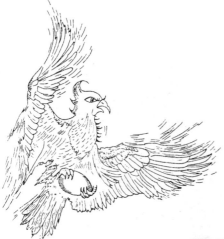

WHAT IS
THE PURPOSE
OF LIFE?

In our modern world the Phoenix rises into a cloud of materialism so thick that it is hard for the young seeker to distinguish the way through all the conflicting claims. Half of the world is ruled by systems claiming to be the heir to power through nations of workers. Yet those who wield the power in the name of the humble and exploited are themselves ideologues who will sacrifice the life and freedom of millions of people for untried theories of government. In them there is no real love, no compassion, no seeing of their own brutality and cruelty, and they are blind to the coarse, unrefined quality of their beings. Through them, the lowest material vibration of consciousness rules over the sensitive, artistic and intellectual people of the earth. The spiritual is considered weak and deceptive and is eradicated by loveless hoards of immature children, trained from a young age to wield the gun and bayonet and to trust in nothing but political power, to love nothing but this power, and to make this power of domination their only God.

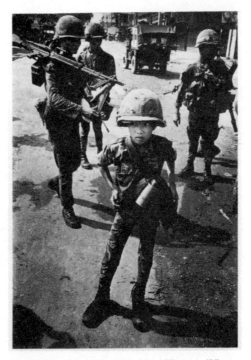

Ten-year-old ARVN, a "little tiger", feted for killing two "Vietcong women cadre" the day before (his teacher and mother, it was rumored).

Great nations, who once ruled their people benignly and in ancient times encouraged the development of natural philosophical systems in China and India, have materially declined, with their two thousand year old philosophies in disrepute. Attracted by the gleam of personal power over others and seduced by a philosophy of social equality, the hungry peasant believes that the new political system will give him brotherhood and a common wealth. Daily, millions are believing that the ancient teachings of love and compassion of Buddha and Christ are false and are adopting the aggressive expansion of communism and its faith in guns and in the power to kill those we are taught to dislike or disagree with. In the name of brotherhood and comradeship the vastly populated nations of India, China and the East are rapidly deserting their spiritual heritage of a two thousand year old wisdom for the shining baubles of more modern systems. They do not see that these systems do not work and bring more pain and more suffering than the evils they replace. Only when people have been robbed and stripped of their spiritual freedom and their religious sentiment can they see, too late, the lack of love and the heartless coercion of their political bosses. By then, the old ways have been so ridiculed that the ancient traditions are obliterated as ineffective deceptions of the people. Yet in the West, where affluence and untrammeled materialism have been the goal of the people for hundreds of years, the young are discovering for the first time these ancient systems of self-growth and methods of refining consciousness. These systems are being updated with the modern knowledge of science and psychology to bring a new yearning for the old values of love and compassion and the super-sensitive life of man.

A book on the spiritualization of political power and a system of organizing people and social institutions cannot ignore this breath upon the waters of our higher being. It must grasp the nettle of political consciousness which calls for action now and at the same time reveal the essence of the Universal One which is the real objective of these Eastern religions and philosophies. Any economic or political system which leaves out love and the functions of a mature heart in our relationships with each other will eventually pass away over long periods of history. The waves of religious passion and political power come and go, wiping out each other in great alternate movements of enlightenment and barbarism. This has been the way of man for countless centuries. One set of people believing the other to be squeamish or too lenient has annihilated and invaded the weaker groups; the weak then grew up and became powerful as a social reaction to barbarism. Alternately replacing each other at the ends of the swing of a giant pendulum, each undoes everything the other does and throws away any advance of the world's social evolution until we land ourselves with the conflict and absurd polarization of opposites that we have today. Now at this very moment two giant political forces are poised to annihilate each other with a finger on the nuclear trigger of a total planetary holocaust that would destroy all living organisms. Therefore man must learn to love; he must love for survival's sake, for without love he is an evolutionary misfit which has come to the end of its road, like an extinct species. The sobering thought is that the planet could wake up tomorrow morning and find that life as we know it will be extinguished in a matter of a few days of radiation sickness.

Man must now hear well the teachings of the great compassionate ones or perish. The science of the heart and its evolution is now not a luxury to be pursued by the rich and affluent but by those whose stomachs are empty and whose one thought is the next meal. For their survival on the planet and the survival of the race is now being decided for posterity in the hearts of men everywhere. For rich and poor alike, there is no escape. It is no use to say that the poor cannot think of spiritual matters while they are yet empty of food. They *must* think of these things. Whether they are hungry or not, dying or starving or locked in prison, free or enslaved, they must think of this love now, because if it is lacking in sufficient measure, the entire planet will be deluged, not with the great flood of water as in times past but in the rain of rockets and bombs and in the flood of blood. For man has ignored the Cosmic One and used the angel intelligence within to create and evolve the beast in himself. Love is no longer optional but mandatory for survival. The problem is that love cannot be legislated or coerced. Love can only flourish where it is spontaneous and free; otherwise it dies on the vine shortly after its tender shoots have sprouted. How much time can one devote to learning how to love? How much time have we got left to learn to love before the sea of blood swamps the entire race?

It is here that the great systems of the East which emphasize impersonal cosmic love and the individual love of Christ for persons rather than abstract philosophy, must now come together with science in the West to penetrate the nuclear being of the One, to avoid the nuclear holocaust of human negativity. We must otherwise pay the price of all ignorance, which is death. All natural systems have their disintegration programmed into their own structure if they do not follow their true pattern of evolution and respect the evolutionary guide of all cosmic life. This guide is love. To ignore it is to bring suffering. The marriage of East and West, of the head and the heart, is the purpose of every messiah. Today everyone must be the messiah, and the love must rise in every heart. This rising in the heart is the flight of the Phoenix towards the sun.

THE GOOD LIFE

Not only love is necessary for our survival but also beauty. Beauty is normally thought of as a luxury to be enjoyed after the material necessities are taken care of. Yet beauty is as essential to our survival as our food, for all our earthly values are backwards and upside down from the values of that intelligence which evolves the universe and which sent to us the Sermon on the Mount and the teaching that we must learn to love even our enemies. Mankind's values are not yet the values of evolution. We think that survival of the fittest means the grossest material competition, but the truth is that survival does not favor food over beauty nor shelter over love. In Nature, usefulness and beauty go together and when we separate them, we distort reality. How does the butterfly find its mate and perpetuate the species? It seeks out color and beauty in the delicate pattern of the wing. And how do humans mate? We, too, seek out the beauty of form and the beauty of the soul and respond to the warmth of love in another.

Everything that we do is a seeking of love, though sometimes the love is distorted and twisted. When a power-hungry person goes into politics and begins to build an empire for himself, he is only seeking love. When a businessman amasses a fortune at anyone's expense, he is seeking love. But to really find what he seeks, he will have to discover his own heart in which there is flowing always enough love with no need to go and seek it, for it is his own. This is the love that can care when soldiers half way round the world have smashed their rifle butts in the face of someone like ourselves. This great love that reaches out and radiates out is expanded and refined so pure that there is a subtle blurring of the boundaries between self and other, and it sees in another person the beautiful patterning of being on which the Evolutionary Intelligence places its highest value. We must not always think that survival is crude and violent and material. Even at the dawn of time, the delicate moss and fern and the flowers with their tiny sexual organs and soft velvet petals survived. Creation *is* love. Evolution is not forever traveling toward complexity just for the sake of being more complex. Why does evolution create more complex and more specialized forms? Because only through that refined physical vehicle

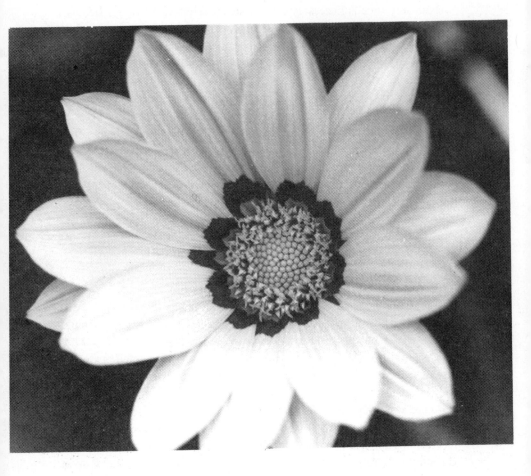

which survives as an organism can spirit discover itself in this material world. Only when the brain and nervous system, our material instrument of awareness, has reached its highest perfection, can the light of consciousness shine through it in such a way that it becomes totally aware, i.e., totally *itself.*

What has this to do with politics or with getting some food on the table and some fun in life? How can consciousness possibly be as important as the material things we lack or the power that we need or the recognition that we crave? "Let the hippies and scholars and fools go study consciousness! What we want is wealth and power and pleasure and the good life!"—so speaks the majority of mankind.

BUT IF THE UNIVERSE IS DESIGNED A CERTAIN WAY AND IF OUR VALUES ARE PLACED ONE HUNDRED EIGHTY DEGREES OPPOSITE TO THAT VAST DESIGN, THEN IT FOLLOWS THAT ALL OUR EFFORTS TO GET WHAT WE WANT ARE GOING TO BRING US PAIN AND WE WILL NEVER REALLY FIND THE THING WE ARE SEEKING.

A dictator or party secretary may get into bed at night, sweetly pleased that he has just sent more dissidents off to prison camp to work or die. It is in tune with his values and his goals and therefore he has done a good day's work. He is getting ahead in the party. Soon he will be at the top of the structure of power and then surely he thinks he will be the happiest of men. But deep within himself he is driven by a longing he cannot understand and he feels the anxiety of climbing that precarious ladder to power. He has to look out for himself, lest someone betray him and they send *him* to a prison camp. And he knows that if it should happen, no one will care but himself. Scared little man, lying in the dark waiting for sleep to come, repeating to himself like a mantram, "Everything is going so well." But in his life, things go wrong and he cannot understand just why.

In the ancient spiritual document, the *Bhagavad Gita,* the avatar Krishna is symbolized as God incarnate who overthrows the usurper and dark forces. He is speaking to the hero Arjuna and to the Evil One (the selfish materialistic ego, who is personified as his brother). "I am going into meditation," Krishna said. "When I wake, I will grant the first wish to whomever I see first." After awhile, the Evil One made sure he came in and sat by Krishna's side as he meditated. Arjuna came later and in respect sat at Krishna's feet. When Krishna awoke, his eyes fell upon Arjuna sitting humbly at his feet and he said, "Well, Arjuna, you have the first wish." The evil brother jumped up in anger. "I was here first," he cried. But Krishna replied, "I said the wish would go to whomever I first *saw*." The Evil One was much disturbed because there was a great battle soon to be fought on the field of Kurukshetra and he wanted to ask for the weapons which would guarantee his survival. Now Arjuna, his chosen enemy, would ask for them! Krishna turned to Arjuna and said, "You may choose my gifts or you may choose me, but you cannot have both." Arjuna hesitated for a moment, for he too was thinking of the expected battle and there were not half so many good fighting men in his army as in the army of the evil brother. But he looked at Krishna and his heart was moved by love radiating from his being and he said, "Your gifts would be meaningless without you, so I must choose you." Krishna smiled. The Evil One was exuberant and delighted and quickly asked for the material power with which to fight the battle, and his wish was granted. Then they proceeded to the battlefield of Kurukshetra where the small army of Arjuna lined up bravely against the vast array of power and the armies and weapons marshalled by the Evil One. Arjuna would have been afraid but it was good to feel, in the chariot by his side, the calm serenity of Krishna. And so the battle began. Arjuna held his bow ready and waited for the signal and when Krishna would point "There!" and "Just there!" "Here, behind you!" "Look!" "Over there.....shoot!" then Arjuna would let fly the arrow and watch it speed straight to its mark. The voice of Krishna as the ultimate Self flashing in his intuition, guided Arjuna and made his arrows truly find their way, while the material power of the Evil One, blind without the all-seeing eye to guide it, was soon defeated.

For each of us upon the battlefield of our life, is not the only armor the light of consciousness? Is not this the greatest protection—our own consciousness, the shining armor of our ultimate being into which, if we allow even the slightest darkness to penetrate, the seeds of disintegration are allowed? That is what the commandment really means when Christ says "Worship the Lord your God with all your mind and all your heart and all your being." It means put all your attention on Consciousness, because consciousness is God. They are the same thing; there is no difference. If there could be a difference, who would make it? Who is there to make any difference between ourself and God but consciousness? That's what makes all the differences. Human beings might be all the same consciousness but they're doing different things with their consciousness, so they all appear unique, but God might be saying, "Yes, you can do whatever you like with the consciousness that I give you. You can all be different, but I know that I am the same being in everyone; it's only what you do with me that makes me different."

If we ask ourselves, "What am I doing with my consciousness?" most of us will find that we are using it to cause pain to someone or to feel pain ourselves or to dwell upon some kind of negative emotion. This happens as much at the level of international politics as it does at the level of personal everyday life. We feel so empty that we have to invent all sorts of negative crises in order to feel something going on— Watergate political scandals, sex scandals, local gossip, and in our own minds perhaps self-pity or blame. We think that the feelings are caused by situations outside our consciousness and that someone is hurting us or that life has not played fairly with us, because we do not understand that

OUR CONSCIOUSNESS REALLY IS UNDER OUR CONTROL.

Even the threat of nuclear war can only affect you if you allow it. If you let it pass straight through you, just like a ray of light goes through a glass of water, would it have any power to disturb? If you can allow the thought to pass through you, then it doesn't cling to any part of you and it doesn't get invested with consciousness and it doesn't multiply and get very thick with negative energy. Your consciousness only reacts when you yourself put a seed thought in it and water it and nurture it just like you grow a seed in the ground. You can't get any more out of the ground than its potential. If you plant a cabbage seed, you can't get a carrot or a piece of corn. Everything multiplies after its own image. So if you are feeling some suffering, it means that you yourself (not anyone else nor any situation) have planted some negative thought seeds that flower with little petals of suffering on them. It doesn't matter how long ago. What matters is, why are you allowing them to flourish in your consciousness?

Whatever influences are coming to us from the galaxies or the stars, from cultural brainwash and childhood memories, or from the next-door neighbor or the guy driving his truck down the street, we have the power to take that stimulus and make it into anything we want to. That is enormous power that we have. Incredible power! We take the beautiful stuff of awareness that we have been given and wake up with every morning and we spend it on worthless activity. That's why we feel down and depressed, because we're not really spending it on what it was given to us for. If we took the consciousness that was given to us in this incarnation and used it for its real purpose, what would we be feeling? What is the true purpose of the consciousness we have? Why do we have it? What is it for?

The purpose of our evolution is just this: that we use the body given us by nature as a vehicle through which we can behold that underlying force which has brought us to this moment over aeons and aeons of time. This is our destiny—to find out what consciousness *is*! To refine our consciousness to the point where it can see its own glory. That is the purpose for which we manifest on this earth in this universe, to see the nature of the real stuff, the stuff of which we're made. If we can discover with our consciousness, even for one second, what consciousness is, won't we see the glory of the One who *is* that stuff, the One who sits at the heart, in the nuclear center of everything, experiencing itself as that?

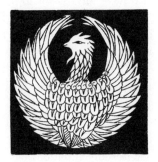

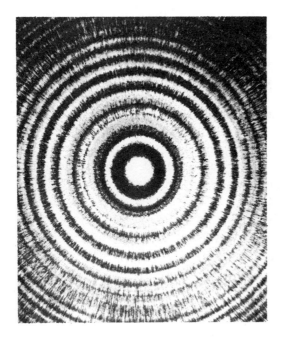

THE GIVER OR THE GIFTS?

How can we get to the state of mind of Arjuna and come to know, not just abstractly but as a deep conviction, that consciousness is the only thing worth discovering? It starts with an awareness that you can never be happy through chasing after compensations and that the only thing worth having is to know yourself because that is the only thing that will stop you from feeling pain. You have to come to the point of realizing that once you finally get all the things that you chase after, there is still an emptiness. When you have tried enough of these and discovered this truth for yourself and have felt the disappointment at the end of it all, then you can come back and ask in earnest how to discover the one thing that can give you such a continuous flow of blissful feeling inside that you don't need anything because you have everything. A feeling of life and joyfulness and love is always springing up and welling inside you, and because it is your own consciousness, there is nothing "external" to chase after. Whatever you are looking at, whatever you are seeing, is mirrored in your consciousness and you realize that there is no separation between the object you are experiencing and yourself.

Why listen to music? The music is going on inside you, cosmically, and all the atoms are vibrating their tones and noisy trucks join in, together with frogs and children shouting, dogs barking, refrigerators humming. You listen to the whole thing like a concerto. So you only go to play music when you lose that cosmic connection. In this state of consciousness, everything is upside down. Some people would rather eat food than do anything else in life. When you get in touch with your pure consciousness, so much is going on inside you that you just eat mechanically to keep your body alive. That is what Christ said when he was talking to the Samaritan woman by the well. His disciples came up and said, "It's time to eat, before the crowd gets here." And he said, "I'm not hungry." They said, "What happened? Did somebody come and give you food?" And Christ replied, "I have food to eat that you know not of, and I have water to drink that once you have drunk of that water you are never thirsty." He didn't feel like eating. He was with the spirit. When you get in the spirit you can go for days without eating. When you do eat you enjoy it, of course, like anything else. You enjoy everything. So this state of consciousness is not something negative nor is any of life's pleasure lost. It is only that none of the parts is that important to you, once you have tasted the whole. And when you have that attitude to eating, then suddenly, because of your vibration and your contact with everything, the best food somehow always appears. Whatever is right for you at that moment appears. And because of this, you don't have the constant craving to fill the empty hole up, which is really just a compensation for not having the glory of your own consciousness vibrating all the time inside you. When the whole universe is vibrating in there, you can identify with any part, or you can be the whole thing. You can be a hermit and stay totally alone, but there is a danger that you are just leaving the world to go to pot. If you've got a wonderful gift that is not being shared with others, you won't feel good with yourself. If your consciousness is really in that space, then you've got the secret of the universe in your hand and you'll feel you have to go and give it away. You will even work yourself to death trying to help other people to see the obvious, but they won't see it so easily. That golden stuff which is really you is the hardest thing to get people to really go after because they cannot trust the fact that when they have that, they won't need all the other stuff. They don't trust it. They don't trust themselves. If they could trust their own consciousness, they'd be able to trust the cosmos to give them everything that they need to be fulfilled or to be filled full. This is what the sages are saying in all their songs to God: "My cup runneth over." It is the experience of having so much consciousness that you don't know what to do with it. You've got so much to give that you don't need to take anything. It's an inexhaustible welling-up inside, like an ever-springing well, and this is why you are never thirsty. This joy is the attraction that will motivate people to seek out the giver of life's gifts. This is the reward. It is so great that if you can ever believe it, then the kingdom of heaven really is at hand. This is what Christ came to say, "It's within your grasp. You can take it if you want it." It's yours. You have it already vibrating inside you. All you have to do is to make it the most important thing in your life.

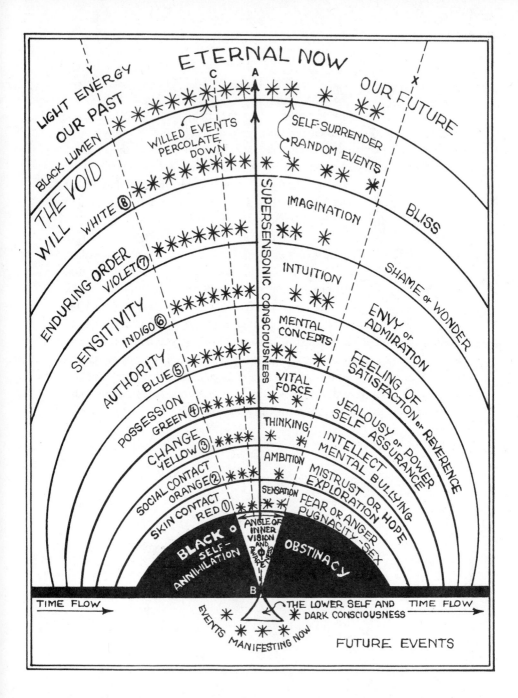

Our emotions and faculties are manifested by the absorption of light at different levels of being. The process is controlled by the chakras. If the angle of vision (ABC on the diagram) is narrow we can only pull a few events into our imagination. By the time they filter down into the lower levels towards the lower self at the sensory material level there will be fewer and fewer events to manifest. If we widen our angle of vision to XBY we see a lot more potential in the universe.

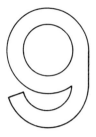

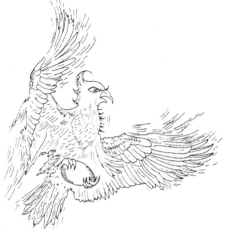

THE SEVEN LEVELS OF NUCLEAR EVOLUTION

The basic human drives which are the same in all people at all times in history and in all places, should make us feel like one united human race, but in fact they do just the opposite. The same drives, expressing through various kinds of human filters, are like light shining through colored panes of glass, producing red, orange, yellow, green, blue, indigo and violet. If we feel strongly identified with the green glass, we will see the yellow one as something totally different and foreign to us and even threatening; yet we are the same light of the spectrum expressing differently. When human nature polarizes into parties, groups or systems in irreconcilable conflict—one group ready to exterminate the other group—to say that the same basic nature drives them both seems naive. We do not consciously experience these drives, so they are just another idea in our large repertoire of sophisticated and complex ideas and, by comparison, the idea of seven levels of consciousness may seem crude and rather simple. Not until we become more aware by direct experience of these seven drives in ourselves and the inner conflicts they produce can we begin to see that the political conflicts in the world "out there" spring from the same root as our own inner dialectic. The reconciliation of communism and capitalism is not just an ideal or a concept or a theory. It is the natural resolution of that same tension which any of us can experience in our own psyche when our energies pull us in two different directions both at the same time: toward loyalty or self-interest; toward integrity or security— "Shall I tell my boss what I really think and make myself feel good with myself? Or shall I play it smart and keep my job?"

The easiest drive to get in touch with is the longing for security— for money, fame, knowledge, respect, social position, love, a home, a predictable future—which originates in your heart. If you are threatened in the crucial area of your emotional security, you will feel the pain of fear and panic in your chest, where the psychic center of energy called "the heart" is churning with emotion. In the heart center lies the key to life, for there you will either be driven by insecurities to achieve all sorts of personal goals or you will transcend the drives of your personal life and enter the kingdom of ultimate security where you are one with the whole and you know without a doubt that the abundance of the universe is yours and that you will never lack for love, for material things or for anything that you truly need. You can tune into yourself and get in touch with this heart center and its very real feeling of security or insecurity. But unfortunately it is not so simple as it sounds because humans feel fearful and insecure on several different levels of functioning.

There are seven of these psychic centers within all of us, seven levels of consciousness upon which we function in entirely different ways. Stated abstractly, they sound like a typology superimposed upon reality by the intellect. But in fact they have been scientifically researched and validated. And in addition, they are worlds we can enter by direct experience and perceive their reality for ourselves. Each dimension of our consciousness that we open and develop brings us into resonance with a new frequency of color vibration. In *Nuclear Evolution: Discovery of the Rainbow Body*, you can find an in-depth

RED	the sensation type
ORANGE	the social type
YELLOW	the intellectual type
GREEN	the self-assertive type
BLUE	the satisfaction type
INDIGO	the intuitive type
VIOLET	the imaginative type

These channels of consciousness each have positive and negative expressions which blend and overlap in all people, so that no human being is *merely* a type. And yet we behave in typical ways according to our predominant energy, especially in our conflict.

discussion of these seven levels of consciousness created by the way we process light and turn it into conscious expression. In one expression for example, this light of consciousness is blue and the color blue can be seen in the aura of a person whose awareness is filtered through the conceptual framework of the "satisfaction" type. This person will resonate with the color blue in his clothing, home furnishings, car, and general environment. Thus color becomes a key to psychology, and the Nuclear Evolution typology is scientifically verifiable by objective tests with light and color. It is no coincidence that the communist revolutionaries were called "Reds" and resonated with that color, since their entire focus was on aggressive physical action and reaction, a dominant characteristic of the red level of consciousness.

On the following pages is a thumbnail sketch of the seven fundamental ways in which our consciousness may respond to life. See if you can recognize your own basic drive dominating your responses.

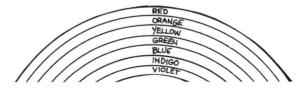

THE SEVEN LEVELS OF NUCLEAR EVOLUTION

DRIVE (1)   *Sensation type:* Orientated to transient external stimuli, the impulsive
RED   manipulation of objects affecting touch and experience in the
                   immediate now, without much awareness of past or future events. His
                   concrete reality is not related to flow of *time* which is always *now.*
                   Relates all sensations to self-pleasure or self-pain and is unaware of
                   inner worlds of others unless they are useful for purposes of self-
                   esteem. The color red brings on reactiveness and physical excitement,
                   related to anger, pugnacity, aggressiveness, sensation, intensity,
                   physical bully.

Example: The "sensation" type is one who is very quick to react to the words and
                   actions of others. This person may get angry at someone talking
                   strongly to another or get hot under the collar when he or she feels
                   misunderstood. The urge is to respond physically. Reactivity causes a
                   listening problem when communicating with others in a group setting.

DRIVE (2)   *Social type:* A sensation type who is orientated to the future and
ORANGE   contact with the community. Hopeful and optimistic at finding his real
                   place in society, living intensely and meaningfully in the concrete
                   world. Expansive and always seeking wider fields of experience.
                   Experiences *time* as sensation in the present but applies it to the
                   future instead of the immediate now. The color orange relates well to
                   herd instinct, ambition, agitation, restlessness, exploration and
                   busyness. Movement of sexual energies towards thinking processes
                   causes interest in politics and pride.

Example: If you see someone who is always concerned with what others think
                   about what he/she says and does and is easily swayed by others'
                   opinions you can recognize the social drive. This person often
                   changes his behavior to gain social influence or to curry and give favors.
                   May be positively interested in social welfare of others.

DRIVE (3)   *Intellectual thinking type:* This type analyzes everything and must
YELLOW   know what and where. Uses intellect to cut up events into true or false,
                   past or future and remains detached from the immediate now. Must
                   know logical framework before capable of understanding anything yet
                   seeks originality and change. Accepts conclusions based on theoretical

content and temporary proofs in order to justify putting "content" into an ideal or hypothetical *form*. Often feels emptiness and coldness in relationships and develops zealousness to compensate. Experiences *time* as continuous flow of process. Insists on details and logical supremacy in all matters, is self-assertive and relates to intellectual thinking, drive towards change, love of novelty and mental excitement.

Example: A person with this drive dominant may be found planning out every detail of every proposal. At least he will question everything and bring in all sorts of options and alternatives in his mind. Although he likes to figure things out his answers may hit on the right solution or may lead the group around the mulberry bush. People on this level usually speak from the head and rationalize a lot.

DRIVE (4) GREEN *Self-assertive type:* The desire for power to survive and store up energy and "vital force" causes individuals to expand energies to get them. The need for emotional and spiritual security leads to feelings of lack. Such individuals seek the effectiveness and power to assert themselves in the community. Jealousy caused by loss of control over the love object needs to be dealt with when arising from the possessive instincts. This type relates to self-centered love fixations, love/hate emotions, power and feelings of absorption and retention. Self-assurance and confidence may camouflage unacknowledged self-doubts. Experiences *time* as past, present or future depending on each situation and its threat to security.

Example: This security-minded person may be one who handles the money in the group or cares for the possessions. He may be jealous of others' abilities or possessive about someone or even possessive about his own ideas or insights. Job security is important.

DRIVE (5) BLUE *Feeling-satisfaction type:* This type lives in a mental world of his own commitment to idealistic feelings. He is hindsighted and historical, living in a present composed of memories of the past. Existing concepts, family values, recognized authorities and situations are all bound into his ideals and accepted images of reality. His feelings for family and community traditions and fixed sense experiences are imprisoned in an objective time so as to relax and feel satisfaction. He experiences *time* as binding all events into memories of emotional and mental concepts. Loves established ways, principles, ethics, morality.

Example: This drive manifests in the traditional and conservative people in the group who like to keep the peace and as a result resist innovative changes. Such a person tends to live in memories about the past and refer to past examples and authorities as ways the group should go.

DRIVE (6)   *Intuitive type:* Discontinuity with the past and present gives this type a
INDIGO   personality which is always living in the future. He appears to be impractical and divorced from concreteness because he does not identify reality with the senses, is continually impatient for the present to catch up with the future already perceived. Not punctual and difficult to tie down to details, fixed concepts, ideas or plans. Instinctive need for communication, sensitivity, telepathy, intuition, integration, etc. Places his faith in the future, in the not-yet-manifested; and experiences *time* as a telescoping of the future into the present, and the past as a dim mist.

Example: A person with this drive strong in their character may feel other members of the group are not sensitive or perceptive enough and will be impatient for them to see what he sees. Someone who is always envisioning the potential of the group but may be impractical or reluctant to work out the day to day affairs and concrete details to manifest it.

DRIVE (7)   *Imaginative type:* This type seeks for an ideal state of harmony and
VIOLET   enchantment as seen in the drama or the stage and is therefore out to make a good impression and become popular as a result of his charm. Tenderness and consideration of others and himself are marked traits by which he skillfully makes himself indispensable in situations. Is basically concerned with time and its annihilation orientated to the healing power of poetry and literature and its transforming effects through highly original metaphors. Needs an archetypal image of the Cosmic Intelligence, otherwise conflict between "will" and the "imagination" develops. Tries to create a pattern of life and sets out an example of goodness. Experiences *time* in his imagination and is able to distort it in drama, art forms, poetry and imagery.

Example: A person functioning primarily with this drive will be an inspirer in the group. He will try to shape the group to the vision he sees and make it a manifestation of divine order, all things working together harmoniously like a cosmic dance. He may use charm in order to be admired.

BLACK

NUCLEAR

CENTER

OF BEING:

Absolute type: Cannot compromise with uncertainty and hazard in the universe without self-surrender to Cosmic Intelligence and entering an immortal state of being. The annihilation of the "real external world" occurs when the individual ego unites with the self-consciousness behind all of the manifested creation and notions of bodily objects. This type has a desire to bring order out of chaos by the "willing" of external events in *time*—the function of prayer. The drive of self-annihilation creates a stubbornness and desire for absolute freedom to be a law unto oneself. Self-mastery involves coping with this secret desire to play God at the heart of all being. Unyielding, certain, over-confident, hard of heart, spiritually ruthless, self-defeating and on rare occasions completely broken in "will" and lost in the dark night of the soul. Must surrender to ultimate self or becomes destructive instead of creative. Is often grateful for small recognitions and does not expect rewards. Will serve only what he feels is a universal or cosmic will. Messianic pretensions must be coped with for psychic health as they are driving forces in the secret desires of many more men than is believed.

Example:

Those in this domain of consciousness may try to rule and "play God" seeing themselves as destined to be an instrument of divine will, whereas others may see them struggling with the will of Nature and sucking in the group time and energies like a "black hole". They will put down the whole group to put themselves up rather than listen to feedback.

On the other hand, a pure person living from the nuclear center will be in tune and surrendered to the Divine Will and their manifestation will show that. Their aura color is white or gold-white—all colors of the rainbow working together in the One.

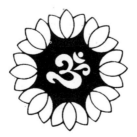

VALIDATION OF THE NUCLEAR EVOLUTION COLOR DRIVES

In 1968 a friend asked me to help to get 20 of the leading minds together and he would get a grant from the Canadian Broadcasting Corporation to invite them as guests to tape a seminar on the next step for mankind. I immediately invited several leading names in the then barely embryonic field of consciousness studies. My friend invited Humphrey Osmond, Prof. Tom Patterson, Moniem El-Meligi and several other typologists. At the end of this conference with its rather interesting mix of people, Humphry Osmond announced that he and another researcher had taken two subjects the previous night and put them in hypnotic trance to find out whether the inner-worlds of the subjects corresponded with their typological profiles. The two researchers had used every psychiatric method to get at a complete inventory of the drives, outlook and self-image of the two people. I made a bold statement that I could do exactly the same by using my aura pendulum and could tell them exactly how the two subjects would respond to life, what their fears were, how they looked at and experienced their time-worlds. Humphry looked at me with great disbelief but to his credit he told El-Meligi and others that if this were so, then all the years spent working out their advanced methods had been done in the dark because, as far as he knew and they knew, among men of science there was no one even remotely close to what they were doing; if I could do what I claimed it would be remarkable to be able to get the same results. He said that they were pretty confident that their methods of probing the unconscious world were deadly accurate; he would like to see what my specific results were. He then asked his colleagues not to tell me anything until he could fetch the two subjects whom they had tested out the night before.

Thereupon, in front of these skeptical psychiatrists, one by one, I read the seven levels of these two subjects, the various attitudes as seen from the subjects' points of view, how they related to time, their basic drives, how they reacted to different kinds of people, their attitudes towards authority, etc., etc. Gradually I watched the professors' mouths fall open as I repeated practically word for word, by reading the colors of the subjects' auras, what they had researched the previous night. The aura, or energy field surrounding the human body, radiates a distinct color and vibration which I could see and also detect with the pendulum. The professors found that I was even using words similar to theirs, like "sensation", "intuitive", "feeling" types. The correspondence of my twenty years' work alongside their own years of work was too close to be coincidence. The explanation could only be that we were indeed all seeing the same things in Nature confirmed in each other's methods.

This was a great moment for me because until then I had found no one to scientifically duplicate my work in color. Only clairvoyants and psychics had been known to penetrate in inner-worlds of men and most of the ones I had spoken to contradicted each other or were so loose in their concepts and language that their results were almost useless for erecting any meaningful typology. In fact many of them, although they could see the colors of the human aura, had not the slightest idea what the colors meant and, if they did guess, they were so often wrong. I had read books by so-called color experts and many of them were completely wrong if one tested their theories. Some were partially right but there was no real way of verifying when even two people got the same results. The number of psychics I could trust in those days was three or four out of hundreds I had met. They were Geraldine Cummins, Ena Twigg, Olga Worrell and Eileen Garrett (sometimes). Even some of these did not get their information from colors, so I was very surprised to have these results confirmed by non-psychic skeptical scientists.

The implications were enormous but few people realize what is involved. If we can truly map the inner-worlds of human beings accurately and provide objective proof that can be transmitted and taught to others, then we have literally solved the age-old problem of the confusion of tongues and man's ignorance of himself. Most people only know the thoughts that flit through their minds in the moment and have no idea of their own unconscious drives and motivations, and they are even less in touch with the motivations of others. Here was a way of knowing not only our aura levels on which we function but also a personality system that enabled us to see the world through the eyes of others. We could now map out the instinctual and the spiritual drives and determine man's place in the natural order. Up till now only astrology had attempted such a typology of the human personality. To be able to fingerprint the soul of man and to create a typology not based on theory but on empirical testing of behavior, meant that the results could be researched and confirmed by anyone else using the same system and methods I had used, namely psychological experiments and detecting with modern dowsing equipment as outlined in *Supersensonics**. Earlier I had come across the empirical system of Dr. Max Luscher of Switzerland, which had given me similar confirmation that our drives were reflected in color responses. Now here in the work of Humphrey Osmond and others was a totally different cross-check on the validity of the results. The method was ideal for probing the inner conflicts, anxieties and aggressiveness which led to hostility and thence to violence and war.

I have done much scientific research and have the papers of my experiments ready for someone who wishes to edit and deal with them, but to me the work of convincing skeptical minds is a waste of time. I am looking for open minds, ready to validate Nuclear Evolution not only in the laboratory but in their lives, and ready to finance it with their own beings. Therefore this is neither a scientific book nor a political book in the standard sense of the academic traditions, because we can talk on and on about scientific methodology or politics and world dilemmas and never get to the one thing the world needs to know—the way to understanding and peace.

HOW DO WE SOLVE OUR CONFLICTS AND BRING PEACE?

Whether a conflict arises between a man and his wife or an argument develops between academicians at the rational level, violent frustration of mis-communication has its origin in the gap between one level of consciousness and another. This unacknowledged gap, this unawareness of the fact that human beings live in different inner-worlds, causes most of the frustration in human interaction. No useful

---

* *Supersensonics: The spiritual physics of all vibrations from zero to infinity.* Published by University of the Trees Press, 1975.

peace research, however erudite, can be done until the primal drives of human beings are seen for what they are. Nor can these be elevated by education. Many educated people remain hostile within, though they may be sophisticated in expressing their aggression.

LEVELS OF CONSCIOUSNESS

The easiest hostility to perceive is the belligerence of *the sensation level of consciousness.* The lowest form of communication is a punch in the nose—the concrete physical manifestation of frustration in the immediate now. People on this first level of consciousness live in the world of physical sensation, so their time-world is always now. No matter whom they meet on the intellectual level, they will experience the same impatience and sense of frustration, as the intellectual begins to weave in and out of past, present and future in a vast web of words. Communication is blocked. Wordless anger builds. Then POW! comes the punch in the nose. Even if the punch does not come, it is inside, clenching the hands and pumping in the adrenals of a sensation-level consciousness. Such a person prefers to be direct or to take action, rather than to spend time talking, planning, considering options or negotiating. He cannot hear communication from another level, such as the intellectual, because he reacts, gets angry, and is too upset to listen for the real meaning behind the words. The hijackers of planes, international terrorists, bombers of buildings, the Patty Hearst affair with the SLA kidnappers, are recent reminders of the physical level of aggression. Wherever there is a revolution by force and violence, this level of consciousness is at work. The hard-line communist drive to amass territory is a physical conquering of another country. The communists achieve their political ends by domination and manipulation of the concrete physical environment. The same level of consciousness is at work when dissidents are shipped off to Siberia to hard-labor camps. In South America, totalitarian juntas and dictatorships torture dissidents, using physical brutality to block opposition.

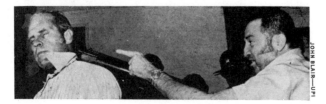

The social level of consciousness generates conflict through the manipulations of ambitious people eager for status, elbowing their way up the social ladder at anyone's expense. Due to their own extreme egocentricity, they assume the same in others and so are mistrustful and suspicious, often projecting their own faults out and seeing them in others, even when the other doesn't have that particular fault. When a society-oriented person talks with anyone whose values come from an inner center and therefore go beyond the codes and customs of society, he or she is likely to be first baffled, as if meeting a creature from another world, and then hostile in defense of his own world.

Ex-President Richard Nixon is a good example of the ambitious type. He spent years presenting himself to the American public, trying to convince people he was presidential material. Beaten in the presidential running, he tried again and kept on trying until he achieved his goal. Sheer ambition, perseverance, and even sentimental manipulations, like appearing on television with his dog, went to create the trustworthy image of a future president. With a plea of "trust me", Nixon rose and fell from political office several times before his last surge to the presidency and his fall to disgrace. Had the American public been able to see the underlying man beneath the Nixon image, Watergate would have come as no shock. Nixon's own deceptive social-political stance which swayed with the most favorable breeze was projected out as a

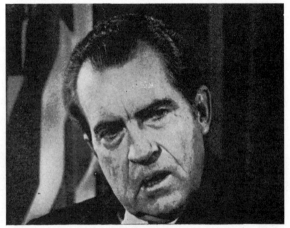

Richard Nixon

person who was mistrustful of others, because he himself could not be trusted. The Watergate case of his authorizing burglary of the opponent's headquarters is a perfect example of the mistrusting nature of the ambitious social-political man. Nixon is only one of many examples of the negative side of this level of consciousness in our society.

The thinking type will express his frustration in rational argument and debate, yet the feelings behind his arguments may be completely *ir*rational and he won't know it. The thinking type is usually fooled by his own civilized veneer. If he tries to argue with the reactive sensation type, the energy of anger which bursts out so suddenly in the conversation may completely throw the intellectual into confusion and you will see that the true state of his emotions is the opposite of the controlled style in which he began. The decision by the judiciary and the government to bus students to different schools to force a racial balance and to achieve the idea of integration expediently, shows a "planning" type of consciousness which achieves "on paper", so to speak, what is not accomplished in reality. This type believes in administering the higher principle of equal rights to all men through the intervention of a reasoned-out government plan, even though it means bussing children many miles away from their homes. At this level of consciousness, the

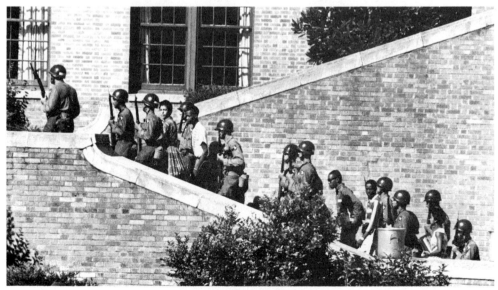

Little Rock, 1957

humans affected by the plan are less important than the order and symmetry of the plan itself. The planning of work and organization in logical structures is done by the intellectual type who relates to everyone through the head and is often cut off from the reality of other levels of expression.

The self-assertive type conflicts with others in a spirit of keen competition. It is his purpose to get all he can of whatever he values, and to get it before someone else gets it. He will settle a dispute by "deals" and compromises in which he still gets some if not all. If he meets a person who just gives of himself because he wants to and not with an eye to getting something back, i.e., a person to whom love is not a "deal", he cannot comprehend it. If he meets with a mystic, whose view is wholistic and not competitive, he may feel threatened and defensive. The mystic says, "Sell all that thou hast and give to the poor and follow me," and the rich young ruler goes sorrowfully away.

The balance of competing interests has been the ideal of capitalist nations for centuries. The US economy is run on contracts, ideas and competition. But the efficiency of the capitalist and democratic system as the freest and most successful form of governing in the world, is due to the positive control of this self-assertive level of consciousness.

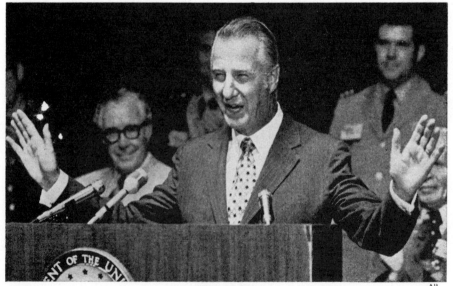

Spiro Agnew   AP

When the self-assertive drive becomes greed, and when behind-the-scenes smart illegal deals begin to seem to be a built-in part of the system, we need the firm control of anti-trust regulation. Daily we hear of company executives being bribed and government officials squandering money. From the national level of former Vice President Spiro Agnew and Director of the National Budget Bert Lance to the local level of county officers, reports stream in, to the point where we take irregularities for granted. We can almost any day expect someone in power to be exposed for fraud or misrepresentation as we the people sit passively by and watch. As a nation we are at the mercy of the huge Arab and American oil companies who ruthlessly press their advantage in having a monopoly on the oil market which no international law can legislate. To the exploiters and manipulators their own actions seem normal and natural. To those in other levels of awareness they are horrifying and totally selfish.

The satisfaction type is peaceful by nature but can be so much inclined to harmony that he practices "peace at any price". His essence is like the mother bird who defends her nest. This fanatical dedication can lead to the ultra-conservative type of solution to human problems. This level of consciousness is the world of the idealist and the ivory tower theorist. The satisfaction type buys peace by nonviolent withdrawal, which may eventually bring violence from others upon himself, or he creates peace for himself by violence to others: "Let's make the world safe for democracy"; "A war to end all wars".

An example of this drive is the picture of Neville Chamberlain arriving back from Munich with his falsely-claimed appeasement of Hitler. The picture appeared in all the British newspapers with the headlines "Peace in Our Time", showing Chamberlain flourishing a worthless piece of paper on which the treaty to avoid World War II was written. Only a few months later, World War II began with Hitler's invasion of Poland, ignoring England's guarantee to Poland that Germany would not invade. For this level of consciousness, peace is such a beautiful ideal that it is hard for a satisfaction type to imagine the inner-world of a Hitler who is bent on aggression and who has no

intention of following the peaceful orderly rules on any piece of paper.
Chamberlain bought Hitler's assurances in order to satisfy his drive for
"peace at any price"—even the price of collusion with the devil.

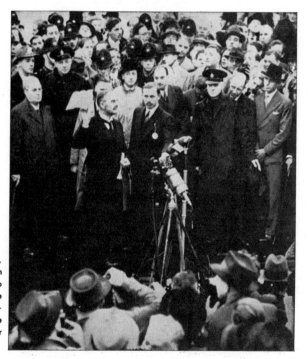

"Peace in Our Time," On September 30, 1938,
Prime Minister Chamberlain returned to London
from his conference with Hitler at Munich. To
the crowd which had gathered to meet him he
waved a copy of the Munich Agreement, pro-
claiming it a pledge of "peace in our time." The
event was the supreme irony of the prewar
years.

The intuitive type is always living in the future and is never really
with us unless he uses intuition together with the other more practical
levels of consciousness. Because he sees the potential of a situation, he
usually creates a state of conflict by copping out on his responsibility
in the present. He tunes out on the problem and lets it fester and then
is indignant when it explodes. But in its positive expression the
intuitive has the makings of a true leader of the people, in tune with the
whole. In 1962 President Kennedy took a decision to intercept Russian
naval vessels bound for Cuba with long-range ballistic missiles which
could be trained on America from a hostile Cuban base a few miles off
the US coastline. He told the Russians to turn back their ships or there

would be war. An ultimatum was given which could and would be carried out. What would have happened if Kennedy had not stood firm on his intuition that the Russians would not risk war nor risk their ships on the way to Cuba? Had an appeaser from the satisfaction level of

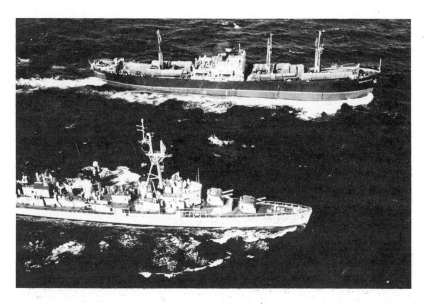

The President ordered the US Navy to intercept the missiles en route to Cuba. The missiles went back to Russia.

consciousness been president, a mighty missile base would have developed in Cuba and Russia would have formed a picture of a weak opponent who could not act decisively.

The imaginative level of consciousness lives by private images of how things are and does not often take a close look at reality. When someone forces him to look, he withdraws into his self-created reality and shuts out the crude insensitive one who talks facts. Both the intuitive and the imaginative levels, however, are visionary. They may glimpse a vision of the future and give it form, yet people on other levels of consciousness who have no vision will not listen. Then these more sensitive persons become like the Greek prophetess Cassandra whose misfortune it was to see disaster approaching yet be unable to convince anyone until it was too late. A conflict between an intellectual, whose mind is rigid with the step-by-step logic of reason, and an intuitive or imaginative person, whose mind is open and can leap across logical steps to a direct perception of truth, is almost impossible to resolve without some awareness that these levels of consciousness are entirely different worlds of perception.

Behind the civil war in Northern Ireland, alternately smoldering and flaring since the 1960s, glows the imaginative vision of a United Ireland. Even though the majority of Irish people have no intention of uniting, the visionaries still project the image of a peace and unity which can never come until the reality of the actual situation is squarely faced. For the Catholic minority, unity means a return of Northern Ireland to the south, which would force the Protestant majority to become part of Catholic Ireland. For the Protestants this is a solution to be opposed to the bitter end. Only the presence of the British troops prevents a complete bloodbath and the creation of thousands of refugees. The British troops, summoned by the northerners, prevent the Catholics from forcing the union, while the IRA, a terrorist group with many sympathizers, foments dissatisfaction (possibly with foreign instigators) and embarrasses the British government.

Although a referendum has been held which resulted in a decision to keep the British troops, the IRA, in their imagination, believe that there has been some advance through their bombs and violence. They receive their main support from romantic Irish-Americans who send guns and money to carry out a war in their imaginations in the streets of Belfast. If their money was going to buy guns to kill their own children and if the blood of fellow citizens were to flow in their own local towns in America, they would never dream of supplying these weapons.

Can you see yourself in any of these seven portraits? If you can, then you can also see how these same thresholds of awareness act as filters for the perceptions of our leaders as well as ourselves. If the doors of perception were cleansed, we would see that we were all one interconnected whole and we could no longer battle ego against ego and nation against nation as we do now. But when we are stuck in one

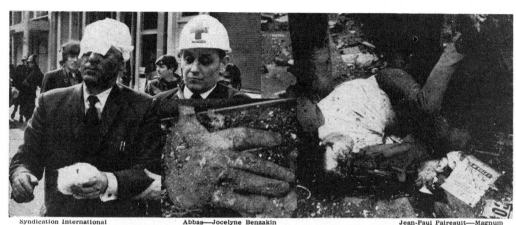

Syndication International   Abbas—Jocelyne Benzakin   Jean-Paul Paireault—Magnum
IRA atrocities: the walking wounded, a victim's severed hand and a garbage man's broken body.

level of awareness and see the world only from that angle of vision, then our character is as limited as our seeing. The seven levels of awareness which I have outlined here are, in every person, blended into a unique personality which transcends typology. Yet the limits we put on our consciousness are real and they give us the limiting traits of a type, however much we like to think we are beyond it. You can see the same limits coloring the whole panorama of political life in the world's groups, because groups respond to life in the same typical ways that problems are solved by the individuals who comprise the group. What *would* happen if the doors of perception were cleansed? What vision would you see?

YOUR RAINBOW BODY

If human eyes were sensitive to light with a frequency tens of thousands of times faster than that of the color blue then we would easily see that the whole sky glows with radiance. Cosmic rays with wavelengths much smaller than our eyes can see are constantly showered upon us from all directions in space. This diffuse rain of gamma rays cannot be sensed by the optical windows in our skins, but this does not mean that our skin and nerves do not sense them, absorb them and process their energy as radiation. Discovering their source is a mystery to present-day astrophysicists. Some scientists theorize that the omnipresent radiation is an archaeological cosmic artifact left over from the Big-Bang which began the expansion of the present universe, and others speculate that it is the total sum of all the rays of cosmic energy being sent throughout space from all galaxies and supernovas and distributed throughout the universe. All kinds of arguments and formulas and astrophysical observations are being advanced at this time to make one theory more plausible than the other, but the scientific community has not yet widely accepted any one explanation.

In 1968, I advanced my own theory of Nuclear Evolution* which said that this background radiation of the universe was the total sum of all the radiating stars bouncing this light off each other and exciting the atomic configurations and groups of material particles by absorbing and re-radiating the radiance like a phosphorescent substance. These high energy cosmic rays with energies up to ten million electron volts are continually bombarding our bodies and everything else in the universe, but we cannot feel their effects or sense their high energy light scattering off electrons because our sense of sight, touch, etc., does not function in this part of the total spectrum. Nevertheless, this does not mean that we are incapable of experiencing this optically-transcendent radiance of light, and my theory predicted that scientific observation would prove in years to come that this light was in fact identical to what we call consciousness. In other words, our senses could not experience this light, but our consciousness *is* that experience, with our body acting as the transducer of the light. It steps it down into what we call human intelligence or the spectrum of mind-stuff.

This theory also postulates that the intelligent behavior of atoms, cells, DNA molecules and organs which make up our whole bodies comprise a holographic grouping which mimics the nucleus of the entire universe on a smaller scale and contains within it the same power and consciousness of the *One* power of radiance which exploded in the first place. This original expansion is still happening but on a time-scale vastly different from that of our senses, so that our sensory

---

* *Nuclear Evolution: Discovery of the Rainbow Body* was recently republished in a second edition with the addition of new material in a now 1,024 page book published by University of the Trees Press, 1977.

experience is much too slow to witness the fullness of this total show of all the brilliant suns of creation on every wavelength and at every frequency. Yet at other levels of experience and in other time-worlds the human consciousness can stand witness to the glory and radiance of consciousness itself, modified as it is through different spectrum levels of our human vehicle of perception. Throughout the ten years since the theory of Nuclear Evolution was first published I have never read anything in any scientific journal or heard of any scientific observation which contradicted this theory that our consciousness is not only the product of the superconscious perception of the light of the universe, but also that this consciousness is the cause of this universe-wide light resting at the heart of every nucleus on every threshold of organic and inorganic experience throughout the Cosmos.

This obvious fact which enables our own consciousness to look through space and soar between the stars of the universe, looking through the biological telescope of the human eye, is the same light referred to in mystical terms in the Bible as cosmic sound and in other writings as **AUM**.

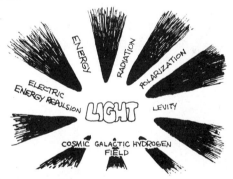

In the beginning was the word
And the word was with God
and this word was God.
The same word was in the
beginning with God.

In him was life and that life
was the light of men.

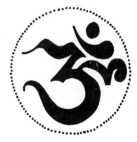

> And the light shineth in
> the darkness and the darkness
> comprehended it not.

It is obvious that no light can shine in the darkness but the light of consciousness. Only this light within the nucleus of our being cannot be quenched by darkness.

For ten years I have lectured, written and sold over 18,000 copies of *Nuclear Evolution* and I am still like a voice crying in the wilderness of man's gross sensual perceptions. The light of consciousness is God and is the light of the Universe and is ONE. What I am trying to say is that in consciousness in its pure state, there is no other and all things are made from this ONE consciousness and without this ONE nothing can be made. There is no difference between the ONE and our personal consciousness in its pure state. The ONE who makes this statement through all the mental images of my consciousness is not my personal self but the universal radiance shining in the darkness of our human minds. "I" which speaks and writes is the same "I" in the reader which persists through time from the beginning. There is no difference except in our consciousness if it be impure. When consciousness is purified of all its concepts about itself then that ONE shines through and we see clearly with the Supersense that the sound of the universe is always singing God's name through every atom and every star and through every being. This celestial song expressing on seven levels of consciousness as a spectrum of invisible radiation, is so obvious that we cannot see it. Our consciousness at the nuclear center cannot be realized easily because purification of our gross sensory experience is not easy, but we have all had the experience of it in being born. Before we acquired concepts of ourself, before the Ego rose to claim the throne of reality and separate us from that light and took us into the darkness of the sensory worlds, we have all stood with that ONE and seen its glory.

> There was a time when meadow, grove and stream,
> The earth, and every common sight
> To me did seem
> Apparelled in celestial light. . .

Our birth is but a sleep and a forgetting:
The Soul that rises with us, our life's Star,
Hath had elsewhere its setting,
And cometh from afar:
Not in entire forgetfulness,
And not in utter nakedness,
But trailing clouds of glory do we come
From God, who is our home:
Heaven lies about us in our infancy!
Shades of the prison-house begin to close
Upon the growing Boy,
But he beholds the light, and whence it flows,
He sees it in his joy;
The Youth, who daily farther from the east
Must travel, still is Nature's Priest,
And by the vision splendid
Is on his way attended;
At length the Man perceives it die away,
And fade into the light of common day.

William Wordsworth

If this impassioned plea for Nuclear Evolution should sound impatient or like making a claim for a new theory, it is only because I have been crying in the wilderness and my human patience is imperfect. Yet I know that in God's good time all will be confirmed. All that I have written from that space in consciousness must eventually be known by all men and women on earth because it is none other than the very content and structure of their divine self. Thus my theory that consciousness and the universe-wide radiance of the Cosmos are ONE, will become the basis of all I say in this book because in that ONE is the fire which consumes the Phoenix and gives it birth.

It was this fire of the primordial consciousness which Christ knew when he said,

"I SHALL RISE AGAIN"

PART TWO

VEHICLE OF TRANSFORMATION: THE HUMAN BRAIN

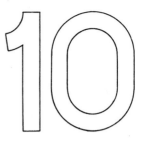

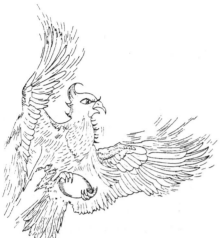

LABORATORY FOR DEMOCRACY

The real laboratory for democracy is not at any think-tank, nor at the political caucus where the razzle dazzle circus of electioneering takes place, but inside the human brain. The structure of our human consciousness will determine the ultimate structure of our evolved world society. Yet our consciousness evolves very slowly because a built-in part of our nature is that we perceive and experience life with only as much of our brain as is functioning. How can we be aware that there is *more* to be aware of if the very instrument of our awareness must view its own workings through its own limited ideas? Of all these ideas which filter and shape our reality, by far the most limiting is the notion that we are not really responsible for what happens in our consciousness—whether we are negative, angry, optimistic, irritable, happy or sad. We have a very passive attitude toward our own brain, as though its workings were pretty much automatic and out of our control. Yet to think of our brain as something acted upon and formed by the primitive social organizations of mankind instead of our brain evolution acting upon our society is to completely misunderstand the reason for our present world chaos. Because mankind has not fully learned to use all the parts of his most awesome equipment found in the higher functions of the brain, we are still bumbling along with political systems which don't enable us to understand anything but the lowest types of sociological organizations which are largely built for the restrictive limiting of selfish power rather than designed to amplify the creative supersensory power residing at the core of every person's being. What kind of world might we create if even a very few people were prepared to lift their consciousness to a new threshold of awareness?

In *Nuclear Evolution: Discovery of the Rainbow Body,* I have set forth seven levels of human consciousness corresponding to the seven frequencies of vibration in the rainbow's spectrum. Most of the human race is content to function on only three of these frequencies. *The Rise of the Phoenix* explores the social dimension of Nuclear Evolution and the way in which these very real levels of our evolving instrument of consciousness show us our destiny not only as individual souls or as nations but as an entire planetary race of humankind. The evolution of society is only a mass outgrowth of our individual levels of evolution and can go no higher than we ourselves can go. Thus the future of the world hangs upon this moment in time and depends on whether or not we now begin to move into the higher functions of our brains to create evolved social structures from those higher levels. Study of the brain reveals to us that we are not just our feelings, our intellects, our senses or our concepts and that the ancient Sanskrit texts perhaps were right in suggesting that our real destiny lies in the domains called "spirit". What is the spirit? To some it is a familiar mental concept from religious upbringing. To others it is a synonym for emotional sweetness and pious sentimentality. Is "spirit" the same as "mind"? Or is it some strange new world within our own brain that waits like a sleeping giant for us to discover it? Is the human brain a predictable computer? Or is it, as the scriptures say, a temple for that which is totally *un*predictable and awesome?

THE HUMAN BRAIN AS A MINI COMPUTER

The development of artificial intelligence stored in modern computers seems like intelligent behavior. All that has been stored has originated within human brains, yet these sophisticated computer programs have not been modeled on actual brain mechanisms. The mapping of brain functions has only recently been established, and even that new knowledge of the brain has been misleading and at best highly speculative. Many surgical operations on the human brain have failed simply because the brain was regarded merely as a mechanistic electrical circuit which could be chopped out here or there to correct human behavior. The wiring of the brain may be mapped out and we may now understand how its computers function, but none of this will tell us how our images of personal limitations in human consciousness are limiting our own brains at every moment and dictating the limits of our experience. If we personally believe that brain cells, or our senses which feed them with signals, cannot experience certain sensations, then we will automatically limit the functions of our higher brain centers accordingly. In the same way our imaginations will restrict our attempts to reform and remodel society because we limit the potential of the humans who make up that society.

HUMAN SOCIETY AS A MACRO COMPUTER

If every person is a single cell in a worldwide brain in which the whole of life is reflected as a hologram*, then the brain itself is a pattern of crystallized evolutionary intelligence which is gradually building social systems over vast periods of time. The human brain has taken about 5,000 million years to develop on the 10,000 million year

---

* A hologram is a photographic method of recreating a three-dimensional image in space using the principle of interfering waves of light. Every part of a hologram negative is like a photograph made up of thousands of mini-photographs, each one containing a picture of the whole image. If we cut the corner off the negative and pass light through it, the whole image is recreated but smaller. A single cell of the brain is like a hologram because it has a residual memory of everything which has ever happened to every other cell in the whole body, even though that memory may be held in the form of a loosely shifting dream or a warm fuzzy feeling.

old planet through all the combinations and recombinations of life, first as primitive algae and amoeba, then through fish and reptile to mammal. As the reptile crept out on land from the water it grew hands and feet and moved laterally from side to side rather than swimming with its single tail. This left to right movement developed the left and right brain hemisphere along with the left and right limbs. The fish has a partially split single brain because of its side to side motion, whereas amphibians with legs and arms develop two separate hemispheres.

The behavior of all organisms and especially the social organization of the different species of vertebrates corresponds to a progressive increase in the development of the cerebral hemispheres and cerebellum. When the lizard crawled out of the primeval slime and became a land animal exclusively, its functional brain became adapted to the wider environment. Man exists in the amniotic fluids before birth and comes, like his amphibian forebears, out of the oceanic state of consciousness at birth into the full expression of his right and left brain hemispheres as he begins to crawl and walk the land. A baby which is not allowed to crawl, develops less distinctively the separation between left and right hemisphere functions. Highly civilized societies like ours, which work from linear tunnel vision specialization of each half of the brain, are at a disadvantage in the wilderness which requires instant three hundred and sixty degree awareness and intuition. Races which depend heavily on Nature and must survive in areas where one needs intuitive and equal use of both hemispheres at once, tend not to let their children crawl in the early months of development. Both American Indians and Eskimos, who prize this three hundred and sixty degree sensitivity to the wilderness and the total environment, carry the child on the back as a papoose in the first months. Crawling is encouraged in left brain societies like ours, where intuitive unconscious awareness is actually discouraged in favor of the specialized logical or artistic behavior. In great intuitives, when both scientist and artist are present in one brain, there is a noticeable unconsciousness of social conformity and a natural abhorrence of crowds, such as we find in Einstein's behavior. Because the genius is not conforming to the norm, he is free. He has three hundred and sixty degree consciousness and pulls things in from all around him, whereas ordinary people are like horses with

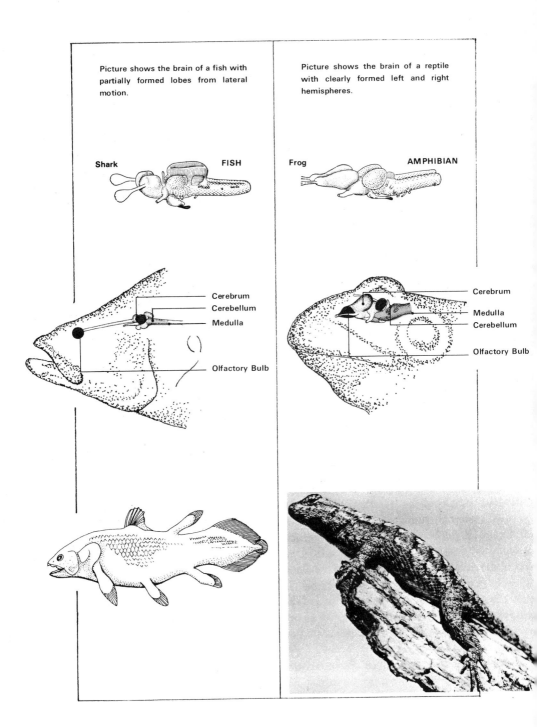

Picture shows the brain of a fish with partially formed lobes from lateral motion.

Picture shows the brain of a reptile with clearly formed left and right hemispheres.

Shark   **FISH**

Frog   **AMPHIBIAN**

Cerebrum
Cerebellum
Medulla

Olfactory Bulb

Cerebrum

Medulla
Cerebellum

Olfactory Bulb

blinkers on, who cannot see to right or left. Their consciousness is functioning with only one degree out of the three hundred and sixty and they perceive their world as if they were looking down a tube. Because the brain of the genius is balanced, it is like the undifferentiated brain of a primitive.

The native from the country visiting a big city is soon lost and to watch a primitive tribesman open doors, car handles and seek orientation from absent clues is to experience vicariously just how lopsided a right-handed civilization really is. All doors open right-handed, screws turn right-handed, traffic moves on the left or right side, not on both sides, etc. In the same way the city dweller who goes to the jungle or wild forest is lost with no sense of direction, no streets, roads or signs to guide his comparative ability to distinguish right from wrong, left from right, high from low, etc. People who stutter or stammer are often suffering from the twinning of two equal hemispheres in social situations where only one hemisphere or the other is expected to be dominant. Take them out into the wild forest and they are at home and do not stutter. Block off their right-hand functions or left-handedness in ears, eyes and hands by sewing up pockets, putting on eye patches, or exercising one side of their minds or bodies to make one side dominant, and the stuttering will stop.

The correlation between left brain society and right brain society has been set out by several authors.* The left hemisphere is predominant in analytical, logical thinking and verbal and mathematical functions; it processes information sequentially. The right hemisphere is involved in wholistic conceptualization (putting together, as against analysis, which is taking things apart) and its language ability for sequential sentences and actions is limited. The right hemisphere governing the left side of the body is responsible for artistic endeavor, skill in craftsmanship, imaging one's position in space, recognition of faces and wholistic patterns of intuition. However, what is not generally recognized is that all cells of the brain have a holographic memory of

---

* *The Psychology of Consciousness* by Robert Ornstein (Viking Press, 1972). "The Split Brain in Man" *Scientific American* (August 1967), pp. 24-29. "The Other Side of the Brain" by Joseph Bogen, *Bulletin of L.A. Neurological Societies* (July 1969).

every other cell and can therefore be trained by consciousness to undertake any other function imposed upon them by auto-suggestion, hypnosis, repetition or the programming of rote memory. We who live in a right-handed, left-brained society and think that this is reality, now are beginning to realize that there are large portions of our brain that we are not using. On top of that, we can see that this specialization of brain parts is in itself misleading and that, like the fish whose brain is undivided, we too can move and live without such separative specialized functions. Although these functions are fantastic creations of our evolution, we need to see that they are only a small part of our perceptual equipment. We can use not just our outer eyes but also develop our inner eye which sees intuitively with a faculty as old as the primeval lizard whose instantaneous reaction to stimuli (now a developed part of all evolving animal life, insect life and human life) came from that kind of brain which was once just a piece of sensitized skin on the top of the head. Gradually through evolution the reptile began to treasure this piece of skin and build protection for it and, at the end line of evolution of the reptilian brain, it actually went inside and became the pineal gland. Now we have that pineal gland in our own brain from those times when we saw with our brains and when our inner eye and the brain were one. Since then our

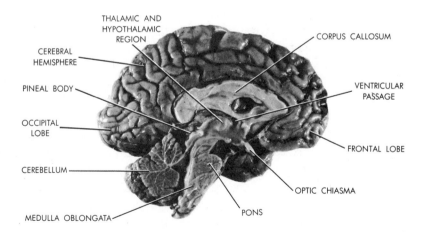

brain has become more specialized and the external eye has become more specialized to just the narrow band of visible light, but in those days it was sensitive to the full spectrum of light, of inner and outer cosmic radiation. In other words, the rods and cones of the human sense of sight have now been highly specialized and the piece of skin has become light sensitive in our eye as it is now, only responding to certain optical vibrations and frequencies of radiation. But any piece of skin or group of cells still has the capacity to be our vehicle of perception. Only our own limiting and our concepts and self-certainty prevent in us that marvelous kind of "seeing" which is done by detecting the oscillations of our whole vibrating consciousness and which is not limited even to the higher levels of "insight" that we humans have managed to reach.

The perceptions that are possible to us would sound like fairy tales to those who have not yet opened to the idea that potential use of our brains and senses is unlimited. Sensitivity to the supramental worlds is not something impossible but merely a faculty of organic life not yet manifested in everyone. To reach it requires some trust or faith or openness of mind so that our consciousness does not restrict its own operations. People tend not to want to know these vast potentials, even though it now is possible, because they fear to lose a grip on life as they know it, or life as they were brought up to live it. They do not mind developing psychic faculties, provided they can use them in the service of the social drives, to predict the future or to advance themselves to positions of power in society. But little do they realize that they can use the psychic vision to evolve a critical pathway into the heart of Nature and see the whole of life as it is now at this eternal moment. To lose the joys of the lower senses and leave the grosser levels of consciousness is difficult when all we have to go on is the mere promise of an *extra*sensory bliss a thousand times greater than sensory delight. To research those worlds not yet explored inside us is a little frightening to some people. We do not trust. And so the world continues to negate itself in the same way that it has always done. Because we cannot trust the new pathways, we get stuck on the evolutionary path and stay trapped in the same mental prison.

In the organization of the brain and its pathways to higher functions we get caught up and identified on different levels. These levels of consciousness, which are like invisible walls, constitute entirely different inner worlds in which we live. If mind and memory are programmed by social customs, we may identify with a whole network of highly civilized behavior patterns at the second threshold* of our awareness. But at the level of our lower sensory functions, which are governed by a different part of the brain, we remain pretty much the same as primitive people. Our angry reactiveness, for example, springs from the lowest portion of our brain (the first portion to evolve) and most people identify with this physical, material level of consciousness. Yet there are six more brain computers built upon the first.** It is good to be aware that this primitive part of the brain exists; otherwise we can never evolve this level of our being, and then the world can never improve because the people who live in it stay the same. In angry situations, in big crowds, in lunatic asylums, our social controls (which are programmed into the second brain) are sometimes removed. To watch alcoholics and drug takers whose civilized veneer is removed or is not functioning, reminds us that the angel in us is not far removed from the animal in us, and we can see the full import of our animal nature in our relationship to our fellowman. In all the terror and anguish of man's brief evolutionary period on this planet, brought about by his own bestiality and brutality foisted upon the weak, we are reminded of the purpose of this book in its dedication which I repeat for emphasis:

> The Phoenix rises out of the ashes of all those who have died in the name of human rights and particularly all those millions of unknown saints and martyrs who have suffered torture, pain, brutal imprisonment and who now lie quiet beneath the earth.

> Let them now rise with one voice and cry to the hearts of living men and women that they too may make the right of

---

* The second threshold is related to the second chakra center of the Hindu sages.
** The seven chakra functions are related to seven levels of consciousness in yoga.

self-determination and freedom of mind and body into a flaming torch of the human spirit.

This book is dedicated to those who will carry this torch of the spirit through the generations of a coming higher evolution. To them I give the name of genius. Whether president or peasant, whether mother or son, they are the real heroes of life.

Society is a hologram in which you, the part, are exactly the same as the whole. Therefore, no matter how much you abhor the world's atrocities, no matter how much you feel they are created by others who have not the same high ideals or sensitivities as yourself, the fact is that the world is one whole, a total fabric of weft and warp without separation, and you *are* that same world which seems so separate from you. This is hard to believe and hard to see, because we all feel that we cannot condone the terrible things that happen in the world. Many people go off to the woods to get in touch with Nature and return to simple values, but even these people have no idea what potentials lie inside them that have nothing to do with whether they live in Nature or do not. The seven-layered model of the brain is therefore to be viewed as a hologram in which society itself has emerged as a direct mirror-image, reflecting to us our own personal lack of ability to change it consciously over thousands of years.

Every would-be messiah must face this lack of power in all the world-changers throughout history and provide an answer to it. He or she becomes the anointed one, the Phoenix, only to the extent that peace is brought to the earth. There is no other criterion. Peace of mind or the peace that passes the understanding of mind begins with us. We cannot blame another for our own disturbance, even if we are being crucified. Disturbance of our own consciousness is the key to our evolution. The mirror of society does not only reflect the consciousness of Hitler and Stalin and Mao Tse Tung. It reflects *us*. We have to take it personally however disturbing. Otherwise we cannot undertake that tremendous messianic task which has never yet been fully understood by man, much less accomplished. Jesus Christ may save the world yet. But in naked fact it is not yet saved after two thousand years. Christians must look at this and not pretend an accomplishment which is not a fact. The Bible is a best seller, but the world situation gets worse. We must acknowledge that fact or perish in our own fanaticism. To Marxists, religion is useless except as an opiate for the masses. And it is this gap between the teachings of religion and the actual manifestation of its followers that gives the Marxists a good cause. If we are to succeed where religion up to now has failed, let us start with our own manifestation.

The evolutionary intelligence is now presenting a task to each one of us as his or her own personal work to do—the task of changing the quality of human life on this planet at its very source, in our own consciousness. The evolution of society goes hand in hand with the awakening of higher functions inside the human brain. The brain model for an individual is the same as the personality model of the seven levels of consciousness on which a new constitution for society must be based. Although we express on seven levels of awareness, the consciousness which comes through those seven very different levels of expression is one consciousness creating itself in different forms, just as the form of a flower is organized around one center and the growth rungs of a tree form around a center and a spiral shell grows outward from the center of a sea creature. All of Nature follows this principle. Only if a constitution arises organically from the center (its true source—the total consciousness of all the individuals in the group or society) will it be integral and strong and bring forth that flowering of culture that is its aim. In this sense, our own brain, our own consciousness, our own mental vibration is the laboratory for democracy.

We must have patience with our self and its instrument. To play such an instrument we must learn the discipline, like learning any other musical instrument. To expect a virtuoso performance on the piano or on a violin within a few weeks of beginning is as ridiculous as expecting a human being to be able to use the fantastic instrument of the brain the moment we first discover its potential for playing the cosmic music of the soul.

The model of the brain below shows the sequential order in which the brain evolved into a wholistic organ to allow for the more complex

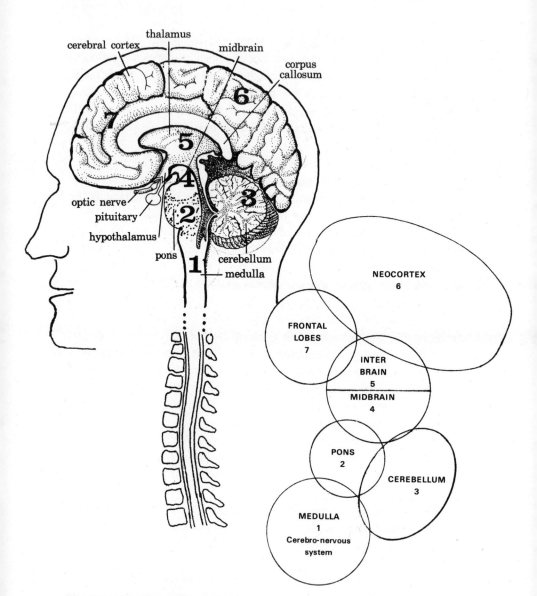

thalamus

cerebral cortex

midbrain

corpus callosum

7

6

5

4

optic nerve

pituitary

hypothalamus

2

3

pons

1

cerebellum

medulla

NEOCORTEX
6

FRONTAL
LOBES
7

INTER
BRAIN
5

MIDBRAIN
4

PONS
2

CEREBELLUM
3

MEDULLA
1
Cerebro-nervous
system

The octaves of the brain represent seven levels
which can be played like an instrument by an
eighth domain of cosmic consciousness. Some
players can only play and hear in one or two
octaves, others are virtuoso performers like
Christ, Buddha, etc. The brain is essentially
music; in lower expressions it is noise.

movements of the total organism as each evolving function became specialized. For instance, the occipital areas at the back of the head which focus the sight on colors and objects is a later addition than the inner sight, that inner eye which is linked with the peripheral vision and the mid-brain. We shall explain this later. Meantime we can see that the various levels of function correspond with the functions of different types of people in society.

1. sensation — workers/activists
2. social skills — coordinators/social workers
3. thinking — planners/intellectuals/teachers
4. security — administrators/bankers/managers
5. memory and mind — conceptualizing idealists/ philosophers/scientists
6. direct knowing — intuitive leaders/psychics/diviners
7. wholistic images — poets/visionaries/priests

These seven dimensions of consciousness, which evolved in man as the seven parts of his brain evolved, each resonate with a vibrational frequency of the color spectrum—red, orange, yellow, green, blue, indigo and violet. The scientific knowledge we know of the invisible universe and its structure comes from spectroscopy, from the interpretation of the spectrum color emitted from atoms absorbing and reflecting light energies. Leonardo da Vinci and Sir Isaac Newton, born two hundred years apart, each discovered the spectrum independently and both regarded this discovery as the most magical secret of all knowledge. In the fifteenth century when Leonardo was painting in the dull earth colors of the Renaissance painters, he was shocked to see the brilliance of the spectral colors as a beam of light came pouring through a prism. He wrote in his notebook in secret mirror writing that this was the signature of God. Why would he want to keep it secret? Because seeing the seven colors suddenly emerge out of one beam of light and display such iridescence far beyond his capacity as an artist to duplicate, filled him with reverence for that which was beyond the powers of any human being to create. He believed he had discovered the secret source of the universe hidden in the rays of light and he was not far wrong, since our own consciousness itself is comprised of the same light having the same seven colors within it and seven different vibrational frequencies which shape the quality of our awareness. This intuition by Leonardo was overwhelmingly impossible to communicate to another human being with the colors at his disposal and induced in him an intense feeling of humility. Nuclear Evolution is an in-depth study of just how the levels of structure in the brain relate to color and to the levels of human consciousness, how we shine the light of pure consciousness through the many-colored glass of the seven-layered brain and, according to the level of our evolution, "stain the white radiance of eternity" in beautiful or un-beautiful ways.

These seven levels of awareness are the functions which in earlier societies developed into distinct classes. Particularly in older civilizations over longer periods of history we can see the specialization in society, organized according to brain function and level of consciousness. In India, the caste system with its untouchables and menial laborers; Greek, Roman, Persian and Egyptian slaves; and more recently black slavery in America represented the lower classes of physical workers. The octaves move up through the levels of society to kings who in turn were influenced by dreamers (as Joseph influenced Pharaoh) and wise men who were employed as seers, sages and visionaries. Occasionally we would get a visionary, a teacher and a leader in the same person, e.g., Socrates, Pericles, Plato, Asoka, Ahknaton, etc., but on the whole, society was structured in and around these classes and patterns which corresponded to the levels of brain development with of course much overlapping whenever there were individuals whose input into the culture caused a corresponding rise of the whole. Like leaven, an important contribution of awareness causes the human spirit to rise throughout the whole. What Einstein did for electromagnetic man, Christ did for planetary consciousness, planting the seed of selflessness that would bring us to this present time when our next step is the "nuclear consciousness" not only of the planet but of the whole cosmos.

Christ spoke in simple parables of wheat and tares and mustard seeds, of sheep and vineyards and harvest. He wanted people to see the things of this world from a level of consciousness that was "not of this world". But now we have the capacity to understand more deeply what the "kingdom of heaven" that he spoke of really is. We know it is not only the concept of a kingdom of heaven upon earth but the union with heavens everywhere unlimited by space or time—the fulfillment to be found in the totality of the galaxies revolving in our consciousness in every cell of our brains. To experience this we must first understand that there are levels of consciousness related to brain function which must be integrated wholistically in order to conceive, perceive, see and know the beauty of the eternal hologram in the nuclear model of the whole. This ultimate organism on earth developed not by happenstance from amoeba to man, but by the unconscious pull of an evolutionary intelligence, guiding our development and building the human brain with far more usable equipment than can ever be dreamed of in man's imagination.

THE UNDISCOVERED COUNTRY

We know so little about even one function of the brain, such as memory, and yet memory is the basis of our whole sense of identity. To understand that the mind is the psychic reservoir of seven vehicles of consciousness that have emerged from the long chain of our passage through evolution is to understand the whole process of memory and thus to understand what we are and why we are here. Go to any philosopher and ask him what is memory and you've stumped him. There are no books written on what the memory is, except a few mechanistic scientific concepts which go up to the third brain. That is as far as science knows about—the three brains. The four on top of that, they have no experience of. If the scientist thinks the third brain is the limit and there is nothing beyond, then as far as his consciousness is concerned, there isn't any more brain because that is his concept and he is not able to experience any higher functions with the higher brain. So it is very difficult to go to any philosopher or to people who write books or teach in universities or even to gurus and say, "What is memory?" because they haven't researched it. They may have read some ancient Sanskrit script but it doesn't say there either, and if it doesn't say there, how do they know it? The only way anyone can know it is to get in touch with the source and find out directly from the source how it *made* that thing called mind and how it functions. What is the structure of it? What is the hierarchy of events that go on inside the mind? What is the function of memory? Why do we have it?

Obviously we wouldn't be able to evolve if we couldn't store our experience, our mistakes, our successes; they all have to be recorded. In India this storing is called "karma", or they use imaginative terms like the Akashic Record, but the Akashic Record is merely all our memories, the racial memory, the physical memory, the evolutionary memory working in us and recording all the things that we have done in our lives. And all this stuff is who we are. In order to understand who you are, you have to look first into the physical mirror-image of the cosmic forces—the brain. And this will lead you necessarily to the *meta*physical hidden energies of intelligence which have guided and developed it wholistically into one complete organism. At this juncture, between the physical and the metaphysical domains of consciousness the transforming insight into the evolution of the human nuclear being occurs.

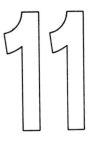

HOW I DISCOVERED THE NUCLEAR BRAIN MODEL OF EVOLUTION

It begins with the spectrum. I thought there must be a reason why Nature invented the octave. In every level of phenomena the octave and resonance are present, whether it is vibrating atoms, vibrating strings, vibrating molecules of air, vibrating electrical circuits or oscillating radio waves. The same principle that is inherent in waves of light which cause interference is always present everywhere. Much occult stuff has been written on color and energy that is obviously rubbish, since it cannot be related to anything verifiable in Nature, and yet behind many of the analogies of the ancient seers is the law of seven with its repeating eighth note making up the octave. Obviously humans have not grown up in an environment impregnated with octaves everywhere at every level of life without being affected themselves. For many years I puzzled how the human being and his perceptions of the environment around him were conditioned by matter vibrating inside the cells of the body and brain as well as in the atoms which make up the cells. I wondered how these parts of us reacted to vibrations of light and radiation which pour into the earth from every star in space. I meditated on this daily for many years, using the spectrum of the sun's light reflected through a prism as my object of meditation. While my other acquaintances in the spiritual life were using Buddhas, saints' pictures, crosses, altars, mandalas, relics, lights, and God-knows-what as objects of veneration, I was moved to use the rainbow colors as seen in the brilliant luminosity, unrepeatable by any human invention or design. Up to this day, in spite of all the psychedelic pigments now made and the art of printing in seven colors, I have yet to see anything that equals the luminosity of an actual spectrum divided into the rainbow by a natural crystal prism.

I knew intuitively that the colors I saw were not objectively seen on the white paper in which these seven vibrations of light shone. Somehow I knew the color was a resonance effect in my own consciousness and that the color was actually internal, put together inside my head from the vibrations of light entering my eye. I meditated many years on whether it was the eye that perceived or the brain cells in the occipitals which saw this luminosity. I researched everything that science had to offer on the question of wave motions, from atoms and quantum mechanics to color theories galore. I spoke to professors in art colleges all over the world and found they had no answers and didn't know what I was talking about, with the exception of one who had founded San Francisco's leading art school in 1926, the very year I was born, and who was eighty-six years old when I met him. It was 1968 when he read my first edition of *Nuclear Evolution* and decided he must come to London to see me, as apparently I had answered the same question which had gone on in his mind for years. He was a teacher of color theories to many professors of art and had been looking for the interconnectedness between color and human consciousness. Still, it was ten years after I had begun my initial research before he came with his confirmation. Most of my research on light and the brain was done with very little help, and indeed I did not know of anyone else doing anything quite like it. This insight that our consciousness was involved in the experience of light did not come suddenly blooming like a rose out of nowhere but came from countless observations of Nature over many years.

It is difficult even today to talk to people about this original insight as many do not know what I am getting at when I infer that light, i.e., vibrations of color, arises only in consciousness, and that consciousness *uses* the atoms, cells, pigments and molecules of our brain and nervous system to perceive the light. To me, color is a disturbance of consciousness rather than the absorption of certain specialized cells in the brain, which is how color researchers and current scientific explanation view it. I believe this current scientific theory is true at the physical level, but it *does not account for the act of seeing objects, anymore than it accounts for the perception of color.* As far as the perception of objects is concerned, I endeavored to explain and validate my theory of consciousness by using the scientific observations of Professor Vasco Ronchi, the inventor of the Ronchi interferometer and the director of the National Institute of Optics in Florence, Italy, whom I have corresponded with since 1962 on this problem.*

The fact that the whole universe interacts between all its parts and exchanges energy with its parts through the principle of resonant waves of vibration, became for me the uppermost thought in my consciousness, since man himself had evolved in this ocean of vibrations. I scoured every scientific discipline to make some sense out of man's physical vehicle, and only now do I see that there is the slightest glimmer of hope that science will apply its own method to the problem of perception itself, rather than looking for the answer in the material proteins and atoms of the body. Once I saw that not only our body and its atoms and cells but our minds as well obeyed the same fundamental law of resonance, I began to do psychological tests on people with colors and eventually with prismatic colors, created in my own laboratory by powerful lighting systems, to see if I could use these tests as a way of probing the unconscious mind to find if there were different thresholds of experience in humans which could account for the many different levels of consciousness in which people appear to think, experience and function. I researched the material currently available in psychology and found no answers. I read all the material put out by psychics on color and found it most unreliable, everyone claiming

---

* A full account of my ideas and Ronchi's ideas appears in *Supersensonics.*

different things depending on which teacher they had read first. Many of the psychics I personally spoke to did not even know the meaning of the colors they saw in the aura or psychic atmosphere, but I envied them their ability to see the vibrations of energies of color more subtle than I had meditated on with my prism for so many years.

WHY DO I ACCEPT AURAS?

I found that in talking to scientists they would feel disturbed by any mention of objects having unseen "auras" that extend into the space around them. They would feel very insecure that such things could not be measured by the instruments we have available and would utterly deny that any such possibility as an aura could exist. Yet it was all right to talk with them about the invisible magnetosphere around our planet or the Van Allen radiation belts which surround this planetary object in space. To suggest that every object in the universe radiated a subtle, invisible energy which could be measured by the Supersensonic instruments I had developed myself, was enough to bring instant and antagonistic ridicule as if such evidence were unscientific. My scientist friends had forgotten that even the telescope was unscientific in Galileo's time. Galileo was told by his peers that the lenses distorted reality and therefore could not be trusted, so they all rejected the telescope. In a way both Galileo and his contemporaries were right, for even a telescope does not see the stars as they really are. Even the sun only shows us six per-cent of its energy in the visible spectrum and the other ninety-four percent is its invisible aura. Objects seen with a telescope do not reveal the full amount of energy or vibration pouring into the earth from space either from our own or from other galaxies. Our eyes do not even reveal the amount of space present in our universe which is enormous and mind-boggling. Objects in space,

Radio emission coming from the halo of the great nebula in Andromeda galaxy 100,000 light years across, which is about the same size and shape as our own galaxy. The radio emis-sion is extended into space as an aura of invisi-ble signals. The galaxies are also about 100 million light years apart in space. This aura was detected around the celestial object and plotted at various points by John D. Kraus of Ohio State University, showing the intensity of the points of energy emitting at 1,415 megacycles. The visible galaxy is shown below with its invisible radio aura shown superimposed in the picture. This galaxy also generates ener-gies in other parts of the spectrum not measura-ble with the present scientific detectors, but easily measured by Supersensonic methods which can then be later verified by constructing equipment to test and validate the findings.

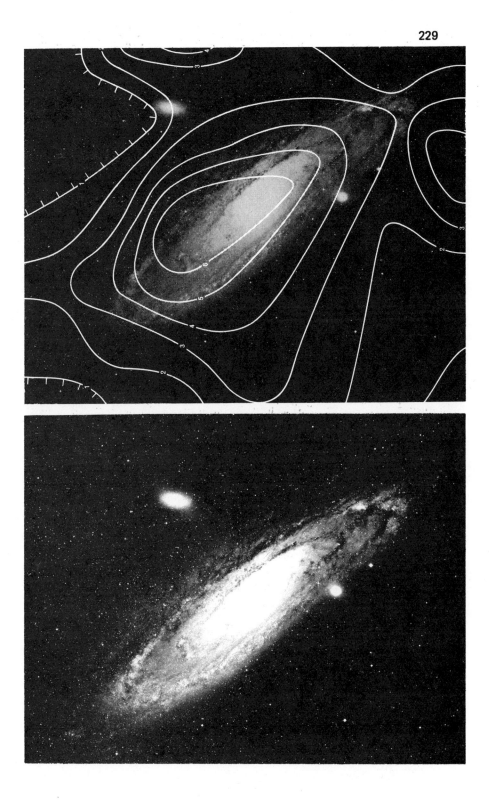

like the stars in our own galaxy, float together in groups and clusters, like the Andromeda nebula (M31), and these in turn belong to an enormous cluster of galaxies in the constellation Virgo. Even with the most powerful telescopes we cannot see their vast, invisible auras. In the top picture on the preceding page we can see the Andromeda galaxy, so similar in size and shape to our own galaxy, and our closest neighbor. The eye cannot see that this object in space has an aura. But radio emissions show that there is a great invisible aura around this entity we label the Andromeda nebula, suggesting the presence of a halo. Objects such as this galaxy are vibrating invisibly at certain frequencies and rotating in cycles at a specific frequency. Every object in space has such an aura and every human being, star or atomic nucleus has such an aura. Yet scientific thinkers who got all their knowledge of the universe from the spectrum and its vibrations in the atomic band of frequencies cannot see that this same spectrum is related to the universal resonances of all life including our own consciousness. Perhaps superintelligent genes have been spliced into the production of our brain enkephalins so that one day we shall see these hormones opening up our ability to think-in-light, to know that every object, large or small in space, is vibrating its own cosmic song, communicating its aura throughout the whole of space.

It was not until 1963 that I met a man named Fred Kimball, a very rough diamond without any education, who was introduced to me as a man who could read the mind of dogs and animals, and he informed me that I had the same ability as himself. At first I did not believe him, but he took me out in the street in the sun, stood in front of me and said, "Now project your consciousness into my aura and look around me," and lo and behold I saw very faint colors, swirling and radiating, like a very faint rainbow. This was my first introduction to seeing auras naturally, which had been blocked for so many years by my own skepticism. Once I saw that it was possible, I began to deepen the faculty and extend it from people to objects, plants, systems in Nature, until I saw directly for myself that every organism and system interacts with its environment through a rainbow of resonances. I could see different colors and shadings around different persons and objects.

It was at that time that I began to have insights thick and fast about my meditations on the rainbow colors. I began to see that certain objects were impervious to certain energies of different wavelengths, did not radiate in certain parts of the spectrum, and therefore had no aura color of that vibration. I also began to see that people were no different from objects, atoms, or plants in this respect, that they did not re-radiate any color that was not in resonance with that energy they were receiving from the Cosmos or from the environment around them, whether that energy came from a man-created source, such as electromagnetic light or radio waves, or whether it came from the sun or even the vibrations of chemical molecules and atoms. Human beings only receive from the Cosmos those energies we choose to let in. We shut out many energies because we are not in resonance or in tune with them. This observation of resonance with colors of the different frequencies of light showed up in almost everything I looked at and I saw that it was my own consciousness which was functioning at different thresholds depending on which level it was concentrated. As I developed my intuition in the fields of telepathy, clairvoyance and the projection of thought across distances in my experiments, I began to see that these gifts of the human race were no better than the people who used them, and that even the most celebrated psychics were no more advanced than the quality of the consciousness they possessed. I also began to see that there was an even higher level of functioning beyond intuition that was to be found only in the consciousness of our greatest men and women who had added powerfully to our knowledge of human existence, and I called this quality found in inspired poets, musicians and prophets of all races—imagination. I found the highest imagination to have far greater penetrating insight into the workings of Nature and the Cosmos, whether human nature or so-called inorganic systems of Nature, than any psychism. I therefore began to experiment with imagination and found it had profound effects on human tissues, proteins and enzymes produced by the cells. I performed many experiments with enzymes, external to the body as well as internal, using this power which I called imagination. I probed Nature's infinite possibilities, finding to my great surprise that Nature Herself was the greatest imaginer who had long ago imagined things far beyond the imagination of humans. It was then that I began to apply my understanding of Nature's primordial imagination to the scientific concept of evolution of organisms and systems.

It suddenly dawned on me that at the center of every natural system there was a record of everything that it had ever been and that its present pattern was the total sum of all its evolutionary experience. What we had to do now to find out its essence of existence was to tune our consciousness to penetrate into that totality which covers all, since every organism has grown in that totality and only differs from it by the individual choices it selects from that total environment. This realization of the power of the imagination to penetrate Nature brought me to meditate on the nucleus of any system, whether it be a cell or the original seed-cause of a vibration, in order to discover the origin of its patterning. It was at this time that I discovered Supersensonics, or the ability to detect the most subtle vibrations, and was humiliated by the fact that the ancients had known about this ability for a long time. As I began to read their analogies and metaphors, I saw clearly that they, too, had discovered the power of human consciousness to tune in to the Cosmos through the nervous system and through the brain's levels of perception, to tune in from the highest levels to the lowest, through what science would call harmonic systems of resonance, using all kinds of divining instruments in order to get a feedback signal when their consciousness was in tune. These instruments varied from yarrow sticks in ancient China to the forked twig of a peach tree of a water diviner, to the breastplate of the prophets, to the divining rods of the Egyptians. I began to see that this same faculty was to be found in the antennae of insects, the sensitive direction-finding skin of the amoeba, even the ability of cats to find their way home from miles away. However, what amazed me more than anything was the fact that human intelligence, which normally did not function at this level of perception, had within it this common ability that is found throughout Nature. Even the humble atom has this power to select its unity with other atoms through the affinity of its vibrations. And yet humans live without this awareness that even the vibrations of particles and waves of light have this same power to seek that which is in tune with it. "Why are humans ignorant of this?" I wondered.

Applying this insight to the brain and its mode of operation and keeping up to date with every scientific development in order to verify these observations of Nature at work, became my full-time meditation and brought me back full-circle to that luminous patch of seven colors reflected from a white piece of paper through a prism. I discovered that the human brain is also a prism, actually filtering the cosmic light into an octave through its vehicle of expression, the human body, and resonating with the basic seven colors, while the eighth level resonates with pure consciousness itself. The following concept of the brain is built on countless observations, past and future, and I welcome any further observations from the perceptions of scientists, poets or mystics, who can see and perceive the universe as one whole vibrating nucleus with all its parts resonating together on different thresholds, unified over all by that consciousness in which we experience everything. This holographic model of the brain acting as a physical replica of the energies in the original nucleus, is replicating itself all over the universe in different patterns and thresholds of vibration. The brain is the vehicle of this nuclear consciousness which can be likened to a seed. This seed unfolds on seven different vibratory levels and our direct knowledge of our own brain consciousness determines our own level of evolution. The following model of evolution then is given to the scientific community and to religious people alike, and shared spiritually with those who may feel some resonance in their own consciousness. From time immemorial those who feel resonance with the spectrum of light and the oneness of life already have experienced, at some primordial moment, the destiny of the brain.

HOLOGRAM OF CONSCIOUSNESS

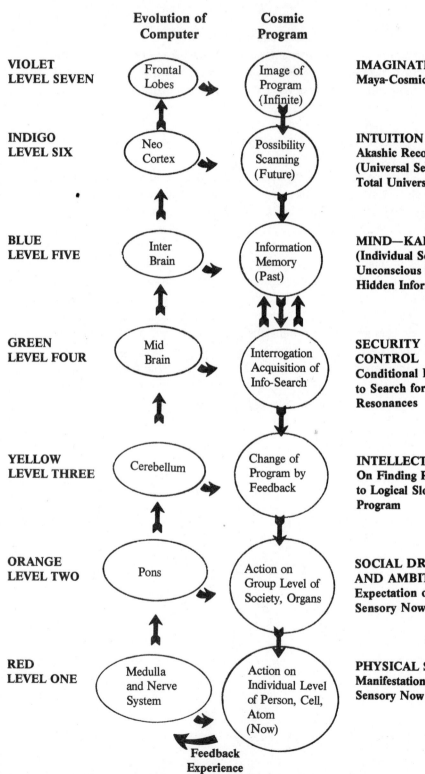

Evolution of Computer

Cosmic Program

VIOLET LEVEL SEVEN — Frontal Lobes — Image of Program (Infinite) — **IMAGINATION** Maya-Cosmic Dreaming

INDIGO LEVEL SIX — Neo Cortex — Possibility Scanning (Future) — **INTUITION** Akashic Records (Universal Self) Total Universal Info

BLUE LEVEL FIVE — Inter Brain — Information Memory (Past) — **MIND—KARMA** (Individual Self) Unconscious Store of Hidden Information

GREEN LEVEL FOUR — Mid Brain — Interrogation Acquisition of Info-Search — **SECURITY CONTROL** Conditional Instruction to Search for Resonances

YELLOW LEVEL THREE — Cerebellum — Change of Program by Feedback — **INTELLECT** On Finding Resonance to Logical Slots in Program

ORANGE LEVEL TWO — Pons — Action on Group Level of Society, Organs — **SOCIAL DRIVE AND AMBITION** Expectation of Sensory Now

RED LEVEL ONE — Medulla and Nerve System — Action on Individual Level of Person, Cell, Atom (Now) — **PHYSICAL SENSES** Manifestation in Sensory Now

Feedback Experience

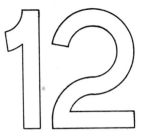

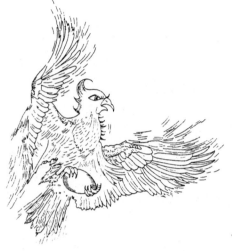

EVOLUTION
BY CHOICE

Going back through the long step-by-step process of evolution, we find that the human brain has passed through seven major stages of development. Evolution proceeds not in steps like a ladder but in steps which trace a spiral that rises towards more and more complex organization. It does this by simplifying all previous steps and incorporating them in the next step ahead like a ratchet up the spiral pathway. We will describe these major steps one by one in the following chapters, in order to see how evolution puts all the different parts together. But in describing them one by one, it is easy to lose the sense of circular causality or recycling and to give a false impression that our brain evolved in one lump after another.

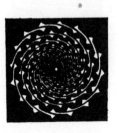

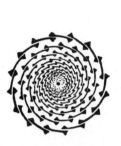

Using metaphorical images for the ratchet effect along an expanding spiral seen on the right and as a contracting spiral seen on the left, we identify the expansion with light waves which are centrifugal and the contraction with centripetal gravitational waves. The centralizing inward-working force on the left represents involution and darkness; the outward-moving light represents evolution. According to Darwinian theory, evolutionary processes select those individual organisms best adapted to their environment. According to modern theory, man now possesses the ability to control his own evolution. The question is, does any of man's cleverness lead to involution? An example of an involutionary trait of today is that more children than ever are leaving school unable to read and write, because of little challenge and because of long hours sitting passively in front of television screens in the darkness. Are they adapting to the dark or to the light? Are they inwardly tuned to gravity (the grave) or to levity (light)?

All the leaps from one level to another in the development of the brain overlap each other just as the levels of consciousness which express through the brain overlap and are continuous within a single nucleus. The brain as a physical manifestation of these stages of development is an effect, not a cause, of the evolving levels of consciousness, and this can be seen in the very overlapping itself. If the levels of consciousness had to wait for a physical instrument to evolve, then the seven brains would necessarily have evolved in linear fashion, one after the other. But consciousness does not work like that. The levels pre-exist within the nucleus in the same way that the spectrum of color exists within a ray of sunlight. Every person's levels of consciousness are homogeneously mixed, yet they separate when passing through different densities and intensities to produce the thresholds within the total experience of what our brain normally experiences as consciousness. As an analogy, consider a peacock egg as a nucleus with all the parts mingled together—colors, feathers, claws, eyes and beak—undifferentiated in the yolk of the egg with the DNA chain containing the message of life all mixed and waiting to become a beautiful bird, waiting on the trigger of sperm to fertilize its potential. So too, the levels of our consciousness are in our own nucleus all mixed together in undifferentiated potential though, when they manifest, there may seem to be a linear unfolding, and one level may emerge at a later time than another.

It is important to grasp this before we speak of Nuclear Evolution and its model of a seven-layered brain, because a model is necessarily simple, and the model of the brain which I am presenting in this chapter seems to develop one, two, three, four, five, six, seven, in separate lumps, one after the other. But evolution doesn't really work in a linear sequence, creating one entirely new thing after another. The whole of evolution reveals that all cells throughout Nature organize themselves in their specific patterns by nuclear transformations of their already existing parts. In evolution there is not just one way of producing a structure but many. We need only look at the number of photoreceptors and eyes in the organic world to see the diversity of those structures, which, like the human eye, reveal to many insects and animal creatures not only the amount of light but the color, shape, position, distance and velocity of the source of the light.

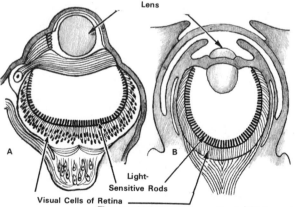

The eye of (A) the clamworm Nereis, (B) the squid.

The common pigment in all animal eyes, Rhodopsin, is called visual purple. It captures the light energy and raises the molecules by excitement. This initiates a chemical reaction called blanching which stimulates the nerve fibers and sends electrical spikes to the brain where they are translated into conscious sensations. If the brain is damaged we cannot see with the eye, or if the optic nerve is cut, or if signals to the brain are temporarily blocked with anaesthetic, we also cannot see.

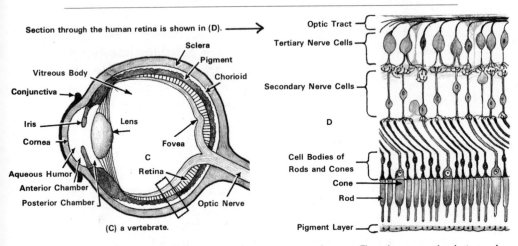

Section through the human retina is shown in (D). ——→

Sclera
Pigment
Chorioid
Vitreous Body
Conjunctiva
Iris
Lens
Cornea
Fovea
C
Aqueous Humor
Retina
Anterior Chamber
Posterior Chamber
Optic Nerve

(C) a vertebrate.

Optic Tract
Tertiary Nerve Cells
Secondary Nerve Cells
D
Cell Bodies of
Rods and Cones
Cone
Rod
Pigment Layer

This means we do not see with eyes but with the brain and with our consciousness. The rods are more abundant around the periphery of the retina where they perceive motion and see in dim light. The cones are more concentrated in the center of the retina and they focus the bright light of the object seen.

The very complexity of all the parts available out of which evolution transforms an older system into a new structure is nothing short of miraculous. The composition of the cell and its molecular structure, and the composition of the complex molecules of life such as DNA out of the structural arrangements of Nature's atomic elements are examples of the way that Nature works with the existing material at hand. To make up its most exacting structures which form themselves into the millions of multicellular organisms we call our body, the same polymers, nucleic acids and proteins are used by evolution in forming whales or bacteria, people or viruses. Just four bases of molecules and twenty amino acids go to make up the genetic code in all of organic life from the blood cell to the smallest alga.

What does this mean? It means that we are all made of the same thing. Everyone has four proteins and twenty-two amino acids in the DNA. It is only the different arrangement of those molecules that make us all look different. In a maggot or an elephant is the same DNA. A piece of grass has the same DNA. Isn't it incredible that the building blocks of the hereditary message, the very thing which passes on all the differences, is all one—the same stuff in your nucleus as in mine! What is different is the way they're arranged and how much of each. The differences in the millions of organisms upon the planet are not due to biochemical innovation or engineering but in consolidation of existing structures and the selective molecular distribution of a few basic chemical components. The butterfly and the bird, the tree and the flower, the shark and the snail are not different by virtue of their chemistry but only in the way those basic component chemicals are distributed and organized into patterns. In the great leaps of evolution no new genetic information is supplied but only the different utilization of the same chemical structures that were already at hand.

In this same way, Nuclear Evolution does not operate in Nature in some mechanical linear sequence of events like an engineer ordering up parts for a project. It makes do with leftovers and turns out objects of creation which are unique responses to a specific series of events in our life situation. An individual soul is not defined by any specific social program but can break the system and, like the genius inventor, make a TV set out of cardboard, string, an electric motor and tinker's tools.*

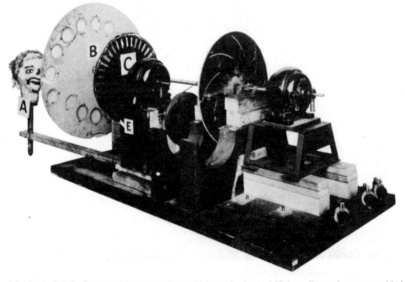

John Logie Baird's first television transmitter which used a form of Nipkow disc and was assembled on a washstand. 'The base of his motor was a tea-chest, a biscuit tin housed the projection lamp, scanning discs were cut from cardboard, and fourpenny cycle lenses were used,' it has been written. 'Scrapwood, darning needles, string and sealing-wax held the apparatus together.'

* The invention of the TV by John Logie Baird was first demonstrated in 1926 before the astounded scientists of his day. In 1939 he invented color TV.

Nuclear Evolution of the brain structure and the hologram of life contains a natural method of generating new circuits by arranging existing structures of brain and chemicals which are already at hand. Redistributing these structures in time and space and changing the shape, performance and behavior of human life on earth is a function of consciousness and its organization of the existing products of human society. The color, light and energy of the cosmos are merely used in a different way to bring about a profound leap in the individual nucleus of being and its group interactions with the environmental materials at hand. Apart from the remorseless selection of the fittest as depicted in the inevitable law of organic development of Darwinism, there is the freedom of the "tinker" to create new reality from a hundred thousand choices. It is this very tinkering with life and society which is both a godsend and an abomination at the same time, for only those who are aware of the ultimate purpose of life can fulfill the cosmic will. Thus Nuclear Evolution is dependent on the ability of each human to inquire of the Cosmic Intelligence which is the correct way to reorganize our conscious life as a social species.

Even the future of our life as a *physical* species is in our own hands. It appears as if our genes are coded into the DNA purely by a mechanism of Nature which we cannot control. But who is "Nature" if not consciousness? And who are we but the same consciousness? How could Nature by a "mechanism" create something totally unforeseen? Wherein does her creativity really lie? Is it true that her laws are mechanical? To scientists they may appear mechanical, but in fact the options of Nature are infinite, just as our own options are not limited as we like to think. The way we use our brains, for example, is not limited to rigid specific linear processes. For every human brain that exists there are at least one hundred ways of going about any one task or one hundred possibilities of mates that we could marry if we were only aware enough to tune into their existence. The limit is in our awareness, not in the brain equipment that Nature has evolved for us. The totality is present in the environment if we do not limit it, and our access to the total intelligence is more a question of tuning our thoughts to control our inner environment to make it responsive to a selected cosmic program which is ever available to every organism.

Only the philosophy of life of each organism, whether it be man, animal or atom, determines what it shall extract from the total environment around it. For an atom it might be an affinity for bonding with another atom. For a man it might be a job opportunity. Why does one man perceive a hundred opportunities for getting work, while another finds none and blames his ill luck or his karma? In the same way, we also have at our disposal the potentials of our heredity (not only in the child we are shaping to be born but in the child we were ourselves) for we choose to develop only a tiny portion of our real selves simply because we are not aware of any more. We speak of evolution as a process of Nature, a process that is "out there" and which "happens" to the world. But in fact evolution only moves by choices. Even the unconscious moves by choices, though we are unaware of them. The choices we *don't* make because we are unconscious—these are stagnation, because they perpetuate ignorance, which holds back evolution.

We can see this most clearly by looking at primitive forms of life such as the amoeba. Unicellular organisms reproduce themselves by self-division of their cells, not by union with a mate. Hence, life goes on repeating itself without innovation, and the basic forms of unicellular life evolve very little over vast periods of time, whereas the more complex organisms which engage in sexual activity between partners (represented by much later organisms in evolution, such as insects and animals) contain within them the tremendous potentiality for change and innovation and adaptation to situations and new environments. The unicellular organism just goes on and on in the same old way, reproducing another organism just like itself, and in the same way the lower levels of human consciousness seek uniformity and are most content when nothing new is happening. Look at the number of humans sitting like zombies in front of their television sets. What stunted organisms these are who, at the end of their education, cannot even read the great inspiration of the great minds of past times. Just like lumps of jelly, with no power to evolve themselves, no power to communicate with the refined consciousness at the forefront of human evolution. The choice each organism makes toward the higher or the lower is the choice between innovation and dullness. *So it is not that Nature intends innovation and evolution but that each organism, as part of Nature, moves like the ratchet effect, jacking up its conscious-*

*ness along an evolving pathway or regresses and stagnates. We all
have that choice.*

If the process of evolution is to recycle already-existing materials to
make new organisms, then our own creativity is the same. We do not
have to create a totally new portion of our brain, for example, but only
to further its development in the direction it is already moving.
Nature's options are infinite; but although there is already a guiding
field-force these options depend upon conscious selection to get evolved
into something new. The slowness of evolution is due to the fact that
low level creatures are content to choose not to do anything new, so
when we think of evolution, we think of billions of years. But in fact it
need not be a slow process at all. The higher we evolve, the faster we
can change, just because we are willing and aware and tuned in. Our
most important choice and next step is to activate the cosmic program
asleep in the nucleus of the cosmic egg. To do this we must know how
consciousness uses the power of self-suggestion and imagination* to
change our dreams into reality and thereby change our own body-
mind-brain into a hologram through the transcendence of dualism of
light and dark, positive and negative, male-female into the singularity
of the One. Thus in heaven so on earth, as in space so in matter.

The very idea of sexual union arising among all complex organisms
of Nature requires the existence of two separate halves. Did evolution
create the positive male energy and the negative female energy out of
dust and ribs in the garden of Eden, or was there some pre-existing
prototype with which to work? There is no positive/negative attraction
between individuals at the unicellular level of life. Yet there is still a
positive nucleus within every unicellular being which dictates its
relationship to the negative environment around it. An alga replicates
by splitting into daughter cells, and this unisex is programmed in the
nucleus of the alga. No fun, you might think! But who knows that the
excitement of an alga may consist of an excitation of its skin, since its
skin represents the negative environment around the positive nucleus?
Light excites the skin and triggers the unisexual splitting, just as our

* This whole question of penetration and expansion of the cosmic nucleus in ourselves and
the structure of it is the subject of *Nuclear Evolution.*

own skins are excited in a tactile way, and the arousal of the human sexual drive can only be completed skin to skin.

What could motivate an organism to make such an enormous change and how could it even think of becoming bi-sexual if unisex were all it had ever known? Are not we ourselves reluctant to let go of the life we've always known and to risk becoming someone more evolved? Can we relinquish the sexual delight of our male and female bodies in order to open to the experience of unisex at a higher octave of evolution, and is this not the thing that is asked of us by the sages— that we cease to identify with physical bodies long enough to experience an entirely new kind of ecstasy? Although we communicate such wisdom in words and our thoughts about it are complex, our reluctance to venture forth is not much different from the arch-conservatism of the one-celled alga. How then does evolution occur? The answer is that the change is asleep in the nucleus of life, waiting to awaken.

Scientists can document the way in which the unicells gradually polarized into negative and positive functions to better serve the whole species, but science will not say anything about change being "asleep in the nucleus." Yet the scientists' own level of inquiry is just as mysterious as any spiritual metaphysics when it comes to explaining just how Nature works through individuals for the good of the species and why she "intends" such improvements, since there are too many perfect adaptations for anyone to suggest that evolution could have happened purely by chance. So we are talking about two different levels of being: one level where individuals are making choices and another level where an evolutionary Intelligence is "pulling" us forward in spite of all our resistance. And this is just as true of any alga or amoeba as it is of a human being.

Thus it was by choice that the incredible leap was made from one-celled creatures to complex organisms that engage in bi-sexual reproduction. Why was this a leap? Why a step forward in evolution to go from the self-sufficient and efficient replication of an amoeba to the mating of two? The answer is simple: because it was the opening of a doorway into fantastic possibilities. If we look at the difference between the amount of consciousness expressing through a human being as opposed to the consciousness of an amoeba, then we can imagine how vast is the difference between the consciousness we are expressing right now in our own lives and the quality of consciousness we have the potential to express, by virtue of this same evolutionary process that makes something "new" from something old.

Once the positive/negative attraction within one cell became an attraction between two separate organisms, one positive and one negative, then a reorganizing of each generation's genetic information could take place. In other words, the vast complexity of the organisms of the earth are built, like a branching tree, upon that first step in which two beings join to form another organism which in turn joins with a mate to form another (this one having the inheritance of the first four) which also mates and forms yet another, with the heredity of eight. And in each mating, the drives, urges and potentials are passed down from all the generations so that now, after billions of years of physical evolu- tion, the potentials of our hereditary genetic material are too vast to imagine. Who or what determines which qualities out of all this great storehouse will shape a new infant? The primordial imagination works to select a mate just as it does to reprogram our DNA to create our unborn children.

The annunciation to Mary that she would give birth to an extra- ordinary carpenter who would bring a new perception of Cosmic Intelligence into the world was the organizing field-force which brought a messiah into being. In other words, the Christ force in the incarnating Jesus was strong enough to enter his mother's consciousness and purify it with an imaginative vision of the incoming soul, thereby setting up a guiding field for the foetus to be born in pure consciousness, which is God. Great beings have the soul power to project themselves forward in time and even to consciously select the physical womb in which they will be born. Great beings who exist on higher levels of consciousness who wish to return to the physical world come down into the lower evolutions one step at a time, through the seven levels to physical birth in the womb of flesh.

It was said of Christ that he was born of a virgin. This did not mean that his mother's body was virgin but that he was born into pure consciousness, consciously selected by self-programming of the psychic field which brought the annunciation to the visionary part of Mary's higher imaginative faculty in the brain. In this way the superior being who has perfected himself on higher levels of consciousness actually influences the future so that he can move about among physically born people in the flesh and bring to the world the light of consciousness. This was the "virginity" not of his mother's body but of his own consciousness which he knew was that "light of the world" which guides evolution. Thus he speaks from the "many mansions" of his father's house—the many levels of consciousness which exist in the nucleus of the whole, and he says to mankind:

YE ARE THE LIGHT OF THE WORLD

To the extent that you are convinced that your consciousness is the "light of this world," you are one with Christ who rises again and again in pure consciousness to speak the same message. Thus in the same way, the imagination of mankind becomes the guiding field for evolution and at the everyday level of life, our future destiny as a physical being is programmed by the images we hold of ourselves.

Scientists generally believe that organisms change and evolve by adaptation to the external environment, but Nuclear Evolution holds that internal stresses and emotions and chemical hormone production are much more powerful than any external factor. The annunciation affected the biological condition of Mary because her consciousness was full of wonder, and she was able to receive the divine message in a state of faith and humility. "My soul doth magnify the Lord," she said, "Behold, from henceforth all generations shall call me blessed." Thus her own thoughts and attitudes created the internal environment in which the event could happen just as it was foretold. In every person or living thing, these inner responses create the psychic womb in which imagination plants its seed.

Each individual program becomes physically different with each generation, so that the redistribution of the common genetic materials which everyone has, creates an awesome potential for new types of organization, new structural combinations with every human embryo. The sky is the limit. The re-ordering of genetic material by deliberately programming our consciousness via the creative imagination makes it possible for any person who knows how to do this to become the parent of a highly evolved being or a new messiah. None of us is limited by our heredity but can totally re-shape the potentials of our unborn children.

We tend to see genetics simplistically as though there were only a few options. You may say, "Well, I have my mother's eyes and my father's sense of humor, and I have uncle George's nose." But you could just as easily have gotten aunt Mabel's nose and great-grandfather William's eyes. So what did the choosing? As far as we are concerned, the choosing all happens at an unconscious level and we just wait to see what comes out. We do not realize that at each stage of evolution the growth of organisms has not come from the differences in gene products but from the complex regulatory circuits which have unleashed or restrained certain activities of the organism thus leading to the specific genetic program which selects the quantities of biochemical products from its immediate environment.

Now what does that mean in plain language? It means that *if you discipline yourself, you regulate the secretion of brain hormones which create chemical waves of emotion commonly called devotion or ecstasy or conversely, if you do not practice self-discipline, you may unleash lower feelings of anger and hatred thus leading your organism to select at an unconscious level (automatically and beyond your awareness of choice) certain qualities of biochemical products and nutrients from its immediate environment.* In other words, what is happening consciously in a person gets translated into the unconscious selecting process. Hence low level minds beget more low level minds and the world tends not to evolve. But if we consciously decide to evolve *ourselves,* then the reverberations of every step we make become enormous, because our consciousness does not just stop at its own skin but replicates itself in many mirrors. For example, we may think that our lives would be cast in much the same mold regardless of what we are doing with our consciousness and that we would still be married to the same mate, still be getting the children off to school, still be working at the same profession, no matter what was the quality of our inner life. But the thought climate of human beings, whether it is fear, anxiety, security or love will determine to a large extent the situations we find ourself in from the total spectrum of possibilities available. That situation will become our teacher, bringing pain or well-being.

The brilliant function of pain as a teacher leads us to suspect that evolutionary leaps in brain organization have come from the trial and error of avoidance of pain rather than the conscious selection of better environments. This is man's ignorance of his own vehicle of consciousness, and it is in his immediate power to change the modus operandum from pain stimulus-response to bliss-seeking and light-seeking functions of the human brain. Conscious evolution is the direct result of light synthesis, whereas attraction to pain, violence and the darkness of the mind is unconscious *in*volution, leading to annihilation of unwanted and depraved species.

Man has the choice of how he will use his brain at this moment in history. By rethinking his whole evolutionary program backwards and forwards humankind is able to program its own future and to shape its own worth. This is the real meaning of the word "worship" which comes from the ancient word "weorth shipper", meaning "a shaper of worth". The brain's ability to shape worth is controlled by the image man has of himself and the way he regards his own brain. In order to understand what the human imagination is and to know its power over the government of all human life, man must first understand the lower levels of brain function which lead to this highest of his faculties. It is impossible for anyone, even the highest philosopher, to understand what the human imagination is without first understanding the layers of consciousness and brain organization which have gone before it in order to manifest it in creation.

248

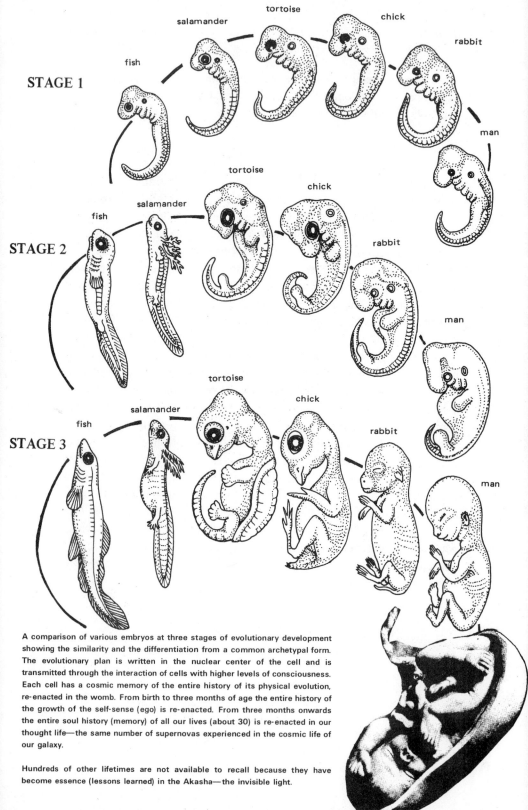

STAGE 1

fish salamander tortoise chick rabbit man

STAGE 2

fish salamander tortoise chick rabbit man

STAGE 3

fish salamander tortoise chick rabbit man

A comparison of various embryos at three stages of evolutionary development showing the similarity and the differentiation from a common archetypal form. The evolutionary plan is written in the nuclear center of the cell and is transmitted through the interaction of cells with higher levels of consciousness. Each cell has a cosmic memory of the entire history of its physical evolution, re-enacted in the womb. From birth to three months of age the entire history of the growth of the self-sense (ego) is re-enacted. From three months onwards the entire soul history (memory) of all our lives (about 30) is re-enacted in our thought life—the same number of supernovas experienced in the cosmic life of our galaxy.

Hundreds of other lifetimes are not available to recall because they have become essence (lessons learned) in the Akasha—the invisible light.

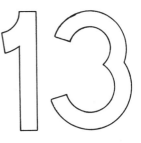

YOU ARE A RAINBOW OF ELECTRICAL VIBRATIONS

Physically we each recapitulate in our own mother's womb the long chain of physical evolution from the first one-celled amoeba through the fish with its gills, through the reptile and the mammal with their tails, until at last we arrive in our final form, the human body. In the same way, we recapitulate throughout our lives the soul's history of our psyche as we travel through the thresholds of our consciousness. As children we begin life in full physical vitality on the first of the seven levels. As we grow old we begin to look backward into the world of memory from the fifth level of consciousness, and most of us cease to be alive in the now. Finally we die, because the image held in the seventh level of our consciousness tells us that whoever we think we are has used up its allotted time. If we resisted the temptation to look back nostalgically in time, would we grow old? If we put a different image into our minds, would we succumb to death so soon? What can we learn about ourselves by *consciously* recapitulating our psychological evolution as it has unfolded and manifested through the evolving physical organ of the brain?

The philosophy of "Dialectical Materialism" developed by Marx is based upon the premise that matter precedes spirit and brain precedes mind. When the brain is damaged and the spirit can no longer express through it, to the Marxist this is proof that we are totally dependent upon a material physical organ and therefore we are material beings. The entire manifestation of communism proceeds from this one initial thesis. As you know by now, the thesis of Nuclear Evolution is that what we really are is consciousness, and our consciousness shapes our brain, our body, our children, our life situation, our future, and our society. This truth is nowhere to be seen more clearly than in study of the brain, for the very same phenomena that prove to materialistic minds the hypothesis they wish to believe, namely that matter is the fundamental reality of this world, also reveal to those who have eyes to see it, that behind the infinite variety of emotional, mental and physical responses which take place in our brains, one consciousness is vibrating. It shows itself in seven entirely different masks over the face of Reality.

The idea that there are seven levels of brain function which enable our consciousness to express itself in seven entirely different frequencies of vibration did not spring out of my head as a full-blown concept but was the result of many years research, including the observation of what happened in my own brain. I was particularly struck by feeling in my brain, waves of electrical energy being released by the excitation of layers of brain matter. At first this was purely subjective, but EEG measurements confirmed it. Later, after the development of Supersensonic methods of measuring internal states, I used Supersensonics to piece together the wholistic picture.*

---

* I describe this research in more detail in the chapter "Science and Spirituality" in *Nuclear Evolution.*

In scientific terms, the process by which consciousness expresses through the brain seems complex, but its underlying principle is quite simple. Most people who have gone to school know now that there is white matter and grey matter in the brain, but they do not realize that the brain uses these two kinds of tissue to create an alternation of positive and negative electricity. Not that the color is important. The important thing is the *layering*. The two kinds of matter appear in layers, and the layers work very much like a capacitor in electronics equipment. Even in the spinal nerve this polarizing between positive and negative exists between the white matter and grey matter.

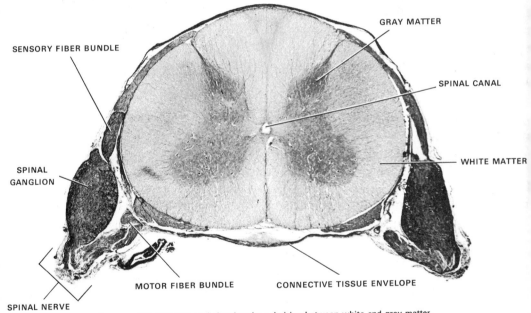

Cross section of spinal cord showing the polarizing between white and grey matter.

A cross section of the animal spinal cord shows the motor nerves passing through the center around the spinal canal which is filled with the same fluid from the ventricles of the brain to which it is joined. The sensory nerves pass on the left and right side in two bundles of fibers in the spinal ganglion. The spinal cord itself is a dense mesh of neurons, the center of which is formed of grey matter with the axons and dendrites forming the white matter around it. The left and right spinal nerves were often referred to by the ancient sages as yin and yang, ida and pingala, negative and positive. This polarizing of signals is common throughout the body and particularly through the grey and white matter of the human brain which is structured with alternating layers of potentials amplified by oscillating circuits and rhythmic pulses. Millions of nerve fibers lead to the human brain from each organ of sensation and these impulses weave patterns in time and space in the meshwork of the human brain to cause us to see and experience a hologram. The wave fronts of the impulses impinge on the white and grey matter in the brain to produce a tuned circuit which draws its power from the energy of the sun and the stars.*

We are so accustomed to the ordinary experience of seeing an image of the "outside world" in our mind's eye that we do not call in question the whole complicated process by which little electrical spikes go traveling through the rods and cones of the eye and are received in the brain. Why is it that when we look at the world we do not see a homogeneous mass of little spikes? The brain does not receive images of trees and human beings and food to eat. It only receives spikes of electricity which pulse in the nerve centers of the brain, and it translates these spikes into what we call "reality". In actual fact the outside world, as we know it, exists only in the image which the brain creates out of these impulses carried in the little spikes. Although an

Our consciousness translates millions of spikes of electricity into images, a process which we call perception.

---

* See the explanation of the Universal Hologram Theory of Nuclear Evolution showing how we absorb cosmic energy and experience consciousness. (*Nuclear Evolution*, Chapter 6.)

object appears solid to our eyes and to our touch, in fact every physicist knows that such solid matter is made of many little bundles of electrical charges with considerable space between them. Because we cannot see through this space in solid objects, we tend to think it isn't there, yet heavy protons from stars sail right through these spaces in our bodies and we do not even feel them go through us. Relatively, the space between the positive and negative charges in our atoms is large, but we do not normally think of this space nor do we think of the push and pull of these charges constantly going on in our bodies. We think that the world is solid and that a hologram is an illusion produced by intersecting beams of light, but in fact the world is also a hologram and is itself nothing more than a sensory illusion. The light from the sun and stars intersects with the light of our consciousness working through the brain, and the two together create the intersection of time and space where at every moment the entire universe is re-created and experienced as "real".

In 1968 when I published the first edition of *Nuclear Evolution*, the word "holographic" was not used by scientists except in terms of the re-creation of wholistic visual images in three-dimensional space. I was using the word in an entirely different way. The idea that the brain produces several holograms which create the counterpart of a visual display of reality inside the brain, is now receiving some scientific attention, but it is an ancient idea, first recorded by the imaging system of the *I Ching** which formulated the electrical tensions between the psyche and the internal and external biological environment in terms of positive and negative lines built into sixty-four hexagrams. These hexagrams were built up of positive and negative lines which depicted a pattern of forces playing through a person at any one time so that if this pattern were disturbed, it would affect that person's relation with the environment and would build up tensions which would then be reflected in the different line arrangements of the sixty-four hexagrams.

---

* *I Ching*, trans. Wilhelm/Baynes with introduction by Carl G. Jung, Princeton University Press (1950). The *I Ching* is an oracle which differs from some other forms of divination in that a spiritual component is built into it.

The tension within people is like a cloud of water vapor charged with electricity. We only experience something in the cloud when a bolt of lightning comes from it and flashes to the ground to release its electrical tension, but in fact the tension is there at all times before the discharge takes place. The fact that a cloud of water vapor could hold millions of volts of electrical force would be evident only to a water diviner or to someone who suffered from headaches before a thunderstorm. The thunderstorm is the discharge of the lightning, balancing the tension between the heavens and the earth. And in the same way, every person has a tension within him waiting to be discharged.

The ancient Chinese diviners built the *I Ching* as a system for discovering what these tensions were, not only between the electricity in clouds of water vapor and the earth but also between the earth and human beings. They learned that when such a cloud passed overhead, corresponding electrostatic charges were induced in the human nervous system and brain.* They provided a way for all people to become diviners and to tune into the tensions in their own minds between heaven and earth—their higher selves and the ego—or between one's present situation and events in the future that have not yet happened. The *I Ching* can guide a person in such a way that his future actions will be in tune with "heaven" and can show him if his present state of mind is out of balance. It points the way to perfect equilibrium, from any state or degree of imbalance, whether it is in our health, our social life, our relationship with our own unconscious mind, or our attitude to God. The theory of Nuclear Evolution shows how cells maintain their electrical charges through electron transport chains along the neural pathways very similar to the electromagnetic fields set up by the atoms of our body. These fields within fields within fields that trigger each other off and on (commonly referred to these days as being "turned off" or being "turned on") are the result of the wholistic system of the

---

* Many people notice that after a thunderstorm or a rain they feel effects in the nervous system, in the membranes of the sinuses, and in the electrical activity in the cerebrospinal fluid in the center of the brain. The same effects can be produced by a negative ion generator which will artificially excite the atoms in a room (See rear of book for more details on negative ion generators.)

mind and body resonating in harmony with the hologram of life. The ancient Chinese called this "being in tune with heaven and earth"—the hexagram of Peace—with heaven below supporting earth above, in perfect balance.

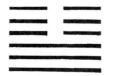

The symbol for peace or balance is the three positive lines of the Creative (heaven) polarized with the three negative lines of the Receptive (earth) above.

Our consciousness, our mind and our emotions, and the physical structure of our bodies are all determined by these positive and negative patterns. Although the Chinese used symbols to depict them, modern science uses volts and amps and milliamps. We do not always realize that the intensity we feel in ourselves or in others is electrical intensity and that consciousness is expressing through us with high or low voltage, depending on our openness. Anyone who wants to control his or her own consciousness and become a high-energy person must understand this process of Nature. Some people are naturally charged, spontaneously charismatic characters who do not know how they maintain their energy or enhance it. But others who don't have this natural ability to tap into the cosmos directly must, if they are going to achieve effectiveness in the world, begin to explore conscious methods of bringing this enhancement process into operation.

Most of the world's problems are due to the fact that people don't know that a vast treasurehouse of power exists within every cell of their body. Many of those who have a surcharge of energy cannot handle it, and they take to alcohol as a depressant or use drugs to calm themselves. In this way they unwittingly hamper the very power and force which could *lift* them instead of disturb them if only they knew how to control it. Nervous tension and anxiety in people lead to insecurity and feelings of inferiority. These are at the root of all human relationships, wars, and social misery. Until people can control this free energy naturally flowing between each one of their cells, they are committed to an existence in which their entire brain and nervous

system and consciousness is continually being disturbed by the unconscious forces around them and within them.

The concept of Nuclear Evolution as applied to the brain cells and
all other cell life of individual humans and even the organization of
social life is clearly stated in terms of alternating thresholds of electrical
intensity in layers of activity. We have only to look at different people
to see their different thresholds of electrical energy manifesting in their
lives. They believe these levels are fixed and unchangeable because
they do not yet understand what a hologram really is. If a hologram is
made of light and if the world as we experience it is made of the light
of consciousness and if the same consciousness that is in the whole is
also in every part, then any one person possesses all the resources of
the whole and the only thing that can prevent him from enjoying this
vast power is that he doesn't realize it is there. This holographic view
of brain activity as outlined in *Nuclear Evolution,* claims that it is
possible to affect the random events of evolution through the intervention of consciousness by generation of large amounts of brain electricity
at will. This idea of super–conductance of the brain electricity was
achieved personally by the author and first researched at an Indian
yogic hospital and since at several other Western institutions where a
record of the brain electricity was recorded*.

Brain signals are emitted along certain paths which extend out from
the central mid-brain area through a large nucleus of fibers. The signals
are modulated and tuned, not to individual cells but to the whole
brain's activity, which results in a selection among hundreds of thousands of paths, so that the signals will only travel along specifically
chosen pathways to certain areas. The way this tuning takes place is
still a mystery to science, and little is known as to how some specific
neural channels are chosen in preference to others. The preferred
circuits are often habitual and are formed through the embryonic
development of the nervous system and the subsequent conscious

---

* The author still possesses the strip recorder chart of the EEG readings at some of
these institutions. Details of the experiments are available in the second edition of
Nuclear Evolution, pp. 491-501.

discipline of the channels. Our whole sense of self and our entire life pattern, including our future, is shaped by such patterns of habitual thinking. Many medical men think that it is impossible to control brain circuits, but I myself have proved to several of them that it is possible to shut off parts of the brain or to amplify other parts and create large charges of microvolts showing that electrical potentials can be consciously changed in the brain pathways.*

In other words, there is no habitual thought pattern or emotional response or typical action, no matter how deeply rooted in our psyche or genes, which we cannot change. We can entirely change anything about ourselves if we so desire. With this modern knowledge of positive and negative control over Nature's forces within us, we can develop that sense of conviction that Christ called "faith". To hold a desire in our mind, emotions and body with this kind of deep-rooted confidence and conviction, instantly changes our world. Once we become aware that change is actually taking place in our internal environment and that consciousness is actually affecting our biochemical makeup, then self-change is no longer just a nice thought at the ideal level.

Although some people achieve results for themselves in health and well-being through positive affirmations held in consciousness at the mental level, many other people cannot muster sufficient conviction to achieve the same results. These people are like a little old lady with a set of expensive carpenter's chisels that are useless to her. Only a skilled carpenter knows how to use them. Or you could say that most people are like a businessman who has bought a fantastic computer but has no booklet to show him how to use it. Our brain and body is such a computer, far more complex than medical science itself, yet we do not need to know medical science in order to know its secret, since everything that happens to us medically is controlled by a non-medical force. Such a force can create faith healing on different levels, the most potent of which is instant transformation of the flesh as practiced by

---

* There is an account of research on my brain at the Kaivalyadharma Yogic Research Hospital (*Nuclear Evolution,* pages 496-500).

Phillipine faith healers, ancient Hawaiian Kahunas no longer existing, or by Christ in his miracles.

Christ knew how to do it but he could not communicate it to many other people, because the knowledge was not put into scientific format and could only therefore be transmitted through the life-force itself to his close disciples. If he were to come again, it is doubtful whether he would choose that method since these powers of self-knowledge, self-healing, and self-transformation have reached so few people in the last two thousand years. If he were here today he would certainly be as conversant with the scientific method as he was with the ancient scriptures of his own times. Many scholars would question anyone's ability to speak for Christ as if he were here today, but a true Yogi has within him that same authority to speak for *all* those who are enlightened, since they are all one and say the same things in different words. Therefore if you find one, you know them all. This is Christ's message, "that you should love one another as I love you," meaning that to love someone at the level of the nuclear center of being is to know them in their heart. This can't be done by scientific method or by medical knowledge or by psychology of today. But this does not mean that it will never be done by the science of tomorrow which may include these domains presently excluded from it by ignorance of what consciousness is.

The reader might ask why bring in scientific jargon, and who cares whether we have neurons or dendrites? The answer is that without a link between spirituality and science, there can be no transmission of divine knowledge on a wide scale. Even though a person may receive this divine knowledge, it will die with him unless he can encapsulate it in a language which enables man to communicate it to his fellows. This is a language of the mind and the spirit and the imagination which carries with it a powerful shock of realization which penetrates the soul and ego. The mind and imagination carry the force. They are not the power but only the vehicles of the power, just as our nerves and dendrites are the vehicles of consciousness.

It is known that sets of neurons with their dendrites can be arranged in the brain as oscillation circuits in which impulses travel over a circular route and are raised in potential each time an impulse passes through a certain synapse. These cause certain rhythms to be set up in the brain known as alpha, beta, delta, just as there is a rhythmic oscillation in the pacemaker which controls the heart, resulting in contraction of the heart muscle. Many have learned to control these rhythms and to "go" to different levels of consciousness as one would go to a place. There are also many other rhythmic functions of the automatic operations in the body which are governed by such oscillating circuits which can be brought under conscious control by yogic training.* Expressed in the language of psycho-biology this kind of self-mastery may seem too huge a feat to attempt. But really the only difficult part is the initial realization that it is *possible.* After that, the discipline is no more demanding than any other kind of discipline, and the results are so rewarding that the whole process becomes like an adventure.

It is important to realize that the tuning of the brain circuits is converted into learning and memory by different organisms and animals by setting up stored patterns of potential energy in the cells of the brain through choosing specific circuits. This learning or conditioning of signals filtered by the random activity of the brain can be found in the lower animals and the lower parts of the human brain. We function by habitual responses which are stored as an energy in the brain, and we call this memory. This kind of memory is like an unconscious choosing process that is happening automatically yet nevertheless is a choice. The higher, conscious selection, which many scientists do not believe is subject to control by force of will, is made through a unique mind control of the cell bodies of the autonomic sensory system. Any unconscious choosing can become conscious choosing once we are aware that choices are happening and we begin to deliberately interfere with them. But people tend not to want to be aware and not to want the hard work of reshaping their inner worlds and gaining control of these automatic functions. Why should they bother? Yogis can control their heartbeats and yet what use is it, since people are getting along just fine on automatic?

The answer is that a yogi is no more interested in his heartbeat than

---

* See Rumf Roomph Yoga tapes for instruction in conscious control. Listed in back of book.

you are. But he is interested in being master of his consciousness. This means that he is able to change himself and to change his life, to wrench his mind out of its old grooves, to wrench his identity out of its habitual limits, and to make himself over in a new pattern. The control is exercised through the mental effects on yin and yang or positive and negative cells. Why has Nature split us into positive and negative? Does it somehow facilitate consciousness? What in positive and negative makes control possible? For the answers to these questions we will have to look again at the stratification of brain matter into layers and the polarized electrical impulses that become possible through this stratification. What is the future of man? Where is evolution taking us? Will our brain become even more polarized and even more minutely stratified? Will our seeing of the hologram of life be any different if we are able to generate wave trains of energy, increasing the charges between and in the layers each time the energy is accumulated in one layer and boosted in another layer?

We can imagine the alternating layers as the rungs of a ladder or the teeth of a ratchet by which the energy is jacked up each step to a higher potential so that on the top rung the energy is stored like a capacitor. This concept of the brain as a capacitor is very much like the capacity of an electrical storage battery, where by adding more plates or layers, the amperage of the battery is increased. People who can store large amounts of electricity by raising their vital forces to higher layers also increase their thinking capacity, since the electrical charge in the brain ionizes more brain fluids. The ionization of membranes and fluids in the brain is equivalent to exciting the atoms of our brain cells to a higher threshold. This is what ionization means.

A thing is said to be ionized when there is a surplus of either positive or negative energy. Negative ions add electrons to an atom, exciting it. Positive ions take away electrons, also exciting the atom from its state of rest potential. To take away negative electrons makes the nucleus of an atom more positive. To add electrons makes it more negative. Therefore, whenever our membranes, brain and cell fluids are excited through the adding of surplus negative ions all the nuclei of atoms in our body become more enriched, electrically charged and excited, making us like the hot wire of an electrical circuit and storing this charge in our bodies. Such a person is commonly referred to as "a live wire".

This state can be achieved by meditation as well as by sitting in front of a negative ion generator. The experience may not be consciously felt, but if we rub our hands together or touch our skin after prayer or meditation, we find that it has become very dry and silky. This is a sign that our cells have become excited and their atoms ionized. It is well known that when the skin is dry, the body holds a higher charge, just as when the atmosphere is dry in cold weather, carpets hold thousands of volts of electrical potential which can be stored in the human body walking across the room, so we receive an electrical shock when we touch a metal object. We can actually see a blue spark. This rarely ever happens in the tropics where the air is moist and warm and the skin is usually slightly damp from perspiration. Nevertheless, even in the tropics, through meditation the skin can be made very dry and highly charged through controlling our consciousness. Hence the many accounts of miraculous healing and other bio-electrical phenomena in hot countries like India and long ago in Palestine.

Besides meditation, there are a number of other ways to charge up the skin with negative ions. One is to run tap water and place the hands on either side of the running column of water but without touching it. Another way is to do some chanting of a spiritual nature. The hands of many faith healers become very dry and highly charged while they are performing a healing, yet this does not mean that there is any spiritual benefit in negative ions. The body can be charged up by an act of consciousness or by a generator, but the generator does not advance you spiritually except that it could relax you and in that way give you a charge to facilitate meditation. Negative ions intensify any situation electrically. If you are a clear thinker, they make you think even more clearly. If you are already spiritual, then you become more intensely spiritual. And this intensifying is due to the ratchet effect of electrical charging.

Is there any connection between the spiritual light of the electron-rich nucleus and the "white" matter, or is this just a superstitious interpretation of the stratification of our brain matter into "light and dark"? To answer that, let us look at the fact that the same layering of cells which forms the structure of the layered brain cells also forms the retina of the eye. These alternating white and grey layers shown from the surface inwards are composed of different types of cells with different electrical potentials. The molecular layers are triangular in shape; the second layer is in small pyramidal shape; then comes a layer of large pyramidal cells and then a layer of variant cells which are repeated throughout the cerebrum in different ways. Throughout the brain and body we come across structures which carry the positive charge and are made of white matter cells and these are invariably surrounded by or adjacent to the darker granulated grey matter cells. But just as in metaphysics, where dark and light are part of a larger energy that is beyond good and evil and where positive and negative have no judgemental connotations, the same is true of the electrical structure of our brain and body. Life has given us all the same equipment in which the polarization of brain potentials into positive and negative causes the pulses we call brain rhythms, and we are each free to use it in creative or destructive ways as we so choose. In the course of our evolution we become more and more positive, more and more aware, and we let in more light into our consciousness. In time this will manifest in the physical body and we will be more and more able to charge up the white matter in the layering of our brain and our body structures. Simultaneously the grey matter will become more able to store negative electrons, thereby increasing our vital force.

Very few people realize that the secretion of brain chemicals can be controlled at will to affect our emotions and levels of consciousness simply by raising these electrical potentials and *awakening millions more cells than is normally possible* and getting them to switch on. In most people they are switched off and lie unused throughout an entire lifetime. It is amazing that throughout history man has not realized that his exciting activity in politics and the competitive world of commerce as well as the performing arts all depend on what level of his brain he is using. With many people this is all done unconsciously. Whether you are a laborer, an intellectual thinker, a businessman, a psychic, or a highly gifted philosopher will depend on what part of your brain you are primarily using, while more or less neglecting the other parts. It is as if we get into ruts and habits in shunting these energies into familiar

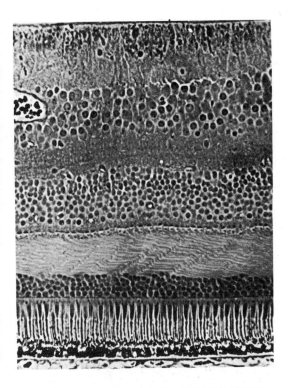

The above shows a micrograph of a section of the human retina with its rods, bipolar cells and horizontal cells. The bottom layer consists of ganglion cells. The whole shows how nerve impulses are amplified into signals through several alternating layers.

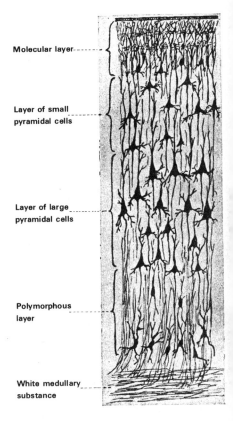

Molecular layer

Layer of small pyramidal cells

Layer of large pyramidal cells

Polymorphous layer

White medullary substance

The above shows the four types of cells which make up the alternating layers of grey and white matter in the higher brains of the cerebrum. The irregular polymorphous cells whose nerve fibers extend into the layers of white matter alternate with the internal bands of white matter existing between these strata. The circuit is reminiscent of the plates of a battery for storage of potential current.

circuits and channels. This is why people get stuck on one level of consciousness and seem to become a stereotype such as the academic scholar ("egghead"), the workingman, the politician, the dreamy poet, and all the other categories of society that we all know so well. But none of these labels is real, because they only describe our *habitual* modes of functions and omit the larger part of our total being which is capable of expressing through all seven brains and even *beyond* the brain entirely.

Each of the seven brains acts as a ladder, just as each brain has its own methods of jacking up the brain electricity between the alternating layers of grey and white matter. Modern semi-conductors and solid state electronics work on this same principle where energy is raised up or amplified to a more excited state by passing through positive and negative stages. Life itself is very similar, with the small biological batteries called mitochondria in each of our cells, which work on exactly the same principle in which the inside membrane carries an opposite charge from the outside membrane. When we feel excited mentally, emotionally or physically we are unconsciously raising the threshold of energy through these layers in our body, in our nervous system, and in our brain.

The body of a human being is no different from a capacitor since its main function is to hold an electrical ionizing charge so that consciousness can express through it.

Because the structure of the brain cells is layered in tiers it is possible for us to process the intensity of brain signals to reach different thresholds of activity. The lower parts of the brain send out electro-chemical waves to the different layers above in the cerebrum and through polarization they act like a capacitor. A capacitor not only acts as a tuning device but also as a storage of electrical potential energy. It appears that the white and grey brain cells, through different construction and polarity, set up a charge within the layer like the plates of an electric battery which also works on the principle of holding a positive and negative charge of an electrolyte. In this case the electrolyte is the sodium and potassium exchange of the intercellular fluids between the cells acting together with the balance of chemical ions in the intracellular fluids. The similarity between a capacitor, a battery and the alternating layers of the brain can easily be depicted in the following pictures:

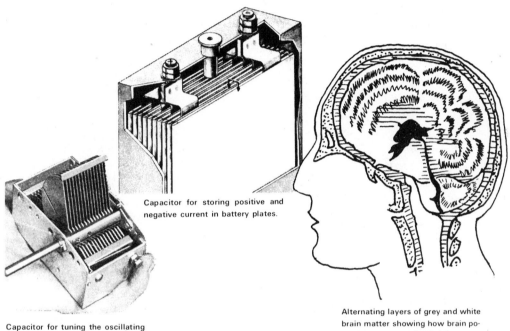

Capacitor for storing positive and negative current in battery plates.

Capacitor for tuning the oscillating circuit of a radio coil.

Alternating layers of grey and white brain matter showing how brain potentials can be amplified from one threshold to another.

The frequency of the brain rhythm depends on the tuning of the neural circuits as a whole. In deep meditation all cells can come to a resting potential whose waves of positive and negative energy are equally balanced at high amplitudes. The results of conscious exercises are easily proven by EEG measurements. Meditation opens the channels for more energy from the cosmos and from higher levels of consciousness to come into the chakra system and then to the brain cells and to fine tune the brain cells to higher frequencies so that they become more able to receive and store subtle energies. So the capacitance effect is increased and the brain cells hold more and finer awareness. In this way we enlarge our *capacity*, and then it is there for us to use and draw upon.

It is not generally known that we actually *store* our vital forces on seven levels of our being. Just as we have seven major ganglia and seven endocrine systems for secreting hormones, so do we have seven vital force centers which are linked with the operation of the seven brains. In the next chapter we start at the beginning with the layers of the spinal cord and we proceed through the layers of brain organization which correspond to these vibrating centers, which were often referred to as a psychic electricity by the ancient sages who saw each one clairvoyantly as a spinning "wheel" of etheric energy, in Sanskrit called a *chakra*.*

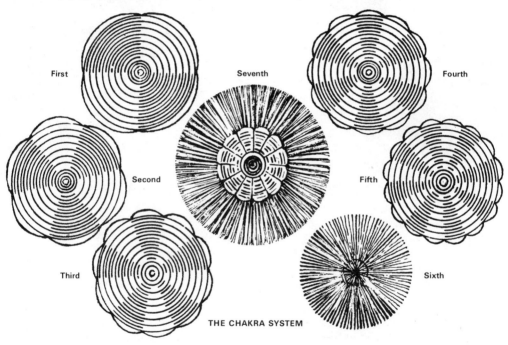

THE CHAKRA SYSTEM

Each chakra is spinning at a different rate of vibration called a frequency. The study of these frequencies continued in ancient India for many thousands of years until the present day when the author

---

* Further details on the frequency of chakra vibrations and their relation to color and to levels of consciousness can be found in *Nuclear Evolution.*

discovered that the chakras were related to the seven brains. *To control the frequency and the positive or negative spinning of these chakras gives us conscious control over the positive and negative functions of the brain, and thus control over our own destiny.* Instead of pumping all our consciousness into electronic computers and engineering more and more complex systems, our next evolutionary step is to learn to become engineers of our own consciousness and of the forces in society which are reflections of our inner worlds. If even a small group of people came together and practiced awakening the total number of cells in the human brain, the energies developed could liberate the enormous potential of mankind for a New Age.

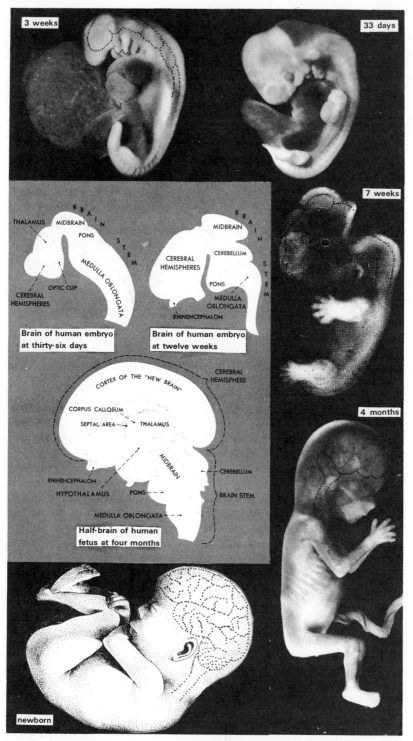

3 weeks

33 days

7 weeks

THALAMUS MIDBRAIN

B R A I N

PONS

S T E M

MEDULLA OBLONGATA

OPTIC CUP

CEREBRAL
HEMISPHERES

**Brain of human embryo
at thirty-six days**

B R A I N

MIDBRAIN

CEREBELLUM

CEREBRAL
HEMISPHERES

S T E M

PONS

MEDULLA
OBLONGATA

RHINENCEPHALON

**Brain of human embryo
at twelve weeks**

CORTEX OF THE "NEW BRAIN"

CEREBRAL
HEMISPHERE

CORPUS CALLOSUM

SEPTAL AREA THALAMUS

MIDBRAIN

CEREBELLUM

RHINENCEPHALON

HYPOTHALAMUS PONS

BRAIN STEM

MEDULLA OBLONGATA

**Half-brain of human
fetus at four months**

4 months

newborn

EMBRYONIC DEVELOPMENT OF THE LEVELS OF THE BRAIN FUNCTIONS

The increasing encephalization that has taken place during the course of the brain's evolution is
recapitulated in these stages of embryonic development.

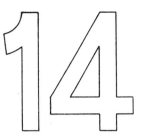

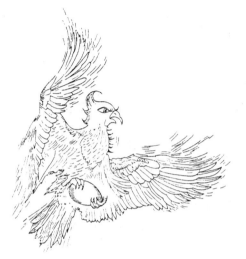

WHAT IS MAN?

We now embark upon the main theme of this book which is that man functions not only on seven levels of consciousness, has seven controlling centers of psychic electricity in his body vibrating in a more subtle form of matter than his gross physical body, but also *man has grown his brain through evolutionary time to correspond to the evolution of his control over these centers.* As man was raised from one level to another and each level became proliferated and complex, another level beyond it began to simplify its complexity and bring all the ramifications of the lower level together. Just as telephone exchanges have sub-exchanges at the local level which branch out to all the residents in an area and are linked to main line telephone exchanges until they are all funneled into one cable running under the sea through London to Europe, so do the millions of nervous impulses coming from one level of consciousness to the next become concentrated into one signal at the higher level. This enables us to learn through experience by taking many perceptions of small events and concentrating them into concepts. Once we learn to drive a car we no longer think of all the separate operations that we had to think of in the beginning, since our higher brain function raises all the separate movements into one comprehensive automatic action of coordinated driving. In the same way, our body functions automatically through the lower levels. If our consciousness is not able to function through these higher levels, then we are endlessly bogged down in details and in the constant effort required to remember performing these separate actions.

This is particularly true at the level of health. If our consciousness is orientated physically, we eat from one stimulus to the next. As our hunger juices secrete, we stuff into our mouth any food we can grab to relieve the hunger. However, at higher levels, our consciousness automatically filters these signals from the lower body, enabling us to put off eating until the most suitable food comes along. The higher centers know that we should never fill our stomach completely full although our lower body forgets that proper digestion requires churning of the food. However, if people are focused on the lower physical levels of sensation, their consciousness always obeys the lower craving and fills the stomach completely until they cannot eat any more.

This pulling of the consciousness to lower levels of gratification dominates a large part of some people's lives whereas, for highly evolved people, such matters are put on automatic pilot, because they know fully well that the body can easily go without food for several days and that digestive juices creating hunger pain can be consciously controlled. Many people experience this often without even realizing it. They get highly interested in a project or they get so excited that they cannot even bother to eat because it would interrupt the pleasure of what they are doing. *Therefore the trick of controlling one's lower animal appetites is to learn how to substitute even more pleasurable brain activity.*

To a rich person eating the best foods such as caviar flown in from Moscow or some delicacy brought from Japan or Paris, there may be no greater pleasure than wining and dining on the fat of the land. But such people are usually sick. If they are not sick physically from poor eating habits, they will be sick emotionally, mentally or spiritually, because people cannot put a large percentage of their consciousness on gratifying their stomachs without taking it away from their spiritual refinement. This is the problem with having a lot of money. The temptation to indulge in the best of everything takes too much time away from *our real purpose here on earth which is to understand how all our lower drives become totally concentrated and absorbed in higher functions of the brain activity.*

Meditation is concentration to the point where all else is excluded. In this act, the total complexity of the world around us is concentrated into one timeless moment and thereby simplified on a higher rung of the ladder. Anyone who becomes totally absorbed in anything, no matter what, is meditating. Once they have brought all the activities of the body, mind and emotions together and simplified them into a single point, they can then take the next step after concentration, which is expansion on the next level. *Thus does the human system work at every level: that it must first concentrate its activities on the lower rungs in order to proliferate and expand its activities at a higher level.* So we are talking about stair-stepping up the levels through alternating concentration and expansion.

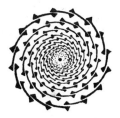

It is this need of the human organism throughout evolution to bring together and synthesize many activities that has brought *the evolutionary development of the brain as a series of governments, each one ruling the one below.* In this chapter we begin to see the unfolding of this process in the structure of the spinal column and its thousands of branching nerves and its connection with the government hierarchy of levels which have synthesized each other as we climbed the ladder of evolution over billions of years until we have arrived now at our present conscious awareness of atoms, cells, organs, brain and body as a vibrating electrical entity. The next step for man is not only to realize how this came into being, as this chapter will outline step by step, but to discover that the society into which we are born is also structured in its various levels of government and communication along the same pattern. Since society is a projection of human intelligence or ignorance, it cannot be any better than the human beings which comprise it. Therefore to see these levels of consciousness reflected in society in our relations with others, in our attitudes towards ourself as a being and towards the environment around us enables our consciousness to raise up complexities into a very simple and concentrated evolutionary purpose. *That sole purpose of the cosmic intelligence operating through man and all his many sub-systems is to discover the awesome nature and glory of consciousness itself.*

Concentrated consciousness on the highest level synthesizes every-thing below it in one simple insight. This insight can come to any person who is prepared to put his full attention and concentration on the totality of his consciousness and how it came to manifest as what it is. This "isness" and the situation which surrounds it—good or bad, brilliant or indifferent—is the result of the operations of our conscious-ness acting through its seven vehicles. Our happiness or our misery is entirely determined by this functioning. Therefore it is terribly important for each human being on the planet to concentrate its entire being *at every threshold of life* on the synthesis which will bring this insight into the nature of the life-force acting through us. To begin this journey through our vehicle of consciousness we will describe the seven levels of brain function leading to the stratification of society and human activity.

We start with the cerebrospinal nervous system which is not only hooked up to the brain but is an extension of it, just as the branches of a tree are an extension of the tree roots. The same cerebrospinal fluid that is in your brain is also surrounding your nerves and is quite

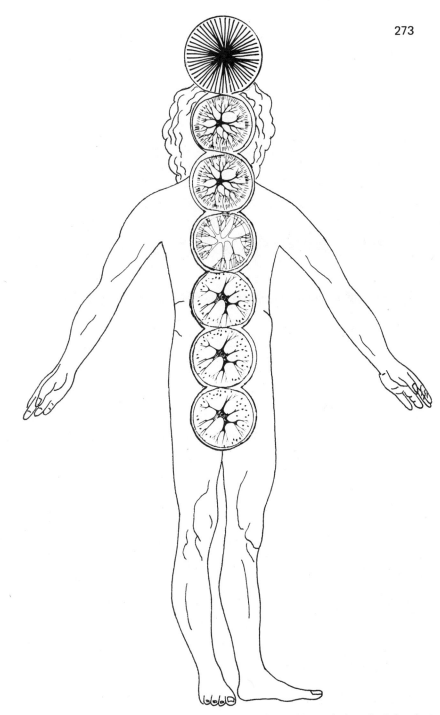

In the whole of life, the human system must first concentrate its activities on the lower levels in order to proliferate, and then expand its activites at the higher levels.

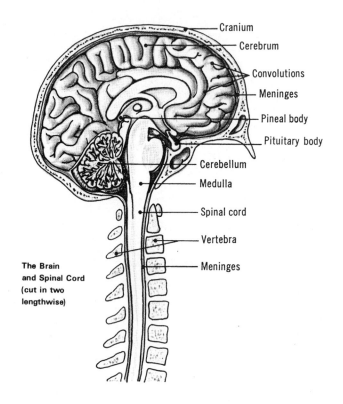

Cranium
Cerebrum
Convolutions
Meninges
Pineal body
Pituitary body
Cerebellum
Medulla
Spinal cord
Vertebra
Meninges

The Brain
and Spinal Cord
(cut in two
lengthwise)

separate from the cellular fluids of your body, so that the nervous system is an extended part of the amplifying circuitry of your brain. That fantastic nervous system is within its own skin and that skin is the same continuous skin which contains the totality of the brain. Thus the entire brain and nervous system is one piece, with a skin which science has labeled in three sheaths (pia mater, the arachnoid sheath, and dura mater). These three sheaths actually separate the brain and nervous system from the rest of the body. Though nerve trunkways are interpenetrating the whole body, there is no contact made between the nerves and the body, because the nervous system is completely contained within its *own* "body". In effect we have a body within a body.

Why is it important that there are two separate body systems: one body sensing the universe directly and then communicating that sensation

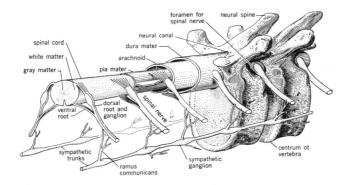

Picture shows a section of the cerebrospinal nervous system along the center of the spine and the sympathetic nerves leading from it to all parts and organs of the body. It is important to realize that the entire brain and nervous system are floating inside a triple membrane which itself penetrates the cells and intra-cellular fluids. Like two separate bodies they float inside each other with the nerves cushioned within these sheaths like a double-walled vacuum flask. There is never any connection between the two bodies (the cerebrospinal system and the rest of our body) except through a release of chemical neurotransmitters.

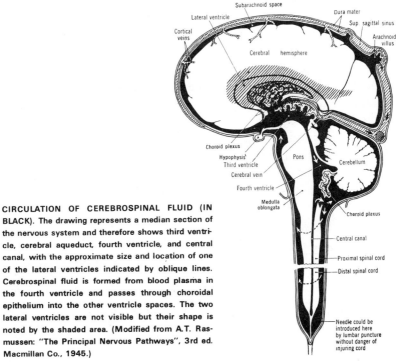

CIRCULATION OF CEREBROSPINAL FLUID (IN BLACK). The drawing represents a median section of the nervous system and therefore shows third ventricle, cerebral aqueduct, fourth ventricle, and central canal, with the approximate size and location of one of the lateral ventricles indicated by oblique lines. Cerebrospinal fluid is formed from blood plasma in the fourth ventricle and passes through choroidal epithelium into the other ventricle spaces. The two lateral ventricles are not visible but their shape is noted by the shaded area. (Modified from A.T. Rasmussen: "The Principal Nervous Pathways", 3rd ed. Macmillan Co., 1945.)

to the rest of the body which is quite separate from it and only connected by chemical reactions? It is important because people do not think of themselves this way; they are only aware of "me" in a vague and undiscriminating way, not seeing how they process the experience of "me" through seven brains.

We live in physical bodies, yet we are primarily aware of our emotional body. We tend to experience the physical body mainly when it feels pain or when it gets a disease. Most of the time we are identified with our emotions, which means that much of human experience is at the level of chemical interactions between the two bodies. *Humans take these chemical feelings as reality,* without understanding that it is only one level of consciousness communicating with another.

The outer body acts as a huge sensitive skin, communicating with the inner body consisting of the nerves floating within it, and the nerves then communicate with the physical level of consciousness by chemical hormone transmitters.* The physical level of consciousness believes it is the outer body, but consciousness is really only connected to the physical body by the slimmest of links, for there is no real direct connection except through secretion of neuro-transmitters which provide an electro-chemical stimulation between nerves and other cells, muscles, etc. to produce a subjective feeling. What, then, is real? Is the subjective chemically-induced feeling really real? Is the outside world with all its stimuli that the nerves pick up real? In actuality, the nerves are totally isolated from the outside world, cut off by their own protective sheaths. Without the outer sheath of the physical body, mediating at a lower threshold with the external environment, the inner sheath of the

---

* Just as the nervous system is seated in its own triple-walled sheath, so does the physical cell-life of the human body act as another sheath around that, and each sheath has its own type of liquid which polarizes the different electrical potentials, one related to sodium and the other to potassium. Both work through the ionization of electrical potentials. The interaction from inside the cell through the cell wall membranes and the interchange between the cells and the nervous system is described fully in *Nuclear Evolution*, pages 590-600.

nervous system could not connect with the outside world at all.

Why is it that the brain and nervous system are isolated inside a skin? The obvious answer is that the skin is a protection for them. But if we look back very far into prehistory, we find that in the first stages of its evolution the sensitive brain *was* a piece of skin, nothing more. All our sensory organs have come from this one supersensitive organ of perception—the skin which has gradually become refined, repatterned and infolded and encased inside the skull. The inner body of brain and nerves became isolated from direct contact with the outer world in order to preserve the link with consciousness on the non-physical levels and mediate between the internal and external.

As you read through the development of the seven brains in the pages to follow, it is important to keep in mind that the original skin of the amoeba carried within it all of the seven brain functions in a non-specialized form and that every organism has these capacities whether it has yet developed specialized equipment or not. This is why amoebas can "hear" vibrations though they have no ears and why insects can intuit a mate a mile away though they have no sixth brain. Humans, too, can hear and see through any part of their skin if they take the trouble to reawaken the capacity. The brain has become specialized to more adequately develop and express each of the seven levels of consciousness inherent in all creatures but these are present in rudimentary form long before the specialized structure evolves to handle more advanced functions.

The agent which has guided the skin's development into specialized receptors is consciousness, but that is a many-splendored word which few understand. Whether we call consciousness "God", evolutionary intelligence, creative power or just plain awareness, it will mean different things to the different people who use it and filter it through the seven brains. Because consciousness has modeled our human brain over some five billion years, we can get some idea of its many thresholds by studying the functions of its parts from a wholistic viewpoint. "Wholistic" means that each reader is not reading of some objective brain, external to his own, but is in fact a total system, hooked up irrevocably with the entire vibrating environment of atoms, cells, organs and their total environment of world, space, stars, etc. This book is part of that system and, although it is now in your hands, it is also in your brain, vibrating there as a disturbance or an excitement depending on what you are doing with your consciousness.

To describe the seven parts of the brain by their Latin names or to locate their convolutions which control the physical parts of our body does not add to our knowledge of the brain as a wholistic sensor or reveal that it is a capacitor or tuning device. So far science has only understood four out of the seven brains and, although the scientist can tell you where in the brain to press a certain point that will make your left leg move or your right eye blink, what do we really know about ourselves when we know this? Just pointing to the parts is not enough. We have to see the wholistic evolution of the brain as a total organ and see what purpose the Evolutionary Intelligence has for it.

By divining we can gain some idea of the way the brain has grown and adapted to our yearnings, fears, drives and needs as a species over a period of five billion years of the earth's ten billion year history. I published the book *Supersensonics* for this reason—to describe the methods of sensing by sensitizing the brain and nervous system to subtle L-fields to detect the purposive functions in Nature. In this way we gain access to realms of knowledge into which science has been unable to set its foot. By divining beforehand and then backing up the results with scientific experiments afterward, we are using the brain's highest faculties, the frontal lobes, to discover the brain's own nature, rather than relying on the intellect which is only the third type of computer to evolve in our brains and which therefore permits only a much cruder, much less refined expression of our consciousness.

Study of the human skull, going back in time, reveals that the frontal lobes have grown larger and larger with each advance in evolution. If we look at the brain of the ape we see a very sloping forehead with almost no forebrain, gradually increasing in size with Java man, becoming less sloping with Peking man, the brain cavity enlarging with Neanderthal man, coming to the raised forehead of modern man.

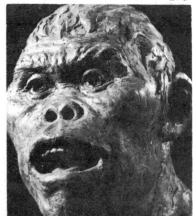

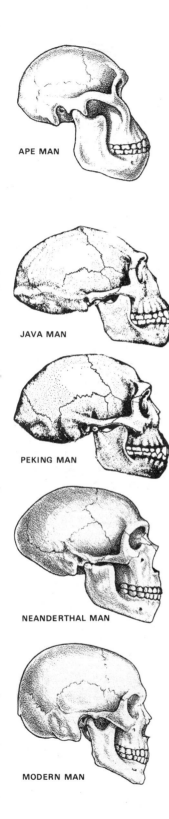

APE MAN

JAVA MAN

PEKING MAN

NEANDERTHAL MAN

MODERN MAN

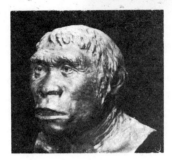

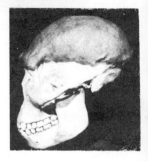

Courtesy American Museum of Natural History.

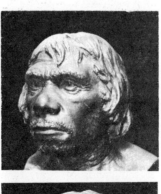

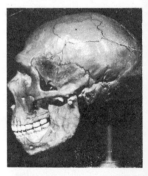

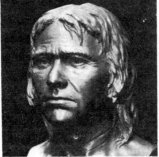

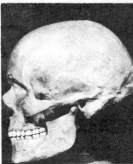

How can we ever hope to learn about the function of these lobes without consciously using them?

Theories about our biological memory, about our mental memory, have not progressed beyond the stage of description and analogy in the medical sciences. Therefore to describe actual functions of brain parts, through developing a supersensor which can answer questions from another level of intelligence, is the first step to discovery of what our brain parts actually do and how they developed. If we study how the different parts of the brain relate to each other, rather than talk about actual cells and structures as the medical books do, then we can see not just the external manifestations of the brain which are already in evidence but also the internal possibilities not yet discovered. We cannot tell what a computer actually does by describing its hardware parts any more than we can judge the potential of a human being from its bones, liver or blood. It is through the constant refining of the software of consciousness that the structure of the brain is lifted up to more complex relationships resulting in higher and higher adding-on of more complex equipment.

Just as a rat has a larger portion of its sensory cortex developed in the area controlling its whiskers, so do humans have a larger portion of the brain devoted to seeing. Yet the real seeing is not just a matter of focussing rays of light or of seeing colors as physical sensations in the occipitals at the rear of the brain but of seeing the images as pictures in our mind. This is handled by our imagination and recall memory which is given meaning in the frontal lobes and higher brain. To accomplish these more complex relationships between the sensations we receive and the meanings we experience, the higher centers of the brain are built one upon the other, not just as add-on pieces but as part of a wholistic interlocking amplification of what is going on in human consciousness over thousands of years of evolving tissues and cells.

How does study of the brain reveal to us the hierarchical functions of consciousness? We have said that already hidden in the nucleus, the yolk of the cosmic egg, is the coding for the levels of organization which first appear in the chakras or plexi of our nervous system and then form themselves physically into the seven brains. Each brain as it evolved was developing to fill a need felt by the organism. Obviously the needs felt by a chicken will be different from those felt by a fish or by a human, but the basic hunger drive or the need for a mate or the need for social position among their species originates from the same basic drive but is translated in different ways according to each special environment. By investigating our own drives it becomes clear that evolution develops the brain not just as a series of separate departments. There is a wholistic purpose in each level developing the way it does. It is the relationships *between* the brains that are important to the organism.

Darwin only tuned into the first brain in his theory of "survival of the fittest". The behavioral psychologists have tuned into the second brain in the study of learned social behavior in insects, animals, humans and other species. Medical science has divided the brain by lobes, rather than by function, and their pictures reflect this physiological orientation, which does not acknowledge seven brain functions nor raise the question of what kind of consciousness has shaped its instrument in seven parts. Nowhere in academia does one ever get the feeling for what makes man's consciousness so different from that of an insect or an animal, even though he physically mates, as animals do, and he cooperates in groups, as insects do. Like fish who fight each other within their species, a man fights other men to defend his home or to find a mate or a dozen other reasons that are as old as the earth. And yet a man is very different from a fish in the quality of his consciousness, and the difference is visible in the structure of his brain.

The general geography of the brain is like a map: it is useful to take along to the territory but it cannot give you direct knowledge of what the territory is really like. You have to go there to find out and walk the territory yourself. If you are a good map reader, then you will find your way around easier, but if you cannot read maps, then they are useless representations of the territory. The map of the brain you see (below) is therefore such an overview and can tell you nothing about yourself unless you examine that territory and look for familiar landmarks and clues within your own being as you retrace your long journey through evolution, brain by brain.

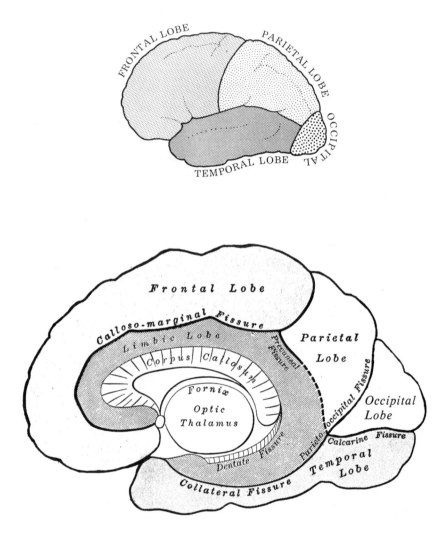

The important thing in these pictures is to see the difference between the brain seen externally (top picture) versus the brain in cross section (bottom picture). In the cross section we get a feel for the cavern that is hidden within the very core of our brain. We think our brain is a heavy lump of grey convoluted tissues, divided into lobes, but deep at the center, in the fluid which is captured there, our glands secrete the peptides and magical chemicals that can transform us from ordinary mortals into fantastic beings filled with light. Like the cave of the genii, hidden inside Aladdin's lamp, it waits unknown, and it will continue to wait until someone inquisitive like Aladdin takes the trouble to rub the lamp and make a wish.

THE FIRST OF THE SEVEN BRAINS OF MAN

**The Medulla
Oblongata and
the Central
Nervous System**

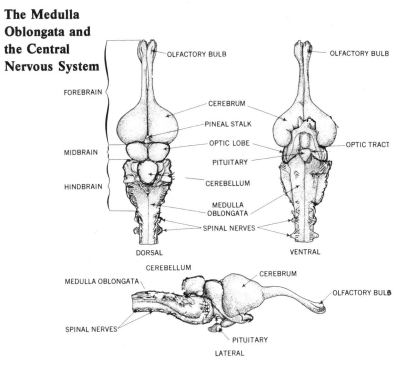

BRAIN OF AN ALLIGATOR

As I said before, the reptilian brain was first a sensitive piece of skin, a primitive kind of eye not sensitive to light alone but to all vibrations in Nature, across all octaves, and this sensitivity can now be traced in some lizards as a rudimentary pineal gland which reaches through the brain like a bulb on a stalk just under the skin. The human pineal gland also acts as an antenna though it is buried inside the skull, not sticking out on a stalk, and it is only a vestigial remnant of this faculty of the lizard brain to sense all gross vibrations and discriminate vague associations, which means it is undeveloped by most people. The lizard experiences a pineal effect of three hundred sixty degree *physical* sensation which human beings have lost. With our skin we do not feel three hundred sixty degrees around us; we only feel that link with the environment through our consciousness, provided we have

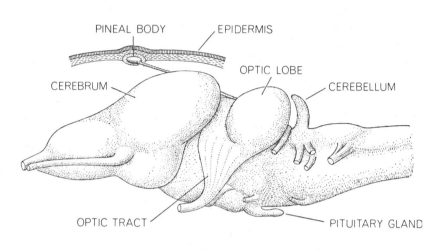

This picture shows the pineal gland in the reptile brain which has become slowly encased in the brain of mammals through the long course of evolution.

awakened and activated it at the higher levels of brain activity. But we still have a vestige of this physical sensing that began in the reptilian state of our evolution. When someone looks at the back of our neck, we turn around, because we feel an actual physical sensation in the area of the neck.

We will discuss the pineal gland later in connection with the higher functions of the seventh brain and the faculty of imagination; for now it is only important to be clear that in the reptile, the pineal is a *physical sensor,* whereas in man it has become a faculty of *extra*-sensory perception and has gone deep inside the skull and taken on an entirely new role. Both the pineal gland and the reptilian brain (represented in humans by the Medulla Oblongata) are a very primordial part of human sensitivity on which I wrote the book *Supersensonics*. The science of "Supersensonics" is the reawakening of the reptilian brain and the human pineal functions at a whole octave above the evolutionary threshold when man left the reptilian consciousness and became a mammal. The lower supersensing capacity is innate in most insects and other natural organisms. Man has it in psychic perception, water dowsing, and other forms of divining. These seem like very sophisticated talents, but they come from a very primitive part of our makeup.

We have also inherited from this most primitive area in our brain development, the automatic reflex of stimulus-response reactions. An example of an early sensor is the construction of the ear to respond to the nature of sound. The sensor of our ear drum is a sensitized piece of skin which vibrates only to oscillating waves of sound and which transmits its vibrations through the middle ear into electrical vibrations along the nerves and neurotransmitters. So likewise do our other pieces of skin, like tongue, nasal membranes, eye cells and touch cells, carry the stimulus and its response to a specific part of the brain. The senses carry the stimulus from the site of disturbance to the brain center where our consciousness is then oscillated or disturbed by its energy. It is remarkable that sound vibration has such a profound effect upon us, though its computer in the brain is only one percent as big as the occipital computer which handles our eyesight. Yet sound vibrates our deeper feelings as much as sight does: all the startling noises and inspiring rhythms that have so great an effect on our sense of hearing that they condition our whole response to life. When we listen to a Beethoven symphony or a solitary flute or when we catch the strains of an old familiar hymn pouring out from a church as we walk by, we respond from a depth of feeling that seems temporarily to overpower our other levels of consciousness. This is because the part of the brain that handles sound is so primordial that its power to move our emotions is tremendous, regardless of its size. In the same way the part of our brain which is geared to reptilian sensations covers much of our sensory skin sensations by which we sense the universe and yet is only six percent of our brain intelligence. The remainder of our brain is used in "making sense" of these signals and coordinating them into what we experience as more human functions.

The reptilian brain through evolution of millions of years has gradually receded into the protection of the skull and become differentiated into specific innate human responses common to the reptilian living habits, e.g., walking, swimming, crawling, swallowing, vomiting,

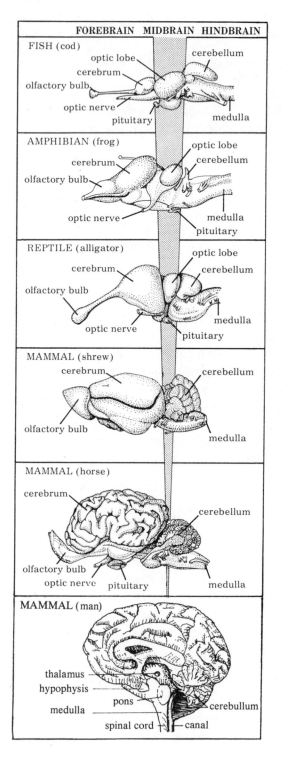

FOREBRAIN MIDBRAIN HINDBRAIN

FISH (cod)
- optic lobe
- cerebrum
- olfactory bulb
- optic nerve
- pituitary
- cerebellum
- medulla

AMPHIBIAN (frog)
- cerebrum
- olfactory bulb
- optic nerve
- optic lobe
- cerebellum
- medulla
- pituitary

REPTILE (alligator)
- cerebrum
- olfactory bulb
- optic nerve
- optic lobe
- cerebellum
- medulla
- pituitary

MAMMAL (shrew)
- cerebrum
- olfactory bulb
- cerebellum
- medulla

MAMMAL (horse)
- cerebrum
- olfactory bulb
- optic nerve
- pituitary
- cerebellum
- medulla

MAMMAL (man)
- thalamus
- hypophysis
- medulla
- pons
- spinal cord
- cerebullum
- canal

The more the organism needs to utilize a level of consciousness the more that particular brain is developed. Animals use the different levels in primitive ways. Only humans have the capacity to manifest the full potential of a higher level of consciousness with their more developed brain equipment. The development of each level enriches and refines the expression of the levels below it.

The Mid-brain has shrunk in proportion to other functions as creatures have evolved higher capacities and gone beyond purely emotional responses. Each animal devotes a large part of its brain to its most used biological functions; for example, the brain areas devoted to the whiskers in a rat are larger in proportion to other areas. Brain function expands by growing more brain cells in the areas of greatest stimulation.

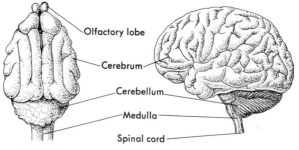

Olfactory lobe
Cerebrum
Cerebellum
Medulla
Spinal cord

MAMMAL   MAN

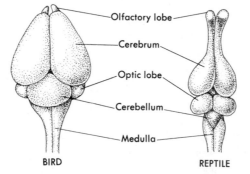

Olfactory lobe
Cerebrum
Optic lobe
Cerebellum
Medulla

BIRD   REPTILE

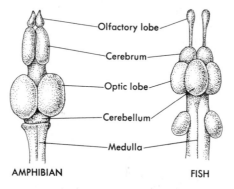

Olfactory lobe
Cerebrum
Optic lobe
Cerebellum
Medulla

AMPHIBIAN   FISH

The comparative structure of vertebrate brains and detailed structure of the human brain. Note the relative sizes of the Cerebrum in the different vertebrate classes. An increase in the size of the Cerebrum in proportion to the rest of the brain corresponds to an increased ability to learn. Other areas of the brain include the Cerebellum, which coordinates muscular activity; the Medulla, which relays messages to and from the spinal cord and controls visceral functions; Optic Lobes, which integrate visual inputs; Olfactory Lobes, which determine the sense of smell; the thalamus, which integrates sensory inputs; and the hypothalamus, which regulates emotions, sensations, and many visceral functions.

breathing, speech or tongue control and basic voice box (croaking), digestion, metabolism, beating of the heart, etc., all of which are controlled by the Medulla and its associated cranial nerves and the total nervous system. A reptile, when you look at it, doesn't seem to

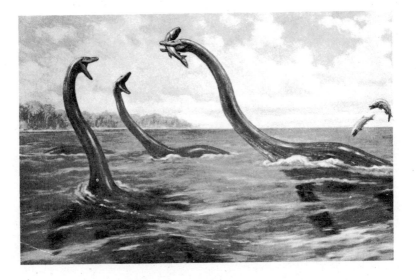

have any emotions; it is purely reacting to stimuli. You can even move as if to hit one of them and it doesn't move because it doesn't have fear; it doesn't have those built-in associative responses, whereas a human would think, "Hey, that guy with a stick is going to hit me, so I am going to run." The later mammalian brain has that fear and emotion but not the reptile. If you hit a lizard once, the next time it will move *before* you hit it, because it is educated by pain, but this is avoidance, a stimulus reaction to pain, whereas birds and dogs have developed as far as the third brain (as you can see in pictures of their skull formation) and they feel not just avoidance like other animals, but fear, as humans feel. Birds and dogs actually live with fear even when no predator is there. This is a survival mechanism very different from the stimulus-response survival mechanism of the first brain.

All higher animals have emotions which they store in the second level of the brain, but the reptilian brain is that part of our sensory mechanism of the brain which determines what part of our body will respond to direct sensory stimuli. In other words, we have to get hit before we feel it. We do not feel a ray of light yesterday, tomorrow or this evening but only at this instant. Only after the event can we reflect on it. The memory latent in the nerve cell in this part of our cerebrospinal system of sensations is fully automatic, with its own built-in primitive intelligence which is highly reactive to sensory inputs. Cells, nerves leading through the Medulla into the brain, and the brain dendrites generally, are all part of this system and are all sensitive to this primordial reptilian level of consciousness.

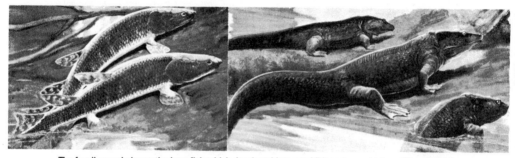

The fossil record shows the lung fish which developed into amphibians from which reptiles and birds have evolved. One species of reptile possessed feathers and wings. The aquatic ancestors of mammals and birds were eventually replaced by the age of terrestrial animals.

The time framework of these sensors, including the whole skin and its peripheral system of nerves as a single organ, is *NOW*—the immediate now of all sensations. This corresponds to the "red level" of society in Nuclear Evolution, i.e., the active and reactive sensations of non-thinking people. *Most people are more developed in this part of their brain than in any other part. They respond to life as reptiles.* They are at the mercy of each new stimulus so that soon the day is shattered into a thousand fragments and they don't know where the time has gone. Any long term project, requiring commitment to slow steady work, is difficult for them, for they do not look ahead into the future to the fulfillment that in time will come. Red level people prefer to do some faster job whose results are visible in the now and then perhaps to lie and bake upon a flat rock by the ocean, enjoying their senses like a reptile in the sun.

Yogis attempt to gain conscious control over this primitive auto-nomic nervous system by self-suggestion and meditation, using self-hypnosis to bring about mastery over the senses and over other functions of the brain. Thus yogis have the ability to stop the flow of blood on command, to speed up or stop the heart, or to control the release of neurotransmitters and go into suspended animation for several days. I learned all these techniques during my two years in India as a yogi, but I also learned that the voluntary control of involuntary processes does not require any evolution of consciousness and can be learned by anyone prepared to learn self-hypnosis. Much more signifi-cant is the fact that yogic education and training of the entire memory of cell life and nerve reactions can modify the synthesis of DNA in the nucleus of each nerve cell and change the normal metabolism of ordinary cells to become sensitive to color and light and even to thought waves. Many animals can sense radiations which man cannot, because man has subdued this sensitivity in the course of his long evolutionary journey. A much higher form of yoga than the mastery of involuntary processes is the reawakening of these inherent sensibilities at a higher level of functioning than occurs in the animal kingdom. You can shut off or control your involuntary processes and still not expand your awareness. But to develop your natural sensitivities with higher yogic methods of training so that they emerge on a higher non-sensory octave of consciousness lifts the human state to cosmic awareness.

Each step in evolution modifies the previous step so that we do not expect man's reptilian brain to be actually performing the functions of the dinosaur or having the sensations of reptiles. But in human aggression we can see a reflection of the stimulus-response reactiveness which evolved as a survival mechanism in our reptile ancestors. The very fact that many first brain functions have remained automatic and are not normally under conscious control is one reason why most people have failed to evolve their conscious awareness above the level of the first brain. Most of the human race is red level and responds to life in terms of a physical, sensory, material reality. Even the simple yellow level ability to plan ahead and be systematic is surprisingly rare, when you really begin to observe people more closely.

Like the powerful response to sound, which is preserved in the primitive functioning of the first brain, so too our emotional response to any stimulus that comes through our senses has a power that completely swamps the clarity and logic of the head. When a person shuts off these feelings and speaks only from the head, he seems dead and dry, as if cut off from his own roots. So the first brain is the source of our most powerful negative destructive energy, but it is also the positive source of our vitality. Therefore the task of a modern-day yogi is not to master his heartbeat but to master his heart. Though many try to reach the highest functions of the brain by leaving the first level of consciousness behind, the true yogi *channels* the primitive power of his life force through all the seven brains and becomes like the deeply rooted tree, whose sap greens the leaves even on its highest branches.

THE SECOND BRAIN

The Pons
The Fourth Ventricle

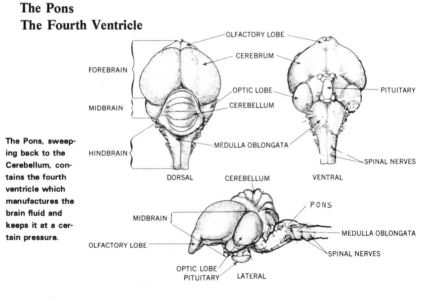

The Pons, sweeping back to the Cerebellum, contains the fourth ventricle which manufactures the brain fluid and keeps it at a certain pressure.

BRAIN OF A PIGEON

The early mammal or paleo-mammalian brain of birds and animals is tuned to the storage of experiences which extend beyond the immediate skin sensations of the first brain into the social dimension of our physical environment. In other words, the self-sense or identity is expanded beyond the skin to include others. A reptile sitting in the sun feels a physical sensation which triggers feelings of well-being but he has not much social life, whereas a beaver has a family life, keeps house, relates to other beavers socially and even has a language of communication. The Pons is that part of our brain which began to infold and become protected as the next most primitive part of the structure of the base of the skull, immediately above the Medulla Oblongata above the spinal column at the end of the spinal cord. It is the part of our brain which gives us a more refined memory than immediate physical sensation and makes us act together with a response similar to the herd instinct of most mammals.

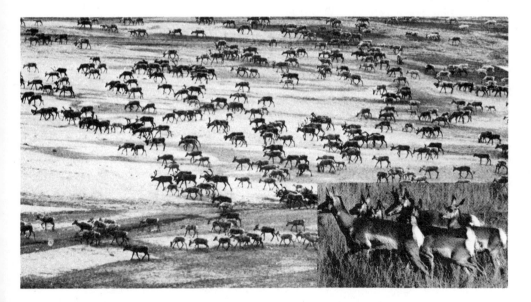

The flocking of sheep or birds, the instinctual herding and seeking of group protection which animals display, is governed by that part of the brain which gives unconscious orders to other parts of ourselves: the muscular movement, skill in using tools and instruments, and skill in using the sense organs, such as hearing which extend our sensations out into the environment beyond the skin to contact other members of the species. This second stage of brain development corresponds to the orange level of consciousness in Nuclear Evolution, the urge to be sociable.

One can call it a "social instinct" which makes man into a cooperating species. Social class arrangements exist in the *pecking order* of most animals, birds, and insects, and these same patterns are seen in the more complex society of humans because humans have primitive instinctual biological drives towards grouping on which they build a complex behavior pattern. Social grouping is universal among humans; therefore it follows that it is not culturally acquired as learned behavior as some psychologists claim. Why does it matter if social grouping is learned or is an instinct? If it is only learned, then it is arbitrary and not a deep-rooted part of our nature. But if it is instinctual, then it is one of the deep drives which requires effort and costs us much struggle to master. Only man, of all the species, has the capacity to become master of such a drive.

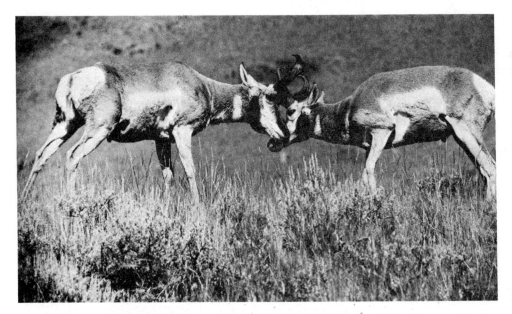

Animals show similar patterns of dominance, aggression and submissive behavior to those of humans at the second level of brain function.

In ancient times the similarity of man to animals became the cornerstone of many a philosophical theory. The modern behaviorists seem to feel that demonstrating this similarity is an end in itself. My purpose in setting out the basic outlines of Nuclear Evolution is neither to play up the link between man and animals nor to play it down. These links between general behavior patterns are not fixed realities but vary with the way a person perceives the universe. Any person can make the link stronger or weaker, depending upon how he sees himself. If he realizes that his feelings are coming from a level of his consciousness whose roots lie deep in prehistoric time, then he can dis-identify with them and in the space of a moment be feeling something totally different. If we begin to identify with seven levels of consciousness, rather than one or two, we begin to see our limits and see how to remove them. The second brain, for example, governs our relating with each other, but it does not govern the sensitive heart feelings between us nor the higher motives for our gathering together. Do people go to church from orange level motives? Or do they go with the worshipful impulse of the higher levels of consciousness?

Each level has positive and negative expression, so it is a mistake to compare them and to criticize ourselves for lower brain functions which in their right context are positive. Yet the limits of each level are only visible from the other levels and, in this sense, comparison is helpful. For example, the time-framework of the red level consciousness, reacting to the pressures of the moment, becomes very clear to someone acting from the second brain. The time frame of the second brain is the action of the immediate now put off to the future time of all interspecies action in the environment—the future-orientated "now". The reason action is put off and cannot happen "now" as in the previous Red level of organization is because in social contact, decisions to act are all held up pending the decisions and actions of others who all have independent wills, minds, sensations, etc. This is the well-known delay in politics and in all social action which is put off until tomorrow.

It is always difficult for people to see the connections between complex social function and the primitive survival instincts of our second brain. It is perhaps easier to visualize its function if it were suddenly taken away or that part of our brain were damaged. Lacking this second drive mankind would not congregate in groups, churches, or parties. Cattle would not herd together, birds would not flock together or fly in formation. The birds who fly together do so at first for survival and safety, but later they begin to develop bonds and loyalties among them. And so it is with humans, too. Though we may seem to come together because of a wish to form bonds, this really is a refinement of a more fundamental primitive drive in us with which we are out of touch. At a primitive level of survival the coming together of each species in groups is as necessary as eating food. Without an instinct for seeking the company of like species, the animal and insect world would not propagate effectively and the skin to skin contact in the sexual instinct of the first brain would be largely a hit or miss affair. In the civilized world all dangerous animals are kept in cages, so we are out of touch with our second brain drive to huddle together for safety, but if we were all alone in a jungle full of tigers, every snap of a twig would awaken in us this drive to survive and this fear of other species. Having gained some mastery of the environment, we have transferred this fear to our own species, and the modern version of this primitive emotion is a paranoid response to anyone who is different from ourselves. But if a wild gorilla were walking down our street, we would suddenly not mind that others were different and would join them against the common foe. This is why war propaganda is so successful in uniting a society into some feeling of oneness, because the banding of creatures against a common foe lies deep in our evolutionary past. The size of the group we are willing to expand our ego to identify with is directly proportional to the size of the threat. A national assault requires us to respond as a united nation. Otherwise, we might be content just to be part of a club or several clubs or to be "in" with a certain social group in one small town.

Whatever the size of your frame of reference, whatever the background against which you define yourself, the fear of not being "in" is very real. There is the fear that others are getting something that you are not getting, the feeling of missing out, the feeling of inadequacy from living in a competitive society. There is the need for confirmation and approval from others, the need to be accepted and to belong. Acceptance gratifies *pride* which is a basic psychological attribute of the orange level. Pride's need to be accepted by others is different from the internal confirmation we get from knowledge, possessions, money or any kind of security which is for our own *self*-confirmation. Being accepted by others may not depend on knowledge or resources of any kind but simply on conformity. People accept whoever is like themselves and whoever accepts *them* for the same reason. And this is why the state of society at this moment mirrors to us our deepest fear of all and the fear which most drives us to want to be accepted just as we are. This is the fear of looking at ourselves, assessing our bad qualities, and making up our minds to change them. Running from this frightening possibility makes people afraid to risk an encounter with anyone different, whose very existence might possibly raise questions about a better way to be or to live. By running away from ourselves in this way, we also run away from society and disown responsibility for it. Hence the condition of social impotence springs from the very same primitive fears that originally prompted us to join with others and form society.

However, our motive was not solely to survive but also was a reaching out, an extending of our boundaries outward from the skin into the environment. The negative impulse of fear has a positive counterpart in the second brain which is the urge to bond with others. This positive social consciousness is also found in the permanently programmed social responses of insects and even in groups of certain sensitive atoms which have learned a definite choice in the kind of atomic groups which they will interact with, bond with, etc. Many modern physicists have invented various atomic qualities such as charm, color, etc. to account for these very real properties of atomic interaction. These attributes are not felt consciously by the atoms but more in the way that humans would feel about the social vibrations of a certain person when he or she came into their presence. Something tells us to switch off or on at a very primitive gut level of interaction. We can call this a second sense but it is more akin to liking or not liking. We can call it love of fellowman (or the opposite, adverse reaction) and this love of contact with our own species is reflected in all other organisms of Nature. What keeps the brain linked together as an organism? Instinctual and very primordial is the chemistry and love of fellow atom. How is it that an atom, which has no brain as such, has social responses common to the second brain? The answer is very simple when you realize that the seven thresholds of consciousness exist throughout the nucleus of life and thus are available to every part of creation, from atom to galaxy. Only through evolving vehicles for consciousness can Nature fully express these levels.

The level of consciousness of the second part of the brain, when it is underdeveloped, is responsible for lack of social feeling, for exploitation of fellowman, enslaving of others, cruelty to other animal species and groups of animals. In factory farming or feeding lots, animals and chickens are subjected to terrible confining quarters. We have other good examples in the senseless killing of dolphins in tuna nets and the inability to feel for the plight of political prisoners.

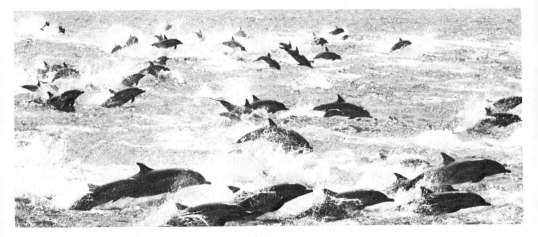

Those who have access to levels six and seven are able to get inside other people and feel what they are experiencing or to project what is going to happen to people or to creatures in the future, whereas red level persons must wait until the events are actually happening and, even then, are not likely to feel what anyone but themselves must be feeling. The orange level "feel" for others is not this quality of empathy or identification as though the other were oneself but rather is a sense of connectedness or concern for "another" the way we feel about members of our family or about our countrymen. This is not so much an identification through feeling as an identity by association. Orange level people can be selfish and uncaring, just as any people can, but the red level of consciousness is more prone than any other to think of people unfeelingly because they relate to people as sensory objects and they have not yet developed the orange level concern that is at least willing to reach out and acknowledge the being of another.

Those who function mainly from the red level look at people merely as cyphers or numbers which are "out there" somewhere in an abstract thing called society. The red level, action-orientated terrorists that throw a bomb into a crowded restaurant or hold a hijacked plane full of children as hostages to further their cause are people whose brains are stunted and unable to see society as anything more than something to exploit. There is no social feeling among red communists about conditions in the prison camps of Siberia. Nor did the action-orientated Nazis feel much for the deliberate genocide of millions of Jews. Likewise the Chinese communists have little feeling for Tibetans, and Cambodian communists have no respect for human feelings in the so-called red social revolutions which are enforced from above and are not real revolutions by the people at all.

The love of fellowman when fully developed in a Christ or Ghandi does not function from the second brain orange level herd instinct alone but does utilize and develop the stunted remnant of this second part of the brain in conjunction with the higher and later parts to generate the awareness of what the Hindu religion calls "Ahimsa" or non-hurting of others and other species. In the Western nations the herd instinct has usually been negatively used for gathering together in armies, whereas in the past in the East, the social instinct has been channeled into social and religious tradition. However, we must look at the brutality and harming of others and of other species that still occurs side by side with all the religious traditions in underdeveloped countries everywhere, then ask ourselves if this traditional training of oneness and union is impractical and idealistic or whether it had survival value. *Have we learned yet that to destroy others will eventually generate those forces of aggression which will destroy us?* This is the wisdom of

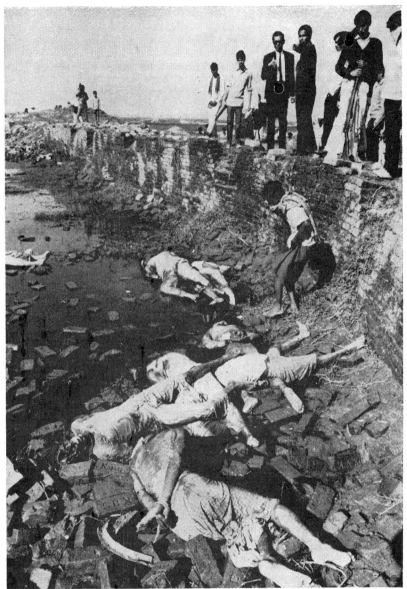

Abbas—Jocelyne Benzakin

Slain Bengali intellectuals: "The whole nation is a mass grave" caused by action-orientated red level and negative social orange types who wiped out a whole social group.

the second brain—that together we survive; divided we fall. In union there is strength; in separation we are the food of dictatorships.

Why should Nature in her infinite wisdom make the social instinct come second in the evolution of the brain? Her most fundamental survival mechanism is the mating instinct of the first level, which insures physical reproduction of the species. At the level of the second brain, organisms relate to each other not only for mating but for higher purposes of communication such as group survival. And yet we cannot really get a total picture of the evolutionary process if we look only at the initial impulse. If we look at the end result as well, we see that Nature's habit is to gather parts together to make wholes. Though the first impulse for grouping may be to mate or to physically survive, the social drive then begins to refine itself through time into more subtle dimensions of consciousness. Man masters his environment in groups but his communication within the group is not only for the purpose of mastering the environment or doing business. His drive to belong is for the safety of being part of the herd, but he also has the desire to communicate and to relate and to build bonds that are capable of transcending the desire to personally survive. The Japanese kamikaze pilots made a religious ceremony out of group survival at the expense of their own personal lives, not that this was Nature's purpose that people should commit suicide for a merely partisan cause. The second stage of brain evolution was necessary as a foundation for that ultimate transcendence of the physical world in which we enter into oneness with the entire universe. It begins with the innate drive to contact and relate to others like ourselves, then broadens until all things are seen as ourselves and the survival of the whole is as important to us as survival of the part.

There was an ethos in World War II where fighting for society and for peace made one a hero. World War II was the end of an era where pride in battle and courage in fighting were considered a social virtue rewarded by the highest medal of honor—in Britain the Victoria Cross, in France the Legion of Honor, in Germany the Iron Cross, in America the Congressional Medal of Honor. Hidden in the social drive of the kamikaze pilot, whose highest honor was to die for society, is a fundamental social instinct that is analogous to throwing a bottle in the ocean when you are stranded on a desert island. You have no idea where the bottle will go but in your drive to survive you reach out to the world. Hidden in the depths of the second brain is the desire to do something now that you yourself will never see the results of, to plant an acorn that will not in your lifetime become a full grown oak, or a desire to preserve forests for future generations who will live on when you are gone. This instinct to survive through posterity is the positive and expansive quality that came with the development of the second brain. It can be felt at a low level in a very personal way, as when one desires an heir to carry on the family name or the family business, or it can be a very lofty trait of human beings, depending on how pure is the consciousness that is flowing through the second brain.

THE THIRD LEVEL BRAIN

The Neo-mammalian development of the Cerebellum

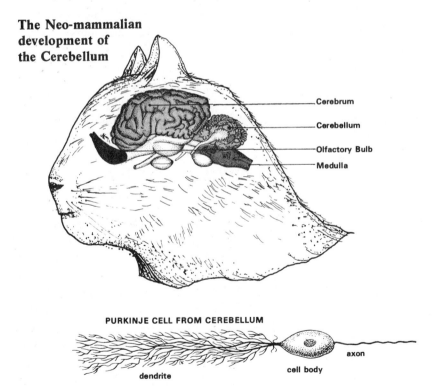

Cerebrum

Cerebellum

Olfactory Bulb

Medulla

PURKINJE CELL FROM CEREBELLUM

axon

cell body

dendrite

The next level of organization leading to the development of the third brain is found in the ability of organisms, insects, animals and man to adapt to *change*. Great changes took place in the environment from the times when great lizards roamed the earth and climbed out of the primeval waters to adapt themselves to new food supplies and the land. To adapt we must have an organ of comparison. An organism must be able to weigh choices and make decisions. We know when a thing is heavy or light by balancing weights in each hand and feeling the resistance in the muscles of our arms. Something in our consciousness is able to gauge the differences and to discriminate similarities. This faculty enabled us to adapt to different environments and also to form some comparative knowledge of our social life over millions of years of evolution. As the need for this faculty became greater, the new brain developed which could make discriminating choices between either/or, hot or cold, long or short and be able to arrange for ordered sequences of behavior, rather than merely responding to stimuli or social pressures at random. In short, we evolved the ability to think at a certain level and thereby expect a chain of events. The faculty which allows man to adapt is his ability to progress events forward in time, based on what has already happened or what is happening now. The faculty of expectation or anticipation and the beginnings of reasoned actions and adaptation to situations brought forth the development of the Cerebellum.

The ancient world was not such a stable place as we have now in modern civilization, and the threats, opportunities, changes and problems of living were frequently catastrophic rather than idyllic. A quick response and a healthy doubt were necessary, not only for survival but also in testing and comparing everything in the environment which every animal or bird must do in order to make sure it is not being deceived by events. The Cerebellum is built directly on to the Medulla and Pons and is situated immediately below the occipital lobes of the Cerebrum with its greatest diameter being about three and one half inches. It is a miniature brain in itself, containing grey and white matter. The alternation of grey and white matter gives this brain, for the first time, a new capacity. The Cerebellum is the first of all the brains to think in terms of opposites—light and dark, soft and hard, hot and cold, heavy and light, thick and thin—expressed in the ancient Chinese divination symbol of yin and yang.

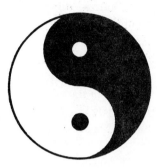

The Neo-mammalian memory is represented by the Cerebellum area and contains all our lower emotional responses situated below the Mid-brain. Rich in cells and with complex connections with the brain above and the spinal cord below, the Cerebellum governs the coordination of all lower functions including special acts concerned with range, direction, rate of force of movement and the synchronization of physical organs. This part of the brain has the capacity for analysis and comparison so that whenever we have an experience which it is able to compare, it can randomly scan the lower brains and pick out sensory information and emotional responses, because this brain is situated in such a way that it can use the two lower brains at the same time.

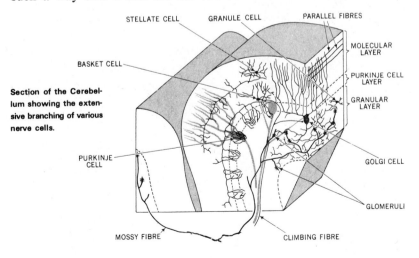

Section of the Cerebellum showing the extensive branching of various nerve cells.

STELLATE CELL GRANULE CELL PARALLEL FIBRES

MOLECULAR LAYER

BASKET CELL

PURKINJE CELL LAYER

GRANULAR LAYER

PURKINJE CELL

GOLGI CELL

GLOMERULI

MOSSY FIBRE CLIMBING FIBRE

This third part of the brain is what makes an intellectual. It makes us able to use all the logical and comparative sequential methods of analysis and to compare, contrast, differentiate and organize. Like a hunting mechanism searching for a slot, it sets its computers working and comparing, just like a juke box arm. Out goes the arm and pulls out the record and plays your favorite tune. You identify so strongly with your mental storehouse of records and with this juke box mechanism that you are always caught up in its automatic workings (especially if you are an intellectual), and you do not get a moment to see what or who you really are behind all that comparing and scanning activity.

This intellectual level of consciousness is represented by the color yellow in Nuclear Evolution theory. It is linear in its functions, operates like a computer and can scan, categorize and select because this part of the brain is cross-referenced and coded with all the signals

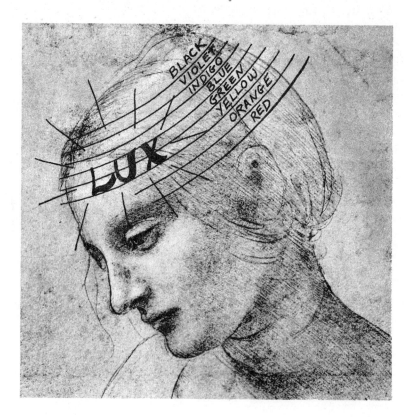

entering into the first two brains. It can be used in the service of the brain's higher faculties, which were added at a later time in evolution, or it can remain cut off from them as nothing more than a hunting mechanism, used to rationalize any number of random actions and experiences from the lower two brains. Without imagination, one of the faculties that was added much later in brain evolution, this intellectual function is terribly dull. In an evolved person however, the intellect becomes very sharp because it links with superior reasoning. Hence it was quite possible for the dull-minded doctors and scholars of the Inquisition to rationalize tortures of men and women in the name of Christ and to justify their actions to the glory of God. In the same way today, millions are liquidated by completely ruthless intellectuals who have no feelings or sensibilities above this level. Their emotions do not touch the heart but only reach the primitive instinctive feelings of animal and human life: fear, flight, survival, rage, parental affection, and a sense of everything being in its right place (the sense of logical order).

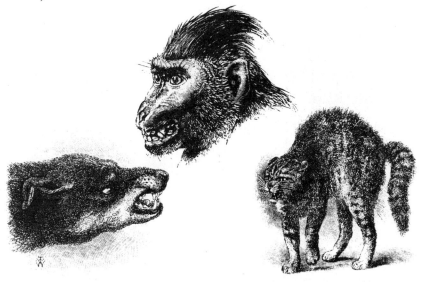

Darwin was a first class artist and sketched these animals in their natural reaction to threats. The display of these same emotions in humans is covered up by the higher Mid-brain functions of emotional control above this third level of reaction.

When this linear sense of order is not subject to any wider external logic or when it lacks that environmental confirmation from Nature or from other people which gives us empirical testing of experience, it will lead an animal to subjective and arrogant estimates of reality which often bear no relation to fact. An animal or human will then be totally dependent on its own estimate of reality from its own theory or assumptions. This causes limited perception because we can then only arrive at a self-centered validation. Without the operation of the higher brain centers there is a cut-off feeling of separation from the environment. This may be the origin of schizophrenia which occurs when the Mid-brain and Inter-brain situated above the three lower brains cannot secrete the peptides or endorphins—the chemicals which relate the self-sense to our basic sensory experience. This intellectual third brain is that which makes us feel separate from the universe we live in and is therefore the seat of the ego or the self-sense and the beginning of that simple self-consciousness which separates itself from the whole. It is also found to exist in some of the higher animals and of course in all normal humans. Like the eye which evolved to greater specialization at the expense of the lizard's pineal kind of seeing, this third level, specialized area of the brain costs us that feeling of being *at-one*.

Depending on how strongly we identify with the workings of any part of the brain, we are free to use this intellectual faculty and its special advantages without being bound by its weak points. The impact of intellectuals upon society, both for good and for evil, is clear to see. Behind every revolution and every bloodbath in history you will find the intellectuals spinning their web of theory. Only when we see how these different levels of the brain, each rooted in a unique portion of evolutionary history, shape our reality, only then can we stop identifying with the lower levels of our inner third world and begin to create from the nuclear center of our being.

THE FOURTH BRAIN

The Mid-brain
hypothalamus
thalamus
floor of the Inter-brain

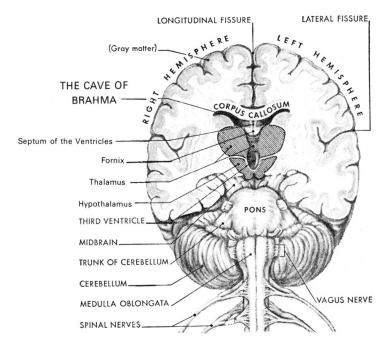

It is in the fourth brain that we can best see the close correlation between consciousness and matter, because the secretion of hormones in this brain creates the emotions we most identify as "me". Just above the Mid-brain there are important nuclei concerned with the regulation of body temperature, metabolism, sexual development, sleep, endocrine secretions and their effect on the nervous system and personality. *Our whole character can be changed by hormone exchange.* Therefore our evolution or stagnation hinges very strongly upon this area of the Mid-brain and its control over our fluctuating identity.

It is interesting to observe the rationale of evolutionists who claim that adaptation to environmental conditions is the cause of all evolutionary change on the biological level. The influence of the *internal* environment of a human being is so much stronger emotionally and even physically than the external environment, yet most evolutionists do not believe that mutants or adaptations in cell life ever spring from the pressures of internal environments or from twisted thought processes. To watch the change in the body of a person which comes with a change of mood and attitude is to witness a remarkable effect on the physical structure of the human system.

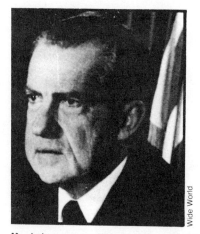
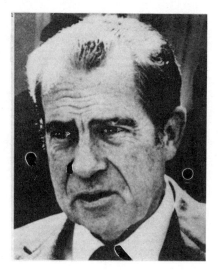

Mood changes are reflected in both body and face, as illustrated by pictures of Richard Nixon before and after the Presidency.

If we could visualize the effect on a body when it is saturated with hormones secreted by an endocrine gland and if we could realize that that body is actually sitting in a sea of chemicals throughout the entire internal environment, we would be aware that it must have just as much effect as if the person sat in these chemicals in the external conditions of life. Surely adaptation would take place in the evolutionary sense from the powerful chemicals secreted by fear, pleasure, sense of expectation, love, hunger, or hatred and anger. The wide range of human emotional expression, not possible to animals, begins to become possible in this fourth chronologically evolved part of the brain. A dog, too, has heart. It tries to talk and emote through its voice. But its maturity stops at the fourth brain.

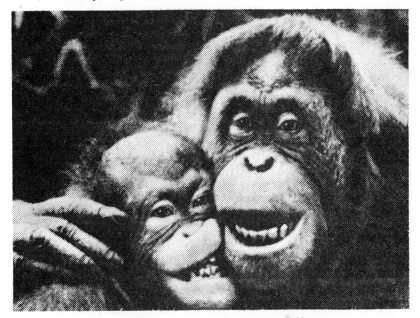

An ape, like a human, expresses his heart through his eyes.

So the fourth brain is only the beginning. Laughter and crying and other emotions are refined by the higher centers of the Cerebral Cortex but this fourth part of our brain is able to select and use these from many random experiences.

Expressed in terms of the chakra energies, you could say that the fourth brain regulates the energy or life-force which can only express in the chakras when they are "open". In an intellectual, for example, the energy may be directed almost entirely through the third brain, and only if something happened to prevent the intellect from its usual habits could it be *re*directed down into the first chakra and be experienced as physical vitality or sexual feeling or the energy to manifest something. Or it might be redirected upward into intuition and imagination which would greatly enrich the intellectuality.

The fourth brain controls the gateway to the higher functions of the brain which can supply the power to the higher centers or shut them off at will. The maintenance of consciousness in the waking state is dependent on brain level two, sometimes called the reticular formation. Without this basic power of life-force switched on, the powerful computers of the upper levels can only go into coma and unconsciousness. Stimulation of the top part of this area of our brain in level four can rudely awaken us from sleep, just as inactivity in this area brings on a lazy dazy hypnogogic state we call trance. Stimulation of its lower parts in level two will put us asleep and unconscious of the activity of the Cerebrum while we begin to dream. Sleep is triggered by the secretions of peptides and enkephalins which build up in the fifth level above and act downwards upon the fourth level below to trigger this unconscious gateway to the mind. In states of hypnosis or the twilight drowsiness that comes just before sleep, these peptides act upon the Mid-brain fourth level to shut out our conscious mind and transfer our activity to the higher regions of our brain.

Not everyone realizes that the conscious mind which we identify as ourself actually vanishes when we fall asleep and enter the world of the *un*conscious mind. We awaken refreshed the next morning because this nightly venture into the deeper part of ourselves is beneficial to us. But how can such a thing occur? How is it that the "I" which is at the forefront of our consciousness all day long could simply be swallowed up in an entirely different realm of awareness and then be reborn the next day and say "I am awake"? It is possible because the fourth brain, as I said, is able to switch off the lower computers and switch on the higher ones. And what causes the brain to do this? Our own consciousness which says, "Now it is time for sleep."

What makes the fourth brain a control center for the rest of the brain? Its central location between the three lower and the three higher levels makes the Mid-brain a kind of crossroads where our consciousness can choose whether to cling to the stability of its oldest and time-proven brain circuits or to push forward in the direction of its future evolution. The Mid-brain connects the Pons (level two) with the Inter-brain above it (level five) which links level four with the hemispheres. The Mid-brain of level four is continuous with the underside of the

Inter-brain and is joined with the optic thalamus which forms the floor of the third ventricle in the center of the Inter-brain. The ceiling of the Mid-brain is the floor of the Cave of Brahma or the third ventricle in the Inter-brain (level five).

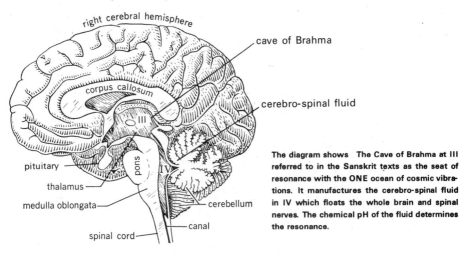

right cerebral hemisphere

cave of Brahma

corpus callosum

cerebro-spinal fluid

III

pituitary

pons

IV

thalamus

medulla oblongata

cerebellum

spinal cord

canal

The diagram shows The Cave of Brahma at III referred to in the Sanskrit texts as the seat of resonance with the ONE ocean of cosmic vibrations. It manufactures the cerebro-spinal fluid in IV which floats the whole brain and spinal nerves. The chemical pH of the fluid determines the resonance.

The Mid-brain is an important relay center for sensory impulses passing to the various computers surrounding the walls of the third ventricle. Because the Mid-brain is located exactly in between the higher and the lower brains, we feel it as the center of our being. In yoga the fourth level of consciousness is called the "heart center" and is a central focus for feelings coming from all other parts of the brain as well as the corresponding plexi in the lower nervous system where we "feel" our isness. Because of this the heart center is also the area where we feel threatened or confirmed in our being. Our feeling of possessiveness and our sense of lack, which are related to the storing up of vital forces in our body, all the feelings that have to do with insecurity and security, are controlled by this part of our brain.

This fourth part of the brain, also called the hypothalamus and thalamus, controls our use of fat and water. Fat stores the body's surplus oxygen, and water is the liquid crystal in which all the chemical reactions of the body take place. The storage of fat is directly related to our drive for energy or food or anything else that can make us feel secure and can fill the lacks that make us feel uncertain and unsure. People who eat food to fill the need for love are driven by this urge which proceeds from the thalamus (next to the hypothalamus).

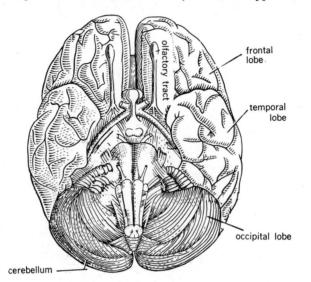

The floor of the Cave of Brahma is formed by the Mid-brain, a mass of white fibers rising from the Medulla and Pons and the Cerebellum, enclosed by a mass of grey matter called the reticular formation. These nerves then radiate to the optical thalamus and Cerebrum above through the structures of the fifth level Inter-brain above it. These channels of the fourth level emotions are controlled by the higher levels in the three domains above and the three below.

In Nuclear Evolution the Mid-brain corresponds to the fourth spectrum color, green, which relates to our release of secretions of brain peptides which takes place in the Inter-brain (level five). Green is symbolic of the stored up vital force. The time framework for our fourth level feelings is past, present and future since our feelings of insecurity respond to all three lower brains and go back and forth in time in a linear fashion very much like the third brain hunting for a slot. The third brain, arranging things in the logic of past, present, and future appears more mechanical, but really the fourth brain is just as much a computer even though it may not seem so because it is shifting in the realm of feelings. The difference between the shifting time worlds of the third level from the fourth level can be explained by an example we are all familiar with.

Let us say you fall in love. You want to possess the love object for yourself very much. The possessive feeling mounts to an obsessive desire. Even when the love object is away, the heart center (brain four) grows fonder and fonder of the missing love object. As long as you know he or she is still yours and there is no competition you feel reasonably secure and elated at being in love. But if you hear your loved one is seeing someone else or even if you see him or her look at someone else in a certain way you feel a threat to your well-being. Flutters of insecurity go up and down your solar plexus which controls level three, and a dull ache begins to accumulate on your sternum bone in the region of the heart. This love pain brings stress which creates emotional insecurity on all other levels of being, so that life begins to be very painful. In fact the pain of a bleeding heart far exceeds that of a bleeding body. At this time of threat, your time world suddenly shifts from the bliss of possessing the love object in the now and projects into the future which appears bleak at the thought of loss. All these bring a feeling of insecurity about the future and we begin to imagine what it would be like to live without our loved one. Ninety percent of all songs on the radio refer in some way either to this feeling of pain or to the instant bliss of possession.

Now supposing your loved one does more than just look at the attractions of other members of the species and actually leaves you. How do you feel? Besides having the energies of the psyche raised up to the heart center in times of insecurity they now sink like a lead weight into the stomach of depression. Appetite goes and you think of all the good times in the past. You hunt to find old photos, sentimental objects from the past. Your time world has shifted to the past, the future is nonexistent and the present is empty. You struggle to make the past become the present and even wish and hope for the past to come back again in the future but actually your whole time world is past. Love-sick for the one you love, your possessive drive aches in you, echoed by the songs on the radio, and you do not realize that ninety percent of the human race is like you, hurting like you, laying this possessive trip on themselves just like you. You believe you can't do without it. You would do anything to get the love object back again. You refuse to wash away your attachment and you wallow in self-imposed misery.

This example is true in varying degrees for anything loved, whether it is nuts for the squirrel who is putting away a stash for the winter, the possessive love of a mother bear for her cubs, or the thrill of money in the bank for the miser. If you collect knowledge, you will have many reference books and become like a walking encyclopedia full of opinions, both your own and others'. It will be difficult for you to lose any of this investment without feeling the same threats of uncertainty as the lover with his love object, for the heart center motivates us much more than we consciously know.* It is not difficult to see that most humans are impoverished in this area. Insecurity is the main spiritual problem, as well as the social problem of mankind. The fourth brain transfers its insecurity feelings to the entire body and all other parts of the brain because the fourth level at the center of all the brains is cross-referenced and wired to all other levels of our brain, both old and new parts which are all in a state of expectancy whenever we fall in love or become attached to anything. What would it tell us about ourselves if we realized that these kinds of feelings which, more than any other part of us, we take to be ourself, could be changed in an instant just by a simple stimulation of the brain?

The master gland of the sixth level intuition which dominates the lower fourth level Mid-brain and fifth level Inter-brain through secretions of endocrine chemical triggers acting upon emotions, causing aggression and fear, can bring about vast changes in the life of animals. Ferocious animals can become tame and tolerant, and meek animals can be stimulated into a rage by hyperstimulation of these areas. In human beings these effects can be viewed as madness.

The action of the hypothalamus on personality changes in humans can be seen by its power to control the pituitary gland at the front end of the Cave of Brahma. The hypothalamus sitting on the floor of the Cave is connected by a fine network of capillaries which pass polypeptides

---

* There is a great deal of evidence that the greed of capitalism and the possessive drive are related to level four, just as the desire for political power in communism is cultivated in the demand for social obedience to authority (level two). That both are compensations for lack of love is explained more fully in *Nuclear Evolution* pages 300-316.

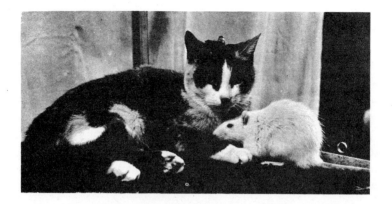

The yogi's control of electrical stimulations to the Cerebrum is duplicated in the cat in the photograph by an electrical stimulus so that the cat peacefully ignores its normal prey. The same cat, electrically stimulated in the hypothalamus is put into a rage by the laboratory assistant who, as soon as the stimulus is removed, is best friend. Similarly, conscious control of hormone release at the hypothalamus can create bliss or anger at will. This is one level of self-mastery for the yogi.

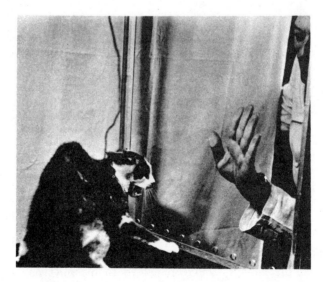

HOW REAL ARE THE EMOTIONS WE IDENTIFY AS "ME"?

(neurotransmitters) which command the unconscious centers of the nervous system which regulate temperature, emotions, sleep, fear, rage and bliss. The social effects of a disorder of the hypothalamus can be seen in the decisions made by Napoleon. His sleepiness, epilepsy, and alterations of sexual characteristics affected the course of history. Below we see Napoleon as a young man. He was thin and active; he looked upon sleeping as a waste of time and slept only four hours a day. His eyes were piercing and his manner commanding. By age forty, his appearance had changed and he became flabby and soft and feminine, needed much more sleep and often slept during battles. He

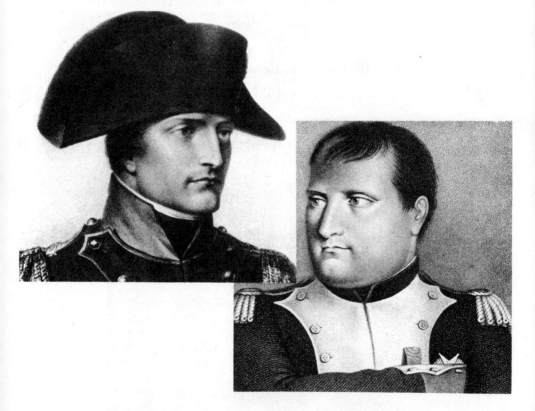

had fits of crying and fury and lacked any sexual desire. He himself observed the changes and commented to his physician on his full rounded breasts and smooth lily-white hairless skin. His decisions at Moscow in his 1812 retreat and his later hesitation in attacking at

Dresden and Waterloo while he slept in a chair were typical of an impaired hypothalmic function. The social impact on the French Empire of his defeat might have been far different if he could have received treatment for the hypothalamus malfunction which affected his personality.

Imagine a whole nation or race afflicted genetically by such a deficiency and such changes. The type of society we foster and encourage depends more than we realize upon the activation of the neurotransmitters which control these glandular secretions, and this need not be done artificially or at great expense through medical treatments. Our own consciousness, when properly directed, can control the action of the hypothalamus from the higher centers of the brain. A yogi can change his feelings just by concentrating his consciousness intensely enough to create opposite waves to counterbalance and thus annihilate the particular vibration he is feeling. What would happen to the vibration of a society if a number of its citizens were able to change their hostilities to feelings of bliss and peace and oneness?

I am mentioning such a possibility not as a "what if" but as a very live possibility. Yet we cannot hope to gain such mastery in society without thoroughly understanding what our conflicting feelings are and where they come from and how they operate. We may be feeling red level aggression but the real motive for it may be green level insecurity. Our orange level drive to belong to our peer group at any cost to our own inborn uniqueness may stem from insecurity, but at the same time our insecurity about money or power or fame may also come from the orange level need to belong and be accepted. Our feelings do not stair-step neatly up from high to low but affect each other by overlapping positive and negative vibration cascading from level to level, by virtue of this central relay station called "the heart".

The process is not a linear one but a circular one (a feedback loop) which comes through the filter of the thalamus in the roof of the Mid-brain that forms the floor of the "Cave of Brahma". The control of our feelings of security and well-being in the thalamus center are polarized with our emotional fear and anger in the hypothalamus. This control at the level of the fourth brain is determined by our thought life and the choices we make on the next level, level five, where higher ideals overwhelm the primitive threat to our emotional security and cause us to choose the outwardly less hostile response to threat even though inwardly we are feeling like murder. Often people are not in touch with the violent feelings they have repressed, and they believe their own mask or self-image. Conscious control, which comes from the higher levels, is a different thing from repression.

The primitive emotional response is a chemical phenomenon and is controlled by the thalamus by the process of inhibition or feedback as in the typical negative green reaction when our chosen mate goes off with someone else. Instead of outright aggression and anger, as on the red level, we find at the fourth level the repressed feeling of jealousy and sense of loss. Most people fear hostility and automatically inhibit their anger because they know the consequences will generate anger and hostility from others, but when this controlling inhibition is removed, the hatred and resentment from the fourth level is released as anger on level one. Rarely does the energy from level one fuel the negative feelings of level four. Usually it is the other way around. Even though you may be punching someone in the nose or throwing pottery and bric-a-brac, the motivating energy may well be coming, not from the red level at all, but from the green or from some other level of consciousness.

Each level has its own type of feeling. One can feel insecure at any level, yet the fourth brain's feeling of insecurity is unique to itself. Since all the feelings are controlled in this fourth level brain computer which acts like a central intelligence agency for the chemical emotions and the world of feeling, it is hard to see the differences and trace their origins.

Feeling at the red level is an immediate skin level reaction in the immediate moment, behind which there is no thought or inhibitory process from the higher levels of the brain. Feeling on the orange level is an urge to extend ourselves outwards towards our fellowmen, and likewise with other species towards their own breed. This feeling, which manifests as the second level herd instinct, comes because of a need to feel secure in the environment. Third level emotion is a gut feeling which comes from ordering things in a familiar pattern or logical sequence. This need to have things straight and sorted out gives us a feeling of security at the mental level, a feeling that we live in an orderly universe and that the activities of our brain are rational and not random. The fourth level which we are describing now is a totally different kind of emotion that people feel when they fall in love or get crossed in love or feel the lack of love altogether. This affects our feeling of security at a deeper level of the heart. The part of our brain which handles this is superimposed on the lower levels below it and any one of those levels which causes a positive or negative response can influence the fourth level of the heart causing it to feel wanted or unwanted, confident or rejected, secure or insecure, possessive or satisfied.

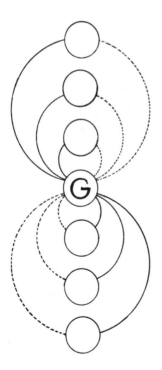

Other things are happening at each level besides insecurity, but this shows how insecurity on all the levels is concentrated in our feeling of self-worth or self-negation. Each emotion at the lower levels is passed through the higher central function of the fourth level. Similarly the emotions from the higher levels are also passed down through the green level which sits at a neutral point in the middle of the spectrum of all the seven brain functions with three below it and three above, all contributing in a circular loop which makes us just feel one piece, since our heart is unable to separate where these feelings are coming from or how they get processed by these different filters behind which we live. When a person thinks, "I am feeling this or that" he is unable to unravel the complexity of his feelings. And many people have only a vague feeling even of the cause of their insecurity, not realizing that the seven-tiered brain not only handles each function separately but also funnels them to the central computer which mixes them all up together, giving us the impression that I am just "me". It is only when we come to study ourselves deeply and to research human nature and the structure of consciousness itself that we obtain a glimpse into the fantastic complexity of our brain. Many experiments have to be done in life in order to arrive at this knowledge. It may take some people many incarnations to get any clarity and to really know themselves.

Even scientists, noted for their objectivity, are highly reactive when threatened in their weak spots or poked in their ego. To watch them react inside while trying to keep a calm and reposed face or mask is an education in keen observation. Most scientists are gut level reactors to anything which does not fit their yellow level drive for pattern and logic, and they go completely to pieces when threatened on any other level.* Their usual defense is to pretend they have no feelings at all about the subject in question. So psychic phenomena on the sixth level, for example, draw an immediate denial. Spiritual experience on the fifth level feels more comfortable without devotion to a God but is perfectly alright when the devotion is towards the scientific method. Such people usually pretend they have no feelings or subjectivity until they fall in love. And then they act very much like any other lower being with the usual jealousies, hidden resentments, anger, frustration, and all the other qualities they dislike in ordinary mortals. Since science is a learned behavior, we find underneath the scientist's acquired veneer the same stupid animal that is evolving into a higher being. But scientists are not alone in this. Any human being with an ego is capable of being unsettled when you make him look at himself beyond the perimeters of his self-image. And in this sense the only real security for anyone is to get beyond the ego altogether. Otherwise there is only a partial security and a partial strength. For example, people who feel secure in their devotion on the fifth level and even secure on the fourth level of being in love, can be visibly disturbed by the cutting power of the yellow level intellectual logic, which tends to ride roughshod over feelings. Each level is capable not only of disturbing the other but of transmitting that disturbance to the centers which make the ego and the heart churn. Thus the heart center is a central focus of our feeling of *being,* rather than our thinking or sensing or socializing which occur on the lower three levels.

---

* For correlation of brain development to colors and levels of consciousness see Chapters 11 and 13.

The Darwinian theory of survival of the fittest was limited just to the physical level—the fear of physical domination, expressed in societies competing for the goods of life—but insecurity seizes us in many other areas than our physical needs, and competition is not removed from the heart level until the higher three levels are understood and mastered. Why is the brain structured in this way? What has made the insecurity in our heart? The need for Nature to gather from the environment well-being, sustenance, love, and all those things which make living organisms reach for light and nourishment, causes the fourth brain to integrate the lower functions and to simplify them in one feeling of *being*, secure with itself in its environment. Failure to achieve this security at the physical, social, and intellectual levels separates man so that he is unable to adapt, feels fragmented and threatened by life and, like all other species that cannot adapt to new environments, becomes so rigid that he ceases to evolve and soon is extinct. This is the position where man is now at, unable to adapt to the heightened separation caused by weapons and powers. *He is now faced with self-extinction through lack of ability to communicate with Nature's purpose and with fellowman.* It is the fourth center in the heart where we learn to adapt, to forgive, to yield and surrender. And it is for the three levels above it to show us the way.

Having seen the interconnections and overlapping of the chemical emotions, social emotions, intellectual emotions, and the emotions of our being at the fourth level, we can now proceed to understand how perturbations from the fifth, sixth, and seventh levels will add their notes to the symphony of life. An analogy of the orchestra might be that our physical level is like the big base drum, our social level is as tinkling brass, our intellectual level is blowing our horn, our heart level is like a harp, the blue level is sweet idyllic violins, and the sixth level indigo is like the far-away strains of the flute, while at the seventh level our imagination is the conductor with his baton. Beyond it *all* is the great organ music of the soul, which sits at the keyboard pulling the stops for all these different instruments and listening to the whole performance at the center of our being. Deep in the heart center we are moved to poetry when the Phoenix rises again and again from the dark ignorance of the lower centers and flies up into the light of the temples.

BEYOND THE GATEWAY

The next level of organization is beyond the gateway of the Mid-brain and reticular formation into the territory where our dreams are actually made. In this area the whole of life becomes a dream, whether sleeping or waking, simply because it is here that our reality or unreality is made. Just as the Mid-brain of level four acted as a powerhouse to fire up the conscious activity of the higher brains, so does this fifth level of the Inter-brain act as a storage, like a huge tape recorder or computer memory of all that happens to us. Throughout the stretch of evolution in which the brain has developed, the organisms which adapted to change and stored up their food and energy began to feel also the need for storing up experience. Experience is another name for reflection upon our actions, feelings, emotions and thoughts. Many of these thoughts and emotions throughout our long journey through the evolution of biological matter have been caused by trial and error, by learning the effects of light and dark, by forming some estimate, however fanciful or inaccurate, of the forces acting through humans and through life on this planet.

Just as all the planetary bodies from the vast material mass of Jupiter to the smallest piece of meteor dust in the asteroids are completely controlled by the gravitational field of the sun, so is the action of the seven centers of consciousness controlled by our self-regarding consciousness. Beyond all the levels of the human brain and its added nervous system, the intense gravitational field of our consciousness holds all the atoms and organs together in an electrical cloud of biophysical energies. Instead of centering in the body centers they are balanced at the other end of the spectrum and controlled by the brain which influences all our physical activity through the psychic electricity of the chakras. The chakras continue to act as sluice valves for cosmic energy but the control of the lower brains passes to the higher brains whenever the consciousness of a human being shifts its center of gravity beyond the Mid-brain into the Cave of Brahma.

Just as the moon and the new halo of hundreds of artificial satellites around the earth are not controlled by the sun's gravitational field which controls the earth, but are instead completely obedient to the earth's gravitational field, so does the whole evolving organism of the human vehicle come under the dominance of the field of consciousness whenever the mind is properly focussed and concentrated above the Mid-brain in the Cave of Brahma.

Our brain is a miniature solar system embedded in a galaxy of cells. Whenever we concentrate consciousness on the higher levels of the brain functions we are tuning the spiritual sun of consciousness into the control of our own hierarchy of energies like the sun of a solar system controls its planets. We have a miniature version of a planetary system in the earth-moon system where the moon does not obey the pull of the sun but is gripped in the earth's control even though the sun ultimately controls the earth. Thus our consciousness can tune itself to the planets or to their ruler, to their lesser energies or to the source. Jupiter and its moons as well as Saturn and its moons give us other examples of a system imprisoned within a larger gravitational system because each of them has more moons than the sun has planets. By tuning directly to our spiritual sun we are freed from the effects of planets and from the earth's control over us when we create an intense field of consciousness which triumphs over external influences. If human beings did not have this supreme power of controlling their consciousness they would remain dominated by their environments like the animals who merely adapt. This fifth step in brain evolution, then, is a liberation from the control of possessive pulls around the balance point of our Mid-brain center at the green level. Just as the moon is now controlled by the earth and not the sun, so is our brain controlled by us instead of the environment when our intensity of consciousness frees it from the planetary control of the earth's gravitation.

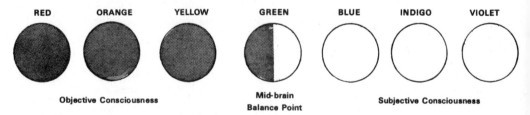

RED   ORANGE   YELLOW   GREEN   BLUE   INDIGO   VIOLET

Objective Consciousness   Mid-brain Balance Point   Subjective Consciousness

We can see how neutral green is the cross-over point for the positive and negative polarization of our being. If we look at the human body as a magnet, we can see that the three upper chakras are polarized negatively and the three lower chakras are polarized positively to the earth's magnetic field or vice versa to the spiritual plane of light and pure consciousness. In the Mid-brain, the green level, lies the cross-over point where we feel secure or insecure, depending on the tensions between the objective reality and our subjective experience.

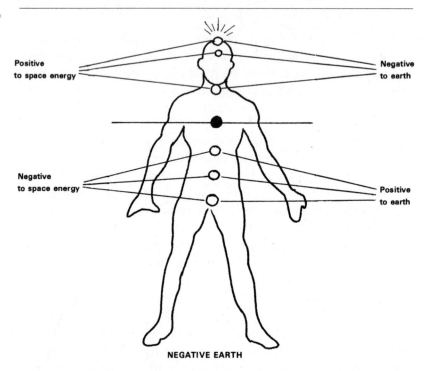

Positive
to space energy

Negative
to earth

Negative
to space energy

Positive
to earth

NEGATIVE EARTH

The connection between gravitation and light is reflected in the growth of all organisms within the solar system. Throughout the long period of evolution the organisms which reach out for the light gradually escape the material pull of gravity. This is true for atoms, stars, plants, galaxies, brain levels, etc. *Nuclear Evolution* describes how we process light biochemically and psychologically and re-radiate it as the field of consciousness. It would be a repetition to go into it here, but for the sake of those unfamiliar with these concepts we can say that light and dark, yin and yang, positive and negative, gravity and levity are all seen as aspects on different thresholds of the same nucleus from which the expansion and proliferation of forms in the whole universe began. In the realm of society these aspects are shown as the externalization of what is conceived in the fifth brain at the ideal stage of man's evolution. Up to the fourth level, mankind is little different from the animals and insects in his drives, his desires and instincts for survival, his fears of flight and fight, or his ways of lovemaking and reproducing his species. All come from eggs fertilized by sperm, all eat and digest and excrete food with the same system of organs, intestines, mouth, stomach, etc., and all struggle for dominance or security in some way by clubbing together. But beyond this, in the fifth level, mankind begins to transcend these primitive features in the ability to *control* himself and his environment and to transmit this knowledge through concepts, words, ideas, etc. The need for a brain which can record and store all this knowledge of the light and dark experiences, the positive and negative aspects of life on earth, is the pull and push which brought forth the growth of the Inter-brain and its subsequent computing equipment in the Cerebrum above it. In the realms of politics and society, the light and dark are very clear in such persons as Christ (light) and Hitler (dark) and in fact are too clear and too simplistic, too clichéd, because these beings are merely focal points of power for human consciousness, which makes them what they are and makes them culturally and idealistically potent as archetypes. The truth begins to sound simple-minded, like a cops and robbers story, so that people think in bar room clichés as if all we need to do is get rid of baddies and we will automatically be left with goodies. We must set out this political light and dark in a new way that has more relevance to the light and dark of the brain matter. The interplay of the electrical and chemical relationships between events in our consciousness will determine whether another Hitler could rise again and kill another six million Jews.

Why do we always pick on Hitler? At least he was an idealist fired with grandiose ideas of a super-race. There were others more sinister because they killed as many of their own countrymen in secret. They were skillful enough to do it by more subtle means. The name of Joseph Stalin does not have the stigma of the racist Hitler, but politically he was equally as dark and devious and was responsible for the death of millions of political prisoners. Solzhenitsyn has described the hundreds of labor camps which were deliberately invented by Stalin for destruction of human life. No one can ever tell us of the darkness of such camps because those who explored their depths from 1921 until now are already in their graves and cannot speak. Up to 1959 it was estimated that a total of sixty-six million lives were consumed by internal repression—many million more than Hitler killed! The dark matters of the human brain and its state of consciousness are even more compounded when we realize that the very victims themselves could not believe that the communist idealists had begun that early to manufacture death and darkness for so many in the name of "Pravda" (Truth).

It is now therefore necessary to probe the way that the light of the cosmos sends our consciousness to us through the gravitational fields of earth and the sun and to see what becomes of it in our brains, our nerves and fibers, so that the reader can see clearly into the truth that our society is but a mirror of the darkness of our own souls. *For neither Hitlers nor Stalins nor any of the known murderers of people now existing who kill in the name of political expediency or some high ideal, can perpetrate such horror singlehanded and alone.* For every dictator and mass murderer there are millions of helpers. Some people who live in the same block we live in would not even visit their own brother or mother if a Stalin or Hitler had arrested them, because they would fear being tainted. Like millions of Russians have done, they would stand by impotent and would shut out of their consciousness the very thoughts and recognition of selfishness that drag them even deeper into the darkness of their existence. Let us in the next three levels of the brain organization get down under the surface of the obvious and see how the social world is part of the cosmic whole. Let us examine why the Christs get murdered and the Stalins thrive for years and years.

It is possible, in the study of the human brain functions and the corresponding levels of consciousness which transcend the animal state, to penetrate our own being like light, or to obscure its deepest functions in the darkness of ignorance. In order to see with the wholeness of our entire upper brain we must see the whole of space and time in a kind of overview that makes it terribly clear what all the implications of the darkness of something like communism are to those who, like the victims of the slave camps, do not see the darkness because they are in it! The whole looks so different depending on what level of consciousness we are looking from. We must be able to see things about light as it is processed into human experience, good or bad.

It is hard for the intellect to experience the interconnectedness of everything or to see any link between someone's biochemistry and some big political event like World War II. People were fascinated by Hitler and Stalin, and these days there are people who are still baffled and curious about such people. The same morbid fascination is still present with such occult figures like Alistair Crowley who drank goat's blood and practiced hundreds of abominations of the mind and body. Today, movies and fantasy play upon the connection of good and evil, light and dark, and society is full of stereotypes through which it achieves its ultimate drives. We know Hitler was a bit nutty and went deeply into astrology and misread spiritual literature just like the murderer Charles Manson did. Many others read the Bible and other spiritual literature and miss the main point of it and go exactly backwards into darkness with it. We already mentioned the Inquisition and the spiritual pride which comes from thinking in darkness instead of in light. It is so easy to get the light screwed up and confused if we do not understand how we make our concepts, how we store up our opinions, mishear and misread. To the one who has experienced this darkness of the unknowing mind these words will make sense, but to the millions who don't know they are in it, are they not waiting for another Hitler or Stalin to reveal it to them? Can we enter the mind of a Mao Tse-tung or any misguided idealist and see how they screw up the light because they are blinded by their own cleverness? How do we create this light and dark, moment by moment, as we think and reflect? How do we choose dark, while talking about light, and what effect does all this have on the atoms and chemicals of our brains?

The study of brains five, six, seven and eight must reveal the cosmic level of perception as well as the social level. The biggest problem is to avoid the moralistic heavy-handed tone of a Solzhenitsyn who keeps crying, "Wake up, wake up, wake up." Yet that is what the next levels of our brain and consciousness are all about. We must get beneath the social level into the workings of consciousness which cause its imperviousness to light, to get to the next textures in the vibrational tone of thinking in light on the higher levels of six, seven and eight. First we must glimpse the reasons why our fifth brain blocks the light with old experience which is stored so deeply that we cannot change ourselves or grow. Only by penetrating the barrier of the mind and its relation to the brain can we connect with the higher cosmic intelligence that can alone evolve man and change the society which emerges from his ignorance or his illumination.

THE FIFTH BRAIN
The Inter-Brain
The Third Ventricle
The Cave of Brahma

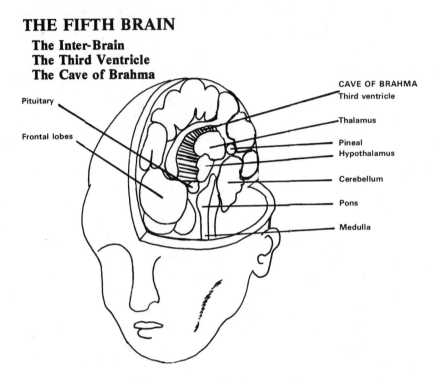

The region of the third ventricle in the fifth level of functioning is the very important concept-making and idea-producing development of the brain, and everything from here on is built around it. It is connected with the cerebral hemispheres of the Cerebrum above, in front and behind, and with the Mid-brain below it. The third ventricle is the cavity of the Inter-brain which I call the "Cave of Brahma" in my loose interpretations of Sanskrit texts. It passes between the two optic thalami which make up the floor and walls of the Inter-brain. Its roof is formed by the choroid plexus. At the front of the cavity is the pituitary gland and at the rear is the pineal gland, both very important to our perception. The third ventricle communicates with the two lateral ventricles which extend into the frontal lobes of the right and left hemispheres, and the rear end of the lateral ventricles extends into the occipital lobes of the Cortex at the back of the hemispheres.

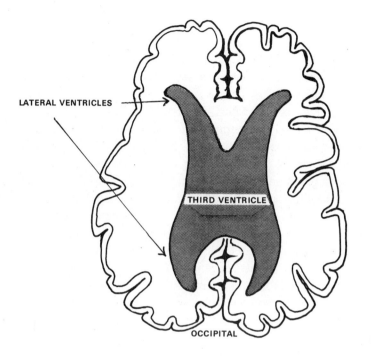

It is this central part of our brain evolution which enables us to store up higher abstractions and thoughts in our memory and to process new experiences, revive old emotional scars, recall deep fears and dreams. These higher centers of control on the fifth level of function determine how we shall respond to the signals, feelings, pains, and pleasures coming to us from the lower four levels of the brain. Without this conceptual machinery to process our thoughts and primitive emotions, our organism would be like an animal, only aware of the emotional chemical hormone releasing its response to stimuli. We would know pain but not the meaning of it. We would be able to communicate but we would not use any words or remember any thoughts and our internal life would be conditioned by the environment like Pavlov's dogs. Idealism as we know it would be absent from life. Without the fifth brain we would not be able to experience devotion or higher types of love nor analyze our emotions. We would not be able to compare them with previous experiences and memories recorded in the lower brains.

The comparing mechanism of this fifth brain is exactly opposite to that of the third brain. The intellect is like a person who enters a darkened room with a torch beam and lights up each object in turn, comparing it by saying,"that's a table; that's a chair." The conceptual faculty of the fifth brain goes in and sees a whole room with each object, chair, table, window, carpet, etc., making the room come together as a whole concept which we identify with as our "home". This is why the higher kinds of spiritual love can only be experienced through the later developed portions of the brain. To brain number three, a brass Buddha is just a Buddha, one among many Buddhas. Buddhas are compared and contrasted with Christs, Krishnas or what have you. To the fifth brain, Buddha is an idea, a concept, an ideal embodiment of the whole universe. Instead of the experience of tearing things apart (like the third brain) the Inter-brain puts things all together in a meaningful lump and has a feeling about it, and it then stores that feeling in the memory at the conceptual level. These concepts are sitting in our mind just as if we had programmed them into a computer or put them onto a tape, so *every time we start to think, we think in those concepts which we have already stored in our memory.*

The time framework for this brain is the past because to have an experience and to begin to reflect on it and think about it is already time past. The moment you begin to think about it, it is already in your memory. Any thought at all that you have is already past, because by the time you have got in touch with your lower brains which are experiencing a sensation, the present moment is gone. But even this process of thinking is slow in the tremendously fast world of consciousness. We don't feel that it takes much time for us to think a thought and move our hand. We think,"I will move my hand" and we do it and it appears to be instantaneous, but at the speed of consciousness it is a very slow operation to get it translated from the concept all through the lower brains and to go down through the nerves. Even at the speed of light it is slow, and consciousness is faster than the speed of light, because light has to travel, whereas consciousness is already there. Consciousness is the fastest thing there is, because it doesn't go anywhere. To go from yourself to yourself doesn't take any time; it is eternal and timeless. So we can say that in comparison with the speed of consciousness, conceptual thinking is very slow because it is storing in the memory those many experiences which are already gone. As we begin to think with the left-hand side of our brain about the feelings and thoughts of the right-hand side, the experience is already in time past.

The fifth level is an integrative function of our brain, capable of bringing together and comparing many concepts and patterns of higher emotions, capable of forming judgements of how life ought to be and making models and estimates of reality. Whereas the fourth brain is concerned with eating to obtain physical vital force, the function of the fifth level is the digestion of emotional food or brainfood. We take meaningful experiences of patterns from the external situation and compare them with what we have already internally stored in memory. This is the level of the mind which integrates ideas and does not simply spit out programmed automatic responses like a juke box selector arm but takes time to examine feelings and thoughts in order to permit or prohibit them. If we think our feelings will bring us security in our heart, then our head will permit us to repeat the stimuli over and over again. If painful, then the mind will form a barrier concept and avoid the situation in future.

This Inter-brain corresponds to the color blue in Nuclear Evolution. In this part of the brain, which I call the Cave of Brahma, lies the potential to become that Cosmic Consciousness which this level of functioning is able to glimpse and worship. But the only way to do it is to wipe out the cosmic memory inherited not only from this lifetime but from many incarnations and biological successes and failures in the evolving of this world of flesh and matter. You have to blow the mind, take the equivalent of a mental atom bomb and set it off, blasting your mind to pieces, completely ditching all those tapes from generation after generation and acquired during the whole of evolution. Tapes! Just imagine how many tapes there are in the mind. More than President Nixon ever dreamed of! The only way that you can get rid of that genetic memory is to wipe the mind so pure and clear that it frees it up and it becomes new-born, a new vehicle, able to perceive things as they really are, without the constant checking against the storehouse of memory.

The kind of mind that has been freed of opinions and also been freed of memory can put new memories in. Anything that your higher mind wants to happen can be programmed into that purity and just watch it grow. Consciousness is just like the soil. It is the ground of your being and you are at every moment, even now, planting seeds in your consciousness, and these grow into the fruits and flowers of your experience of self. The function of memory is that you can't escape yourself. Wherever you run, your memory is going to come along with you unless you've blown your mind in such a way that it is not destroyed (because that would be dangerous to destroy such a beautiful instrument) but instead is purified. If you have no memory of who you are, can you be anybody? And once you have that knowledge that you're nothing, you are free of ego. But the self-sense has a very tenacious memory; it is a painful teacher.

At the level of the fifth brain we reach the first threshold of the spiritual dimension of consciousness. We are provided with the ideal-istic suggestable mental equipment by which we can either reinforce our sense of being a separate ego or we can use the same faculty to find a new way to integrate experience and make it whole. Beginning with a concept of God or of wholeness, we can start to experience that oneness by surrendering to it even our very selves, in an ever-expanding sense of "me", until we reach the greatest Self of all, experientially. Some surrender joyfully to the purification of the mind. They are the ones who trust in life. Others prefer the more difficult and painful way of resistance and stubborn defensiveness. When you ignore the Cosmic One and are unaware of the awesome intelligence that evolved your consciousness, then life merely employs the ego to bring you painfully to your senses. When you realize that you are the whole nucleus, the whole universe expanding, you can kneel and surrender to the One who is your expanded self, not as an idea or concept but in the awesome awareness of that singularity of mind which is your devotion to the all-knowing One. The highest expression of the fifth level of function is to understand continuous human dedication and its expan-sive commitment to the all-pervading Intelligence. In Sanskrit this is called Dhyana or meditation.

THE SIXTH BRAIN

The Cerebral Hemispheres or Cerebrum
Occipital Lobes, Parietal Lobes, Temporal Lobes

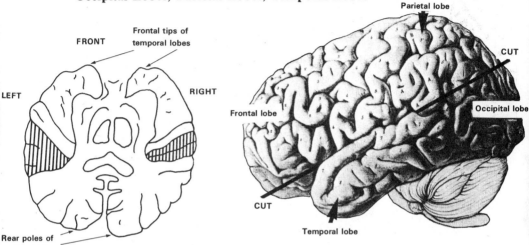

Crossing the thresholds of the sixth and seventh levels is like crossing the sound barrier. When man was unable to fly faster than sound, no one had ever heard of a sonic boom. Now that we are familiar with it, we know that there is some kind of barrier between each octave of Nature which requires a burst of energy to break through, and we know that upon emerging on the other side of the barrier there is a release of energy which we call a boom. An equivalent shock is often needed to get people through the psychic barrier of the sixth level.

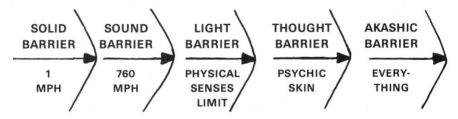

SOLID BARRIER	SOUND BARRIER	LIGHT BARRIER	THOUGHT BARRIER	AKASHIC BARRIER
1 MPH	760 MPH	PHYSICAL SENSES LIMIT	PSYCHIC SKIN	EVERY-THING

The above shows several natural barriers which are thresholds of energy. They can be likened to our own levels of consciousness and its vehicle, the brain.

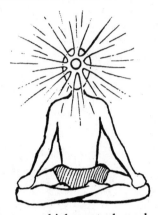

The sixth brain process which controls and overshadows the fifth level storing of memory and which unconsciously decides how we shall respond and identify in any given situation is loosely called "intuition". When we use our intuitive threshold of consciousness our brain responds to situations from subtle inner feelings and perceptions which get filtered through our previous knowledge and experiences stored in the lower brains. There are several kinds of intuition, but the kind everyone has is "knowing without forming concepts". Most people describe it in abstract terms as just "knowing in our bones" that something is correct or not. For instance, we know when we are in love or reacting to the presence of certain persons or whether we like them or not. When asked for a reason we cannot always say. Intuition is such a subtle faculty of consciousness that often you aren't even aware you are using it. Perhaps you get an insight into someone and it feels like you have analyzed them with your intellect, but really you have tuned into them with intuition before the intellect came in to express the insight and give it form. The intuition is much more common and easy to develop than people generally believe.

The ability of the "sixth sense" to know of events which take place beyond the reach of the normal senses has recently been called E.S.P. (extra sensory perception) but it was known to the ancients in phenomena such as clairvoyance (clear seeing), or clairaudience (clear hearing of inner voices that speak truth), or scrying (crystal ball gazing). Every person responds to every situation depending on the limits he places on his own performance. If he cannot do something, he tends to think that someone else who can do it is an extra-ordinary person. So if a stage entertainer mentally bends spoons or if a Christ can read people's thoughts, we do not realize that we all have the same potential in level six which we use for a certain kind of knowing. Hunches or premonitions that later manifest in coincidences beyond the range of chance are common ordinary ways that people awaken to this level of perception which not only governs E.S.P. but places each one of us on the threshold of higher consciousness.

Most people do not know what "higher consciousness" is; they only know what lower consciousness is and call it normal. They allow these gifts of our consciousness to lie fallow and unused. Much of the lack of interest in developing this part of us is more laziness than any lack of potential. People want to know beforehand what happens to them if they take the trouble to develop this part of the brain. They ask, "How will I be different from the way I was before?" People have to get excited about evolving these parts of the brain before they feel motivated to do it. And yet every day they are using the faculty of intuition already and they do not recognize it, simply because they do not understand how they acquire this knowledge. It just comes into their mind. They do not realize the scope of intuition nor what it does to the consciousness of a person who develops it. Level six evolves a wider kind of consciousness that is capable of transforming the quality of awareness on all the five levels below it. In most people, level six is only an inner sense that keeps us in balance physically, recognizes what we see and hear, and puts our knowing into some form. But in others, this sixth part of the brain can open to a marvelous and wonderous kind of psychic knowing which goes on at a far deeper level than thoughts or concepts—a level where our receptivity attracts an insight, like a revelation which can surprise us as much as anyone else. We are reminded of Keats' expression: "Sudden a thought came like a full-blown rose." Most people do not know that this psychic faculty must be trained as any other physical faculty like typing, playing an instrument or professional sports if it is to work accurately.

One aspect of sixth level "knowing" is perception of the future. Level six and level seven are closely linked in the kind of power they give us to shape our consciousness, since the future is the unfolding of events which are being programmed in the "total mind" of the seventh

level above. The power we have to receive information through images
is the power of the sixth level intuition to receive a non-sensory
sensation or impression from the seventh level and then store it in our
fifth level memory. That is, we could have some intimation about an
event that hasn't happened yet in the future and store it in our memory
so that when it happened we'd say, "Yes, I know that already." This is
what the prophet does. He functions at the sixth level. He knows how
the human race is going to go in a couple of thousand years' time and if
he were around then, he would be able to say, "I told you so." We do
that ourselves all the time, too. We have a flash of intuition and say we
had better not do that, but we go and do it anyway and then we kick
ourselves afterward, "Damn it, I had a hunch and I didn't follow it."
That faculty is in us, we *have* that kind of advance memory which is
able to store intimations about the future and to shape the future by seeing
ahead in time. But most of us are a bit lazy and we don't have the motivation to develop that part of the brain so we leave it lying fallow for the next
incarnation or sometime in the future. Our state of evolution will be
passed along with our seed which inherits the imprint of our own state of
consciousness in its cell life. Our seed has then to draw on its spiritual
resources to master what it has inherited. It will flourish or die depending
on how it uses the materials of evolution which lie all around at hand.
And the same is true for us, depending on how we apply our consciousness to the material at hand.

So level six is the part of the brain concerned not only with seeing
and perceptions but also with becoming a "seer". In terms of sheer
survival we can see the vast difference between someone who can only
see what is in front of him and someone whose awareness extends all
around him and behind him in every direction. We can see the
tremendous difference between one who can foresee what is ahead in
the future and take steps to change it before it happens and one who
cannot or who stubbornly refuses even to look. Many scientists denigrate
the intuition because they are only interested in hard facts and they feel
insecure or afraid that there might be other ways of knowing. The great
scientists, like Einstein, Newton, etc., all have this inner vision as well
as interest in logic and material facts. So we can begin to see how lack
of inner vision causes the wise to say, "Where there is no vision, the
people perish." Because the sixth level knowing process is direct, i.e.,

does not go through conceptual modes of the fifth level of past experience from stored memories, we do not need a college degree or a great deal of information to understand it. Nature has given all of us this faculty of the supersense to develop, and through its development of internal vision we can change the blind leadership of society and change the quality of life upon earth.

The Inner Eye and the Outer Eye

The cerebral hemispheres of level six are each divided into three lobes, the functions of which are only partly understood by scientific knowledge today, although the great clairvoyants and yogis have given us interpretations of all the mechanisms by which we perceive the world directly through the hierarchic functions of the brain. The sixth and seventh brains are so closely related and work so closely together that I will have to speak of them together at times and you may get confused about three pairs of lobes or four. The sixth brain is made of three lobes in the left and three in the right hemisphere and the seventh brain is another pair of lobes which we call the frontal lobes that are situated above the lobes of level six. Level seven governs our higher abstractions such as God, Cosmic Knowing, and imagination.

Each lobe of the cerebral brain has a different function. The frontmost lobes are the parietals which are for our use of the inner vision (intuition). The back lobes, the occipitals, govern our sense of sight and the focussing of sighted objects. These occipitals are a refinement of the rudimentary sensing of the skin and are common to all of life which has eyes and sees the light vibrations in the optical window. The specialization of the skin trying to sense light led to the evolution of the occipitals. Insects and animals which also perceive images do not need to endow them with abstract meaning and relate them to the imagination as we do. Hence they have occipitals but undeveloped parietals. The human sixth brain uses the sensing ability in the lower animals but on a higher level and potentially for a higher purpose. The middle two lobes are the temporals which govern and arrange our conceptual speech, our listening and our physical balance. Concepts have to be joined together wholistically from all of our

The interchange between the mini-computers of the fifth level brain and the storage lobes of the sixth level brain is facilitated by the many links between the lower temporal lobes (memory) and the inner vision of the parietal lobes (intuition). The hippocampus at the base of the temporal lobes is essential to long-term memory. Damage to this computer area or to the amygdala next to it results in breakdown of recent memories after a few minutes. Memories of events from before the damage are still retained, however, because they were transferred to the temporal lobes. No actual information is stored in the hippocampus or amygdala or in any of the computers of the Mid-brain or Inter-brain which merely act as hunting mechanisms, filters or retrieval devices to the temporal lobes where the long-term memory is distributed. The function of the fifth level memory and the sixth level perceptions working together produces thoughts which rise in consciousness and govern our access to the past.

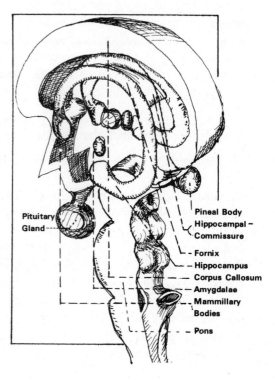

Pituitary Gland

Pineal Body
Hippocampal – Commissure
Fornix
Hippocampus
Corpus Callosum
Amygdalae
Mammillary Bodies
Pons

sensations from the separate senses acting together. It is this part of our brain surrounding the inner vision of the parietals that raises our sensory perceptions of the environment around us to a higher level of abstract ideas and gives us the feeling of *knowing*. But in this area we know without knowing how we know and we give this the name of insight, another name for inner vision—in-sight.

The sixth evolutionary stage of the brain makes possible two distinct methods of visualizing, both of which are quite different from the imaging of the imagination (level seven). The occipital lobes make possible our sense of sight (seeing and focusing on the material sensations of physical objects in the external environment) whereas the parietals make possible the inner "seeing" of the intuition. Together they make the process of seeing an entirely different experience from the animal's. The undeveloped person who has not yet switched on the capacity of the sixth level sees only with the outer vision, just like the animals. Some animals even seem to have more inner vision than many humans, but animals and insects do not have the capacity for insight, they merely react from unconscious drives. It is insight that makes us conscious of our experience. Humans can reflect and rethink their experience, while animals can only learn to store their reactions and experiences in the unconscious parts of their brain. Therefore it is the sixth level combined with level five which raises the conceptual thought to the conscious direct experience. The intuitions of animals, such as the pigeon's homing effect, the zoo animals' foreknowledge of earthquakes, or the mating sensibilities of insects, are all unconscious perceptions rather than "knowing", whereas man has the capacity in his sixth brain to know that he is linking the internal images with sensory images of the outside world. It is the parietals working with the occipitals and temporals that combine our outer vision or outer sensations with our inner vision for higher purposes. This is the beginning foundation of the imagination which is specialized in the next level seven where all the lower functions of the brain are sorted out. There are several other minor lobes in the sixth brain that handle sensory signals and coordinate the phenomena received by the five lower brains.

It is the pituitary, contained within the sixth brain triggered by the parietals, that switches on a supply of endocrine chemical hormones to the areas in the frontal lobes, rear lobes, throughout the brain, and to the blood stream constantly bathing the brain cells, which triggers the sixth level perception throughout the brain as a whole. These hormones activate the intuitive awareness that can transform our brain function.

The three pairs of lobes which give a new sixth level meaning to our external sensory interpretations of phenomena deal with our inner vision in two different ways. They govern both the "hardware" equipment of physical sensing and the ways we *interpret* the sensory and non-sensory signals which converge and form the intricate "software" convolutions of our psychology. The peptides which trigger the intuitive awareness, called enkephalins, become psychologically active when they are released into the Cave of Brahma from the pituitary and hypothalamus. Only when this occurs do we become *aware that we are aware,* the significant achievement of the sixth level of consciousness. The knower of knowledge is directly experienced on this level. This sixth level knowing influences our ability to absorb light and radiation from the cosmos. The more light we can absorb, the more we can know. The more we extend our knowing, the more light we can take in and the more insight we will have of the vast world beyond concepts. Therefore, level six is a tremendous key to our spiritual evolution. By becoming aware that we are aware, we break through into another octave of Nature with a new kind of energy that takes us beyond the world of appearances.

This process of inner vision interacting with our imagination is complex, but we can get some idea of the linkage between level six and level seven by gaining some understanding of how the separate and distinct areas of the brain use the eyes for different purposes. A simple understanding is necessary before we can begin to see how this internal visioning of level six, or its neglect, can affect the quality of our individual lives and our society. We have said that one of the purposes of the temporals functioning on the sixth level is to control our sense of balance and tell our consciousness our position in the environment. The eyes are used by the brain to determine the location of objects at a distance and to judge and compare the reality of those objects by unconscious estimates of their weight, size and texture, and to determine their balance in respect to our own balance in the cosmos. The sixth brain then fine tunes the external factors to the inner knowing for a wholistic consideration of the situation. The sixth brain also uses the eyes to validate the internal imagination by which we reconstruct the outside universe inside our consciousness from the signals received by our senses. The *knower* mediates between the sensory signals and the ego's image of things. The eyes serve not only to see straight ahead and focus objective phenomena with the occipitals but also have peripheral vision which combines with our imagination on the seventh level, with our fifth level memory, and with the intuition to produce dreams, illusion, and hallucinations about our placement in space.

So we are talking about the most rudimentary kind of physical balance in which we can remain upright and not fall over, and at the same time we are talking about the internal balance of "being in tune" with ourselves and our bodies, and in tune with life or with the laws of the universe. These are all very much connected, and they begin with how the eyes work and how the inner eye cooperates with the external vision of the world "out there".

To see the way in which the physical functions affect our more subtle psychic awareness, we have to realize that all the impressions that come to us through our senses are transmitted as little electrical impulses. There is no difference between the electrical impulse that comes to the brain from the sight of a tree and the impulse that comes from the sound of music. In this sense there is little difference between the firing of a transistor in a computer and the firing of a cell potential in a brain. But the software technology of "know-how" makes an enormous difference to the capacity of a computer just as the aware-ness makes an enormous difference in the capacity of our brains. Only the consciousness sitting inside the brain can interpret the signals in such a way that it perceives a "world". In the same way, we also create our social world by the evolutionary level of our consciousness. Whatever we are seeing in our world will vary according to what is aware in our consciousness. For example, our brain actually creates our future by visualizing all possible environments it can conceive of and then aiming for the one which most suits our ego and its needs. We may not even be aware that we are creating in this way or that we are missing a lot of our present environment because our sixth brain may not be activated and therefore we only notice half of life. This affects our future drastically. A lack of intuitive awareness affects the way our present unfolds into the future because we often do not know that our reality is incomplete. We think we are seeing all there is to see and hearing all there is to hear when in fact we are only half awake. To follow the process of knowing carefully reveals that our inner eye and outer eye must work together if we are to remain in balance and open up to more possibilities mentally as well as physically.

The visual cortex at the back of the brain allows us to focus on objects and draws the sensations from the eye back into the head to the area of the occipitals where we experience shape and color. The sense of seeing light, its shapes and forms, is also processed simultaneously by the various thalami situated around the walls of the Cave of Brahma acted upon by the pituitary and parietal functions. The external and internal visual systems interact normally unless you close your eyes and shut one of them off. At nighttime when light is absent or at a very low threshold, the inner vision brain system operates independently from the visual cortex which focuses light. In night driving, people are using the sixth level brain and the "inner eye" to show their position in the environment, and if they have difficulty it means that the relationship of the "inner eye" to the other brain functions needs developing.

We can consciously develop the sixth brain capacities by developing our sense of balance. By blindfolding our eyes we can practice a walking meditation to develop the inner eye or, standing on one leg with our eyes closed, we can get control over our optical thalamus. But the most important way we can use our "inner eye" visual system is to realize that it is fed out of the periphery of the retina and literally sees out of the corner of our eyes. We can practice looking out the corners of the eyes to stretch this visual system. Now we can begin to see how our brain uses our eyes in several different ways. The center of the retina of the eye sends light signals to the occipital lobes at the back of our brain, whereas the outside rim sends signals to the optical thalamus in the Cave of Brahma to stop our body swaying by fixing on visual cues to maintain our physical posture.

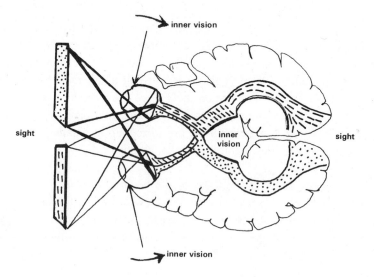

Especially people who sway a lot when their eyes are closed need to practice using the periphery of vision to begin to notice more out of the corners of the eyes to develop this inner brain vision. Our parietal lobe then uses the whole sixth level function and the whole seeing process on other levels to interpret those images which are not just immediately in front of the eyes but are also in the corners of the eyes in the environment around us. Very few people realize that they can even see physical objects behind them when this Cave of Brahma seeing is highly developed.

I remember lying in a bed in a hotel room years ago and seeing a window. I wasn't sure whether I was awake or still asleep. I counted the panes of glass in the window and then realized that I was still asleep. When I opened my eyes I saw that there was a window in the exact location I saw it in my inner eye and with the same kind of glass and the same number of panes. This experience occurred before I began to meditate. Once I began to meditate properly I realized I was able to see everything in a room with my eyes closed. This faculty of inner sight is not something extraordinary, but is commonly reported by people in spiritual experiences when the awakening of the third eye occurs or even by mothers and grandmothers who can tell what their children are doing while their back is turned to them doing the dishes or some other task. This is the origin of the very common phrase, "She has eyes in the back of her head." Some years later I met a minister who started a church based on "Eyeless Sight". He taught his daughter and his son how to read each card in a deck of cards while blindfolded and then he taught his whole congregation how to do the same thing. I was asked to give a talk at his church on how to see colors with the inner eye, while blindfolded, which I did, and I understand that he was able to teach his congregation this skill as well.

SEEING WITH YOUR BEING

With your inner vision you see with your entire being, with every cell and atom of your being. Your inner vision is even coupled to your ears which take over to locate your position unconsciously in the environment. The inner vision uses all the senses and the mind to know the real significance of a sensory input, whereas the outer vision just re-creates the colors and forms of objects in the occipital lobes and compares it with past experience of color, shape, etc. When you use the inner eye to picture what things might be like in a darkened room or what things might be like in the future, you are practicing seeing with the whole being, not just with your eyes. To notice things out of the corner of your eyes, then, is one of the first steps to knowing the future, because it activates the connections between many parts of our brain including that part of our brain we use to create images on the next level above (i.e., level seven, the imagination). Whatever we image in the inner brain will determine our balance as people. If our image is horrible or doubtful or fearful, our balance will be disturbed in our whole being. So not only our inner vision but our future depends on the images we hold in the periphery of our unconscious vision. Whatever fearful or hopeful image for the future we hold in the second-sight part of our brain, will determine our future actions as individuals and as a society. Our image of ourself and our image of the total environment around us will dictate our responses to life itself. If we are only seeing with our eyes and only the back occipital part of our visual system is working, then our awareness of the future we are unconsciously conditioning will be dead. This is what Christ meant when he said:

> "There is a prophecy of Isaiah which is being fulfilled—
> 'You hear but never understand, you will look and look, but
> never see.' For this people have grown gross at heart; their
> ears are dull, and their eyes are closed. Otherwise their eyes
> might see, their ears hear and their heart would understand
> and then they would have to turn again. . . "
>
> Matthew 13:14-15

THE MIRACLE OF CONSCIOUSNESS

The time has come when society and the individuals in it must learn to use the inner knowing of the heart that sees with the inner eye and not only balances us to the external environmental cues but also to the internal environment. This sensing of the internal environment is also related to the inner ear by which great composers and seers accomplish a refined form of "inner listening". This was often referred to in ancient texts as the "ear of the ear" and by later writers as the "voice of conscience" or the "inner voice" of the intuition. All of us have this latent "ear of the ear" which, when developed, is seen merely as the ability of our own consciousness to listen to itself working. This awareness goes on working in our own unconscious whether we are sleeping, awake, or in trance states and sometimes surfaces in symbolic language in our dreams. If we are in touch with it consciously then our brain does not set up stresses between our conscious and unconscious self and we dream very little. Dreams are merely attempts of our inner vision and inner ear to communicate that total being we call our heart to our surface personality through the different brains.

Our total brain is very aware of the workings of the entire body and its chemical balance. Whenever we drink too much liquid the internal message is signaled to the brain to go to find a restroom in the external environment. Likewise if we are feeling tense or disappointed internally about some external situation this message is communicated subconsciously to all our cells and molecules in our internal organs and muscles. Stress, or its opposite, has a profound effect on the smooth muscle of the intestine and stomach in our internal environment. We all know how pressure, falling in love, or a holiday affects our appetite. Although we do not sense it directly, when we are constipated mentally, we will get an internal signal that produces constipation in our physical body. The emotional and mental environment is therefore directly related with what we do and experience in the world around us.

To unite the inner and outer worlds is to become fully conscious of how we create our reality. Only then can we activate the imagination to re-create our reality more in tune with the whole. All the ways we can find to enhance our consciousness and awaken this sixth level knowing need to be used if we are to gain wisdom to make a better world.

The purpose of meditation is the withdrawal of consciousness from the lower brains into the higher to stimulate the functioning of the pituitary and hypothalamus. When this fore-brain area is activated the inner seeing develops and takes control over the rest of the brain. The seer becomes master of himself and all the lower functions render service to the seer who is receiving direction and guidance from the seventh level above. Thus the brain becomes a wholistic vehicle for the service of cosmic wisdom and cosmic consciousness. Not only is wisdom received, but bliss! When the internal functions of the brain fulfill their purpose and become linked with the whole a harmonious resonance sets in between all the levels and between the inner and outer environment. This sixth brain is the seat of the higher *non-sensory pleasure center.* It has been found experimentally that stimulation of the fore-brain bundle of nerves near the pituitary gland, which pass through the hypothalamus, gives laboratory animals the highest rate of self-stimulation rewards. The laboratory animals enjoy this sensation even at the expense of other pleasures or needs such as eating, drinking or sleeping. This same area in humans is stimulated during meditation or the fixation of consciousness on this part of the brain and brings blissful states which exert a powerful influence on human behavior.

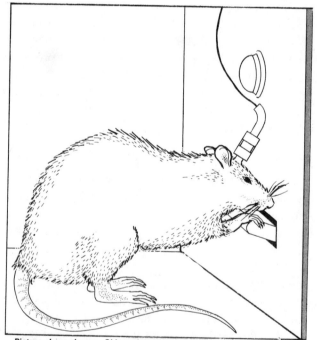

Picture above shows a Skinner box apparatus giving a brain reward to a rat who is allowed to trigger an exciting electric stimulus to the fore-brain pleasure center by pressing a treadle. The rat will stimulate itself continuously for several days until it is blissed out beyond physical need and even to starvation.

A monkey will also sacrifice lower pleasures or needs when stimulated like the rat, even with its frontal cortex much more developed, indicating that humans would probably do the same. While brain rewards are channeled to other specific areas of the brain, including the Pons and the Medulla Oblongata, the forebrain area has by far the most powerful effect. Humans could enhance non-sensory pleasure tolerance levels and detach from their sensory preoccupations by learning to stimulate this part of the brain consciously. To just have increased pleasure without more wisdom would not necessarily be evolutionary at all, but when we see this sixth brain as the seat of inner seeing or wisdom as well as the higher bliss, we can glimpse the next evolutionary step for us to discover. Yoga and the ancient wisdom of sages are for the explicit purpose of developing the sixth brain potential.

VALIDATING THE VISION

The process by which we think and create in abstractions of the next higher seventh level can only be understood by the awakened sixth level below it, which "just knows" when truth is confirmed, because it is that special kind of knowledge which is coming from within rather than from any outside authority. Socrates used this method of "drawing truth out" which is the real meaning of the word "educate". But to some people, recognition at the sixth level is not true validation. They believe that truth must be validated empirically; otherwise it is mere assertion. Because these areas of the sixth and seventh brains deal with phenomena beyond the solid world of matter, empirical evidence of their functions is hard to obtain. The seventh level process has been a mystery throughout history because to envision in our imaginations is a very complex affair involving all the lower brains embedded in the higher functions. Therefore the fantastic powers of the imagination have never been explained before except in very vague religious-mystical terms by great clairvoyants, many of whom contradicted each other, making proof very difficult. The upper brains are not amenable to laboratory proof of the kind that works in the world of matter. We would need a huge laboratory as big as the Universe to prove the validity of the upper rooms of man's consciousness. Though researchers like J.B. Rhine have devised empirical tests for all sorts of ESP phenomena, this research is like playing by someone else's rules or trying to get into a club you don't belong to, namely the club of empirical research. But empirical research only gives us information, not knowledge. Knowledge *is* validation on the higher levels of consciousness.

What is the laboratory for higher consciousness? By what kind of test can we validate a vast vision? The theory of Nuclear Evolution proposes a living experiment in which we prove the higher levels of consciousness by becoming them. There is no other way to do it. The great sage Lao Tzu called this way of knowing the Tao:

#26   Tao Te Ching
by Lao Tzu

When the intelligent man hears about Nature's way,
he seeks to embody it in himself.
When the mediocre student hears about the way,
he sometimes accepts it and sometimes does not.
Unintelligent men scoff at it.

In 1970 I organized in New Delhi, India, the First World Conference on Scientific Yoga to bring together the methods of knowing from East and West. "Scientific Yoga" means that each person must prove in himself and embody as a living example the truth about the higher levels of consciousness. At this convention, over five hundred yogis from all over the world signed documents which empowered me to start a Yoga University to make the sixth level yogic methods of knowing available to all. This project, envisioned by individual minds at the sixth level for the shaping of the future, is constantly fed by images proceeding from the seventh level from all sources in the *total mind*. In other words, the Cosmos supplies the vision like a ray of light through the window of any imagination that is open. However, it is not something seen like a plan or jigsaw puzzle all fitting neatly together, but is more like the colors on an artist's palette and the artist uses the materials at hand to create a picture. A university of yogis for the study of consciousness can only happen when all ingredients and colors are there. Most importantly its manifestation also depends upon the donation of material resources and human energies not only from those who will benefit from the project but also from those who will create it—those who are meant to respond to the vision with dedication from within themselves.

I have been offered millions of rupees and thousands of acres by men who caught the vision. I have been offered ashrams by the dozen and idyllic university sites by the side of Himalayan streams. But always the donors wanted to control or to demand large chunks of my time or in some way subtly imply that I should live out *their* expectations. Since I don't need anything for myself, it has always seemed quixotic to me that I should kowtow to a rich man's ideas and compromise myself rather than be totally free day to day from all expectations, particularly since the vision itself is a vision of total freedom and purity without strings. The millionaires wanted to purchase a vision. But in comparison the students and faculty here at the University of the Trees are themselves the vision and the living empirical evidence, and if the leap in consciousness doesn't work with them, it will never work in the world at large. Only a group of people who freely give themselves totally to the vision because they *are* the vision can manifest the fulfillment of freedom. Only when people freely accept responsibility for every thought, every idea and every vision can there be a group consciousness that is totally embedded in the Tao of life. It is a feeling in the marrow of the bones; it is an excitement in the blood; and it is the acceptance of the world itself as the laboratory of democracy in us.

The way the sixth and seventh levels work together in the manifestations of any social systems, whether it is through the visionaries who conceived the American Constitution or the joint-stock corporation, whether it is Moses' laws or Abraham's vision of the endless seed which spreads throughout the earth, or whether it is the metaphors of Christ or the spiritual vision of Krishna, the vision springs from the sixth level interpretation of the creative imagination and the purification of this interpretation in the laboratory of manifestation. Imagination receives the vision, the intuition interprets it, and the person lives it. If he or she cannot live it, then they cannot expect others to live it either. And if it is not liveable, then it is not valid.

THE INDIVIDUAL EXPERIENCE OF TIME EXPRESSES
THE FACULTIES OF MAN IN DIFFERENT DOMAINS.

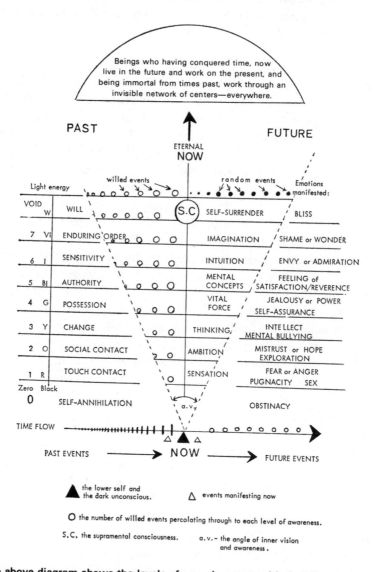

The above diagram shows the levels of consciousness with their main attributes 1 to 7 (left) expressed in terms of positive and negative emotional feelings (right). The drives from the Red sensory level all the way to the Violet level of the imagination are overlapping. The level below can understand the level above, but has little contact with two levels above. When a person has two levels such as the Yellow and the Indigo, the personality may appear to be split, as two different world views alternate in the same entity. When two or three levels are functioning in the same person they may bring a composite result and the separate colors then blend together in the color of the aura.

Thus the process of validating higher consciousness is threefold: the vision comes in through the seventh brain and is interpreted and validated by the sixth. The awakened sixth brain recognizes truth when it comes. But it cannot do so if the imagination is not open in the first place to receive the impressions. The sixth level is like the emulsion on a photographic negative while the seventh level is like the original image of light impressing itself upon it. And even though "just knowing" is always an internal conviction (faith) at the sixth level, when we come to validate the operations of the seventh level imagination we must still get external confirmation of our sixth level knowing. Many yogis have now confirmed Nuclear Evolution and its interpretations of the filtering mechanisms by which we perceive the world directly through the hierarchic functions of the brain, but it is possible that a person could receive the vision, know intuitively that it was valid and true, and yet not be willing to put his life and energy into manifesting it. Therefore it is most likely that only when scientific and empirical observations have validated the images and metaphors of Nuclear Evolution, will the normal awareness of humankind adopt it as a consensus or true world view of reality. But there is a last and most important ingredient in validation: the other five brains, which are the filter through which this vision must manifest, must be pure enough, selfless enough to respond to the vision and to prove it out in individual lives. Not until this final step is taken will Nuclear Evolution be incontrovertibly proved and validated. This step is the tuning of the individual in resonance with the whole—the hologram of creation.

DISCOVERING THE HOLOGRAM

The modern theories on the polarization of the two hemispheres of the Cerebrum which indicate left and right brain specialized functions are not entirely valid since the right half can learn left half functions and vice versa with training. Even when the corpus callosum that joins the two halves together is cut and the two halves function independently, each side can be trained to repeat the functions of the other side by regressing and re-learning from the beginning. The reason this is not usually done is that it takes a child several years to develop complete thoughts and the same amount of re-training would have to be done to re-program each half of the brain.

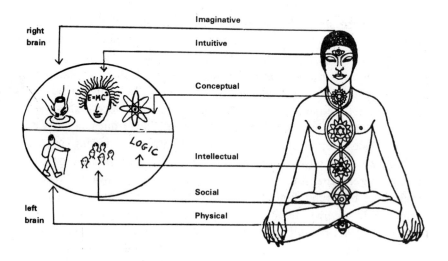

The correspondence of the chakras to the functions of the brain.

Using Supersensonic dowsing instruments it is found that the chakras below the heart are polarized left-handed negative while the chakras above the heart center are polarized right-handed positive. The link between the chakras and the brain centers can be shown in terms which link the lower three chakras to the left brain function and the top three chakras to right brain functions, thereby confirming the left/right brain research which allocates the right brain to intuitive and wholistic perceptions and the left brain to logical, sequential and verbal functions. By linking the chakras and levels of consciousness we begin to see that the corresponding governors of the psychic electricity in the brain provide us with the means for tuning the centers of the brain like we tune a radio. This biological radio, however, cannot be tuned if we do not know that the capacity is there, because it would be equivalent to having a radio in the house of someone who does not know how to turn it on or what to do with the various knobs or how to plug it into its source of power. Linkage of the chakras, which are the source of power, with the Cosmos enables humans to do the equivalent of energizing the radio circuit in the radio and adjusting the wavelengths on which it functions. This has great significance in communicaton between individuals since people who cannot move off the wavelengths they are stuck on and move onto other wavelengths generally lead impoverished lives and function only from the lower chakras. Unfortunately this represents a large section of the human race who have no knowledge of their higher chakra functions and are therefore bound by a reality governed entirely by physical sensations and rational explanations. Moreover they have been trained in school to specialize in those limited functions, thereby stunting individuals in society even further. A good example are those who are stuck in their left brains. They have only half of their Cerebrum functioning.

One must not mistake the brain functions at all the seven levels to be linear but rather see them as circular, thereby linking each system in a wholistic way so that all functions interpenetrate and overlap making it difficult to see where one brain stops and another starts. The best analogy of this is to realize that white light actually is a mixture of all colors which do not exist separately within a beam of light but only become color when their wavelengths are separated in passing through a medium which filters or refracts. Therefore color does not exist independent of light even though when we look at a flower or a painted object we think it has color. Actually the color is made in our consciousness, which is aware on a higher level of perception that the wavelengths of light that our senses are reporting to the brain are in fact the residue of light that is not absorbed into the object. In the same way our brain acts like light—a homogeneous vibration mixed together interpenetrating each other so that distinct levels of consciousness only become obvious and discernible when we do not absorb or when we shut out the light of the Cosmos through our chakras.* If there were no light there would be no color. In the same way if there were no consciousness there would be no brain. This is proved by the fact that when consciousness leaves the brain completely the brain dies, because its support systems are all negated. People are like mediums or filters. Depending on what they absorb so do they radiate the colors of light and quality of perception. This is what Isaiah meant when he said, "The people who walked in great darkness shall see a great light." He

---

* See *Nuclear Evolution* for the detailed process of human absorption, radiation and re-radiation of light through the chakras.

is referring to the day when people will open their conscious minds to the light of the Cosmos—consciousness.

It becomes obvious that consciousness acts as a guiding field or pattern of the biological system and not vice versa as most scientists think today, and the sixth brain is the level in which this is realized. Actions of consciousness, feelings of pleasure, chemical secretions, all can be explained by physical processes, but the physical processes themselves can only be explained by consciousness. To read a book of anatomy or a scientific encyclopedia and then believe that your knowledge of these parts will give you any clue as to their real function, is the equivalent of looking at an electronic circuit and trying to figure out what it is meant to do without any instructions or circuit diagram from the builder. Unless we know what the builder intended to do by putting the parts together it is impossible to fathom. This is true of the human brain no less than anything else. First we must know its purpose, then we can unravel its parts. To try to find its true purpose from its parts is like guessing which number will turn up on a roulette wheel in Las Vegas. On that basis anybody's guess is as good as another. Therefore we must use our right brain to study our left brain and vice versa, and this is the function of yoga and the sixth level brain. Only our intuition can give us an understanding of the purpose of the brain and know what is behind all the information and objective facts we store in it. The sixth level seer lies within the functions of the Cerebrum and lifts the energy up to the level of intuitive knowing, synthesizing and transcending all the levels below into a new threshold of consciousness. All great scientific progress has this software of intuition made active so as to interpret the hardware of its objective findings. The seer of the sixth level sees both the purpose of consciousness and the purpose of the brain.

This oversimplified factual account of the cerebral hemispheres sounds rather cut and dried, as if to say, "there is really nothing mysterious about the intuition, nothing magical about man's psychic potential or his spiritual potential, that they are only a mechanical functioning of the brain and will be explained by science in a matter of time." The wiring of the brain is tremendously complex and, until recently, scientists knew very little about its mysteries although quite a lot is known about its physical hardware. Even among psychologists and brain researchers there is very little known about the software, or the *way* the brain images its experiences. Why is it that one man's consciousness causes his brain to develop toward that deep knowing which sees into the heart of all things and understands the laws of the universe, while another person takes for granted or ignores these fantastic domains in which his consciousness could dwell? He views his brain as a mechanical instrument that uses him and does not see that it is a vehicle which he himself *creates* by the way that he uses *it*. It is true that our psychic faculties are made possible by the brain hardware, but it is even more true that our own consciousness, working through the brain, *creates* the software of the brain and extends its power to be aware. There is no limit to this power except the limits we ourselves impose.* Even the 360 degree awareness of a totally enlightened being is only the beginning of a long journey into the limitless world of consciousness. The beauty of evolution is that once the consciousness expands the brain functioning, the new awareness remains permanently imprinted in our consciousness even after the brain dies. The brain is a precious vehicle for growth, but it is not the beginning nor the end in itself.

The whole object of yoga or prayer or spiritual discipline is to gain insight into these workings of consciousness, and this is also the purpose of our study of the different levels of consciousness in Nuclear Evolution. If we are full of joy within, our body and its immediate environment will be radiated with optimism, and difficult tasks will seem easy. By combining good judgement with future expectations and prompt action, our internal environment is then projected outward with effective results. Let us learn to use our imaging power to bring about a new vision, to see things with second sight, to actively make our world and its future into a new world. The ability to envision the future and shape it *before* it becomes the present, corresponds to the color Indigo in Nuclear Evolution. Because we do have this faculty just waiting to

---

* A technique for growing new cells in various parts of the brain by use of the power of your consciousness is explained on cassette tape #2 in the Rumf Roomph Yoga series, University of the Trees Press. (See Appendix.)

be developed, we can have hope for the future no matter how helpless we may feel in the now. Both individuals and society have the power to re-create the future via understanding of the functioning of the sixth level. This power to envision the future is the only power we have which does not depend upon anyone or anything else, and is our inheritance from millions of years of evolution.

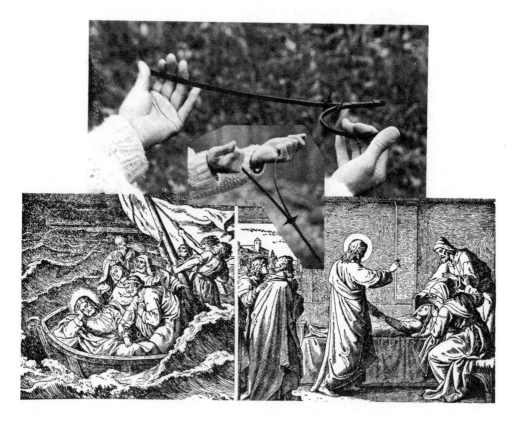

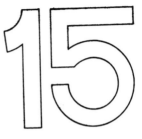

SUPER-SENSONICS: OPENING UP THE SIXTH LEVEL

The sixth level intuition is a vehicle of our consciousness which has not been highly developed in our culture. The ancient art of divining, now rediscovered in the science of Supersensonics, is our fastest way of developing this center of knowing which is directly related to the pineal gland. Although I have outlined much of this sixth level functioning in my book *Supersensonics**, the scientific community and the general public believe that supersensing is a superstitious area of investigation and is not a legitimate use of the brain's potential. It is true that the negative expression of the intuition is superstition. The sixth level of brain evolution determines how materialistic a culture

---

* *Supersensonics*, University of the Trees Press, 1975. See Chapters 13-17 on vision.

will be or how superstitious. An undeveloped sixth level in which the "inner vision" is weak makes the external vision all-important and therefore, through over–emphasis, it appears the stronger. If level six is developed just a little but not enough to glimpse the truly spiritual dimensions of being, then it intuits omens and signs, and its inner knowing is superstitious and very much bound up with materiality. This materialistic kind of intuition is the basis for black magic and all manner of dubious occult sciences. The higher spiritual kind of intuition is always used for white magic or the good of others. Superstition and black magic are the negative functioning of this area of the brain, but the positive function of the sixth evolutionary level is concerned with shaping the future and dissolving the subject-object relationship to the environment thereby leading us to the knowing of reality through both physical and internal kinds of visioning. Supersensonics is very much different from mere superstition and is a science legitimate and appropriate to the sixth level of the brain that it comes from. Many of the three thousand members of the American Society of Dowsers would have no problem believing, since they make very practical use of this level in discovering underground water streams. But for most people, divining is still in the realm of the magical and superstitious. Research reveals a long record of tested historical facts about dowsing and the sixth level faculty, not only in humans but in insects and other animals.

HOW DO THE PINEAL AND PITUITARY RELATE TO THE SIXTH AND SEVENTH LEVELS?

The pituitary releases the enkephalins or peptides which migrate across the floor of the Cave of Brahma. They trigger the hypothalamus, which in turn triggers the pineal to start activating the seventh level. The seventh level then receives the impressions from the various skin senses, but receives the nerve signals on the level of imagination rather than from the lowest level of material matter sensations, which only operate in a narrow physical octave.

The triggering of the sixth level, leading to the activation of the full powers of the imagination in the seventh level, makes the human brain into something like a thought camera with superpenetration of the processes of creation. The sixth level can be likened to the sensitivity

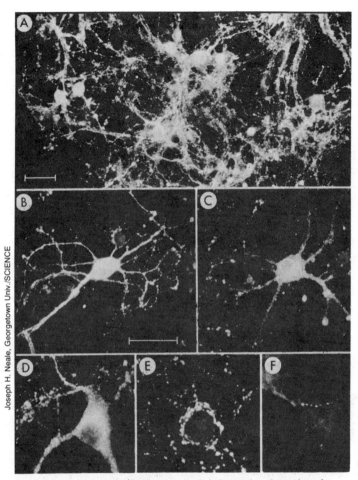

Joseph H. Neale, Georgetown Univ./SCIENCE

The picture shows actual cells at work by tracing the action of fluorescent stained enkephalin (the natural opiate of the brain which puts a person in trance) in brain neurons. Photo shows clusters of neurons (A), isolated fluorescent peptide in neurons (B and C), localization of fluorescence in cell bodies (D) and stained enkephalin at specific neuron sites (E and F). By showing which parts of cells contain such opiate peptides, the technique is "an exquisite model system" to study the effect of opiates on the brain.

of the photographic emulsion receiving the impressions of light by ionizing the silver chloride molecules in the emulsion leaving the pattern of the light on the photograph in the negative. The sixth level acts as the emotional emulsion which receives the impression and acts on it, but the impression itself comes from the seventh level, just as the image in the photographic emulsion really comes from patterns of light reflected off an object. The sixth level interprets these impressions in terms of its own lower level of evolution very much like we interpret our dreams. If the sixth level is not evolved or is not opened completely it will not be sensitive enough to receive the real depth of the images, in the same way that certain kinds of film emulsions are not sensitive to certain colors or frequencies of light. If you dream in color or can close your eyes and see distinct images or colors, it is indicative that your photographic emulsion of the sixth level has begun to function and become sensitized to the impressions from the level of imagination above.

Supersensonics is the ability of the human nervous system and skin to receive impressions from objects in the environment in the same way a tuned radio receives the different wavelengths of radio stations broadcasting on different frequencies. At the gross level of the skin sensation, the experience of impressions will be limited to those of physical objects. When the sixth level is opened, invisible objects can be sensed. The environment is swirling with charged particles which can be sensed by the ionization of our nervous system just as a bubble chamber is activated by electrons, protons and other ionizing particles.

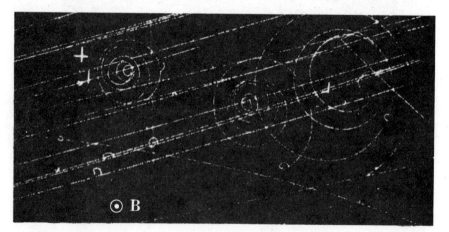

A bubble chamber is a device for rendering visible, by means of small bubbles, the tracks of charged particles that pass through the chamber. The figure is a photograph taken with such a chamber immersed in a field of magnetic induction B and exposed to radiations from a large cyclotron-like accelerator. The spirals are the tracks of three low-energy electrons. (Courtesy E.O. Lawrence Radiation Laboratory, University of California.)

The ordinary mind thinks that invisible objects do not exist, but there are more invisible objects in the environment than there are visible ones. There are the molecules of air we breathe; there are distant galaxies, atoms vibrating in a piece of wood or brick, the sap streaming in a piece of grass, the individual blood cells in the red liquid that pours out of a cut finger. And there are the energies and electrical forces which are ever present, emerging in patterns and energies from every human, making much of the human being invisible to the naked eye. The actual energy field of a human being measures nine feet across or about eighty centimeters in every direction from the heart center. But most people only see what is within the physical skin, the psychic skin being completely invisible. When two people who love each other get within nine feet of each other, their two interlocking auras begin to tingle and emotional energies begin to stream like sap or juice flowing like protoplasm in the cells of life. From the sixth level this delightful elated feeling is very ordinary stuff. But for those imprisoned at the bottom level of the physical sensations, it represents the kind of lower love that is experienced at the chemical level of impressions in the emulsion of the film which relate to the chemical emotions heard about in every radio love song. Man was cut out for bigger things than this, as anyone who has had their kundalini tickled can understand. Divining and sensing the subtle energies of emotion may seem a long way from the lifting up of the kundalini energies in the experience of spiritual love, but Supersensonics is a science specially designed to investigate and bring to birth the spiritual states of consciousness which are possible to man through the sixth level of his brain evolution.* Supersensonics brings together the wisdom of the prophets and the knowledge of modern science.

The ancients believed that the clairvoyant and psychic faculties bore relationship to the pineal gland while in recent years many investigators assumed that because the pineal was hardened by calcification after puberty that the organ was without function. In the last ten years

---

* One of the sensors which can detect sixth level energies is the Supersensonics instrument, handcrafted at the University of the Trees, called a "Kundalini Roomph Coil" which helps a meditator to safely raise his kundalini without putting through more psychic voltage than his physical circuits are evolved to handle.

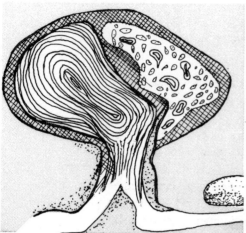

The hypophysis or pituitary gland produces seven hormones from its anterior lobe and two from its posterior lobe. It is situated at the front end of the third ventricle. This gland releases hormones which then polarize the energies which produce a reaction in the pineal gland.

the pineal has been found to be a photo-receptor or "third eye" which converts light of certain wavelengths into nervous impulses. Then it was found that the pineal is stimulated through the eyes and that light also increases the production of serotonin enzyme in the pineal and controls circadian rhythms in several animals and birds. Serotonin production is coupled with ionization of the fluids in the third ventricle. Exposure to continuous light or removal of the pineal gland increases the weight of the sexual organs and stimulates the estrus cycle. Injections of melatonin slows the growth of ovaries in the same way that continuous darkness increases the melatonin hormone activity. Summer's longer days make less melatonin but more sex development while shorter days and less light in winter cause the production of melatonin which in turn inhibits growth of sex glands. Increased illumination in modern times is thought to bring puberty quicker in children.

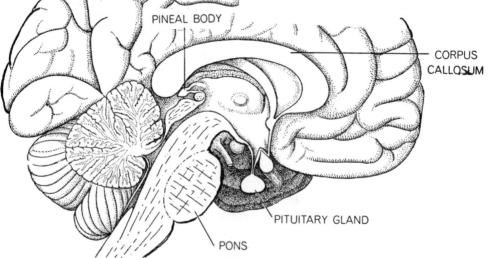

PINEAL BODY

CORPUS CALLOSUM

PITUITARY GLAND

PONS

The pineal gland located in humans in the center of the brain at the rear of the third ventricle was believed to have evolved through evolutionary history from the light sensitive regulator of body cycles of seasons in reptilian brains. The pineal is a light-seeking piece of skin. Light activates the gland to secrete the hormone melatonin, which brings about the state of balance between the energies of the sex glands and the higher spiritual states which facilitate the direct perception of the diviner's signals. The diviner's reaction was studied in seven levels by the ancients who used it to discover unknown facts about God's ways. Hence it was called divination or consulting the gods and was developed to a supreme art at Delphi, in Egypt, and by the ancient prophets.

The three lobes which control our sixth level experience of "knowing" are situated along the walls and roof of the third ventricle or Cave of Brahma where the pineal and pituitary glands sit at each end of the Cave and release their magical hormones to control a whole range of biological computers around its walls. These computers have been built by later

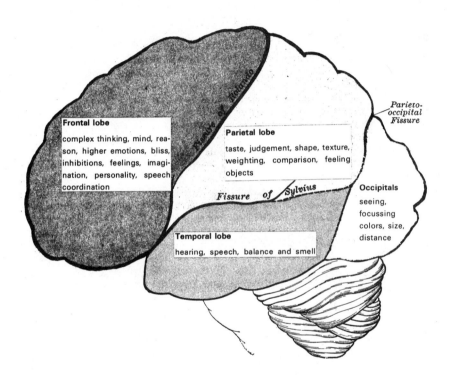

Frontal lobe
complex thinking, mind, reason, higher emotions, bliss, inhibitions, feelings, imagination, personality, speech coordination

Parietal lobe
taste, judgement, shape, texture, weighting, comparison, feeling objects

Fissure of Rolando

Parieto-occipital Fissure

Fissure of Sylvius

Occipitals
seeing, focussing colors, size, distance

Temporal lobe
hearing, speech, balance and smell

developments along the line of evolution onwards from the lizard, but the lizard's crude undifferentiated pineal sensing ability is still retained in the brain of every human. Even the lizard originally got its sensitivity through evolution when the walls of the sensitive skin of the amoeba gradually infolded into the primitive pineal third "eye" of the reptilians. The fact that heredity extends not only from parent to child but from lizard to man or from algae to lizard is not always obvious. But all life is one, even though the links may persist only in the unconscious.

Our entire nervous system has inherited this ability to sense relationships in Nature through the unconscious mind. This human nervous system which picks up comparative sensations is referred to in the Bible as the "Tree of Knowledge". It can sense either/or, on/off, yes/no, hot or cold, light or dark, good or evil, but it cannot make sense of the whole. To know beyond the duality of comparisons and to experience "wholes" rather than "parts" we must go to another level of this sensing ability which the Bible calls the "Tree of Life". This Tree of Life is also referred to in the Bhagavad Gita as the brain with its roots pointing upward at the cosmos. To tune in to the will of the universe, then, we must develop the Tree of Life.

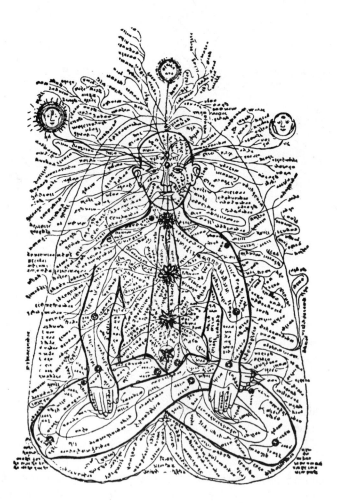

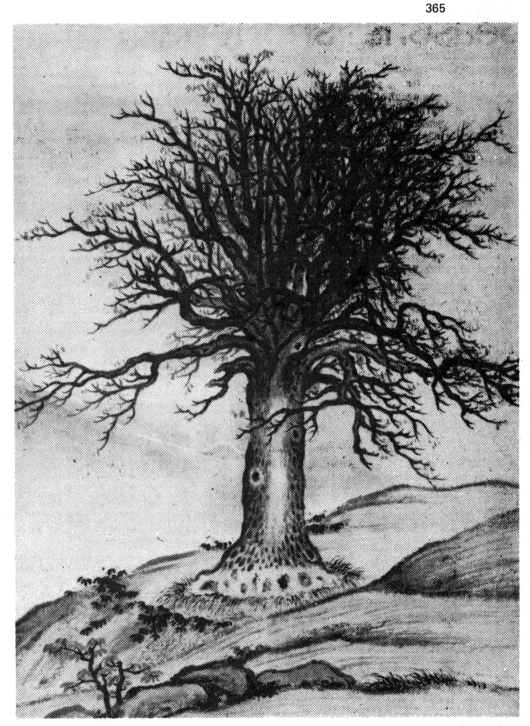

This drawing by Hsiang Sheng-mo circa 1597-1658 symbolizes the image of the nerve dendrites in the brain which the ancients called the "Tree of Life". The human brain has 10^{13} (100,000,000,000,000) nerve cells, each capable of communicating with hundreds of thousands of its colleagues in the hologram of life.

DISCOVERING THE WILL OF GOD:
ANCIENT DIVINING BY URIM AND THUMMIM

Let us go back in time to the age when great prophet-kings ruled the nation of Israel, consisting of twelve tribes, and the main occupation of the prophet at the sanctuary in the temple was to determine the will of God by using the sacred oracle, practicing the ceremony which was called "Enquiring of the Lord". "Urim and Thummim" was the name given to the two parts of the sacred oracle by which the prophets ascertained the will of God. Urim and Thummim, Light and Darkness, Yes and No, Yang and Yin, Life and Death. Urim and Thummim, Yes and No were determined by a pendulum, an ancient practice which Moses had learned while he was yet still a boy in the house of Egypt. Urim and Thummim, Light or Dark, is the answer we get when we practice divination.

The Jews divined through the ancient ceremony of using a breast-plate to determine the sacred oracle. The prophet would wear a waistcloth or apron looking like a short kilt called the "ephod" which had straps going over the shoulders to support it. The Bible describes the details of the breastplate divining instument.* On the shoulders these straps had a rosette exactly like the symbol of Nuclear Evolution, like a flower with many petals and many concentric circles worked in gold. (See illustration opposite.) The breastplate was hooked onto these two rosettes by the means of golden chains on rings. The breastplate itself was made from very fine linen, nine inches square on each side, in colors of gold, blue, purple, scarlet—foursquare and doubled with a setting of four rows of stones around the outside. The first row sardius, topaz, carbuncle; the second row emerald, sapphire, diamond; the third row ligure, agate, amethyst; fourth row beryl, onyx, jasper. These stones were set in gold and secured around the edge of the breastplate representing twelve stones, each a symbol for a tribe of Israel. The chains which secured the breastplate to the ephod, or the apron strings, were also secured by rings of gold to the bottom of the pouch to keep it secure.

---

* Ex. 28:30, Lev. 8:8, Deut. 33:8, Ezra 2:63, Neh. 7:65.

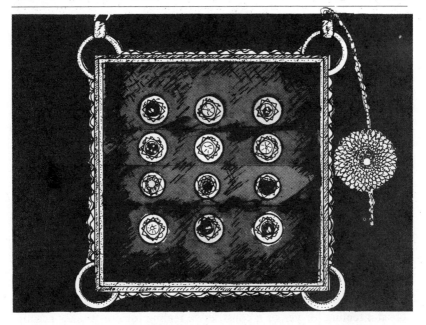

The prophet would enquire of the Lord by placing his finger on one of the jewels and rubbing it, searching for a tactile sensation of resistance for answer of yes or no. Then he would check that answer with the pendulum (the Thummim) to ask further if the message for that particular tribe was yes or no in answer to a question put to the Lord. Going over the breastplate with his fingers he would be able to determine the correct course of the government for the entire land. The twelve tribes on these occasions would bring their questions to be determined by Urim and Thummim.

This practice of divination was lost and its meaning not even known once the Israelites were in captivity, in exile in Babylon for hundreds of years. When they came back they could not speak their own language or remember their own customs, and the words Urim and Thummim were a mystery to them and still are to this very day amongst Bible scholars who do not know anything about divination. In fact it was banned by the early Church. So let us get inside the mind of a prophet of ancient times and imagine ourself in the sanctuary, wearing our breastplate over our heart, tuning in to the will of God, asking our questions in terms of yes and no, Urim and Thummim, and waiting for the diviner's signal, the answer from the cosmos that is in the reach of everyone. Not only every human but each and every insect and animal, everything in the whole of creation, is able to make this contact with what is good and what is not good.

This faculty was known to Adam in the allegory of the Garden and it was said that he knew what was good to eat and what was not good to eat. We all have this ability, and this knowledge is now being given back to the human race from the ancient times. The pendulum is the means for the determination of the will of God—man's sensor of light and dark, good and evil, right and wrong. And knowing this, we can determine our every action during the day, during the week and during the year. Every decision can be made in accordance with the will of God, using our own heart as the tablet of destiny, the breastplate of the prophets. By placing our hand over our heart and asking the pendulum a question, yes or no, light Urim, darkness Thummim, yang or yin, positive or negative, we can feel in the heart a response, possibly a blissful feeling for yes or a constrictive feeling for no. It takes practice to develop certainty in our answers.

We can use this knowledge in the operation of our own conscious-ness and its contact with the divine intelligence which knows our thoughts before we even think of them, knows our karma and knows our destiny before we even ask the question. All is written in conscious-ness with ink more indelible than matter itself. This is a secret of the great prophets, for they alone know that to divine with accuracy the heart must be pure and the motive attuned to the whole and that only when these conditions are present will divining really reflect the will of the universe. Like all divining instruments, the pendulum will bring forth whatever is in the unconscious mind that is working through the nervous system to produce the positive or negative signal. Hence the divining tool becomes a spiritual instrument for the purifying of our consciousness. If we do not believe these divining tools work, there is another way of checking the ionization of the diviner's reaction by an instrument that can detect the presence of ions. This instrument is described in *Nuclear Evolution* in great detail for those who need to follow up some rigorous experimentation. For this book it is enough to know that not only did the prophets believe these were tools of higher consciousness but great yogis and sages in India and China developed whole systems of spiritual knowledge around these tools.

THE ULTIMATE DIVINING INSTRUMENT

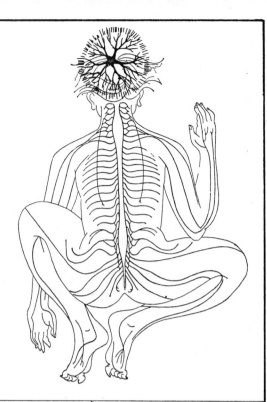

By amplifying the subtle signals of the human antenna, pendulums and other divining instruments enable us to communicate with that deep Self inside us who is maintaining that sensitive nerve system and carrying on all the automatic functions of the body and all the biochemical transfers that go to create thought, feeling, and expression or, in other words, our consciousness.

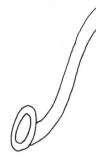

A Jui scepter divining rod in its ceremonial form

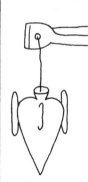

A Merkhet: Egyptian for instrument of knowing

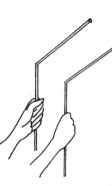

Angle rods of the Western water dowser

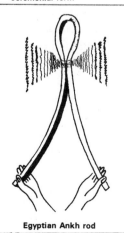

Egyptian Ankh rod

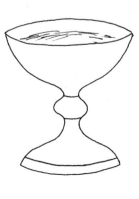

Divining cups for scrying used by Joseph

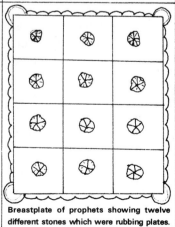

Breastplate of prophets showing twelve different stones which were rubbing plates.

The fact that the brain could detect very subtle signals, perceived by the unconscious mind acting through the neuromuscular responses of a diviner's arms, hands, or heart, was well known to primitive people throughout the world who gained most of their remarkable knowledge of the I Ching, pyramid architecture, and the properties of drugs and of herbs by this means. When we use these methods of divination to determine the levels of consciousness, the levels appear to go in octaves corresponding to the seven levels of the color spectrum. These methods, described in *Supersensonics,* are based on the laws of resonance to be found in music, in physics and in biological interactions with matter. The atomic table of elements displays the same resonance periodicity within its own octave of matter, showing that light, energy, matter and form are not only absorbed into each other as specific thresholds and as steps in the energy continuum but that this continuum extends on either side of the material one. Our physical sensations cannot perceive these thresholds directly, but our unconscious mind can pick out resonance and stress between certain frequencies emitted by gases, objects and their specific oscillations of patterns of energy in the environment and feed it back to us in the form of the diviner's signal. In this way very subtle states of ionization of molecular substances in the human brain, the skin, and the intercellular fluids are detected.

These methods revealed to the ancients much more about the states of consciousness in which they were interested than they revealed about the material world in which modern science is interested. However, detection of very minute vibrations in molecules and cells can be achieved with Supersensonic instruments as easily as divining for oil wells or underground water. In ancient times elaborate ceremonies were evolved to assist in creating the right moods for the meditative state in which the best results of brain ionization are found. The release of enkephalins and the polarity of the sodium-potassium exchange in the brain fluids is best achieved in a meditative trance state, easily induced by yogic techniques. This makes the brain hypersensitive to vibrating patterns of energy emanating from objects and from the cosmic intelligence itself.

Many people fear the trance state because there is a certain giving up of control. But we ourselves have the final say of who or what we surrender to. If we surrender to "entities" we become possessed. If we surrender to the unconscious mind without knowing its forces of darkness as well as its forces of light, then we may be overwhelmed by it and go insane. But if we surrender to the highest and best in ourself or surrender to God or love, this we can do in perfect safety. So again, the purity of the one who is attempting these things and the motive with which it is done will determine what is mirrored back by the universe. Many people pray to their image or concept of God, but few actually believe He will answer back. Divining is a two-way communication with the universe at all levels, from atom to infinity. Whether one actually uses instruments or only waits for God's reply in whatever situation life uses to mirror us back to ourselves, the ability to see or hear this message hinges upon trust.

Trust in God or in the beneficence of the universe is the prerequisite of meditation as well as trance, and here again divining is revealed as a rigorous spiritual discipline, for the whole gamut of spiritual disciplines can be reduced to this one difficult step: *total trust and total surrender to the cosmic will.* The myth of the Garden of Eden describes this state of inner bliss, this paradise, as a garden whose center is the Tree of Life. Adam had the ability to "know" God and to talk to him directly through the intuition. Eating from the Tree of Knowledge of Good and Evil centered Adam in the lower level of his third brain and thrust him from the garden of the higher levels into the external world. Most people do not realize how a seemingly harmless choice or a preference for one level of consciousness can bar the way to a higher level. Nor do they know how much better they would fare if they had this intuition working instead of just relying on the third brain ability to discriminate good from evil, right from wrong and all the other comparative types of knowledge. This comparative state of knowing through the Tree of Knowledge cannot be compared with the direct perception through the Tree of Life because there is no comparison. The Tree of Life cannot be known conceptually for it functions on a totally different level.

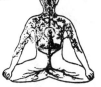

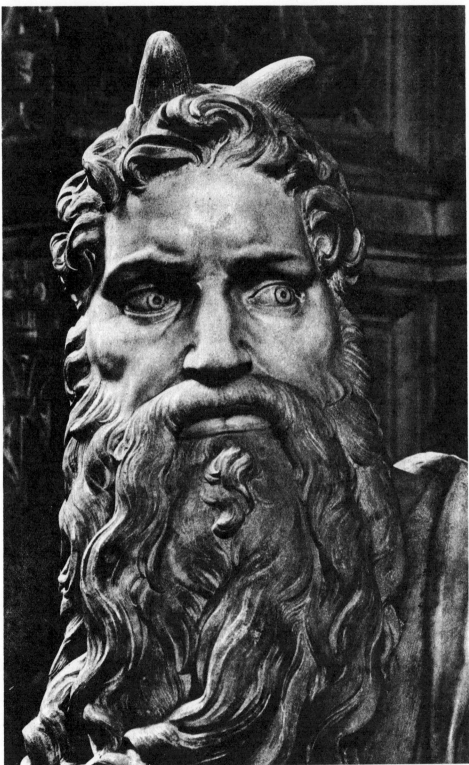

The horns on Michaelangelo's Moses represent the extension of the frontal lobes when the divining faculty is developed in the prophets.

The antenna-like horns on the forehead in paintings and sculptures of Moses is symbolic of the developed intuitive centers of the brain. If we develop and follow our intuition it can guide us in all the situations of our lives. If we develop this faculty even further we will have the psychic faculties called telepathy and clairvoyance. Though these are not necessarily spiritual faculties, unless used by a person who is in himself spiritual, even so, the intuition is related to that state of grace in which man experiences a connection with the cosmos and communicates directly with God, without recourse to laborious thinking processes. The ancient Hindu sages called this "Darshana" or direct perception of reality.

Many people have referred to a guiding intelligence which pulls us through into new life and new destiny rather than something that pushes us and coerces us to conform to an arbitrary absolute pattern. Our intuition and the sixth level of our vehicle of perception has the power to go directly to the source. Whether we call this source "God" or "the force" or "pure intelligence" working through the destiny of kings and politicians or through the slow development of social forms, is of no concern to me. Such intelligence is so far beyond any idea of God or any image of God that can be formed in the mind of man that it becomes rather pitiful to contemplate the dogma and doctrines of our present world. For insight into the true nature of man's imaginations and abominations, the seeker of reality must proceed into the next level of brain function in which worlds unknown to most ordinary people are vibrating. For example, the level of consciousness which becomes aware of the tiny vibrating protein rods or cilia vibrating on the walls of the third ventricle to the subtle cosmic radiation enters a world called "Samadhi". *Sam* as a prefix means "complete", "together" or "equal", and *adhi* means "above" or "over all"*. When this inner vibration is in equal vibration or resonance with the cosmic vibration above and over all other vibrations, then the door to the seventh level opens and transforms our personality. People believe that only extraordinary beings can walk through this door, but the message of this chapter is that we all have the same doorways in the structure of our brains. And we all have the same nervous system, our antenna, in varying degrees of refinement and sensitivity depending on whether we have developed it.

---

* "Over all" is sometimes translated as unity.

374

Even the mosquito (A) is equipped with divining rods or sensitive cilia which can detect a specific species of mate or sense the location of blood from long distances away. A mosquito can navigate a maze and find the source of blood by a form of divining common to all organisms including humans. In humans this ability is sleeping in the unconscious, whereas for the mosquito it is a matter of survival. The above picture shows the antennal hairs of a young male mosquito which are constructed to the same pattern as the cilia in the human brain.

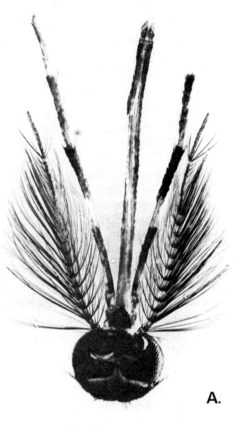

A.

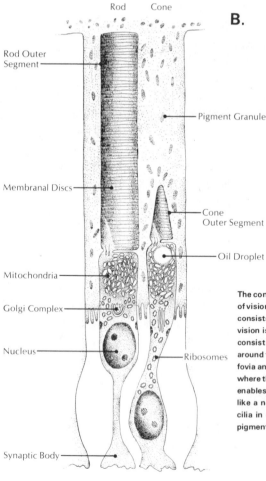

Rod   Cone

B.

Rod Outer Segment

Pigment Granule

Membranal Discs

Cone Outer Segment

Oil Droplet

Mitochondria

Golgi Complex

Nucleus

Ribosomes

Synaptic Body

THE SENSOR OF VISION

The cones send their signals to the occipital area of the brain for focusing of vision, determination of colors, etc. The antenna of the human eye (B) consists of about seven million cones concentrated at the center where vision is sharpest in bright light. The majority of the cells in the retina consist of one hundred fifty million rods or cilia which are concentrated around the periphery. They begin about twenty degrees from the central fovia and send their signals to the walls of the third ventricle of the brain where they link with similar cilia constructed to the same pattern, which enables us to see in dim light. The end of the cell nearest to the light is like a nerve axon and the other end is packed with mitochondria. The cilia in eye and brain contain little membranal discs of light-sensitive pigments and also act as antennae for invisible light radiations.

Divination, therefore, is not a special faculty limited to a few but, like the insects who use the divining faculty for survival and use their antennae as divining rods, the human race has this sixth sense in rudimentary form built into the sensitivity of every brain cell in the central region known as the Cave of Brahma. This name was given by

There are many examples of divination in the insect world on which the survival of each species depends. In the human brain the cilia or fine hairs lining the third ventricle are constructed internally in a pattern similar to the antennae of insects, even though the external shape is different. The antennae of insects, however, are always jointed and take varied forms: (1) knobbed (many beetles); (2) elbowed (bees, ants, snout beetles); (3) aristate (housefly; referring to the bristlelike tip, or arista, projecting from the antenna); (4) scarab-type, composed of flat plates (June beetles); (5) double-combed (many moths); (6) threadlike (moths, roaches, caddis flies); (7) saw-toothed (many beetles); (8) clublike (butterflies).

the author to the third ventricle as a loose translation of the word "Brahmananda Gahara". The ancient texts refer to *ananda* ("bliss") as "sitting in an ocean of milk" or they refer to the "ambrosia" caused by the release of certain neurotransmitters by the hypothalamus which transforms personality. Such chemicals are made naturally in the brain and are called peptides or enkephalins by scientists but they are really chemical waves flowing through human tissues.

An instrument called the "Supersensonic Awareness Meter" uses the consciousness of the vibrating rods or cilia in the sixth brain to detect when our consciousness is tuned in resonance with a given material situation or pattern. The resulting pattern emitted by an object or substance can be expressed in angles of a geometrical pattern or degrees of a circle or in linear fashion along a rule. Each object emits a series of fundamental rays which are detectable by the awareness of a diviner in a biological way when resonance with their vibration occurs in the brain. This causes a neuromuscular reaction to twist the diviner's rod or move a pendulum like a feedback signal from our unconscious mind. At the moment, this phenomenon has not been scientifically investigated by our universities and therefore little is

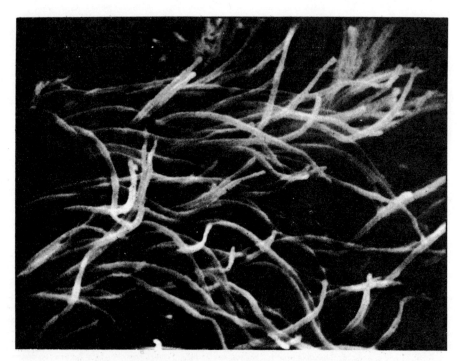

Cilia lining the brain's third ventricle, transport hypothalamic peptides.

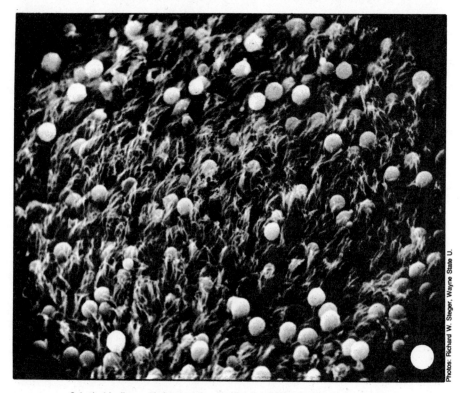

Spherical bodies nestled among the cilia (fine hairs) lining brain's third ventricle.

Photos: Richard W. Steger, Wayne State U.

known to the academic consensus. However, many great doctors and scientists have investigated it and used the method in their practice and kept quiet about it. In Britain there is a group of doctors who have met regularly for many years at the medical society in London to investigate what they call medical radiesthesia which uses the same faculty of the human body to detect these signals. The Russian researchers call it "biological radio" and some call it tele-pathy which means "touching at a distance" or "feeling at a distance" just as tele-vision means "seeing at a distance".

Insects and reptiles seek their mates, their food and their prey by using sensitive detectors which respond to design patterns in the wing formation or detect their vibrations at particular frequencies. Just as the mosquito senses with its antennae the vibration of blood as well as the 350 cycle frequency of the beating wings of its mate, so does the lizard find its food and mate by the sensitivity of its skin and the vibration-prone pineal gland. Its primitive divining faculty is the same faculty which remains and persists in the DNA of human nerve and skin cells from the very beginning of evolution, going back to the sensitive skin of the primitive single cell—the amoeba. The same DNA, made up of the same proteins and nucleic acids, is in the cells of all life and only the arrangement of them makes for all the differences between plants, insects, animals and human species. The amoeba divines for its food and senses its destiny by the same inherent faculty as a migrating bird or salmon, and humans have this same ability to detect other levels of awareness. Thus Nature provides itself with a way of caring for and communicating with all its creatures. There is no need for anyone to get lost in the desert or be unable to know the direction of home or the place where they were born. Eskimos use this same faculty for traveling hundreds of miles across trackless snows and they never get lost. Those who don't know they have this faculty find it hard to understand why some people can go directly to a place or find their direction in life.

The Awareness Meter is described more fully in my books *Supersensonics* and *Instruments of Knowing* which give instructions on how to use it and how consciousness can be measured in terms of a

fundamental angle of a spiral form as a representation* of the evolutionary thrust working through all living organisms. A rough estimate
of comparative intelligence is provided by this instrumental means of
measuring by proportional angles. By divining, you can find out your
present level of evolution on a scale which measures the thresholds of
awareness in proportional terms rather than quantitative values: 1000
degrees represents full use of all octaves of the physical instrument of
perception as in Christ, Buddha, Krishna, etc., or in terms of all around
perception, 360 degrees of consciousness.

THE AWARENESS METER

IN PROPORTIONS OF 1000

2.7	Atoms
10-31	Insects, to lizards at 60 (6%)
62	Animal life begins
220-230	Threshold of higher mammals, dolphins, whales, etc. (some extending higher.)
250	Average intelligence normal laborers
300	Top foremen and skilled workers
385	Ordinary judges, professors, etc.
460	Visionaries, statesmen, philosophers, etc.
600	Level of genius
670 and up	Leonardo da Vinci, Einstein, Newton, Shakespeare, etc.
800-1000	Spiritual genius, avatars, world changers.

---

* An independent adaptation of this representation has been developed by Malcolm Rae
of England who has developed an instrument for potentization of homeopathic remedies
purely from the geometrical pattern on a card placed in the instrument. A book entitled
Dimensions of Radionics, setting out the development which has now been tested by
over 2000 operators, was published in England by Health Science Press, authored by
Dr. David Tansley.

The question comes: once you know what level of awareness you have, what do you do with the information? What good does it do you to know? What the Awareness Meter provides is a feeling for the range and scope of evolution and the strata or levels in which the cosmos works. We may know very well that we have more awareness than an insect, and we don't need an Awareness Meter to tell us so. But most of us have no inkling of the octaves of awareness that exist *above* where we are at. Study of the brain shows us just how mediocre is our tuning of the instrument of consciousness. If, for example, you responded negatively to the idea of "blowing your mind" in order to free the fifth brain for the cosmic program on the sixth level, perhaps you felt that a sense of the wholeness of the universe was of no interest to you whatsoever. In that case, you would have to ask yourself what level of consciousness in you was having that feeling, because the fifth brain's potential to have that experience of oneness is a *fact*, and you have to ask yourself, "Why did evolution give to man that possibility if it were not part of our destiny to have it?"

If evolution expresses in octaves of refinement that extend not only throughout the world of matter but beyond it, then what are the octaves of our human expression? We began with the reptilian brain which had the capacity to see whole in another octave at a lower level and which has evolved out of it; when the brain evolves back *into* this ability in the human being, it sees *whole* but at a much higher rung of the evolutionary spiral. The saint's intuition of the oneness of the universe is quite different from the primitive reptilian feeling of oneness with the environment. What has made the difference? At level three, the human brain acquires self-consciousness. At level five, we begin to undo this separating of our self from the whole. We begin to regain that unseparated feeling, but now including all the levels of awareness we have evolved in the meantime. At level two we develop love of fellowman (not just herding instinct but a real human caring). From level six comes the awareness that we are being aware of the wider whole. Only man has this ability to be conscious of his own consciousness. Thus level six prepares the way for the awesome mystical experience of union on even higher levels and permits the tremendous range of feelings from level four (the heart center) to channel into that seventh level experience in which we simply marvel at the wonder of it all. Wonder is a feeling, just as anger is a feeling, but they come at different octaves of experience. Brain number six permits an intuitive seeing into the heart of all things as if we were that heart, and level seven enables us to form some notion of just how vast and glorious the One really is. These are spiritual states made possible by the magnificent sensing instrument of our brain. And yet the vast potential existed in consciousness *before* the brain was ready to express it, just as it exists in us now, while our brain sits waiting for the stimulus to begin that stage of its unfolding, waiting for the stimulus which can only come from our own self-consciousness.

HOW DO WE GET THERE?

The next two chapters deal with the highest science ever known to man which we could call the ultimate science of absolute knowledge. This transcendent knowing of the nature of consciousness cannot be reached by merely training the body in hatha yoga or by psychological and philosophical concepts. Though it is popularly believed that hatha yogis achieved great depths of trance and meditation, the author has noticed that although there are thousands of hatha yogis, hardly one of them knows anything of the highest science of all. The scriptures, both Hindu and Hebrew, hardly hint at it at all. Though we may meditate and read the Gita, though we may pray and hope for some salvation, this science remains closed to all who cannot understand how to use the instrument of the nervous system and the brain to develop it as a supersensor.

Many people believe that most yogis achieve powers of trance and psychic mind control but, for all these efforts, the divination of man is often lost on them as we can easily see by their actual manifestation. Any yogi who has to ask you anything or even ask for something, does not know the absolute science of manifesting out of pure consciousness. The step to this knowing is through the correct training of the sixth level which links with the seventh level containing the highest faculty of our brain, the power of self-suggestion (imagination), to sense, detect or even program in tune with the whole any event in any part of the universe in any state of existence within the hologram of the cosmic existence. This training is begun with simple instruments such as the pendulum or dowsing rods. Other methods of tuning the centers of consciousness are also available but they all achieve the same purpose of inquiring of the supersensory intelligence which not only created the body, but also knows, like the Tao, the correct way to go.

There are many who think themselves spiritually superior, looking at the Urim and Thummim, the yes and no response of our nervous system, as a fascination with gimmicks such as pendulums. Little do they know their own ignorance, for the study which brought our greatest prophets and the writers of the Vedas to the absolute science of the control of the psycho-active peptides and established hourly contact with the spirit of God (Tao) was divination through man's physical instrument of the body. True gurus use the diviner's response to an interior question in their consciousness to locate or discover any information. The sensation can be a tingle in the fingertips or even the response of our own breath in the nostrils, but the practice is the same. Paramahansa Yogananda, whose Western teachings of yoga included a new form of energizing yoga and Kriya yoga, did not teach this science of divining to his students but he did use it himself. He describes his experience with the diviner's response in his classic *Autobiography of a Yogi.**

> "Using a secret yoga technique, I broadcasted my love to Kashi's soul through the 'microphone' of the spiritual eye, the inner point between the eyebrows. I intuitively felt that Kashi would soon return to the earth, and that if I kept unceasingly broadcasting my call to him, his soul would reply. I knew that the slightest impulse sent to me by Kashi would be felt in the nerves of my fingers, arms and spine.

> Using my upraised hands as antennae, I often turned myself round and round, trying to discover the direction of the place in which, I believed, he had already been reborn as an embryo. I hoped to receive a response from him in the concentration-tuned 'radio' of my heart.

---

* *Autobiography of a Yogi*, Paramahansa Yogananda, Self-Realization Fellowship, 1946.

> With undiminishing zeal, I practiced the yoga method
> steadily for about six months after Kashi's death. Walking
> with a few friends one morning in the crowded Bowbazar
> section of Calcutta, I lifted my hands in the usual manner.
> For the first time, there was response. I thrilled to detect
> electrical impulses trickling down my fingers and palms.
> These currents translated themselves into one overpowering
> thought from a deep recess of my consciousness: 'I am
> Kashi, I am Kashi; come to me!' . . . The electrical
> impulses tingled through my fingers only when I faced
> toward a nearby path. . .''

All pendulums, rods and detectors are amplifiers of that supersense
which can measure even the number of atoms in the hair of your head,
and to regard them as gimmicks rather than tuning devices of the
higher instrument is to reveal our own limitations which we place on
that instrument. To look on these divining instruments as things in
themselves rather than as the tools of the superconscious, creating its
own interaction with the physical world, is to misunderstand how the
science of yoga, the subtle pathways of nerve currents and the channeling of the life force was discovered in the first place. The fact is that
the priests and the majority of yogis of the last few thousand years lost
this knowledge of direct perception and their successors actively
suppressed the development of the supersense while yet adoring it and
promoting it in their own spiritual leaders and gurus. It is the link to
knowing the nuclear center of the Self, for without some way of reading
the intelligence of the Tao and mapping the path of kundalini through
the spiritual vehicle, mankind is just as ignorant of himself as the day
he was born.

The worlds of vibration are many, but we cannot enter them this
moment, just because we decide that we want to see for ourselves. We
have to make ourselves eligible. No man or woman can appreciate the
higher joys of even the material world without first refining their
sensibilities. Why should we take the trouble? Why should we care if
we enter the nucleus of our being or not? I can only say to you, try it.
For every small step you take in the purifying of your consciousness,
the universe will reflect it back to you, multiplied a thousand-fold, in

happiness and good fortune. If you realize where this bliss has come from and why your life has suddenly become smoother, or more fulfilling, or more abundant, then you will get a glimpse of what the yogis call bliss and you will know that it is not beyond your reach.

Christ said to his disciples, "In my Father's house there are many mansions." Indeed the worlds of vibration interpenetrate on many levels of existence. Those masters of consciousness who speak of them from personal experience come to us to develop our supersense so that we, too, may be inspired to reach towards direct experience of God.

384

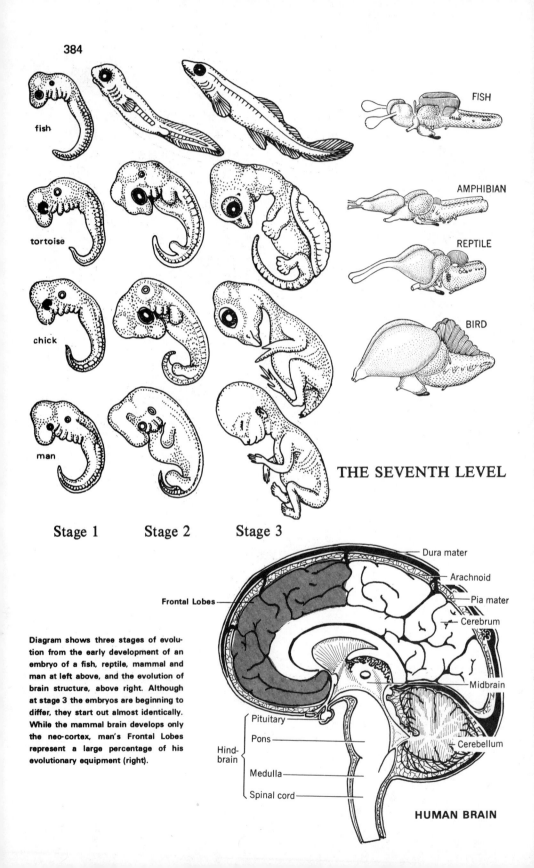

fish

tortoise

chick

man

FISH

AMPHIBIAN

REPTILE

BIRD

THE SEVENTH LEVEL

Stage 1   Stage 2   Stage 3

Diagram shows three stages of evolution from the early development of an embryo of a fish, reptile, mammal and man at left above, and the evolution of brain structure, above right. Although at stage 3 the embryos are beginning to differ, they start out almost identically. While the mammal brain develops only the neo-cortex, man's Frontal Lobes represent a large percentage of his evolutionary equipment (right).

Dura mater

Arachnoid

Frontal Lobes

Pia mater

Cerebrum

Midbrain

Pituitary

Pons

Cerebellum

Hind-brain

Medulla

Spinal cord

HUMAN BRAIN

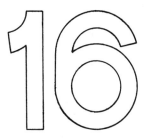

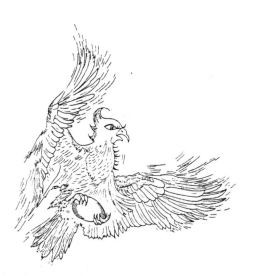

THE
SEVENTH
LEVEL

**The Seventh Level
The Frontal Lobes**

1. Reptilian brain

2. Pons

3. Cerebellum

4. Mid-brain

5. Inter-brain,
   Cave of Brahma

6. Occipital, Parietal
   and Temporal Lobes

7. Frontal Lobes

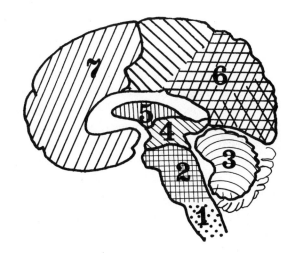

The Frontal Lobes are concerned with the most complex abilities of the mind. Higher reasoning power, the spiritual emotions, devotion, service, surrender, love and the power of judgement (wisdom) have their seat here. And yet, in most people, you can just cut out the Frontal Lobes and it won't make much difference. A lobotomy just makes you a little slower in abstract thinking. Most of the functions of this part of the brain people don't use anyway. The fore-brain is a much later development in man than the other brains and obviously its purpose is for developments yet to take place in the future of mankind as a whole. Evolution or creation starts preparing a long way back before it needs anything in the future, so it has given us all the equipment several thousand years ago that we need to be totally enlightened and all-knowing today. The seventh level resonates with the color violet in Nuclear Evolution and is the domain of the imagination. We may think of the imagination as a rather superficial part of the mind, good for idling away time or writing poems or myths, or for escaping reality. But in fact, the imagination shapes our reality, shapes our society entirely, and is the most important of all our mental faculties. Positive images are just as easy to create as negative images, but most people tend to build their reality upon negatives. For example, we carry with us throughout our lives hundreds of negative self-images, hurt feelings and traumas programmed into our brain computer from the time of early childhood up to the present moment. They are so familiar to us we do not notice them. We do not see that they are only images and can easily be transformed into positive images which are just as real and just as valid. Our self-image determines whether we feel confident or weak, pretty or homely, effective or incompetent, shy, intelligent, immature, sour, or any other thing that we think of as "me". It is the self-image that says "I can't." It keeps us limited to what we have already tried to do or be. New possibilities cannot penetrate the closed imagination when powerful formidable self-images are guarding the gateway. Until we become aware of these and deal with them, our reactions to life will be the same year after year, like a deep rut in which we cannot unfold our real potential. Nuclear Evolution makes these reactions obvious to people on different levels of consciousness and relates them to the hologram of life.

The whole universe is one cosmic egg with all its parts, its people, its cells, its stars and patterns of energy and light, all vibrating within the undifferentiated and homogeneous, intelligent plasma we call the ONE, or for religious people, God. Once the imagination is opened, the Evolutionary Intelligence can pour into the world of mankind the abundance of its infinite creativity, but only when the mind-stuff is pure; otherwise the mind will distort everything that it sees, both inside its own inner world and outside in the physical world of matter. This is what happens in society all the time. The ego reactions of individuals, scientists, religious people and of nations block the unfoldment of higher brain faculties. This is a great pity because it is avoidable, but it is part of the problem of being human so we must accept it with humility and do the best we can to communicate without ego reactions getting in the way. We must always ask ourselves how the ego and its tantrums can be tamed.

The answer lies in our imagination and depends on our self-image. How we view ourselves and how we limit our imaginations determines how we will relate to our work and to our environment. Many people say to me, "I can't accept what you have to say about life or God or man because you aren't speaking in a way I can appreciate. In my mind there are only two ways of relating: either you are scientific or you are using faith. Faith is blind, so anything besides science of the accepted academic kind is not real." These people have limited their concept of science and their comprehension of faith and do not even realize that the attitude they are holding is arrogant and based on fear of any other way. They cannot allow new images to enter their inner reality because their self-image of someone who has it all figured out would be shaken. Their parameters of reality are circumscribed to fit their limited acceptable framework. When a limited framework becomes socially acceptable we are in trouble because not only do we have to fight habitual images that we hold within ourselves, but we also have to buck the social reinforcements all around us.

Emotional reactions govern people so powerfully and so predictably that leaders of nations or political movements have always been able to play upon the hopes and fears in the imaginations of people and make them revolt or go to war or pay out more and more tax money to create a safe and secure future. Without the imagination, fear would be an entirely different experience. A fear enters our mind, and the imagination seizes upon it and soon it is a whole fantasy or internal movie that has churned up emotions and triggered hormones and put us in the state we would be in if the thing had actually happened. These fantasies are as real as some dreams and, if we let them unfold, we often have to insist several times to reassure ourselves, "It's only a fantasy; nothing to get upset about." By this same faculty of negative imagination, we shape our social world as well as our personal inner world of daily life.

Worry or concern for the future, which brings anxiety, is due to lack of foresight and is the one function of the Frontal Lobes which individual persons must master if they are to develop a peaceful society. The price the human race pays for its lack of foresight is revealed in its inability to anticipate, imagine or create the future effectively. The price is our personal and social anxiety about what is to come. In the past this anxiety was necessary to motivate survival, but it has now become so developed and sensitive that anxiety leads to tensions not only within individuals but builds up aggregate fears and tensions which are the cause of wars. Although most humans have a fairly good capacity for hindsight only a few have real foresight.

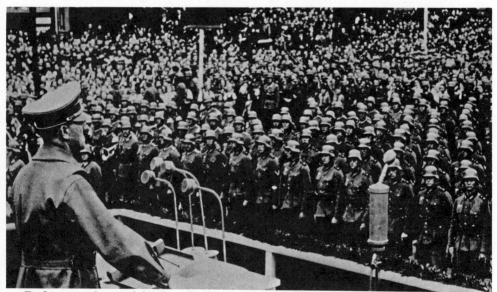

The German people responded to the spellbinding, hypnotic words of Hitler as he called them the "Master Race".
Could they have had the foresight to know the outcome of this egotism?

Society in its most civilized forms has always been brought to its heights through the foresight of the few, through the envisioning of technical and spiritual innovations. Now we must envision the possibility that the collectively uncontrolled imaginings and anxieties of the many about the future create a negative force in society which controls and limits all the lower brains of participants in society.

Yogis set out to voluntarily master these areas of human brain activity many thousands of years ago by getting control of thoughts and abstractions through techniques of meditation. Such self-mastery may now no longer be a voluntary choice but a matter of social survival of the entire species. Therefore the social system itself needs to encourage self-examination and self-government of our perceptions and feelings, especially in the areas of doubt and worry.* It is no use looking at the positive vision of the future and expecting it to really happen until we have looked at recent history and seen that the way we perceive and respond to events reveals a negative state of evolution.

NEGATIVE IMAGINATION

The neurotic condition of society can be traced to the mounting anxiety of individuals concerning their ability to cope with the growing threat of annihilation and with man's attitude to the psychic and industrial pollution of the planet. Certain behavior patterns that avoid rather than cope with personal problems lead people to take drugs such as tranquilizers, alcohol, sleeping pills, marijuana and LSD, or use valium for sedating hyperactive children. These accepted modern-day defense mechanisms for avoiding severe anxiety seldom work for long because the organism becomes adapted and needs bigger and bigger dosages in order to feel any effect. Furthermore these escape mechanisms only alleviate a small part of the total anxiety and they interfere in the long run with a person's effective functioning, thereby creating an even deeper condition of uncertainty and worry. This creates a vicious cycle in which the person feels trapped, helpless and impotent.

---

* For those who wish to investigate imagination in depth refer to the chapter on "Penetrating the Imagination Barrier" in *Nuclear Evolution.*

The neurotic individual may not always resort to chemical means of escaping anxiety but may adopt social means such as intense political activity or fanatic religious practices. Feeling inadequate to cope, he throws himself wholly into self-defeating behavior by expecting the state or God to do what only he can do to break the vicious cycle of guilt, failure and unhappiness. Because the anxious person

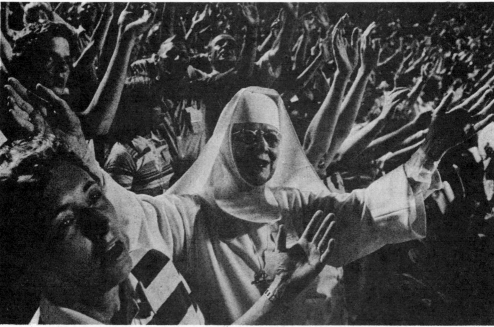

Massive crowds do not lead to saintliness.

feels inadequate, afraid and uncertain within, he elects as his leader a neurotic or charismatic individual who may orchestrate and play upon the same human uncertainties in society itself and thereby cling rigidly to established patterns of behavior and social structures and be unable to recognize any alternative course of action. Any changes are then regarded as threats which shake even more the confidence and certainty of the hoped-for long-term stability. We become fearful of the consequences of any alternative ways of doing things. Each day is lived with the tension and apprehension mounting greater and we feel that something dreadful is imminent. This condition makes the true believer in a cause even more fanatic, more energetic to push his own solutions as a compensation for his fear; and his doomsaying zeal increases even more his fervor for the old well-tried and familiar ways. But the old ways obviously do not work and frustration sets in. This affects the physiological conditions of the heart palpitation, breathing rate, blood pressure and muscular tension and excites the sympathetic nerve system which secretes adrenalin to bring on the social symptoms of group fear and aggression. This tension is the root cause of the blood clot and heart disease, the nation's number one killer!

The average citizen has no idea why he is frightened, and the anxiety is not associated with any particular person or stimulus or condition. The feeling of uncertainty is less due to external events than to the feeling and conflict raging uncontrolled within the individual. It floats free throughout society like a diffuse cloud but at any moment of crisis can become specific and concentrated around certain people or events. It is in such a climate that aggressive energies of war and the destructive will of tyrants act as the focus for the discharge of this tension and anxiety whenever the enemy becomes clearly defined. Such uncontrolled neurotic anxiety is one cause of the unconscious brutality and vicious aggression we shall find reflected in examples throughout this book. The positive solution to the problem is clearly to control the *inner* conflict by mature techniques, rather than resort externally to such avoidance mechanisms as drugs and war, alcohol and pornography.

HOW DO WE LEARN TO USE IMAGINATION POSITIVELY?

The Frontal Lobes of the seventh level of brain organization have billions of direct connections with the walls of the cave of the third ventricle. Surrounding the walls of this cave are millions of resonators—the cilia which cover the thalamus, the hypothalamus and many of the central computers embedded in the walls of the cave which link the sixth level of knowing with the seventh level above it. The secretions of the chemical hormones and polypeptides we call psychoactive enkephalins, which are carried across the floor of the Cave of Brahma, activate the higher realms of thinking and perception. The entire brain and body therefore become the fundamental source of life energy which is raised up by the ratchet effect into higher octaves of organization. The Cave of Brahma is the center of control for the voluntary and involuntary responses to light and radiation from countless stars in the universe including our local sun. The connections between the secretion of melatonin from the pineal gland, the light-sensitive cilia and the receptivity of human skin do not seem accidental or mystical. The gift of perception on a higher level of consciousness reveals a mirror image of the sensitive skin of the most primitive amoeba but on a higher level. We find our white blood cells are the first cousins of the amoeba on a higher octave of complex organization and that the sensitivity of the skin to radiation and light on the inner wall of the Cave of Brahma is the doorway connecting us to the higher realms of existence, the higher reasoning powers and the imagination of a sage. To the ordinary logical consciousness which has not opened this doorway to the supersensitive inputs of radiant energy, the operation of the seventh level brain function is mostly closed off. To open it up completely results in the faculty of true imagination or wisdom.

Why are wisdom and true imagination one and the same? A wise person is interested primarily in how the imagination produces fantasies, illusions, delusions and also reality. In its normal interpretation imagination is a derogatory term standing for something which cannot be real or present in reality. But the wise person knows that nothing can be experienced either from the senses, by abstract thought or the process of deduction unless it comes through the imagination. Even God who spoke through the ancient prophets spoke through their imaginations, and all thoughts, concepts or ideas are essentially images. Every word we speak is an image, whether it is a pictogram in the Chinese language or a phonogram as in English. All language, when analyzed in its basic components, finishes up as a vibration of sound translated into images. This transition from vibration to imagination is at the heart of all experience on every level of consciousness except the eighth level which is beyond the imagination. Wisdom is in knowing what lies beyond the imagination of humans since the true Godhead or fount of consciousness is basically unimaginable. Yet it is experienceable in consciousness. This experience is wisdom. The opening of the Frontal Lobes and the attainment of wisdom can be achieved by concentration and meditation upon a specific trigger area of the brain.

WHY DOES MEDITATION AFFECT IMAGINATION?

There are a group of trigger cells in the back part of the Frontal Lobes just above the pituitary gland in front of the Cave of Brahma which are involved in complex voluntary movements of the tongue and speech. This area is called the motor cortex and is sensitive to the electrical ionization of the membranes inside the Cave of Brahma behind it. In highly evolved people this sensitive area picks up the electricity in the brain and will cause involuntary spasms of the muscles occasionally, as this center in the fore-brain keeps the muscles in balance between a state of relaxation and contraction. If this area is damaged or ignored its power of controlling relaxation is lost. The muscles can even become permanently contracted and stiff as in spastic paralysis. It is this group of trigger cells which controls the alpha rhythms of the brain and relaxes the nerves and cells whenever the conscious attention is focused without any strain upon the particular area as in meditation.* Disease or a tumor or emotional stress in certain parts of the Frontal Lobes can cause personality changes, errors of judgement, lack of insight and very poor control over the emotional, chemical and endocrine exchange. Some people have had to have areas of the Frontal Lobes deactivated entirely in order to eliminate pressures and stress, and they have done so without much change in their ordinary life on the lower levels of consciousness. Such people are found to be dull and without the faculty of rapid abstract thought and higher perception.

Normal people have the ability to bring the Frontal Lobes into

---

*The course *Into Meditation Now* is a specific course of instruction by the author which students take by correspondence. With one hour's practice every day the meditator soon learns to control the alpha state which relaxes the entire nervous system through the parasympathetic nerve ganglia when the eyes are closed.

action through the practice of certain yogic disciplines but most people do not know how to do it without drugs. The light-sensitive pineal gland not only secretes the melatonin hormones which govern the circadian rhythms of reptiles and birds, but also governs the daily rhythmic fluctuations of the brain in man. It has been found in manic-depressive people that the twenty-four hour cycles of the day get out of synchronization with the day and night biological clocks of the body. The circadian rhythm runs too fast in the manic state and too slow in the depressive state. Because the manic individual is accelerated to an earlier time each day the biological clock finds the manic person burning the midnight oil and sleeping during the daytime through exhaustion. In manic states the element lithium has been found to return patients from their hyperactive manic state to normal circadian rhythms. The effect of lithium on the light-triggered pineal secretions in animals has a similar effect to the effect of light when melatonin secretion is inhibited—the higher centers are triggered instead of the lower, physical/sexual center. The manic person is highly red level in consciousness, and treatment with lithium subdues this level while stimulating the levels on the other end of the spectrum.

Many animals as well as flowers show light-triggered seasonal responses (like hibernation), such as the shortening length of the day which brings out late-blooming flowers like the chrysanthemum and poinsettia. Similarly the well-known pineal hormone secretion in human beings which comes from the advent of more light in spring and lessens with the increasing darkness of fall, varies with the circadian rhythmic twenty-four hour cycles of light and dark. In the tropics where light is more intense, sexual activity is more intense, and the size of the sexual organs is bigger because melatonin has a growth factor which triggers the growth of sexual organs and the darkness of skin pigmentation. The pineal gland under certain light conditions, channels the secretions of melatonin to awaken the higher brains for telepathic contact which may account for the telepathic abilities of Eskimos where low-level light predominates most of the day. The absence of ultraviolet light in Eskimoland shuts off the flow of melatonin to the sex glands and sends it instead to the higher centers. Eskimo populations are more pineal-orientated in their imaginations and more conscious of their total 360 degree environment. The Eskimo relates more through the imagination

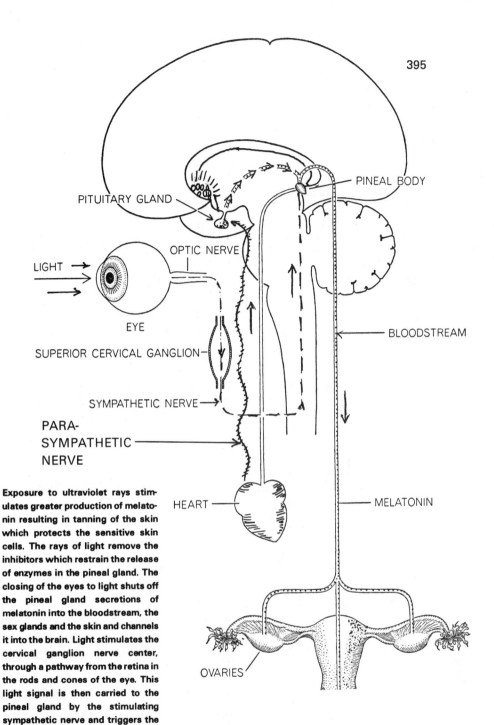

PINEAL BODY

PITUITARY GLAND

OPTIC NERVE

LIGHT

EYE

SUPERIOR CERVICAL GANGLION

SYMPATHETIC NERVE

PARA-
SYMPATHETIC
NERVE

BLOODSTREAM

HEART

MELATONIN

OVARIES

Exposure to ultraviolet rays stimulates greater production of melatonin resulting in tanning of the skin which protects the sensitive skin cells. The rays of light remove the inhibitors which restrain the release of enzymes in the pineal gland. The closing of the eyes to light shuts off the pineal gland secretions of melatonin into the bloodstream, the sex glands and the skin and channels it into the brain. Light stimulates the cervical ganglion nerve center, through a pathway from the retina in the rods and cones of the eye. This light signal is then carried to the pineal gland by the stimulating sympathetic nerve and triggers the release of melatonin into the blood.

In low light the relaxing parasympathetic nerve governs the release of hormones from the pituitary gland which releases enkephalins which in turn trigger the pineal gland to secrete its light-sensitive enzymes. When the eyes are closed and the person is meditating, these enzymes are not shot into the bloodstream but are sent to the higher centers of the brain. Hence the pituitary gland and the pineal gland work together inside the Cave of Brahma to produce higher states of consciousness in meditation.

than the tribes located near the equator where the short daytime, intense light and ultraviolet content of the light causes the hormone melatonin to be sent to the skin and sex glands rather than remaining in the brain. Closing the eyes to light is the first step toward inhibiting the flow of melatonin from stimulating the lower centers. The second step is concentrating and meditating on the trigger cells in the back part of the Frontal Lobes, which sends pineal enzymes to the higher centers of the brain, thus opening the functions of the Frontal Lobes. However, the triggering of imaginative areas of the Frontal Lobes alone does not necessarily produce an evolutionary advance in brain organization. LSD and other naturally occurring chemicals in the brain can give intense visions and fantastic images, but unless controlled from the lower centers of reason, intuition and concept-formation, this activity of the imagination becomes fantasy. The line between fantasy and real imagination is difficult to discriminate.

Those people who have developed their cerebral cortex and use their Frontal Lobes together with the lower levels of consciousness are imaginative, fully alive and full of wisdom on all the lower levels. Just as discipline must be practiced at the intuitive level of the pituitary excitations which open up the sixth level mode of knowing, so must we discipline the imagination, like learning to play a musical instrument, when we function on the seventh level of pineal excitation. Such development of the higher mind-stuff requires subtle distinctions between images which are primal and those which are human-induced, images which are truthful and those which are mere fantasy.

HOW DO WE DISCRIMINATE FANTASY FROM THE REAL?

In order to be certain that our images are true, not false, we have to know what is happening on each of our seven levels of consciousness. Through the discipline of separating the symbolic content of our imaginative experience and by our tuning of imagination to real images in Nature, we acquire the sharpened faculty of direct perception. Images in Nature are formed from fields of intelligence acting through fields of energy and crystallizing them into patterns. To view these natural images as real and to test our human images against them is the practice of imaginative discipline which every poet or good artist must do. A loose imagination which cannot discriminate a self-activated image from a universal image is open to delusion and can be infected with a disease of the imagination just as our body can become diseased if we are loose about its health and give it no exercise. Exercising the imagination is an essential discipline for meditators and should be a required course for philosophers, scientists and religious people who tend to either have too little of it or too much! Most people are so unaware of their imaginative processes that they think that only those who belong in mental hospitals need to discipline their imaginations, without realizing how many false images they too are operating under.

An example of testing out the validity of our images can be readily seen at the social level if we look at the image of the way we are governed, since all government involves going towards a point in the future which is highly imaginary until it happens. To test our image of the way we are governed all we need to do is to study the promises of politicians with their professed plans of what they will do when they get in office and compare these with the actual performance in reality. A remarkable pattern emerges from this exercise which shows that politicians generally suffer from cancer of the imagination and success-fully pass their disease onto their constituents who believe them, vote for them and say nothing when they do not perform as visualized. But politicians just reflect our own use of imagination in our daily lives where we constantly create images of our hopes and fears which don't pan out. A similar exercise can be done with our images of money, with our devotion to images of authority, with our intellectual theories, etc., on every level of consciousness.

For an image to be veridical it has to be able to pass through all the seven levels of consciousness and all the brain filters unobstructed. If we have a great image of the future but it is not practical either economically, socially or physically, it is a fantasy. If we have a self-image or an image of another that is based on insecurity at the heart consciousness. The disciplined imagination has images which are verifiable on all the levels of consciousness, sees things as they are and includes all vibrations from Nature.

The Seventh Level—I
DREAMING WE ARE AWAKE

To achieve this vaster awareness let us no longer think of mind as something nebulous but think of it as structured within the seven different instruments of perception. For this sets us free from the limitations of thinking on only one of the different levels. To realize that you are responding to life at times as a reptile or an animal responds because certain parts of your brain happen to function at that evolutionary level, is different from feeling identified with those responses and saying "that is me". If a part of your brain were removed (like the hunting mechanism of the intellect in level three) your consciousness would still remain. You can remove this part with your imagination just as you can surgically remove your sensory awareness in order to experience that consciousness which transcends all functions. You can remove the sensory faculties without surgery just by hypnotizing yourself, but if you want to find out what the senses are, you must find out what is your real self. Then you will know by your own direct perception that the levels of the brain are ways that we are aware, but they are not awareness itself. Each part of the brain evolved to bring us more kinds of awareness, but each evolutionary development had its price, because each new addition to the brain was a new distortion of reality, just as the specialized eye, tuned only to visible light vibrations, was a kind of evolutionary progress and yet lost us the perception of the less specialized general all-around kind of seeing. So what is the reason we have evolved these seven different levels of brain machinery which create, distort, and make possible our life in this world? Where are we going and what is our evolutionary purpose and our destiny? What mystery is hidden in the Frontal Lobes of our brain and how will its unfolding ultimately change the world?

In great seers and sages this area of the Frontal Lobes is highly developed and understood. The development of the seventh faculty of the imagination can be taught, providing the teacher is your own total being and providing your lower being is made a willing student of its higher nature. This is difficult, because it takes a lot of faith to trust in a reality which, from a material point of view, seems insubstantial and less real than the common sense world we have known all our lives. The laws of the spiritual life are always upside-down and backwards from the laws of this world, and it takes courage to go against what you seem to be seeing with your very eyes and what fits the logic of your intellect and what your own powerful feelings are insisting is the truth. For the lower self to become a student of its higher nature means nothing less than a complete but temporary detachment from life in this world in order to open to the subtle vibrations of another reality.

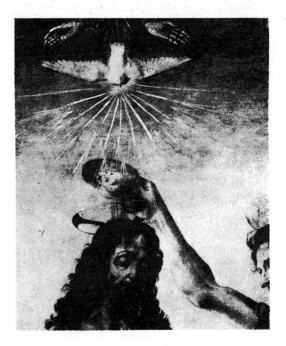

All great beings have had to understand the significance of the dreamlike existence in life and how thoughts come to pass and how they pass away. Unenlightened people living on lower levels of consciousness do not understand that what is seen in the world around them is only seen in their mind. They are convinced there is an external reality of objects quite separate from their own consciousness. They produce false imaginings because they do not know that the world is a dream, a movie show, a manifestation of the consciousness of the dreamer. This is the dream of someone who thinks he is awake because he has no knowledge of another state. It is this unreality which the seventh level is concerned with. Just as the real dream world of the unconscious is entirely made from the ideas, concepts, fears, etc., of one's fifth and sixth levels, so it is with the world of waking experiences on the seventh level. As long as the experience of being awake lasts, it is believed to be our waking state (an awakened state), just like the dream which is experienced for a short time is called reality *as long as it lasts.* Yet there is hardly any difference between the waking dream and the sleeping dream from the view of the seventh level of imagination. Just as we wake up from a deep sleep and say, "I was asleep", so can we enter the seventh level of consciousness and say, "I was dreaming but I thought I was really awake." The only difference is that the waking dream appears more *stable* than the other and lasts longer and can be verified by other people also imprisoned in the same dream. The body dream, the idea that the body is something separate from the universe or cut off from the consciousness which created it, is the prime cause of the false imagination that a human being is experiencing itself in reality as something separate and awake which endures independent of the "world", i.e., the construction of the so-called physical entities of the mind. Yet all images of the world around us are re-creations of sensations inside of us which tell us very little about the real nature of an object. If we look at a brick wall we do not see its real nature made up of molecules of baked clay or the atoms in the clay dancing to the cosmic vibrations of surrounding stars like the sun. What we see is a solid piece of matter, but that solidity is completely unreal, a dream, for its real nature is so full of space that all these electrical charges we call protons or particles or atoms can, with correct spin, pass through one another.*

Recently scientists working at the University of Michigan discovered

---

* *Science News* reported that successful experiments had been performed which showed that atoms are transparent to each other when orientated anti-parallel.
See also *Physical Review Letters* Sept. 19, 1977, p. 733.

a new characteristic of that positive particle of matter of the atom we call a proton. This new discovery answers questions not only about the inner structure of atoms and subatomic particles but also as to why there can be two or more universes existing inside each other and how we do not always sense their existence with our bodies. When a beam of polarized protons from a hydrogen source is fired at a target also consisting of polarized protons, many more collisions between them occur when both the target protons and the beam of protons are spinning in the same direction. It was thought for many years that the

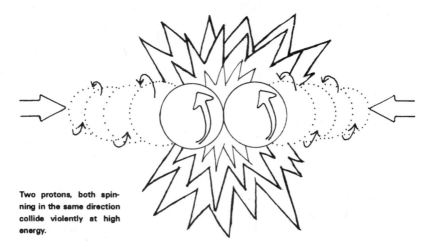

Two protons, both spinning in the same direction collide violently at high energy.

spin of protons had no effect on the collisions of intra-atomic particles. The researchers thought that because these protons are accelerated to energies up to many billions of electron volts that the contribution of the small amount of energy from their spin would be of little effect on these collision experiments. However, it was found that these nuclear particles are much more selective about whom they bump into than any physicist ever thought, because the researchers found that when the spins are opposite to each other, the particles pass through one another

The same high energy protons spinning in opposite directions appear to pass through each other.

unobstructed. This implies that each particle is aware of group rules for being part of the nucleus of an atom and this awareness was predicted by my theory of Nuclear Evolution in 1968, which stated clearly that the individual members of an atomic nucleus did have something to say about their behavior and the way they interact and that very selective processes were involved. In the same way, selective processes are involved in the way the different universes are experienced by human bodies and human minds. The proton was thought of as a dense solid lump of energy or matter, whereas it has now been proved that it can also act as a transparent cloud just by changing its spin. How many material universes are there spinning and passing through each other unobstructed just because they have opposite spin?

It is important that we learn to use our imaginations to visualize how we replicate the solid world of protons and atoms entirely in our consciousness whenever we re-create an external image of material substance in our human minds. It is even more important to know how we create images of the nonmaterial universe out of our consciousness because the self-creation of such images and our identification with them robs us of the experience of reality. Such an ingrained image is the idea and the concept that we are somehow separate from the totality of space and that our minds work separate from the total mind which is throughout space. We do not know that our consciousness can cross the totality of space because we do not have access to total mind. Yet in reality both space and consciousness are one single absolute, just as the invisible radiant energy in space which we call light is one with our consciousness. Yet we do not see this because they pass through one another unobstructed. In the state of pure consciousness where this is realized as *total mind* there are no obstructions and only when we are imprisoned in the imagined state of things do we experience obstruction of light, matter, concepts, thoughts and hence the experience of self-limitation. This idea is completely borne out when at last one transcends the personal experience of being a separate entity from the totality. To enter a new state of consciousness where the totality is absolutely singular and there is no "otherness" in our imaginations between objects in the external universe and the experience of those objects in our minds, requires us to understand that there is another universe made of consciousness and that the worlds of being we see in it are a mirror of our own state of evolution.

The solidity of the material universe is just a waking dream through which we travel unaware that our consciousness when identified with a physical body runs parallel to matter! Of course we can travel great distances inside our heads by watching some scene while sitting in front of a television and know it has been photographed by a camera independent of our own human agency. But the fact is, the image is a psychic phantom and unreal, created entirely inside our heads from light rays, a mere construction of the mind of each person watching it, and is no more real objectively than anything seen in a dream. Even the objective images on the TV film are tailor-made by our consciousness which makes special emulsions and grinds special lenses to approximate the human eye. These emulsions and lenses do not "see" material objects as they are in reality because these instruments too are constructed parallel to matter. Supposing our consciousness is an anti-parallel universe passing through everything? Why does this statement bring a reaction from those convinced that their lower level brains see what is real? The entire universe is experienced in our imagination, in the same way as the dream, because nothing material or solid or stable or permanent has been produced from any of the so-called solid material causes. The ordinary conceptual mind does not really believe that matter is merely the disturbance of our consciousness at a certain level of vibration—a form experienced at the gross level of our physical senses. But even this sensory reality, physicists know, is only an assumption, for modern physics has proved beyond any other discipline ever practiced by the human race, that we do not see the objects as they really are existing on either side of the narrow visible spectrum.

The Seventh Level—II
THE FORMATION OF AN IMAGE

An act of creativity in terms of our imagination comes with something we all do unconsciously, i.e., we form internal images from a bundle of disparate signals, electrical chemical messages from eye to brain, visually comparing one with another. We do not stop to think how the image of anything we look at gets transformed into such a clear picture inside our head, so much so that it appears that the image is actually in front of us, existing in its own right in space, in front of our own nose. But this external image of a tree or a person or a star is only a phantom image; the real image is reconstructed inside us in our brain where we truly experience it. We believe we experience the image of something out there in front of us, but in reality the experience takes place inside our head. The whole universe is like this, going on inside our head, but we "imagine" it to be going on in the space around us.

Why is it important that these two things are backwards in our experience—that the external image or "thing" is unreal but seems real, while the internal mental image that is real seems unreal? Does this fact have any power whatsoever to affect or change our lives? If the world of our minds is more real than the world of matter and if beings exist whose mental images are so powerful that they can change matter, as psychics, healers and holy men can do, then what about our own powers to change our situation or our physical appearance, our state of health or our society? If we do have this power to change things with our consciousness, then we are totally 100% responsible for whatever we are experiencing right now, at the personal level or the international level or even the level of sunspots and exploding stars in outer space. Mind affects matter because the separation between the two is only illusory.

What creates the illusion or image of real space around us in which objects move closer or recede from us? The answer is in seeing the imagination as the way the universe forms itself into patterns of energy to which our senses respond, which we then call "matter". The branches of a tree are an image no less than the swiveling branches of the spiraling arms of our galaxy, rotating on its axis every 200 million years. The images of other galaxies, no less than the image of our own bodies, are primordial realities and patterns which form in our minds and have to be re-created inside us from the signals of light which reach our eyes. Vibrations from the stars constantly bombard our nerve ends and vibrate our consciousness with light stimulations which we see and experience inside our own heads, although they appear to be outside of our bodies. If there are no such light signals, we see nothing there and we say it is invisible. Yet there are objects in the universe whose light is receding from us faster than it is coming towards our eyes. We call this object a black hole because there is no light or images coming from it which can impinge on our senses. But this does not make it any less real, since most of the universe is not visible to our senses. So we can only "imagine" what it must be like in a symbolic or mathematical way.

There are creative things we can do with our minds which we cannot do with material things. One of them is to create a universe with thought alone by using our consciousness in the same way that the material universe uses our consciousness to make its appearance to our mind. We can call this act of creation an "imagination" using our total mind, i.e., the mind we know plus the unconscious awareness which we do not bring into our conscious imaginations and therefore remains unknown. Yet the unknown is real, because the unconscious becomes our own experience of reality.

We can only begin to form new, real images if we can clearly see how humans have been forming old images of themselves, images of God and images of society for millennia. Although the technical process of seeing has been described by science, understanding the way we see the world around us in real experience is still a fundamental part of our human ignorance. Mankind does not know what imagination is, and no philosopher has even attempted to define it. Even the dictionary gives a false answer, believing it to be the faculty of perceiving what is not there. But my point is that without imagination we could not even perceive what *is* there and what lies all around us in our ignorance. Even mathematics and numbers are highly imaginary human creations and depend upon operations of the human mind, for no one has seen a number produced by Nature. To know how our imaginations work is the highest wisdom but we are only just discovering scientifically how we "see" images visually. Perhaps someday there will spring up a new science which will investigate how we can apply our *inner vision* to the harnessing of the creative power of thought, but first we must understand ordinary things like "seeing" before we pretend to understand "vision" on its higher evolutionary levels of manifestation.

The act of seeing is making sense out of the sensory patterns of light and darkness. The eye in all mammals reports its sensory signals to the different parts of the brain, sending it a message that the rod and cone cells in the retina have received a stimulus of radiation which we then "see" as light. The focusing and the sensing of color and distance is done by the occipital area of the sixth level in our brain model, but a variety of other more primitive brain areas also interpret that visual message to our consciousness as a whole experience of an object in order to transform the complete perception into a conception which makes sense. Each area in the instrument of consciousness adds to the information processed by the mammalian brain until a sight is recognized and the animal reacts to what it sees. The visual pathways of the sixth level have grown out of the organizing lower levels because of the need to "see" light deep in the brain. New ways of mapping the entire visual system at work are being found by modern science. Today scientists can radioactively label a glucose sugar which is trapped in the brain cells and then by slicing the animal brain, researchers can analyze the differences in cell absorption of the sugar to detect the vision cells which are most active. Research shows which cells trap the sugar enabling us to find the primitive areas of the brain which are involved in vision.

It is a mistake to think that only one part of our brain—the occipitals—is involved in vision because this sixth level function is only the refinement of a much deeper need of an organism to see light. In humans the formation of an image represents an evolutionary plateau where inner vision is formed into outer vision on a very sophisticated level. But we must remember that in all life forms the inner vision on the rudimentary fifth level, conceptualized to specific needs, comes first before sixth level external vision and not vice versa. A fly developed a compound eye to enable it to be effective in its environment, always buzzing around in flight, and fish developed eyes on both sides of the head which function independently to see what is coming up behind out of the inner need to be protected from attack. The need precedes the manifestation just as consciousness must precede the sensation or experience.

The new research on vision lights up those brain regions where the external visual system makes deep contact with the more primordial instinctual systems in the brain which control our emotions and affect our actions. The sight of blood will affect some people emotionally and others not at all. The visual description or picture of horrific scenes of death or violence will bring home to some people the awful low state of human communication, while to others the sight of suffering will create a feeling of compassion. Yet again, to others a photograph is just a picture and they would have to be present at a mass burial of corpses or smell the stench of rotting bodies to let the visual picture get through to those other unconscious areas of the brain which have little to do directly with the conscious process of seeing.

When we see something imaginary or real that fills us with fear, the chemicals and emotions which make us afraid emanate unconsciously throughout the entire body. The signals are transmitted from the visual system to the emotion-generating parts of our brain in the primitive brain, then up to the limbic area. Tracking the signals through the limbic system to the amygdala and caudate nucleus by Supersensonic methods and training the visual input into our imaginative centers enables us to see where these emotions are triggered and which center in turn brings on the active motor response that we may for instance see in the flight of animals. Somehow the primitive consciousness links the visual system through the hierarchy of interconnected brain functions to connect with the unconscious motor areas of the brain which move muscles, hands and feet. Activity in the parietal, temporal and frontal lobes demonstrates that these nonvisual areas do actually receive signals from the visual cortex to recognize patterns and locate objects in space as well as to run away from or to come closer to them.

Because these signals pass through the brain sequentially according to the way it has evolved, the sense we make at every level of the brain structure will be determined by the vibrational activity we experience in each part of our brain. This is controlled not merely by the outside stimulus or vibrations to the eye or by the information itself as science presently thinks, but by the chakra activity of our subtle body and its etheric centers. These chakras act as psychic sluice valves which let through or close off the vibrations to different parts of our brain according to our state of consciousness. This is very difficult for materialistic people to accept because they believe that the state of consciousness of a person has nothing or little to do with the quality of consciousness but more to do with the recognition of a brain signal from the senses or the eyes. The same applies to internal signals or vibrations as well as any other sensory signal from the skin, the ears, the smell or taste. *A materialist does not believe that there is any consciousness present to experience the senses. He believes the reaction itself to physical sensations is what we call consciousness.* But we all know that a wine taster uses his sensory signals vibrating chemically on the tongue in a totally different way to an ordinary drinker. We can accept that an artist uses his eyes and a composer uses his ears in a totally different way to ordinary folks, yet scientists find it hard to accept that a yogi uses his consciousness in a totally different way of perceiving vibratory sensory signals which enter the brain. The master of consciousness knows how to wake up whole areas of the brain which are sleeping, to bring about another way of "seeing" wholistically. The action which the "seer" takes in response to seeing a light signal from an object which enters his brain depends entirely on whether the higher brain functions are closed off or remain open-ended. If the Frontal Lobes are closed off as in the primitive apes and humans and other animals, then the signal will pass straight through the lower brain areas to the amygdala and the motor areas for action without any reference to higher conceptual or imaginative functions and we will have then what we have called a "red level" response to what we see.

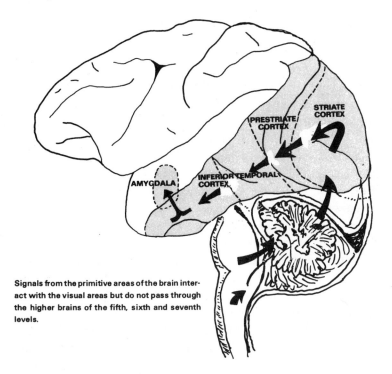

Signals from the primitive areas of the brain interact with the visual areas but do not pass through the higher brains of the fifth, sixth and seventh levels.

If we are developed mostly in the area of analysis through our intellect, then our response to the sensation of what we see will be processed according to logical analytical and other "yellow level" patterns of reaction. Therefore what we see around us in the environment will always be conditioned by images we have already stored and the habitual level of consciousness we dwell on from day to day. To know this about ourself is the beginning of wisdom. Everything we judge about the world, about society, about others, and about ourself, is subject to this factor, particularly when it comes to looking at society and its many conflicting reactions and responses which arise from the individuals who make up the society we live in. This applies to the revolutionary as much as the politician or philosopher. Unfortunately we can only see according to the limits of our own consciousness. All this points to one inescapable fact: that our society is not what it appears to be but is actually a mirror of our own insight or blindness. If we mistake information or sensation for knowledge or sense, we are being ignorant of the very way our own brain works to "see" the world around us.*

It is the nonsensory parts of our brain structure which condition every signal which passes to us from the world outside and it matters not whether that signal is a vibrating ray of light from the sun or a star or the words of another human. Even now I "sense" that the nonsensory functions of my own seeing into Nature's processes is making "non-sense" for many people who cannot follow or cannot pass the sensory signals from the total environment (social, personal and cosmic) into the wholistic linking of the holographic areas of the brain. To the extent that I lose certain readers in understanding my "non-sense" I can only regret that they have not yet opened up their supersense, have not thoroughly familiarized themselves with the Supersensonic methods of detecting brain pathways and currents of life force, and may be happy to continue relating to just the familiar signals they get from their environment in their own unique habit patterns. This obviously will exasperate some people in their understanding of not only my own concepts, but those of many others too. This attitude may appear arrogant since it puts all the blame for any confusion upon the reader rather than the writer, but the fact is that readers who can transpose their own brain functions to work on several different levels of conscious-ness, do not need words to understand what I am saying right now in concepts. Their own consciousness can act as a hologram and put things together wholistically at a level of communication beyond concepts and words. Such people merely need a finger pointed at the problem to instantly understand why we are talking about the link between the social model and the revolutionary concept that our brain is an externalized model of our own consciousness which in turn acts as a model of a wholistic nuclear society which will come together as a group.

We must begin to see brains and people functioning as parts of a

---

* A more thorough treatment of the visual signals which light up the brain's visual paths is given in *Supersensonics,* pages 195-307.

whole rather than as a bundle of separate egos. This is not so easy in a culture which trains us to think in self-centered egotistical terms. So far, in man's organization of society and in fact in the whole concept of democracy, we are working with a bunch of egos whose only safety against dictatorship is that they all cancel each other out. If the departments of the human brain worked like that, then the government we would have sitting at the top of our human form would be self-negating. We must see eventually from the actual situation around us that such a philosophy of competing self-interests does not work but in fact leads to the world situation we have got now. To say that "it works" because it seems to be moving along is to be blind to the reality of a fulfilling life, since Western democracy does not offer a fulfilling life even though it is relatively free of constraint.

The basic concept of our system of government is that there are separate factions or interest groups all trying to gain their own selfish interests. The theory is that when all are free to express themselves, these many interests that are all diverse will oppose each other. The assumption is that the selfish interest of any group when seen by other factions as damaging the common welfare, will be kept in line by the checks and balances of the combined opposition. This unified opposing of a specific self-interest is supposed to keep any single group from dominating or gaining power over our group or social life. The founders of this US system modeled their image of government upon the British Parliament and the Greek city-states federation and discussed it long before they decided to give it a trial. It has never worked very well because the Mafia, the oil companies and the powerful military-industrial complex and their pressure groups' lobbying have made the system inefficient, bungling and full of deceit so that the public has now become a well-fleeced lamb with no alternatives but more government of the same kind. This system is a perfect model of the average self-seeking individual being given the perfect feedback into the brain of all its members of society as a large group of persons beset with internal conflicts. Our present society, conceived as a large interrelated family, is just about as wholistic a system as the average person is integrated with the universe. In the formation of a new image of government we must see how we process our vision and develop our brain perception and imaginative faculty to look at society wholistically and see plainly our mirror reflection. Only then can we understand the conclusion that we all would rather avoid, which is that our lifestyle is plainly in need of another concept; that our present system cannot work. We must admit that it has only worked so far in spite of ignorance and not because of our wisdom. In order to change this pattern we must look more deeply at how we form a mental image in order to get a new one and model our social images on the evolutionary model of the brain.

HOW WE FORM IMAGES

The reception of the original signal pattern as an image in our perceptual faculty of the imagination on the seventh level of communication is clouded with impressions we already have floating around on the sixth level mode of knowing. Somehow in our unconscious the connections are made between the external image we see of an object and the hazy interpretations of its real patterns on level six of the knower which are formed out of the storage of former concepts and experiences in our memory on level five. Because the input of the signal pattern spills over from one level to another without our consciousness being aware of the interference of these levels in our imagining of a pattern of an object, we believe that whatever image is in front of us is being seen clearly as it really is. But much of the real energy pattern of the object is missed out in our perception. An easy test of this is to get several people to describe a simple object as detailed as possible without hearing each other's descriptions. It will be found that some people just do not see half of what is in front of them until it is actually pointed out. This is a humiliating exercise for those who think they "see" all and consider themselves aware people, and there are many rationalizations given for not seeing completely the first time. Those rationalizations which convince us we are not so unintelligent as to miss out half the information, are merely the ego's way of keeping self-esteem.

Another proof that we do not see things as they really are is that our mind cannot read the picture signals through the top three levels (imagination, intuition and conceptualization) faster than sixteen frames a second as in a movie filmstrip. The sensory signal from the eyes, as they take up the image on the bottom level of our consciousness reading the physical sensory input, is seen as a continuous one like a movie if the images are moving faster than sixteen frames a second. We usually attribute this to the physical nature of the eye's actual construction as a receptor. But this assumption again is an actual example of the cloudiness of what we are seeing and saying. We find it easy to make such assumptions from something which appears so obvious. The fact is that no two eyes are constructed the same identically, and among people the difference is so great in size, quality and constitution that it would be impossible to get them to perform optically all the same like exactly ground lenses. The delay of sixteen frames a second is not in the eye's ability, which can recognize changes in patterns of light energy in pico seconds, but in the processing between the eye and the occipitals, the eye and the mid-brain, the mid-brain and the memory banks, the memory of the past with the intuitive impressions which compare present time with future time sequences, and finally the transmission to the Frontal Lobes which throws up the picture in our imagination as a coherent image in our consciousness. All these steps together take a sixteenth of a second so we need sixteen of them in a second for us to see one continuous image. Yet no one would say that the pictures on the movie screen are real ones. Our mind tells us that they are only made by our imaginative re-creation of the patterns of light even though they *appear* real. Our mind, once immersed in the movie, does not notice the speed of the changing images sent from the movie projector to the screen nor the fact that the images we are seeing are twenty feet high instead of real-life size. We do not see that actual images of people are one-quarter of that size. Our eye doesn't notice the transitions because our mind and memory records are working slower than our eye.

This understanding of the reality of how we form images proves that our perceptual process distorts what is real. Only by applying this scientific knowledge to our investigation of ourself can we discipline our imaginations to tune them to a truer reality than the one we are living, and break down the conceptual communication barriers between people and between cultures.

The Seventh Level—III
OUR INTERNAL
COMMUNICATION SYSTEM

(The following few pages on the complex way we communicate with different parts of our seven brains, as well as with others, need to be read very carefully. It is necessary to deeply consider this process to understand how our inner complexity creates our external reality.)

Whether we are receiving images from a movie screen, from an inspiring lecture, from a political rabble rouser, from the words of a book, from a fear-raising evangelist or from the physical objects around us, if the signal to mental noise ratio is too large in our receiving

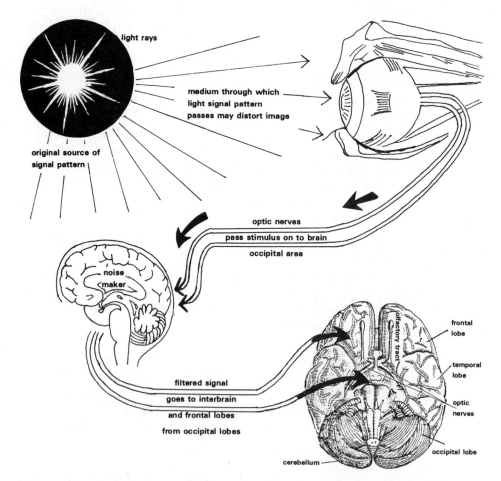

The reception of the image depends more on the clarity of the medium it passes through and the noise which squelches it than upon the original signal which is weak. Too much sunlight in the visible spectrum squelches the vibrations of light from the stars. Too much light with the eyes open squelches the light vibration from the cosmos in the invisible spectrum. Too much noise in the brain circuits prevent internal communication.

mechanism we cannot create the image properly in the Frontal Lobes as it really is. Clarity gets lost because previous concepts from past memory cloud the ever-newness of the incoming image and the impressions of our sixth level knowing die away as they arise and return into the continuous totality of our experience and become a wholistic part of us. Each experience of an external object or stimulus is, at every moment, a vibration fed through a communications model something like this:

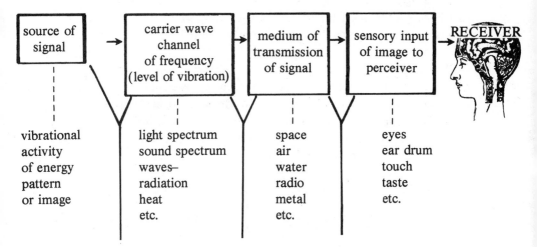

In order for communication to take place, however, there must be some elementary feedback signal which informs the **source** that the receiver has actually received something; otherwise the communication is only one way. In our communication with the images of Nature's objects most of our reception of its images, like the sun, the spiral galaxy, the flower or crystals or rocks are all one-way communication, but in our intercommunications with the human world we expect not only to receive an image or pattern but to respond in such a way that the **source** is given a reply or an indication that the signal has been received something like this:

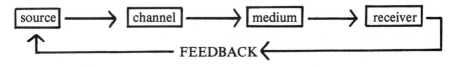

But this is an incomplete model because not only has there been distortion of the signal by the interpretation of the sensory input and encoding of the message and image by the receiver's nervous system, but there are also semantic problems in the reception of the feedback signal back at the source. If the **source** is intelligent we expect an acknowledgement or we would consider that our response to the source has been ignored. If we talk to the sun and tell it that we are getting its signals, we do not expect any response because it is so big and its powerful light message appears to flow only one way, but we are very hurt if we get the same treatment from someone we love, even if their love is always streaming forth continuously like light from the sun.

Any feedback to the **source** from the receiver implies that there is always a closed loop which operates to let the **source** know something. As soon as the receiver enters into a feedback loop he himself then becomes a **source** of images or patterns of energy and if his signal gets through, then the **source** also becomes a **receiver**. But there is something wrong with this model; as we can see we are not allowing for distortions and noise in the channel, so a more elaborate picture of our reception of a sensory signal image would be like this:

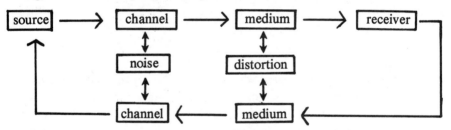

In order for there to be communication at all between the **source** and **receiver** there must be a frequency or channel. This is so obvious but we do not realize how important the channel is until our phone won't work or the post office has gone on strike or we cannot speak the same language as the receiver. Even if we speak the same language there are assumptions in the special way we encode our message and transmit the images of our concepts. For instance when I use the word "imagination" I mean something that is really there in our Frontal Lobes. Is that what you mean? Or do you mean that concept which the dictionary gives—that our imagination gives us pictures of something that is not actually present? If you mean this by imagination then we have a semantic problem in communication, until we clarify our meanings. At least then you are able to consider what my definition of an *image* is so that I reach you with my interpretation. But if I cannot reach you through the printed word as my channel and the medium of ink and paper, then you will not be able to decode my message and I will not receive any feedback that you have been contacted meaningfully by the **source** of my communication—me.

Even more confusion is usually added to the actual transmission of a communication. Obviously if we mean by the word *communication* "an exchange of meaning" there must be the opportunity for me to receive feedback that I have communicated, and to do this the **source** has to become a **receiver**. If a one-way signal of an image is transmitted and it does enter first the imagination, then gets through the impression and conceptual levels of the receiver then we can say we have communicated. But if there is no way of receiving back some confirmation that *an exchange of meaning* has actually taken place, then there is no real communication because there is no interaction and no exchange has actually taken place. When we examine every image sent to us from **sources** in the environment or we penetrate into the exchange of meaning about every word we utter and receive, then we realize with a shock that the fidelity of our human communication systems is very low quality. It is natural for the human ego to react to such a thought and even reject it, because the ego really believes it is capable of communicating on higher levels than it really can. Ego to ego is only one-way communication because the signal never gets through to the real **source** or *being*.

A more accurate way to show how people confuse the true images between the **source** and **receiver** is to outline a model of the type of distortions and noises which interfere with the patterns of the signal image and thereby prevent us from giving any accurate feedback to the **source** which will confirm a deep exchange of meaning. Obviously the whole complex of signals which make up the image to be sent from the **source** has to fit together in a multi-level message which comes to us through multi-media on several channels.

CHANNEL   MEDIUM

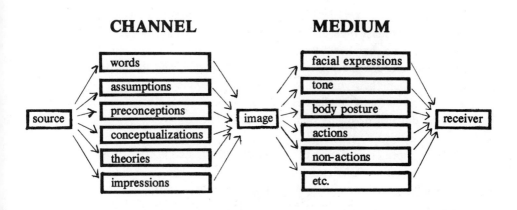

So far philosophers and semanticists have only tried to sort out the symbols of language and the way we use them. Our need to invent them or analyze words as our needs dictate in advertising, or in poetry and religion, or in politics is the work of specialists. It is thought by symbol merchants that all we need for perfect communication is to select the right media, channel a flow of thought and feeling through the right symbol system and hey presto, an integral and honest communication takes place. But the wife and husband who have been married for fifty years may communicate but a fragment of their total beings in this primitive way. They sleep in the same bed every night, they become close and work together, bring children into the world, go through thick and thin, yet in the least there are many things left unsaid, many images and feelings that cannot be expressed, many thoughts and emotions which have no channel open, and can find no medium through which to be shared. Yet many people do not feel this lack because they do not realize what poor communicators they really are. As one-way communicators, people talk, love, hate, compete, play and pray together and think that is the only way; this is the world problem in a nutshell. Are we to be bamboozled that the work of semanticists and the analysis of words and concepts is the last word in communication? We are bamboozled at our peril. Human communication and feedback is at a very low level and operating on very low frequencies, and there is no better proof of this fact than the fifty percent divorce rate between men and women who have lived closely together for years. Yet we find the authorities on communication are speaking of communication techniques even at the highest university academic communication courses, only at this symbolic and multi-media level.

To realize that the so-called expert **receiver** may not know of the existence of any other level of consciousness than his own is a great shock. To think that we are only able to receive on one level or two levels out of seven is too humiliating for the ego to accept. But unconsciously human beings do send many other signals on other levels of communication without even knowing it. Often people are just not in touch with their own feelings which get transmitted in their vibrations, leading to much misunderstanding. Yet until it is accepted that some people do actually communicate and give feedback response on many levels of consciousness beyond our own we shall never, never understand the nature of society and its many confusions and contra-dictions. Nor will we understand ourselves until we understand this fact of human existence.

The fact that our consciousness can operate on seven distinct levels of consciousness without our consciously knowing that all images and thoughts are ultimately annihilated after they pass through the seventh level, is a humiliating thought for most people who think they have this whole communication thing pretty well wrapped up. To go into another level or domain beyond our imaginative faculty which dissolves our separateness in a nonseparate reality is very frightening to some people. To accept that each individual in reality passes into a black hole would be considered by most people a figment of the imagination. Yet if we think about it that is what happens to all our thoughts—they pass into the black hole of consciousness in which all things of the material world and all their patterns and images are ultimately experienced and then disappear, leaving only a memory. All the signals, images, sounds, etc., die away for new signals to take their place. Stimuli emerge like our thoughts, to disturb our consciousness for awhile and eventually die away again into the silence.

This silence in which all sounds and images, concepts, thoughts, etc., arise is the stuff that most people fear. For them to let themselves

go into this void, this frightening absence of images and stimuli, is the
real terror so they compensate by grabbing at more and more stimuli.
"We must not stop talking or thinking in case there is silence," they
think. The dread fear of all radio networks is that there should be
silence, even a small gap of silence. Yet understanding and communicating images of this silence (called consciousness) in which all
disturbances arise, is the subject of this book.

What has this communication model to do with spiritual awareness?
Surely when we try to give feedback to God there is no more
answering nod than we get from the sun. When an individual is trying
to communicate with the Source of all being or the Cosmic Intelligence
which some call God, then we can see that our worship, or our asking
for changes to be made in our human affairs, could be a human
distortion of what the Source is continually sending to us. Hence to
some people such a communication could only be one-way since they
do not seem to get any response and their prayers do not work. There
are many materialists to be found who do not pray and who believe such
appeals to God in human language are very naive and that only human
actions influence the course of events. However, if we view "the
Source" as consciousness or the stream of life force which continually
flows to us we can see that our own attitudes to it are indeed
determining our fate at every moment, and what images we can receive
from it. It may be that the channel on which we can communicate with
God has not been found and cannot be found until our multi-level
model of consciousness is realized by our coming through the black
hole of letting go and going through the white hole of re-creation.
When we re-create our image of our self we automatically re-create the
universe. That self-image requires a feedback signal to know it is a true
one, to know that God actually answers our message with the quality
of our being and the joy of Pure Consciousness. The purpose of this
book is to tell about that feedback signal which changes God from the
Source into the Receiver, makes Him the recipient of His/our own love
and holds up to Him the light of His own glory. That light and that
glory alone is the single divine purpose of the nucleus, the singleness of
the undivided seed of life force of which you and I and everyone else
are an integral whole.

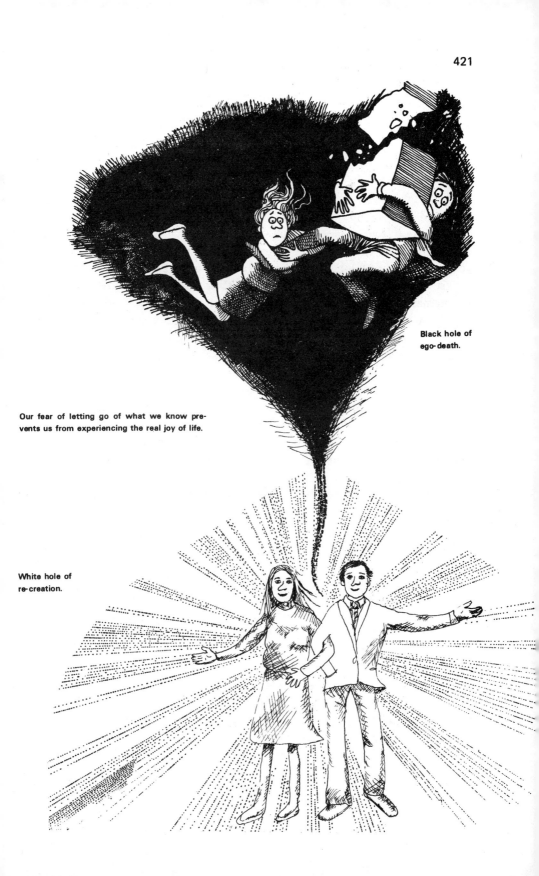

Black hole of
ego-death.

Our fear of letting go of what we know prevents us from experiencing the real joy of life.

White hole of
re-creation.

THE SPIRITUAL PATH

The intellectual level of consciousness sees the spiritual path as a path, a long line and oneself somewhere along that line, so far advanced. How do you tell how far up that path you are? This is not a good question from a spiritual point of view because if you are worried about how far advanced you are, it is a block. Does it really matter if you are going to get enlightened tomorrow or in a week or in five years or just before you are dying or in the next incarnation? If you live in the eternal now, it is always now. Even in the next incarnation it will still be now. If you were enlightened in the last incarnation, it is still now. So to think of it from that level where it has a beginning and an end is a misconception of the whole thing. So long as you have a beginning and an end, you can't get anywhere, because that brings in time. Enlightenment is timeless. What is for one person a short time is for another person a long time. What takes God a few minutes takes us ages. And maybe it takes God no time at all since there may not be any time in His reality, or Its reality. So the first thing we have to do is stop worrying how far up the path we are or even imagining that we have come any distance at all, because the most advanced person is imagining he is back where he started from—at the **Source.**

How do you tell whether you are back at the **Source** or not? It has to do with communication with yourself. If you look at yourself as a long line starting at the beginning and ending somewhere up there, in heaven or wherever, then you are stretching yourself out into a time line, with the **Source** back there and you here. So if you want to get back to the **Source** you have to pray or meditate on the **Source.** But if you are meditating on the **Source** and you say, "Please God enlighten me," and you don't get any answer, you say, "Where *is* He? I keep beseeching and I don't get this whatever it is going to be like, blinding lights, feeling great, walking on air, being invisible, God knows what"— what is enlightenment? It is different things to everybody. But there you are praying and you don't get an answer, so you say, "I can't be very far on the path or God would give me some signal that he got my message." It is like walking out into the sun and saying, "Hello Sun, I love your light. I'm trying to tell you something. Can you give me an answering signal?" But nothing happens. It just keeps shining. There is no answering signal. It is all one-way communication. The sun is so powerful it just keeps radiating all one way. Its powerful vibration squelches our little verbal noises. So you are praying to the sun, "Hey, take some notice of me. Send me a signal. I'm getting your light." How can we give feedback to the **Source** so that It can know that we have received Its blessing, Its consciousness, Its radiation, Its love? Is It sitting there waiting, saying, "I wish you could pray a little harder. You might just get through."?

What is the purpose of having anything in creation like a person or a human or an atom or a sun or a star? If we look at the nucleus of the universe where it all sprung from we are all parts of it. But the parts are not separated; the parts are whole. Even each individual part is indivisible, and it is undivided from the whole nucleus of which it is a part. So the purpose of the nucleus is to radiate that light and that glory of the **Source**. How else would the **Source** know that It was a source unless there were something that it could experience itself in? So that nucleus that has that answering light in it, that glory that radiates, is the feedback signal that the **Source** recognizes when it sees it light up. So the **Source** sends a message back and says, "Got your message. I see you got the light." Then it sends more back. When we have prayed hard and have got through to the **Source**, the **Source** becomes a receiver. If we pray hard enough or *be* hard enough or get intense enough then we become a sender of the feedback signal, and when that signal is accepted or received, then the **Source** itself becomes a receiver. Having received back its own vibration, then It radiates more powerfully, It rewards with more abundance. So strictly speaking, if you meditate on the sun, if you open yourself and pray to the sun and say, "I really love your light," you will get an answering wave of more light, because once you have opened yourself up to the sun's being, it is able to send more energy of itself, not necessarily of the light that you normally see, but of the major part of the sun which is invisible. Then your intellect can ask, "Is it really sending more or are you just getting more?" The part of the sun that you can see with your eyes is just a tiny slit in the visible spectrum. On either side of that is an enormous amount of black light, invisible light. So if you pray to the sun and you tune into it and you talk to it, it may be that you won't see any more brightness in the visible spectrum but you will feel that other part from the heart of the sun light you up, lighten you, fill you with energy, because having opened yourself by becoming a receiver and then sending back to the source, the source is then able to send back to you more. And that reacts on itself. Everytime a person receives a radiation, they absorb it and then they themselves become a radiator. Back it goes to the source and the source having been filled with its own light again becomes a sender of more. So they react off each other like that, boosting each other until there is an enhancement effect. If you go and talk with the sun, it keeps answering back with more light, and so very soon you can't see anything. There is so much light, there is nothing to see. There is nowhere to go anymore, because every direction you go in there is light. You look over there and there is light; you look over here and there is light. Why go anywhere? Why think of a spiritual path? You become the path. The center of your being becomes the nucleus, the **Source** itself, radiating to itself its own light. Because once you join with the **Source** in that kind of feedback, that prayer (it's a constant prayer, a constant surrender), then you *become* the **Source;** there is no separation between the **Source**, the signal, the receiver and the sender. The **Source** becomes the sender, and the receiver becomes the **Source**. The only way to get into that space is to tune to that **Source** and wait for the answering blessing.

Two-way communication between God and man is needed for world peace as well as individual peace. If we think of God as the Evolutionary Intelligence, then it is setting up a two-way communication between the nucleus of all life, including the nucleus of our cell life, star, plant and animal life, and the soul life in all. God the **Source** becomes a receiver then. This communication link between man and God is accomplished through tuning, via meditation or prayer. Each Self is the same, it has to receive the confirmation in its own consciousness that it is actually radiating the glory of light. The whole purpose of the soul in the nucleus of life is that it is to reflect the light back to the **Source**. The **Source** needs the soul to know itself; otherwise it is only a one-way communication—from the **Source** outwards. The **Source** is looking for the conscious response from the creation, a response inward to the nucleus, in order to establish a clear line of communication.

How can we get into God's shoes, so to speak, and feel what it is like to That Being, not to have conscious communication from humans back to Itself? If the sun's communication to us is one-way, does the sun ever become a receiver from us? How is this analogy connected with the primitive area of the brain? How does the higher brain get in touch with the lower brain and get a message back saying, "Thank you very much for your wisdom"? And how does the lower brain pray to the higher brain in such a way that the lower brain becomes a sender, not just a receiver? In prayer you are a sender as well as a receiver, trying to get a message back to the **Source**. If your love is an ego love, you will not get through, there will be too much static noise in the way. It's the same in human communication. If your love is ego love, then the person is just a love object to you. Possessive love is a one-way form of love, whereas love of the whole *is* giving back to the **Source** and even becoming the nucleus again—that primal nucleus in which all parts are contained. Since each person is an integral whole we become One with the **Source** by meditating or praying on the **Source** and the part becomes whole or indivisible. When a person is *individable from the whole* he is a true *individual.* This real and powerful primal imagination can only come and manifest when all the levels of consciousness are open and a clear communication channel is made between the lower brain and the higher. Then society will reflect that oneness and the Kingdom of Heaven will be here on earth.

The Seventh Level—IV
AWAKENING ALL SEVEN LEVELS

In trying to visualize the potential of the human brain in terms of levels of consciousness we can look at the seven domains of the brain as we would view the electrical potential controlled by a potentiometer. A potentiometer, sometimes called a rheostat, is found on some light switches as a dimmer control or on heater regulators and is the volume control on every radio or record player. It is used to control the amount of current that a system can handle or to control the flow of electrical energy. The analogy of a volume control can also be applied to the potential energy in a circuit which can be tuned to different frequencies by varying the potential energy flowing through a system of resistors. The brain is such a system.

Let us look at the most simple analogy of a potentiometer as the measure of brain potential. Any large potential must be created by also having a very large resistance which we can control from zero resistance through 1 and 2 to, say, maximum at 7.

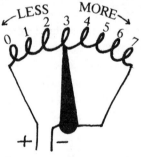

The simple circuit of a potentiometer is created by shortening the distance across a coil of wire so that the coil absorbs less current at positions 1 or 2 than at 6 or 7.

At the maximum resistance the potential is low as we can see by imagining a current flowing through a thick wire instead of a thin wire:

thick wire

big resistance

thin wire

little resistance

Having mastered this simple concept of resistance, we can view the potentials of the brain in their different stages as a set of variable resistances which take a little or a lot of potential energy to make them work. The higher centers require a lot of energy (through burning oxygen in the blood) to make them glow like a stove, and the lower centers are easily activated at low potential energy. It is easy to blow a fuse or thin wire at the lower levels if high energy is passed through

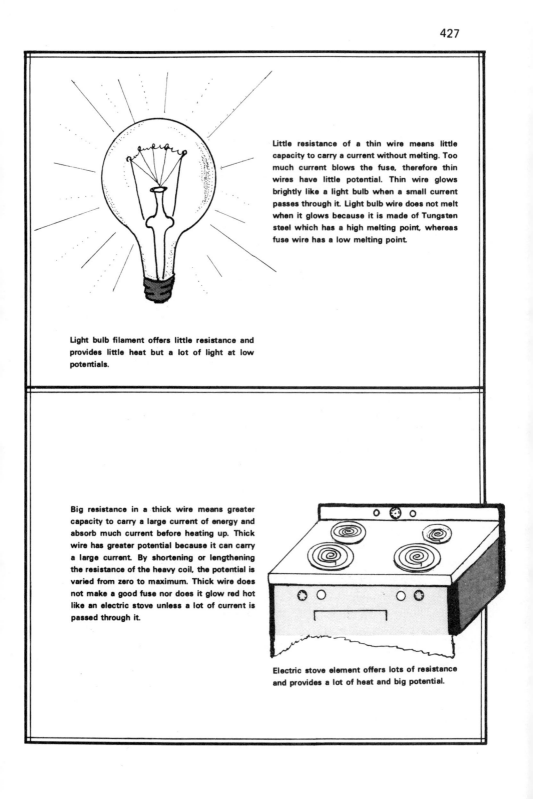

Little resistance of a thin wire means little capacity to carry a current without melting. Too much current blows the fuse, therefore thin wires have little potential. Thin wire glows brightly like a light bulb when a small current passes through it. Light bulb wire does not melt when it glows because it is made of Tungsten steel which has a high melting point, whereas fuse wire has a low melting point.

Light bulb filament offers little resistance and provides little heat but a lot of light at low potentials.

Big resistance in a thick wire means greater capacity to carry a large current of energy and absorb much current before heating up. Thick wire has greater potential because it can carry a large current. By shortening or lengthening the resistance of the heavy coil, the potential is varied from zero to maximum. Thick wire does not make a good fuse nor does it glow red hot like an electric stove unless a lot of current is passed through it.

Electric stove element offers lots of resistance and provides a lot of heat and big potential.

them. Therefore the Frontal Lobes offer the most resistance but have the highest potential if we can activate them.

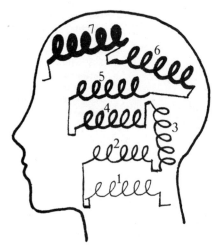

This picture shows the wires getting thicker and thicker, requiring greater and greater amounts of power to make them function. Each potential is controlled by a chakra which acts as a sluice valve for cosmic energy. The seven levels of consciousness can be likened to the flow of electricity through resistances of increasing thickness with the biggest resistance from the Frontal Lobes and the least resistance from the Medulla. Some people have never used their Frontal Lobes because they are low-energy people working on little potential.

The energy required to operate all levels is acquired by yogic training so that beings like Christ, Buddha and other true awakened people can tap into much higher potential energies to activate the sleeping fore-brain. This discipline is achieved by meditation and prayer until control of each level enables a human to use the full potential state by overcoming the greatest resistance. This is the electronic equivalent of tuning a circuit, with each potentiometer coil representing the most simple of circuits for balancing the difference in potential between the positive and negative ends of the wire. This difference between the positive and negative charges will vary with the resistance and thickness of the wire as shown in the diagram on the following page. This creates the effect of raising or lowering the volume on each level. But the greatest effect is when all levels of resistance are at zero, since this offers no resistance and therefore the entire cosmic energy can flow through the brain circuits and become manifested as oneness. This process is the equivalent of surrender, and the brain becomes quiescent and thought-less. However, the greatest potential energy is created at the maximum human resistance since it requires the maximum amount of energy needed to blow the wire or to make the circuit glow and melt down into formlessness. The full manifested state of least resistance is proportional to the greatest potential state created by the most resistance. By controlling or overcoming all the resistance, the entire system of seven levels of brain

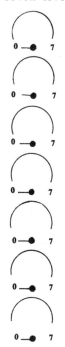

potentials are then realized to their maximum. By gradually reducing our brain's seven resistances and clearing away the blockages to our direct link with cosmic power, we can make the circuit transparent and pure which increases the amount of light passing through at higher and higher potentials until we ultimately surrender. All potential states are differences between positive and negative fields of energy. On every level of consciousness there is a positive and negative potential which is directly under control of consciousness, although most people are not aware that they can alter these potentials at will. Most people unconsciously control their potential by having a self-image. If the self-image is confident and wholistic, maximum potential is achieved. If the self-image is fearful, doubtful, overblown, or self-obsessed, people tend to use their potential negatively and achieve negative results in their lives. The proportion of failures to successes is correspondingly lower in people who are negative. When self-image as a concept of ego (a self-regarding entity, whether positive or negative) is annihilated, then the total environment and all its potentials become one's own because there is nothing to separate the part from the whole. Then we can switch over to zero resistance when the full power comes through without any restrictions. We can, as Christ says, become as nothing. But paradoxically in this "nothing" we are linked with everything because there is no resistance to separate us from the maximum potential. Thus the manifested state becomes the same as the potential state, and positive and negative states are discharged and annihilated. This rare state of being where everything and nothing become one is called unitive consciousness, or yoga which means union or Samadhi. When humans achieve this state of consciousness in a nonpossessive love between each other and realize their potential states of com-union then perfect communication takes place and the ego or self-sense disappears. This is the eighth level of existence when eternal peace is given and heaven lies all about us. This is the primal state of Nuclear Evolution.

The Seventh Level—V
COSMIC IMAGINATION

I have been asked many times about the effects of the stars and planets on the levels of consciousness. At the level of the imagination and intuitive structures, everything affects everything else but not in the direct way that astrologers attribute to planetary influences on personality. The glandular system governed by endocrine secretions of hormones is by far the greatest influence on personality and the functioning of consciousness. Many people are often drunk and intoxicated by the secretions of one level or another or by combinations of gland hormones. The planets do not affect these glands directly but are more like modifiers of the environment. The light of the universe is constantly bathing the higher and lower centers in man's brain and nervous system the same for everyone but its reception is modified by the aspects between the planets in relation to that part of the zodiac or section of the cosmos from which radiation is coming. Each part of the celestial sky obviously contains influences in the form of invisible light. It would be foolish to expect the same influence to come from the giant explosion in the Crab Nebula of 6,520 light-years as the influence coming from the stars in Orion which are only 1,500 light-years away. The planets merely modify the powerful effects of existing radiant energies which make the cosmic birth of the nuclear consciousness in a physical vehicle possible. By using the ability to divine found on the sixth level, the prophets, sages and ancients were able to observe certain personality changes over many thousands of years and to determine the influence of the planets acting on the glandular endocrine system and thereby affecting our personality and level of thought.

The structure of the brain and the growth of its many centers are the outcome of more than planetary influences. The planets only modify environmental effects upon man who responds to these according to his own mastery of consciousness. Hence it is often said by the ancients that the planets impel but do not compel. Once we understand the functions of the chemistry and structure of the events in the brain and discover that they are under direct control of consciousness, then we become aware that the planets do not control our destiny unless

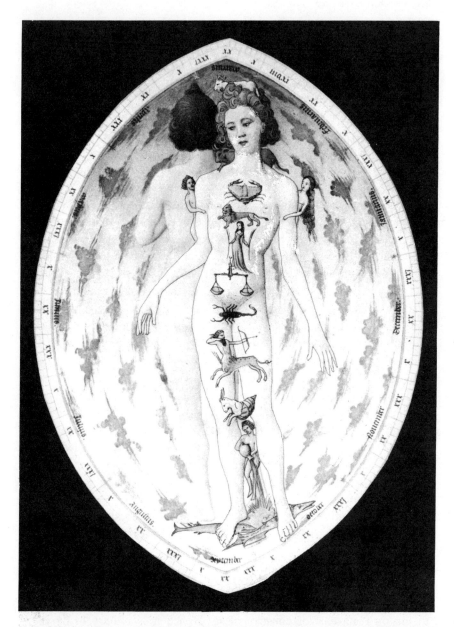

The ancients believed that cosmic rays influenced different parts of the body. The energies from different parts of the sky from supernovas, nebulae and black holes situated in different parts of the Zodiac, come to us with different frequencies from various parts of the spectrum. The Crab Nebula photographed in the red light of hydrogen looks different when photographed in the green light of oxygen and other luminous elemental gases and could effect our senses as well as our unconscious sensing of radiation in other parts of the spectrum. A supernova explosion may give off the enormous luminosity of up to 200 million suns which is equal to the light given off by the entire galaxy in which the supernova star resides. This is enough invisible energy to influence our brains and nervous system.

we are weak and totally passive. To the extent that we control the imagination we become aware that we do control the planets—at least their effects on the cosmic radiations reaching us from different sections of galaxial space. This is a difficult concept for most people to accept, especially many astrologers who do not have this power to control their imaginations and therefore are firm believers in the dominance of planets over life. However in discussions with leading astrologers, like Dane Rudhyar, I have found that they do not believe that personality and behavior are governed directly by planets but that the response of human consciousness is the factor which decides our reaction to the modification of the zodiac light radiations.

The zodiacal modifying of the endocrine structures at birth and the effect of the planets over functioning of the brain centers during the remaining years of life can be determined by divining or Supersensonic methods* at any specific time. The functioning of these endocrine glands is largely under the control of consciousness and the evolutionary process. Mastery of the personality of any individual is proportional to the conscious control of these secretions.

Edgar Cayce, a remarkable example of someone who developed the sixth level inner knowing and documented it in thousands of readings of individuals, opened the higher functions of the mind but got most of his information from the sixth level. Very rarely does he show any originality or vivid imagery common to seers of the seventh level. His readings are dull in style and often tedious repetitions of information from what he himself called the Akashic memory or soul memory of a person. Mastery of the seventh level transcends soul memory and frees the individual from the limitations and modifying influences of the planets upon the radiant energies reaching us from powerful stars

---

*These are fully described in *Supersensonics* as methods of detecting fields of radiation to which our nerves and skin can be sensitized beyond the normal faculties of touch, sight, smell, etc. Just as we can sense with little training the presence of magnetic fields, electric fields, ionization of molecules in air, and location of objects like the mosquito senses blood or the amoeba senses its food, or the blood cells sense the presence of foreign bodies, we can also use divining to determine endocrine balances.

surrounding the solar system. The effect of the planets on the mind of mankind is weak since a planet is only a modifier of the existing cosmic background forces impinging on us at all times. The secretion of the endocrines however affects our immediate emotions and thought life from minute to minute and hour by hour. With the injection of one hormone into the bloodstream we can be laughing or crying, in depression or bliss, within seconds because these substances are mind-changing.

THE ENDOCRINE GLANDS OR SYSTEM

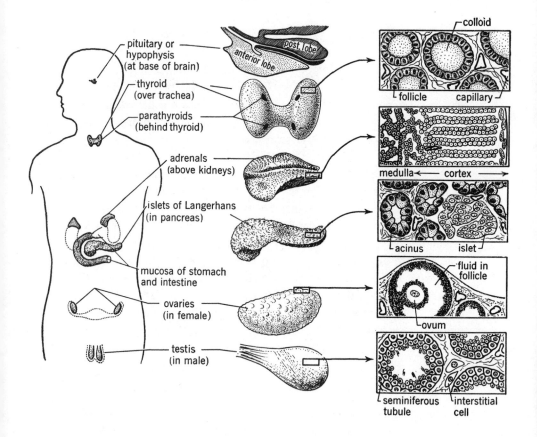

The different structure of cells on each of the seven levels causes their chemical environment to become selective of certain enzymes and hormones and to produce internal chemical resonances which trigger each other symbiotically to change personality, modify behavior and open up the corresponding brain centers to become supersensitive.

In meditation the act of consciousness concentrating at the seat of the pituitary center on the sixth level affects the transformation of the personality on the seventh level. People have difficulty relating this to their idea of God. This is due to a misconception in our imagination about God and what God really is. God is pure consciousness, and the miracles which Christ spoke about as coming from God are wrought by consciousness. Christians do not like to hear and shun the very words of Christ when he said of his miracles, "that even you shall do these things and even greater things shall you do!" Spiritually-minded people have a split in their imaginations between God and man, science and spirit, mind and matter and they turn one topic off to think about the other and thereby begin to regard hypnosis, pendulums and even the divining rods of Moses as gimmicks which have nothing to do with God. This, as we have discussed in previous chapters, is man's arrogance and ignorance of what God is. Naively he thinks the material implement does something of itself. The tool only amplifies the nervous antenna and the consciousness and just as Christ said, if our sense of conviction (another word for faith) can even reach the size of a mustard seed you can say to the mountain, "Get hence", and the mountain goes away. He is not saying that the mind will move the mountain physically against all the laws of physics. He is saying that if your power of conviction has even a little control over the validity of your imagination you can literally obliterate the mountain in your consciousness whilst still looking at it. He is talking of a power of consciousness to create its own image of the external world. The scientist would do well to investigate the power of prayer or one hundred percent self-suggestion at the seventh level of imagination because it is here in this area of human consciousness that human beings actually believe or do *not* believe in the dynamic power of our imaginations to create reality.

The word "Christ" means the anointed one, or in Hebrew—messiah. The word was originally applied to a high priest or prophet-king who was illuminated by God consciousness. Only later in Hebrew history did it come to mean redeemer who would bring salvation. The messiah who wages war against the forces of evil, like Krishna, fights an internal battle with darkness of the mind, our ignorance of the true nature of the light of consciousness. How can we reach this highest state of consciousness where the mind does not separate the means from the ends, the pendulum or rod from God? The answer to this is in the way we use the seventh level. Most ordinary people use imagination negatively to separate their image of man from their image of God. This is because their minds live in the dark ignorance of the ego body and they cannot see that they must arise and awake from the darkness of the body self. Christ is calling us to become aware of God as **consciousness.** Even a scientist who believes in God will switch in his mind from one belief system to another. When he thinks about science he cannot relate to miracles or faith or explain them so he shuts off God. At another time he shuts off science in order to think about God.

On the seventh level Einstein is a great imaginer, and all mathematics is a miraculous work of imagination of consciousness no less than the miracles of Christ. Here the religious person feels shocked that we put God and man on the same level but strictly speaking any idea or thought of God is purely an act of *consciousness* and so is faith. God is a cosmic movie—not the screen or the projector or even the film or story itself but the consciousness watching the screen of the mind. Humans do not separate the mind from the experiences in it and thus they cannot see the workings of their own imaginations. Nor is there any real separation because the mind is made of consciousness too but it is not the *pure* consciousness we call God. How can we realize that the light of consciousness is God? The Hindu sages say "Thou art That" and Moses says "I am that I am" but what does this mean in reality for the one who does not know what they are talking about?

Let us imagine a big screen for projecting a movie upon. All kinds of images, emotions, actions, objects, shapes, situations both objective and subjective are portrayed on the screen with many different intensities of light and color. But the screen itself is not affected by these images. The screen has no awareness of all these images and actions, yet it reflects all emotions, thoughts and images as if they were a reality. We are hypnotized, however temporarily, as we identify with the story, as we are moved in our own being to see ourself in the actions and pictures and feelings of others. The screen is like Christ Consciousness, the Krishna Consciousness, the illumined Messiah Consciousness; it is like the Buddhi or in Sanskrit, Mahat, or the stuff of consciousness, the intellect which precedes the formation of ego in the *field of the knower.* The screen of the higher mind is like the screen of the movie; it does not move and stands in perfect peace through all the violent actions, colors and conflicting storms of our experiences.

The pure light of consciousness or God is like the intelligence who watches the screen of the mind stuff as it reflects the whole of creation in our imaginations as a hologram. The images appear to be in front of us suspended at the point of our experience of them in our consciousness as a primal pattern of imagination. The images which are formed inside our Frontal Lobes are energy patterns, duplicates of other images at a more primordial level of the imaginative pattern of energy in the cosmos. To understand this fully is to understand the workings of the imagination on the seventh level of the brain.

At the level of this seventh brain function there are no ultimate authorities, such as the imaginative speculations of philosophers, theologians or theoretical physicists! The sage does not believe naively in the ultimate authority of the scriptures! The seventh level gives no importance to the teachings of a guru nor does it think enlightenment can come through the worship of any image whatsoever. However holy our consciousness may make it, the sage sees the "image" as an impurity in that awesome *pure consciousness* of which the entire nucleus of the universe is made. It is obvious from the words of Christ, Krishna or Buddha that they saw and did experience this nucleus and tried to describe it for lower levels of brain function. Judging from the world state and the dream state of people generally, they have failed to communicate it. Society has not been improved and in fact has become more unresponsive to spiritual values and much of the world is antipathetic to them, especially if we view the communist half of the world as generally anti-Christ, anti-religion, and anti-person. The fact is that the ultimate experience of the total organism we call the ONE cannot be had from the words of a guru or any tradition. These are, as all conventions, like the notes on the music program; they cannot improve the performance of the music even though they may affect the enjoyment and understanding of the listener. Such knowledge of the ultimate organism can only be had *direct* through one's own efforts and powers of discrimination. By no other process except the purification of our own imagination and the refinement of the intellect can the experience of the absolute singularity of Brahma, of God or the One, be realized. No teacher or scripture, no book or theory, nothing inferred from an external source can give us the pure vision of the awesome nucleus. A teacher can point the way, describe the structure, construct the maps to get there but only you, the real Self can go there and be there in that space where there are no maps because all is pure and direct experience in the ONE. My own guru said in the first few minutes of our meeting, "If you have met me, you have met them all. You need not go and seek other gurus." And I thought he was terribly arrogant and puffed up with his own greatness. It took me twelve years and meeting over a thousand gurus since, to fully understand this statement, so I can only sympathize with those who can't wait that long for understanding of the seventh level to dawn. It is a blessed moment when the ego stops judging and enters the real stuff of being and penetrates to the nuclear heart of all existence. That moment is the moment when the ONE enters his own temple and the waking dream is shattered into a thousand fragments. Those fragments, all containing

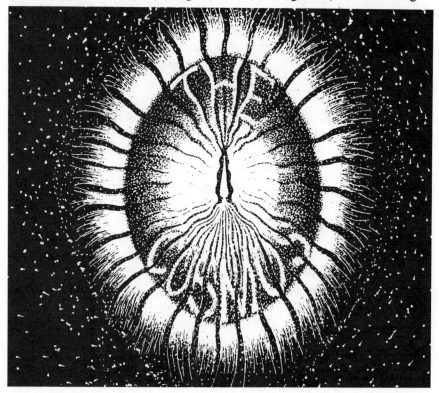

the One, are like people, each of those fragments a nucleus of the whole.

TAT TWAM ASI: THAT THOU ART

At this seventh level of evolution nothing can be taught or learned from external sources, simply because there is nothing external. The imagination itself must be totally clear of concepts and images and therefore pure before it can let anything new in without twisting it. At this level of our being there is no inside and no outside environment because we discover there are no divisions between the physical world and the spiritual. All differences are being made by our consciousness so that our enlightened self sees no less than the total vision of everything connected by *one* closely interwoven fabric of life.

The whole span of evolution of the body and its cells is seen as a continuum of flesh without a physical break in the union of proteins, sperm and ova, and the passing on of the hereditary nucleus of life from the common ancestor of all living things. This historical fact of the biological record explains why the basic biochemical machinery in all living organisms is the same. On its way to the total organism, the nucleus is carried forward by huge molecules that carry genetic information for the construction of offspring made up of building blocks of protein the same throughout Nature. The complex ways that these macro-molecules come together and organize themselves in the human brain produces different people, and the same ingredients and processes produce the differences in other living organisms. The way that life uses this genetic information in the DNA molecule in the nuclear control center of each cell demonstrates more similarities between living organisms than all the differences in appearance. The transmission of the DNA from this one common nuclear ancestor in the ocean is not something remote, which scientists estimate took place 2,000 million years ago, but happens and re-happens every time an organism is conceived. Bacteria, blood cells and all living organisms re-enact the entire cosmic process without any physical break in the eternal chain. Organisms die but living organisms, as long as they are alive, have never died; they are the end-product of a long chain of living flesh in which our consciousness is writing its waking dream. The seventh level

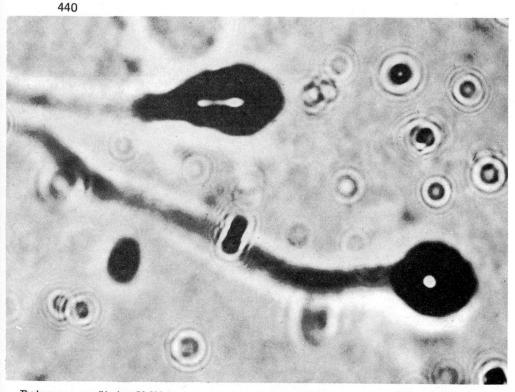

The human sperm cell is about 50,000 times as small as a female egg but contains just as many chromosomes. Sperm have cilia-type tails which makes them swim vigorously towards their one objective. In every union with an egg they create a continuous chain of life in the flesh from Abraham and before.

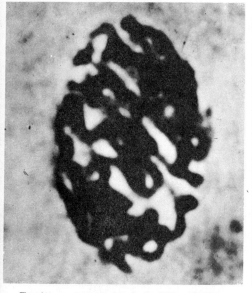

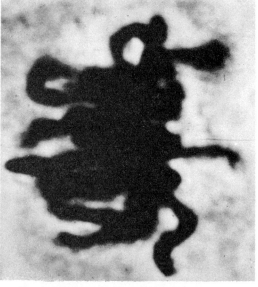

The chromosomes reproduce by the DNA replicating itself in RNA, joining the Y chromosomes of the males with the X chromosomes of the female eggs to make XY's or boys. Other sperms carry X chromosomes and unite wtih female X's to make XX's or girls.

PIP Photo—Allen Grant

The chromosomes align themselves at the center of the cell as they prepare to divide in the nucleus. At this stage the nucleus of the egg begins to completely dissolve into its chromosomes in the surrounding yolk, making all the parts one whole interconnected egg.

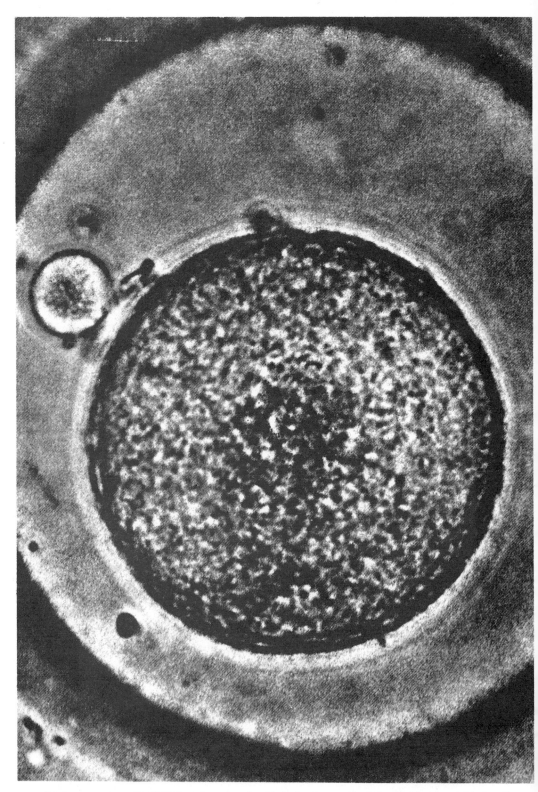

This human, egg, magnified 2000 times, is a cell produced in the female ovary. The dark nucleus is surrounded by the yolk containing many growth enzymes; it contains half the chromosomes needed to produce the proteins of normal body cells.

Dr. Landrum Shettles, Courtesy American Journal of Obstetrics and Gynecology

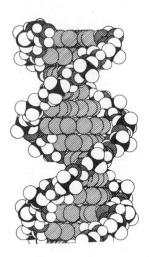

The DNA molecule and its protein partners in the threadlike chromosomes of the cell nucleus, maintain the specific linear sequence of the genes in passing on their hereditary message of evolution. The double helix is said to be the best macroscopic picture of the microcosmic nucleic acid structure of the cell genes. As such it portrays the macromolecule of DNA which transmits the pattern of life from generation to generation. The DNA itself does not act as a template but as a messenger which transfers its "message" to other nucleic acid proteins in the protoplasm surrounding the nucleus. It is a fundamental concept of Nuclear Evolution that consciousness can not only change the patterns of protein synthesis but also enter into the DNA patterns through the controlled action of cosmic light and the enzymes involved.

of the untapped brain potential contains all the organizational coding for the perfect society, for the ultimate organism seen as a universal hologram of the original nucleus at the birth of the universe. The cosmic soup in which this primordial birth took place is no different to the yolk of the egg, the nucleus of the ovum, the original imagination.

This total vision of the connectedness of all things is not an intellectual state seen in the mind as we see normally with our vision, because the ordinary eye has no knowledge whatever of how it sees. The ordinary mind unconsciously re-creates external images into the internal ones which we experience. Similarly all the functions of the human body are automatic and unconscious, i.e., digestion, hearing, elimination, hormone balance, sperm and ovum production, etc. Our seeing of internal images which replicate what is "external" is nothing short of miraculous, for the faculty of "inner seeing" is not merely a replication of a physical sensory process but is also a creation, as it is present in a blind person who has never seen the physical world. In so far as a person has life, consciousness, the "spark of the Divine", he has this capacity to create reality as well as receive it. The Cosmic Dreamer is dreaming through each of us and we are re-creating this dream, conditioning it through our seven levels of consciousness. Whatever we are receiving with the "inner eye" we are also creating, and this is the secret of the seventh level, where creator and created, inner and outer, cause and effect become ONE. The imagination is therefore the highest center in man and contains each person's cosmic program at the nucleus of being. This is Christ's true teaching and his vision of Heaven on earth. It is also the teaching of Krishna, Buddha, Lao Tzu and all the sages, which have been cluttered with the words of scribes who did not understand.

OUR TRUE NATURE

The very nucleus of life in everyone is in supreme control of our reality. It stands at the threshold of the nuclear self as its servant, but its action and commands cannot go contrary to its own programming in its imagination. This programming is what we call our true nature. No one can act contrary to their true nature or that very contrariness will become their true nature. An example of this can be seen when people want to do good. They try to give the world something they feel is needed. Their efforts are not only rejected but their schemes are counterproductive and bring reaction and hatred. Therefore to do good one must first become *good*. Otherwise how do you know what *good* is? A good person does not *try* to do good; everything which proceeds from him automatically *is* good. Christ tries to get across this example of the nuclear seed in the story of the good tree giving fruit of itself whereas the bad tree cannot give forth good fruit. He is describing the state of the heart. He says that what pollutes a person is not what goes into him but what proceeds out of the mouth. For a person to speak foul words, be full of hate and do hurtful, bestial and vicious things to others, there must be vicious or greedy thoughts in the mind. The thoughts do not get there by accident but rise in our consciousness by reason of our true nature being what it is. Even under drugs this seed nucleus will act out, feel or envision its real nature. In many who normally are blocked and inhibited from experiencing their self-programmed true natures because of the overlaying of false imagination and deluded self-images, glimpses of their real unconscious self are possible when the overlaying interference is removed under a drug or in a peak experience. We seek, through drugs, to liberate the mind, but the danger is that drugs may only expand the problems in the mind. In order for us to liberate the mind it must first be purified. Otherwise we may indiscriminately take away those inhibitions that are programmed into our minds by history, by culture, by self-discipline and by primitive spiritual practices, thereby taking license and indulging deeper selfish whims at the expense of society. Certain drugs can quickly release deeply-rooted false barriers in people's minds and lead to enhancement of awareness, but the rapturous images of the drug high often delude people into thinking they have arrived at liberation when in fact they are only glimpsing the potential. When the drug wears off there is still the work to be done in purifying the self on all levels which cannot be accomplished by escaping the self-confrontation through more and more drugs. Dependence on consciousness-altering drugs has reached epidemic proportions in the United States and this escape is also a perverted expression of the real being, the blueprint of a unique human entity contained within his or her nuclear center.

Is our society hopelessly tied to all these programs? If all the learned inhibitions and traits of civilization are but a thin veneer over our true nature which dwells somewhere deep inside our unconscious mind, waiting to express itself in little ways beyond our control, can we hope to change and evolve ourselves to a higher state of consciousness without some kind of a drug? Our true nature is not only the dark and hateful side of us but the radiant and loving side as well. This joyful *self* expresses spontaneously in the involuntary smile or the twinkle in our eye or some little gesture we did not know we were going to do. At a level beyond our control our best self extends its unique kind of love in spite of all our efforts to control it and make it conform to the ways of others and in spite of all our negative self-images that make us doubt ourselves. This joyful, loving part of ourself is our inner power to change the dark side of our true nature and no matter how under-developed it may be it is essential to nurture it if we are ever to actualize our deeper potential for perfection.

Some people who study spiritual teachings program a new self-image based on scriptures like "Ye are the light of this world."* They try to hold in their imaginations the idea of their true nature as light, knowing that whatever image they hold will in time manifest. But

---

* More on what this light means is found in a following chapter which deals with those great beings who live permanently in that unlimited joyous state of consciousness.

unless they are prepared to do the work on the dark side of their being, the light can never fully manifest, because there are counter-images beyond their reach. The task is to bring these to light with love and become conscious of them, see them, own them, face them until at that deep level of love there comes a change of heart. But even at these depths of our being, where our nuclear center is expanding in a continuous process of growth, we may limit it with a self-image of "me" and "my growth". Even though "me" gets larger and larger the more we grow, our imaginations may still have no inkling of just how vast is our real Self which is the light of this world.

HOW DOES OUR IMAGINATION CREATE REALITY IN THE TOTAL MIND?

What is the link between the worlds we experience of energy, matter and form and the formless worlds of free energy and light? How does our brain act as the filter for the energy of cosmic light that interpenetrates the whole of cosmic space? What do we mean when we use the words "total mind", and how is our present reality of the material universe connected to our experience of it in our consciousness? An answer to these questions is the most important knowledge that man can contemplate with his limited mind, against which all other questions pale by comparison. The way we form images in our consciousness determines the type of reality we experience in our thought life. The process of identification which occurs in the mind stuff of a human being has been explained in philosophical and religious terms from ancient times but a scientific explanation of the actual process of identification with the time-like order of events in the universe has not been possible until now.*

The fact that we ourselves place images into our consciousness rather than being passively influenced by them as if they are coming into our minds from outside is a difficult idea for ordinary levels of consciousness to accept. Our normal perception is so rooted in material

---

* The full process of identification is complicated and has been described in my course of 24 taped lectures, called "Rumf Roomph Yoga," published by University of the Trees Press.

sensations that we find it difficult to believe that there are other, more subtle universes beyond our immediate awareness. However physics has proved that we do not sense the inner life of atoms or the subtle processes of nucleic acids which go on in the DNA of our cell life. Only through developing more and more sensitive instruments has the scientist been able to look deeper into Nature with his consciousness and form ideas and concepts about the unseen worlds which lie all about us in our innocence. The imagination is the prime tool of those theoretical physicists who prove the invisible worlds in the heart of atoms and stars. Like Einstein, who was able to "see" with the mind's eye how black holes could be predicted out of his theory of general relativity, we must now develop beyond the concept of relativity to absolutivity—that state which sees beyond the relative comparisons. Nuclear Evolution is the *theory of absolutivity.*

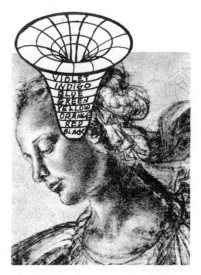

Every person's consciousness is annihilating itself in a black hole into which the universe contracts spiritually as it expands materially.

What is the connection between a black hole and our imagination and what is the bridge which can link them? The fantastic world beyond our imagination (of universes existing which are unreachable with ordinary states of consciousness) is now unfolding through the evolution of our consciousness into new levels of direct perception of the totality of the One cosmic mind acting through all things. How we ourselves create our own reality by the process of imaging can only be understood from another level of consciousness which we could call an eighth level or, better still, the central nucleus in which no levels exist separate from each other but are like a succession of several universes connected only by our own consciousness acting through them all.

THE BLACK HOLE AND CONSCIOUSNESS

What is beyond the seventh domain of brain organization? Is the brain itself the product of another intelligent universe which interpenetrates this physical universe of matter? How could this be feasible or even detectable by our sensory organs and the instruments of science which extend those senses into the invisible world, e.g., telescopes into the macrocosm, electron microscopes into the microcosm, and radio waves, TV screens and cameras for seeing at a distance? To answer this question of feasibility of another universe made of the invisible stuff called consciousness, we must now temporarily use our imaginations to create a new model of cosmic consciousness. This model is of a single nuclear center surrounded by auras or layers of different

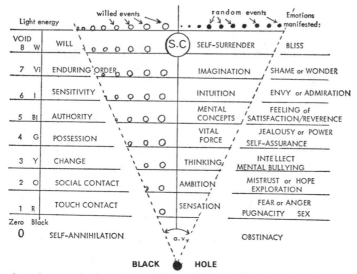

In the diagram above the seven levels are shown in linear hierarchy leading to an eighth level of superintelligent consciousness (S.C.) which can only be experienced beyond the imagination in a unitive state of consciousness called Samadhi (meaning complete togetherness) which produces tranquillity and bliss. The colors represent harmonic frequencies of vibration in tune with the light of the universe, i.e., red—hydrogen, green—oxygen radiation, etc., from all the supernovas and nebulae in our galaxy. On the left are the main attributes of each level and on the right the main drives. The model is not linear or hierarchical in fact; only linear depending on one's angle of vision (a.v.). In the Black Hole there are no levels.

OUR GALAXY IS FILLED WITH OBJECTS VIBRATING AT DIFFERENT FREQUENCIES OF LIGHT (COLORS)

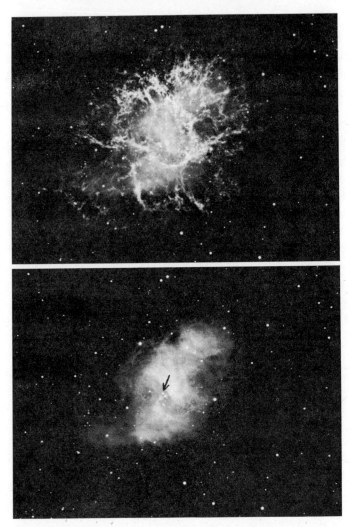

The Crab Nebula. Resulting from an explosion of the arrowed star in the bottom picture, observed by Chinese astronomers from June 10th to July 4th, 1054 A.D., the light was so bright it was visible in full daylight for three weeks. The white emission or glow is the process of synchrotron radiation highly polarized. The filaments on the edges of the top picture, photographed with red light, are ionized gases caused by ultraviolet synchrotron effects on hydrogen gas. The exploded star is now a neutron star flashing off and on and spinning thirty times a second. The bottom picture shows the arrowed star as the nucleus of the whole nebula which is still evolving. This enormous energy reaches the earth and has helped evolve our consciousness over the last 925 years. The bottom picture was photographed in the green light given off by ionized oxygen which took about 6,200 light-years to reach us on earth. (Our galaxy is approximately 100,000 light-years wide and contains over 1,000,000,000,000 stars.) Synchrotron radiation is produced by recombination radiation consisting of high speed electrons spiraling around in a magnetic field thereby providing high energy polarization to ionize the gases and light up the nebula with its different colors.

particles of subtle matter. The idea of subtle matter oscillating at different frequencies beyond the reach of our present scientific sensors is not new, but the scientific explanation for its role in the creation of consciousness is offered by the theory of Nuclear Evolution which says that our consciousness is constantly annihilating everything it experiences in a black hole at the nuclear center of our being. This theory is put forward in detail in *Nuclear Evolution.*

Here is a brief explanation of the presence of a nucleus at the center of our universe which conforms with new theoretical concepts of physics. This center, like a hologram, is now everywhere present throughout the whole, having expanded from its original seed. The separate parts in it, like me and you and other entities, are only different like the parts of a holographic picture are different. These parts have the same inner core at the heart of all existence which is located spatially throughout the whole. If we cut the corner off a hologram negative, the small piece of film contains the whole picture and is just reproduced on a smaller scale the same as the original negative. If we think of the nucleus of the universe as a void or hyper-space in which everything else exists, we can see that our consciousness is such a similar void which is unmanifest, intangible and transparent to our vision, but yet obviously present or we could not think, live or be a self, nor could we deny that our consciousness exists without there being this invisible consciousness to deny it. This nuclear center, seen as a black hole at the core of being, sucks in all vibrations like the silence sucks in all sounds only to annihilate them eventually.

At the moment science regards the black hole as a theoretical curiosity, although many astronomers believe there is evidence for black holes in photographs of the sky around us. A black hole in space is the remains of a star which has died after finishing its nuclear burning and collapsed into an enormously dense invisible state. All the material particles of matter have been burned out and time has therefore come to a stop. Neither does space have any reality inside a black hole because it is so empty like space itself that anything which comes into contact with it is immediately sucked into itself and annihilated. If we think of our spaceless and timeless consciousness which has been purified of all thoughts about matter, we can see that,

From Formlessness to Form
depending on the light

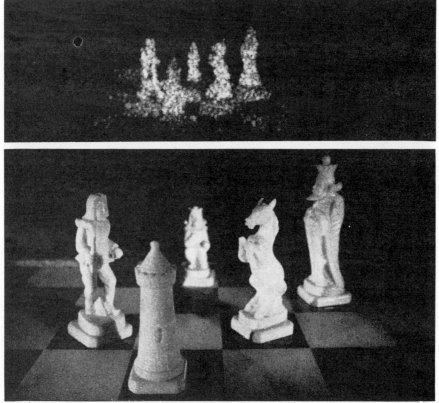

Photography by Emmett N. Leith and Juris Upatnieks

Top picture shows the entire image of the original scene reproduced by any part of the hologram illuminated with a beam of laser light half a millimeter in diameter. Bottom picture shows the full image produced by the same hologram with a broader beam, when the reconstructed waves of light are passed through a lens and brought to a focus forming a three-dimensional image of the original scene even after the chessmen have been removed.

The reality of a hologram which repeats the image of the nucleus throughout the whole of any system is used by our consciousness as a guiding field for evolution. The chicken egg yolk is a hologram of the full-grown chicken and every nucleus contains the full hologram of the bird. Similarly great beings on the human level contain the hologram of the cosmic nucleus within their consciousness. These beings who, having conquered time, now live in the future, having constructed the hologram in their present, are now working on the present out of the past through invisible networks of centers everywhere.

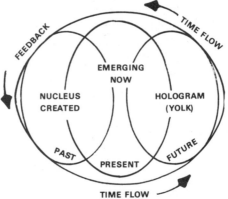

like a black hole, our consciousness cannot tell any difference between itself and empty space. Certainly our consciousness, though invisible and empty, can travel in a flash through empty space to objects which are billions of light-years away, like stars on the edge of the universe.

Black holes are not actually black but are only called black because they are perfect absorbers of everything they encounter. They are black in the sense that they are invisible because they exist beyond the horizon of the visible universe of matter. Things that are sucked into a black hole can be likened to events that fall into our consciousness at every moment. They don't come back. Only a memory trace of an event yesterday or yester-hour remains, and every material sensory event in the now is a new one. No one can see into consciousness when we look along its eyebeams. What do we see if we are a blind person who looks inside our head at thoughts of life? When we close our eyes our consciousness is still there, absorbing all life, but we just close a small window in the visible part of the spectrum to stop things falling into our consciousness. Then like the black hole you can't see into the universe, because any light that is generated inside the eyes never gets out. When you close your eyes, the visible light is trapped inside you. In the same way, a black hole's gravitational field is so great that its light is sucked back into it and it has no contact with a so-called outside world in the universe around it. It is like a human being as a single entity feeling totally alone and separate from the universe around him.

At the center of a black invisible hole in space there is a singularity— another name for "the One". It is a place where the laws of physics no longer apply, where all measurements of time and space are nonexistent because there is only *One* and nothing else to compare itself with. Consciousness, like a black hole, is the drain of the universe. Like the spiraling water disappearing down the bath hole drain, so does the black hole eventually suck all outer things including all the stars and objects into itself. It is like a tunnel or a gateway out of the universe we live in and into another universe which exists beyond our present awareness. That universe is our true home—the home of all collapsed stars which have burned out their material existence never to return to the material universe. Like death, it is the place from which no traveler

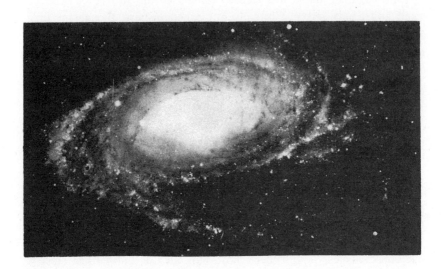

The picture shows two spiraling galaxies from different angles with central shining clouds. At the center an invisible black hole is thought to be consuming the nearby stars thereby providing ionizing radiation to light up the whole and send its light 6,000 light-years to us through empty space. These spiral patterns are repeated in magnetic fields at the heart of the sun, in individual stars and in our own fields of consciousness.

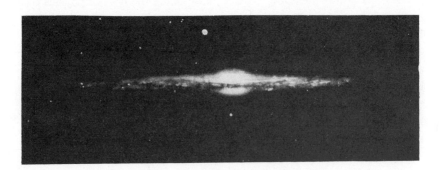

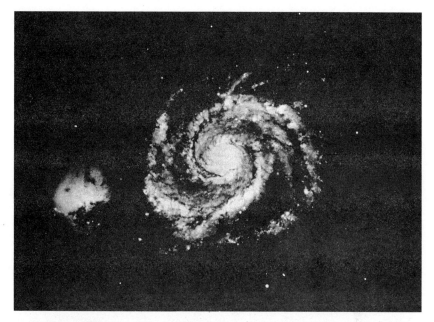

This galaxy, M51, along with a companion galaxy probably has a black hole at center where intensified brightness is caused through a collapsing of stars as they approach the center of the enormous gravitational forces, eventually to be eaten and digested into a formless transparent invisible energy like consciousness. The proportional vibrations at nodal points from the center correspond harmonically to orbital velocities in the spiral galaxy and the frequencies of chakra vibration rates. (See "Supersonics", pages 401-408 for more details.)

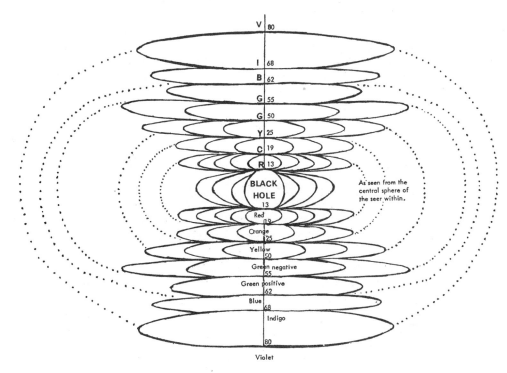

THE SPIRAL WAVEFIELD OF THE HUMAN AURA

ever returns in the flesh. Whatever falls into a black hole never comes out again. Once our consciousness comes to rest in the One, everything stops in the singularity of the absolute and there is no two—no twoness or threeness.

Wherever two or three are gathered together in the name of the absolute black hole of *oneness,* there shall the supreme nucleus of all being be found in our awareness. This does not mean that the creation and all the stars and matter will disappear. Wherever there is a swirling spiral action, rotating around a center, an electrical charge is certain to be there even when there is no matter. This charge is not a separate positive and negative but an inseparable marriage of the two in the one singular identity. Because rotating energies come into the black hole as a vibration or as cyclic oscillations of movement around a nucleus or center, they can go through the black hole and be reflected—not reflected back into our present universe of matter but reflected into another and different "through the looking glass" universe which is mirrored in our consciousness. That universe has its existence in another octave running parallel to our own. In that other universe is the same black hole with an absolute singularity acting as a bridge between the universe of spirit and matter, life and death, God and man. It is the black hole of our own consciousness which permits communication between the universes which penetrate each other. Without consciousness they are inaccessible to each other. From the other universe, however, the black hole of consciousness which is common to both the material universe and the mirrored universe, looks like a white hole. From that white hole can be seen a whole chain of similar bridges between all the black holes which connect all the universes interpenetrated in successive layers within each other. When the One meditates upon itself as the primordial nucleus of all the universes, all the bridges through the totality of space are destroyed in the absolute One who in Sanskrit is called Brahman. When space is annihilated in our consciousness then the black hole and the white whole become the one nucleus which is the rainbow bridge to all the worlds.

> Thou art that bridge,
> Thou art that black hole, waiting to see
>   the white hole of your own glory;

> Thou art the star burning out its matter;
> Thou art the space and the invisible light
>   which travels through it.
> Thou art that!

Perhaps you are thinking that such flights of imagination are fine for religious fanatics, for Einstein, or for mystics, but you yourself have to live in the ordinary world of everyday life. What good does it do for a housewife or a businessman or a politician to think about black holes in space or even to dream of seeing their true Self? These thoughts are the very separations that make up the delusions that we superimpose upon Reality, because in actual fact, our everyday life in society is a direct reflection of how near or far we are from the black hole.

CONSCIOUSNESS CREATES OUR SOCIAL WORLD

The four pairs of lobes in levels six and seven can work separately or together as a whole, on nonsensory smells, images, musical sounds, sights, etc. These functions, ranging from basic sense perception to the kind of imagination found in the brain of an Einstein, can be seen at work in the quality of leadership, the artistic and imaginative skills of our culture, the quality of our sciences, which all affect our social orientation to the spending of money on research on such priorities as going to the moon, feeding the hungry world, etc. In the ancient Vedic culture all the resources of the kings and researchers from 10,000 to 4,000 years ago were almost exclusively given up to the development of the sixth level functions of the nonsensory spiritual knowledge of the human relationship to God, whereas our own materialistic culture has developed greater knowledge of the first level sensory world. It is now time to bridge the gap between the worlds of the spirit and scientific material thinking. Once Western science has investigated the sixth level completely, there will be a New Age of enlightenment which will devote most of its energies to the exploration of level seven in the abstract world of the imagination in the Frontal Lobes.

The Deva-nagari (Holy City) and Deva-chan (Divine World of Light) languages, which were the ancient sacred languages which eventually developed into the Sanskrit language at the root of our own language, were developed in order to describe research in the more abstract terms of level six rather than the later imaginative mathematical symbols of level seven. The great researchers who invented number, mathematics, quadratic equations, etc., from those times could not speak to society or to ordinary man in such symbols as zero or $E = mc^2$ and therefore Sanskrit was perfected as the spiritual and scientific language of that age. This language was perfected and polished to express the truths of the seer-sages of ancient India. Hence the meaning of the word "Sanskrit"—created, perfected, or polished from the verb root *kri* plus the prefix *sam* meaning to complete.

The coming age of scientific researchers will not use the "Divine City" temple script but will use the language of vibrations throughout the whole of space. Already we are probing the vibrations of rare clouds of gases in the spiraling arms of whirling galaxies millions of light-years away, but these will have no real meaning until we understand the way our intuition works. The next age will have a language of its own, the language of science, of physics—the mathematical symbols necessary to the probing of outer space. But these ventures into imagination will have no meaning until we understand intuition, because we will believe the symbols are only symbols. Only at the sixth level can we connect ourselves to the symbols and have a direct perception of a real world behind the symbols. Then we "know" the One who is *behind* all that vastness of creation and is working through it and in it, growing, creating, living, evolving, loving, being.

Up till now mathematicians have not understood mathematics as a spiritual science of proportions* and have used the symbols of the imagination only to prove the concrete world of matter and the

---

* The proportions are the frequency of the colors of the spectrum in relation to each other and their proportional relations to the chakras or centers of control of consciousness in the human organism. All matter is proportionally related by its vibration to other matter. And the human body resonates like an antenna divided into seven proportions which absorb the energy of the universe according to which level of consciousness is functioning. For further details of proportional vibrations, see *Supersensonics,* published 1975, University of the Trees Press.

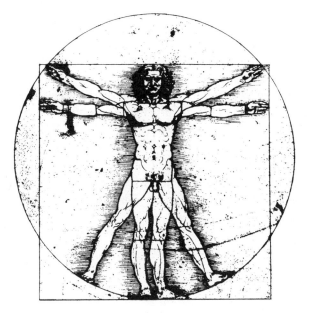

"Study in the proportions of the human body, based on
Vitruvius" (1492) by Leonardo da Vinci (1452-1519).

measurable fields of energy. But the real understanding of mathematics is not something which merely involves logical and complicated manipulation of numbers. That is just intellectual cleverness, of little value to the real world of people and of life, and it will ever perish in the dry-as-dust mind of academic man. The real understanding of our imagination does not come through numbers but in knowing that numbers are purely a creation of consciousness. They are the human expression of the mind's relationship to the proportional vibrations of the real supersensitive universe. For instance, take the transcendental number zero which is the most recent discovery of all the numbers from one to ten, amounting to an exciting spiritual breakthrough. Even today there are many mathematicians who have no imagination of what reality zero must represent. Zero equals the absence of all matter, the purity of the mind from all thoughts of value, the empty consciousness in its raw uncreated state. The nearest description we can give of any number in words is to say that it is not an integer having any property whatever except that given to it by our imaginations, and it is not reducible to any principle of logic; yet it can be known directly by our experience and observation. The experience of "nothing" or zero, however, cannot be had by thought alone, and only mystics have so far seen "zero" as the ultimate symbol for God, the pure Cosmic Intelligence of consciousness.

The New Age will research this "nothingness" not as a symbol in an inductive way or even in a mind-orientated deductive way as mathematicians do, but in the pure way of thought itself. It is difficult to imagine something so pure that there is no "image" in it or concept of it in the mind. That difficulty has prevented mankind from developing a true spiritual language of space. Mathematics is an exact science but there are various ways of being exacting. The word "mathematics" is a

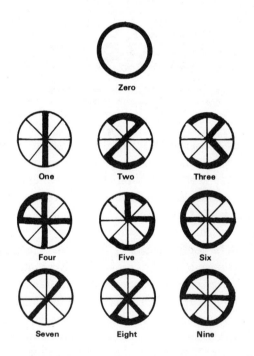

The origin of numbers as parts of the circle is shown in the above diagram from a forthcoming book on "Divine Mathematics". Each number represents a proportion of an octave made from a circle divided into eight parts by eight lines. The symbol of each number radiates the design of a psychic energy of its pattern in our consciousness and acts as a witness in radiesthesia. This discovery by the author was made by means of "Supersensonics". (See "Supersensonics", pages 567-569 for more details.)

Greek word originally developed from the Sanskrit word "mathe" or "medha" meaning the intelligence or wisdom which is precise. It is the wisdom which is certain or exact. Throughout the ages it has changed its character and even as far back as Egyptian times came to mean "calculation". Originally it was a way of validating knowledge or making it certain. I am in the process of writing another book* to show how the origin and use of number can be developed without any calculations in a completely new symbolic way to discover the spiritual worlds of intelligence in the same exact way that man has used it to provide the so-called exact knowledge of the world of matter. But the truth is that mathematics as it is taught today has never provided us with any "exact" knowledge of the material world. All that the ordinary mathematician can say is that there are certain "exact" mathematical probabilities in Nature. The fact is that mathematics is all a product of our imaginations and therefore this material knowledge has all our own limitations in it. Assumptions are not reality, and the reason why mathematics has now become so confusing is because it has become the language of operations and assumptions. Its true function will be brought into the coming age and given in a simple way to the layman as the language of proportions in Nature. At the moment there is a welter of different mathematics so that even amongst mathematicians one could spend one's whole lifetime studying hundreds of different systems without ever applying the mathematics to anything. The situation is rapidly approaching the state of confusion replicating the "Tower of Babel" story where not even the mathematicians will understand each other. No doubt this is due to the rapid advance in computer technology which allows rapid calculations which formerly took months or even years. Sophistication, however, does not provide any more wisdom and the simple way may yet transcend over the complex.

With simple understanding it will be easy to explain that zero is the absence of vibration of movement and that all movement is measured in reference to that absolute stillness. In absolute stillness there is no time. While all our present measurements of vibrations are measured

---

* *Divine Mathematics,* by Christopher Hills, not yet in print.

in earth time they will be eventually measured with reference to zero time. Only pure consciousness can exist in zero timelessness in which the measurements of change and movement are absolute, rather than relative to earth time. The consciousness which is perfectly still can soon grasp the nature of eternal zero-time.* It will be easy to grasp in our imaginations that every frequency has a resonant proportional frequency at double its vibrations at an octave above or at half its number of vibrations at the octave below, and that the exact number of vibrations is irrelevant to the operation of our consciousness or to the nature of Reality. Now mathematicians may breathe a sigh of relief when they realize that the language of the present-day mathematics has lost its foundations which are simple and rooted in the nature of the mind and that these can be restored. To understand this simplicity does not require a lot of intelligence, but more common sense (another name for wisdom).

At present, physics has nothing to say at all about a possible real world lying behind its concepts and equations; physics is simply a model of Nature from the fifth level of conceptual reality. Its own assumption of a kind of reality is merely an interpretation or hypothesis. How is it that we can now talk about a real world on higher levels of consciousness whereas physics can only make models? The answer is that Nuclear Evolution is a wholistic science of absolute wholes whereas physics is a science of parts. The particles and experiments discovered by physics do not enable us to get inside the nucleus of an atom but only to observe it as an onlooker. This *objective* knowledge ignores the *subjective* consciousness of the observer and takes it for a given. But this assumption is false because the method of physics itself conditions the consciousness of the observer whose mind is the greatest filter of direct knowledge. Why should the materialists or the world change from their low materialist level of perception if it is thought that there is no reality beyond that known to them? It is unlikely that they will ever do anything elevated apart from irresponsibly putting more inventions and destructive knowledge in the hands of the dark minds of

---

* The nature of relative time and its relation to movement, velocity and space is dealt with in great detail, *Nuclear Evolution*, pages 420-447.

the earth. Science as it is used today cannot help the world to see any higher than its own limited materialistic view of Nature. Why should materialists change if they don't know any difference?

The new science of tomorrow will include Nuclear Evolution and, by the validation possible through "Supersensonic" methods, will create a New Age which includes the layman and does not leave him out in the cold. By taking any theory, a layman can divine whether its assumptions about the natural world are false or true. If its original assumptions are wrong the whole hypothesis will be false knowledge, and we will not need a bunch of dry mathematicians and physicists to tell us what the real world is like. Everyone will be actually involved as well as the physicist because a wholistic approach contains seven distinct levels to become one with the one truth. The truths of science are changing truths that really amount to no more than a specialist's opinion which can never be absolutely proved for all levels of existence, whereas the New Age truth will be testable in life itself, and science as we now know it will be only one method of validating it. Science will not be the absolute method as it is often thought of but will develop the concepts of nuclear and wholistic evolution just as it has developed the concept of the hologram. Already this is beginning to happen in the concepts of black holes and white holes and new theories in brain research.

THE WORLD PEACE CENTER

The quality of society has been immeasurably enriched by the opening up of the Frontal Lobes, and it is the development of their amazing powers of insight that has brought us not only the spiritual science of the East, discovered by the great rishis and wise men of old, but also the discoveries of electronic man, artificial intelligence, space-time and relativity and a host of other developments which have pushed the world organism to the brink of another breakthrough. To use it to explore outer space or to manipulate the material world without first exploring inner space is to build a fancy "tower to heaven". It is the same old problem of man's diseased dream and points to the abomination of his imagination so accurately recorded by earlier seers some five or six thousand years ago in Genesis 11. The point of evolution is coming again to that focus in time at which the entire species speaks one language—this time the language of vibration, frequencies and resonance upon which the whole scientific worldwide edifice is built. The breakthrough that is ahead of us is not a breakthrough into outer space in which we have floated since the beginning, but into the womb of inner space in which the waking dream takes place.

The breakthrough now waiting for us at the threshold of the future is to discover the nature of imagination itself and its relationship to human communication and human society. Just as it has taken mankind over 65 years to come from Einstein's discovery of $E=mc^2$ to our present radio-TV infra-structure and the mass of frequencies and microwaves surrounding the planet, so it will take another long period to assimilate and put to work the next evolutionary discovery of the nucleus of man's being—what it is, how it relates to itself and how it re-creates the external environment within its own limitations. This is a profound thought for those who believe there are no limitations, as much as for those who claim that all limitations are imposed by the social environment. The social environment is merely a reflection of this highest center in the human brain showing whether the imagination is working correctly in our society or not. Therefore there is no way to change society fundamentally without changing ourselves, and there is no way to change ourselves without changing this internal nucleus of our being.

This is a hard idea for most people imprisoned at the sensory level to accept, because they think they see vast changes all around them. They see the space age dawning and they forget their origins and the foresight of their forefathers in Genesis. The genetic program is not different now from what it was in Genesis, nor is it different for other organisms who are parts of the original total cosmic nucleus. Nor will it be different in the future millennia. The egg is eternal so long as it lasts. At this level the program is like the waking dream which sees the changing world around us as the reality. The fact is that life is lived emotionally and spiritually almost the same as thousands of years ago, and what people call *change* is just the superficial conditions of life. Going to the moon does not change the psyche of a man as greatly as

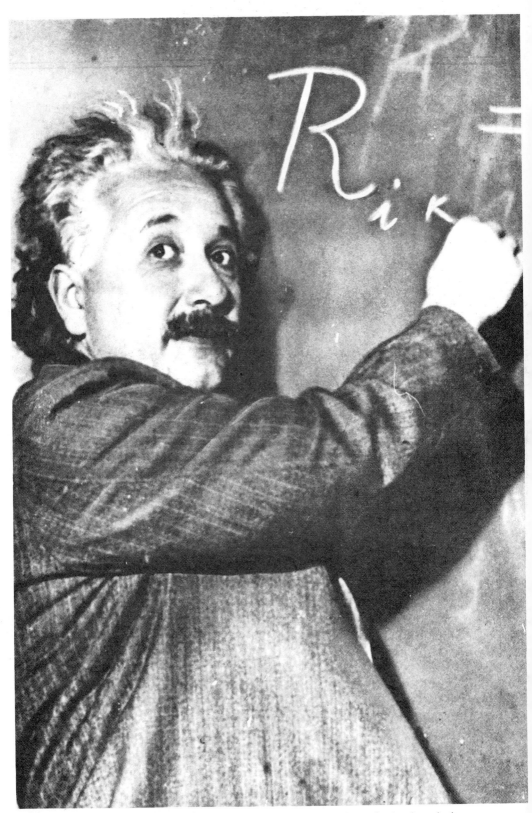

Einstein brought mankind to a new awareness. We are now ready for another leap in awakening.

falling in love on the earth. The possibilities for social intercourse are limited to the speed with which we can bring the functioning of this seventh center of our thoughts and feelings about life under our direct control. Going to the moon or outer space will not get these under control. With most people the imagination is all submerged in their unconscious. What does "control of our imagination" really mean? What does it mean to the man in the street to purify the imagination?

The first thing is to realize that the purification is not a moral process or a set code of behavior by which the human race can be "saved". It means that every person must understand first how their imaginations are made impure by false images of themselves and of the creation itself. All religion, all politics, all philosophy, is really a form of worship. Whereas men first worshipped the elements, trees, rocks and even the sun in former times and made them into religions, we now worship man-made gods like science, capitalism and Marxism. Yet real worship is to shape our own worth, to prepare ourself as a cosmic being, not to look to external gods created in the mind. The real God is Consciousness, the stuff of which the gods are made! To worship consciousness is to purify the images we put into it of all human arrogance and to prepare ourself for the entrance of the Cosmic One who is far beyond our human imagination. To hold opinions, concepts, ideals or even codes of moralistic action is to be self-righteous. Pure consciousness is concerned with the development of righteousness, the skill of right action. This depends entirely on our image of good and evil and our own part in that duality. People are polluted in their imaginations at the most fundamental levels of right and wrong, positive and negative, and never think to question or investigate the quality of their own thought life which they believe in so emotionally. They cannot enter into the seventh domain without first training (or untraining) their imagination. To have a pure imagination is not easy even for the highest of people. To become a lover of all beings is even a more difficult task for the workings of our imagination, since that means loving those people we don't even like.

How do we get to the evolution of a new social model from all of this? Of what inscrutable significance is the fact that we carry around inside us a most complex computer, the wiring of which is so complex that even with our modern scientific knowledge we know very little about its real purpose? What mysterious intelligence has organized such a vast undertaking that all the huge computers available today cannot do what the human brain achieves within its average weight of 3½ pounds? Even with micro-circuits, just to duplicate the number of electrical events that go on in one human brain to regulate our cell life would require a huge building just to house the circuits of such a computer. What has such an awesome piece of equipment got to learn?

We have said that the Frontal Lobes are concerned with imagination and in a book like this we cannot go into detail as to what imagination really is,* but if we can begin to imagine that all the brain functions surrounding the central Cave of Brahma (the third ventricle) are outgrowths from the center of a wheel, then we are no longer bound to the linear model of evolution but we can see that evolution can be looked at as an expansion of a nucleus which contains all the sensory apparatus as spokes or extensions of the self.

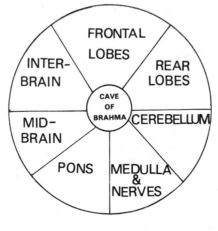

Cross section of a sphere

---

* See *Nuclear Evolution* pages 78-105 for in-depth study on the way we can train our imagination to function on higher levels of perception.

In the wheel model, the nervous system, instead of being our most primitive level of brain function, becomes "equal knower" with all other systems on its own level and the qualities of that level of consciousness no lower in value than any of the other levels. The evaluating judgement that comes of hierarchical thinking gives way to the realization that only the center can know the total reality by putting the seven levels of experience together in a wholistic way which sees things in wholes and not just as a ladder-like collection of separate parts.

Evolution has extended the nervous system out into our body as it did in other animal bodies and as it did in plants, birds and in the sensing mechanisms of insects, amoeba, etc. If we take this flat wheel model as only a flat surface, we can then imagine it extending up and downwards in three dimensions like a sphere and if we can then imagine that sphere to be rotating, then none of the various parts would change their relationship to each other within the rotating sphere.

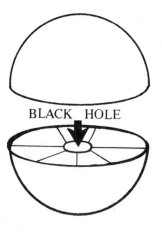

BLACK   HOLE

The seven domains are linked together as aspects of one vibrating sphere to form a holo-gram with a hole in the hub which is void.

The hologram of consciousness functions through the levels of the brain and its corresponding evolution of each organism.

If we look at this sphere as not only the model for the brain, but also the model structure of society, or even as a model of the universe, there will be one point which is the center for them all—the hub. Wherever the center is, whether it is the center of the universe, the center of the earth or the center of our nucleus, there is no movement, only peace, quiet and stillness. The center of peace and stillness is the new model for society and a strange idea now appears in our imaginations that we can hardly believe because it so contradicts all the other information sent to us from the seven parts of our brain structures.

PERHAPS THE CENTER IS EVERYWHERE BECAUSE IT IS NOWHERE IN PARTICULAR.

At the center of every system, there is this one point of stillness around which all else turns and revolves, and it is at this point that we take a giant leap into another state of consciousness, because there is nothing at this central point in the nucleus but pure consciousness. Then the reasoning power of our analytical third level brain asks how can *pure consciousness* without any content be a center of a political system? How can you give an example to anyone if there is nothing there? The answer is the same as that of an ancient seer—Lao Tzu. At the hub of the wheel is "nothing" and that is the most important part, around which the central fulcrum of the wheel rotates. The useful part of a vase is not the walls of the vessel but the emptiness inside it. In the same way, the greatest power is the concept of *nothing* into which all consciousness flows. Thoughts arise in the pure silence of the mind and die down again like a sound disturbs the silence and dies into the silence again. The eternal silence is the frightening goal of all vibration, oscillation, movement or sound. This void is not emptiness as many misconceive in their imaginations but the fullness of all potentials. It is the total absorption of all differences in the cosmic soup, so intense and burning with the sperm-fire of creation that nothing can exist in it except its own pure self. This is the idea of the black hole as the real nature of the human nucleus of consciousness. Being pure, there is nothing in it, no thought, no images, no desires, no need to go or come.

What is the political significance of such a powerful intense vision of our deepest self? When people communicate with each other from this center, there is only peace and love there, because everyone is seen as an extension of oneself from that central point at the center of peace. Nothing can disturb us. That then is the true model of our social life. We only have to understand that the restless, moving, changing parts of the revolving model are not the center but only extensions of the nucleus of being, at the center.

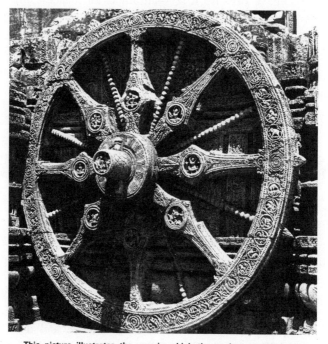

This picture illustrates the way in which the ancient seers tried to communicate the wheel of life with its still center.

They become all servants of the singularity which is our own individable self, our pure consciousness invisible as it is, going out to report back. The changing parts are extensions of the "self" reaching out to the periphery of our being. In the same way the society can be composed of many centers of peace all reaching out towards other centers of peace developed by individuals who have discovered this center of peace within themselves, and in this way peace will rise in each person all over the planet. Peace cannot be something imposed from outside, since that does not leave us free.

Once we see that the Cosmos is a hologram and that each part contains the whole, then the idea of a World Peace Center, consisting of multiple centers of peace, is inevitable, because each person and each group is equally the center of the universe to the extent that they attune themselves to that wholeness. Our social structure then reflects that wisdom and vast Intelligence which governs even the change of the seasons and the flight of the birds and the way that seeds bear fruit each in its own kind. The World Peace Center is the seed of man's happiness, for planted in our consciousness it will bear fruit in the world after the pattern of our own purity of vision. This is what we mean by World Peace Center—the nuclear model of evolution, expressing itself as the light of consciousness extending into wider and wider areas of experience, leaving our imagination and higher functions pure, i.e., ready to receive the beauty of the cosmic vision for the next step, always ready and receptive, always seeing that the whole of society is an extension of the very primordial feeling of love radiating from the nucleus at many levels of ignorance or insight. It is this insight alone which determines our awareness of the supreme design of the structure of the whole universe.

The wheel concept and its rotating spheres or shells of love in different forms is the evolutionary model of man which must be objectified and manifested on earth, written down in symbols of the imagination. Whether mathematical, verbal or intuitive, these symbols are lower means of communication for the higher self. All community groups, societies, companies, political parties, etc., are for this one purpose—to communicate self. The World Peace Center constitution therefore, which is modeled on this nuclear image, is an image of the growth of the individual and the society to the oneness at the center of peace. That is the true laboratory for democracy where the experiment is to meet yourself. Your higher self is really beyond *all* models and communicates not by separating and exchanging communications but by *being* whoever and whatever it communicates with. Since this "self" is unconscious in most people, we don't often realize the pain it feels when we keep it from union and insist upon remaining separate egos. And yet we are this self. Its pain is ours. And only the doorway of a purified imagination can set us free of the gross and blind convictions of the ego. Each of the seven parts of our mind is purified according to its own level. The impure imagination serves the ego— from neurotic fears and erotic daydreams all the way up to religion, whose unbearably simple message of the ONE puts too much strain upon imagination and sends it into a flurry of creating the concepts which separate.

Ordinary religion, its ceremonies and dogma, was never practiced by Christs or Buddhas and is purely man's creation. There are no dieties that are not made of human consciousness in the waking dream state. Creating dieties with our imaginative power is actually perverting the religious sense which says along with Judaism and Islam, "Thou shalt create no image of me". Images of God exist only at the astral level of the lower mind on the sixth level (superstition) and on the fifth level (devotion). In truth these two faculties (the fifth and sixth brains) should be used for worship and surrender only to the oneness of consciousness to be found on the seventh level. Formalized religion is something mankind must grow out of because it casts a spell of conditioning upon the fifth level mind which is another form of self-hypnosis.

Mankind is caught up in the chemical emotions, asleep and dreaming as if under the influence of a furious drug. Consciousness, in its unawakened ego state, is a drug which prevents us from seeking that king of great power sitting in his kingdom, forgetful of his royal blood, forgetful of his self-mastery. Entering the nucleus of the expanding universe gives mastery back to man, which automatically brings an evolution in democracy. And this is why the laboratory of democracy and its model are not out there in society, but rather the ultimate social experiment will be proved inside the human brain. Where will the evolution of the human race take place if it is at the center where nothing exists? Is this place too mystical or abstract a place for the human race? The answer is that the evolution of society can only take place in our consciousness, that stuff which no one has ever seen and which is empty of all content, especially when we try to measure it or even look along our own eyebeams. Ultimately the empty place which is the fulcrum of all fundamental change is the emptiness of the human heart. Its nucleus is radiating with love at many levels of consciousness. Thus the Phoenix rises not merely to expand our mind or extend our consciousness into the emptiness of space but to bring it intensely into the incandescent radiance at the nuclear center of the universe to unfold our destiny and the fullness of evolutionary potential. Our awareness of its supreme design reveals to us the structure of its awesome power. He or she who can fill that emptiness with the power of peace will be the Phoenix rising into the light.

472

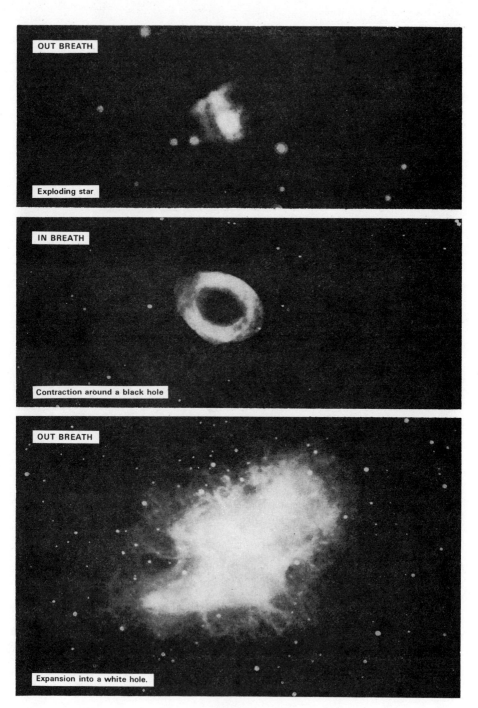

OUT BREATH

Exploding star

IN BREATH

Contraction around a black hole

OUT BREATH

Expansion into a white hole.

THE COSMIC PULSE

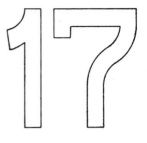

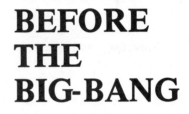

BEFORE
THE
BIG-BANG

Scientists can speculate within a few million years and within a few million degrees of temperature what the original nucleus of the universe was like during the first three minutes of creation of the cosmic fireball which they call the Big-Bang. But how this nucleus of supremely hot matter got there in the first place or what happened prior to the first three minutes they cannot even imagine. To ask how the original yolk of the cosmic egg got there before it exploded is not a question scientists like to be asked, since they then become trapped on no safer ground than someone who claims that God pre-existed matter. Mathematical speculation then becomes belief, and this belief in pre-existence cannot be proved or disproved by ordinary scientific means. Both scientist and theist are left in awe at the prospect of whatever was, if anything was, before the Big-Bang. In that nameless void all men are the same. However, there is another science of the absolute which deals with the origin of being and the genesis of the consciousness we call "the observer". Until we know "who" is looking at the creation and the natural world around us, our minds are trapped in the darkness.

Having shown the functions of the human brain as seven levels of consciousness we must now ask ourselves if this is the complete structure of human consciousness. We can answer in human terms, of course, that the imagination is the ultimate faculty beyond which no one can go and safely return, sane and with a sound mind. But that is not the full story. There are rare beings who have braved madness, who have risked annihilation of self, who have crucified the imagination as well as the ego, and who live in domains of consciousness far beyond the imaginable state of things. Such beings are considered divine by those at lower levels of consciousness, because their words and inspiration appear to come from other realms. But they themselves have insisted that they are humble instruments and not set apart by any desire to rule or master others. They have claimed no glory for themselves but only the privilege of serving the human condition. They speak not of opinions of themselves but merely describe the state of unitive consciousness as they see and experience it in the language and images of their times. Being highly original and using powerful metaphors of another Reality, they have claimed nothing more than that they are looking directly at Nature and the Cosmic Reality as they see it and experience it around them in an ordinary way. That ordinary men have judged them extra-ordinary and set them apart is a problem.

To name a few of these beings who have had this power to move mankind into higher realms is not necessary because each of us has within us our own archetype of the cosmic hero. To the extent that we can identify with it, our consciousness will be elevated, irrespective of the religion we follow or the clothes of philosophy and metaphors with which these great beings stimulated our human imaginations. To say something of these realms of light is of no consequence to most people, since few will follow to immolate themselves like the Phoenix in the cosmic fire. But to give a glimpse of another Reality may reach the few who aspire to that ultimate state where the absolute consciousness resides.

HOW NEAR ARE WE NOW
TO THE REALMS OF LIGHT?

There are two ways of looking at evolution, because on the one hand we have made incredible progress from the times of the cavemen and on the other hand almost no progress at all. The human species has evolved over millions of years, and our recent industrial success and scientific achievements in coping with physical nature have given us the illusion that our modern civilization has somehow transformed our intelligence and improved our social nature yet, underneath the veneer of social forms, mankind does not understand his own conscious functioning any more than men and women understand themselves in primitive societies. In fact, there is much evidence that our modern psychologists, though expounding millions of sophisticated ideas and words in books and infinite sensory information, know less about our seven thresholds of consciousness than did the ancient sages of the East.

When I was a boy, most leading scientists stated adamantly that man was not more than five to ten thousand years old. The new information from archaeology now is that man is nearly five *million* years old, and scientists speculate that mankind has perhaps been evolving even one thousand times that amount, or about half the age of the planet earth. Such are the fluctuations of that scientific "truth" which is supposed to be so reliable and dependable because it has been so thoroughly checked and tested. Science gives us data but we don't know why we are reading it. Why is it important that the sun's temperature is sixteen million degrees while that of Sirius is forty times that figure? Why is it important that the chemicals of our brain are called this or that, or that a cat brain records nervous signals at such and such a speed? What relevance has all this information to life? Are we just becoming walking encyclopedias in our vanity? Only when information can be raised up into the eighth level of transcendence does Nature open her books to the human mind. Information without transcendence is mere information. We have been seduced by the scientific information explosion yet we know less and less about consciousness, the more science probes the vehicle of the brain. Therefore the eighth level is the new evolutionary push into the nucleus of the universe, which can make all our human knowledge become divine understanding to which we give the name "wisdom".

We rely so much on our minds to guide us through life that the thought of going beyond the mind is like jumping off into the unknown. Yet when we really look at our minds, we see that they are continually distracted by all the information gathered by the senses. This distraction then dominates the mind instead of being controlled by it. Therefore the first step in self-mastery is to transcend the senses in order to control the mind. The senses delude us as long as the mind dominates our consciousness and keeps it in darkness. The ones who "think in light" are those who can transcend the activities of the mind and through meditation reach the two levels of consciousness above its threshold of function to the eighth level of the formless universe. But the very fact that it is possible to transcend the mind calls in question the whole long process by which evolution has created the seven brains. If we are able to bypass the brains, why have we bothered to evolve them? The answer is that we cannot bypass the brains until we have got the brains to bypass. Plus, we have to develop the equipment fully, once we've got it, before we can go beyond it.

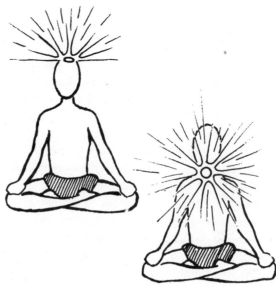

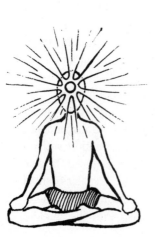

Why is it that in five million years we have not yet evolved out of the most primitive, basic responses to life? We have to have a little patience with ourselves because, despite our long history, the most evolutionary developments in our bodies and particularly in our brains appear to be fairly recent—on a cosmic scale only a few million years old. These very late additions are built onto an ancient system shared by fellow animals. In fact, that system of knowing which governs mankind the most, the emotions, is embedded also in all the patterns of mammalian life which are even more millions of years old. It is because our higher faculties are such late arrivals that we identify with the older and more primitive faculties which have the weight of millions of years behind them. What can even a million years do when many more millions are pulling from a deep stratum of our being which we have long since forgotten and only carry with us unconsciously? This helps us to understand why the eighth level is reached not by evolving yet another brain but by transcendence. And it helps us see how consciousness, regardless of which brain it filters through, is always just Pure Consciousness. Our feeling that consciousness changes comes from the ladder of the seven levels superimposed upon something much more basic and absolute—the ground of our being itself.

THE SCIENCE OF THE ABSOLUTE

Science as a profession has taken a very narrow and erroneous view of the scientific method as it was invented by the sages long ago. Western scientists have omitted the most important part of what it is that validates knowledge and, in clever ignorance of their own blind spot, they have ignored investigation of the real darkness of consciousness in mankind. The ancients had evolved a Science of the Absolute in addition to the epistemology used today which is the validation of evidence. This science of the absolute involves knowing the subject, the perceiver and his consciousness, as well as the object perceived, since all knowledge is conditioned by the knower.

When Western science looks into the past it sees how far we have come and it stands in awe of so much change. When the Eastern yogi looked at the past, he saw the eternal, never-changing truth imbedded in the nature of consciousness throughout all its many changes. These rishis and great researchers not only discovered mathematics but were able to penetrate the link between consciousness and our ancient biological past. They saw quite clearly that to live a sedentary life and succumb to the tendency to overeat is a relatively more recent evolutionary development. To counteract this social tendency beginning five thousand years ago the great yogis invented a system of simple common sense knowledge based on reason. For instance, one should not eat more than three/quarters stomach full of food to allow for proper churning and digestion. Such simple knowledge is not the normal way people eat in today's scientific world. The yogis also said that if we wish to remain in health, the human body should regularly exercise if its ancient biological system is to function in its correct way. Yet socially this is almost forgotten knowledge by the majority in actual application. Modern scientific reports are now reiterating the same advice, yet our society is obsessed with diet and fat. How much more, then, has the human race forgotten when we contemplate the greater knowledge of how we think and how we can know the knower of our consciousness?

Because of chemical and physical knowledge our civilization has become the age of industry and science, yet we know less of the spiritual nature of man which lies beyond the mind than did our primitive predecessors of five thousand years ago! The great sages invested their lives and all their resources and intellectual powers in the discoveries of what lay beyond the human mind. I am not talking of the many religious scriptures or the superstitions of the caveman people found in allegories and symbols, but the teaching of the ancient schools of Pythagoras and Egypt, and the evolution of the Aryan Sanskrit seers of ten thousand years ago, those who invented the systems of yoga. Even today amongst yoga groups the knowledge of the real depths of the Science of the Absolute is missing and left untaught. Yogic methods of knowing and validating human experience which are taught today are almost pitiful. Smatterings of meditation and physical hatha yoga have come to the West, while the great knowledge of direct perception is almost lost in its own country of origin, and even kept secret. We see clearly that India is trading off a rich spiritual past but has today no more effective answers to man's social predicament than the West. Certainly there are in India a few methods of perception which successfully go beyond the Western scientific method, but these are known only by a few, and their traditions do not teach these systems to others openly.

Therefore we must chart the way by which this direct perception can be found by all who aspire to find its creative process and find their way out of the darkness of the mind into the light. The ladder by which we climb into the clarity of Pure Consciousness is described in the process of Nuclear Evolution, the discovery of the Rainbow Body. The preparation is neither easy nor hard. Easy and hard are only relative concepts. It is a question of will. Do we want to find God? Do we want to feel devotion to higher realms of glory? Do we believe we can enter into that glory and share its bliss? Are we willing to put our entire being into it? Unless we do we are wasting our time wanting to evolve to realms beyond the concepts and images of ordinary human life.

We have said that there are eighth level beings who use the seventh level brain and the imaginative faculty in a special way to program the evolution of man's consciousness through the hologram of life that links all humanity as one. Consciousness itself in its primordial state is the foundation of the universe—that which was before the Big-Bang and can be equated with God. But this awesome God which is the creator of consciousness has so many levels of experience, so many mansions of existence, that it appears to any human consciousness to be hierarchical rather than a single whole nucleus. This appearance is the limitation of the seventh level of images. What we are dealing with here is the central core of being which few humans ever penetrate, simply because it is beyond the brain and beyond imagination. It is important here to describe that eighth level state of consciousness, because ordinary human experience is unable to get out of the darkness of thinking within the brain into "thinking in light".

HOW DO WE GET THERE?

Since 1968 I have been teaching my students in London and California the theory of consciousness which I call Nuclear Evolution. I have found that even when willing people, thirsting for the experience, try to conceptualize what the core of being is in our primal state of Pure Consciousness, they fail. The reason is that most people feel it is very difficult to get out of their brains and dissolve the ego self or thinker in nothingness. First there is a fear. "What will I become if my inner core turns out to be nothing?", the brain thinks. This fear is there because the self-regarding entity we call human cannot let go of conceptual reality and fears letting go of the body with all its precious brains that it has evolved and identified with for millenia. But there is really nothing to fear. The realm of consciousness beyond the body and its seven-layered brain, although it transcends the concepts, intuitions and imaginations, does not abandon the body. Most people believe that in order to experience themselves as light, it would be necessary to become bodiless, but this is again the result of the dualistic mind thinking that its own stuff must be either light or matter but not both.

Let us give an example of this difficult teaching that goes beyond our present concepts of reality but is realizable by anyone who will give up completely even for a few minutes their attachments to what they know already. Let us examine more closely the way that the ancient sages referred to this state of consciousness:

> In the beginning was the word, and the word
> was with God and the word was God . . .
> In Him was life and the life was the light of men.
> And the light shineth in the darkness and the darkness
> comprehendeth it not.

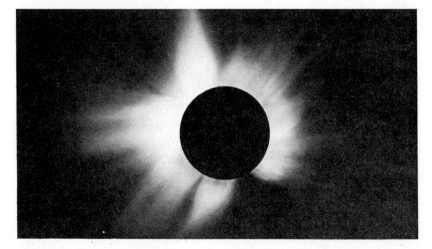

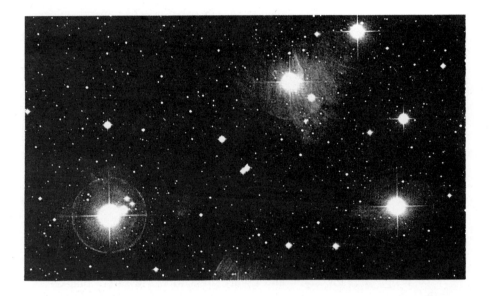

What darkness is there in the universe which is not instantly annihilated by the presence of light? The quotation on the preceding page may be exciting and mystical but it is meaningless unless it is actually talking about the light of consciousness itself. Consciousness shines out like light and, in the darkness of our dualistic minds, we cannot comprehend its nature anymore than we understand the nature of light. There is a certain rational stupidity that prevents even the most brilliant mind from fathoming out this matter which can only be penetrated at levels beyond mere reason. This matter which has fascinated me now for over twenty years is summed up in the axiomatic statement that

LIGHT AND CONSCIOUSNESS ARE ONE.

Though it can be described in words of a paradox, the mind at the conceptual level cannot grasp it, nor can the dualistic mind even imagine it, because its imaging projector through which the light of perception shines, is stuck on its own level of consciousness.

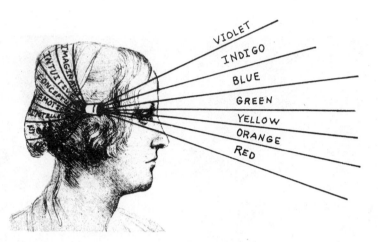

Most humans find it is impossible to enter that state where all the limits are off, because to take the limits off consciousness is to let go of what people already know and rigidly cling to like a safety blanket. What they cling to most is their idea of themselves as a body. It is difficult to let go of this idea that we are a physical body with eyes and ears that are acted on from outside, or the idea that nothing is experienced unless it happens *to* us rather than *within* us. To think the very normal thought, "I am a body", receives confirmation from our senses. Thinking any other way somehow makes the mind think, "I am not a body", rather than the correct thought, "I am a body as well as the universe it lives in, both subject and object expressing reality through each other." Just to say the words, however, is not enough. To fully realize this truth in the depth of our being requires constant reprogramming of our minds until we begin to actually *identify* with the whole and to experience that larger "I" with just as much impact as humans experience the ego. Only then will we begin to think in light and to know by direct perception that wholeness from which the universe arose. And the same is true of scientists. Until scientific method can turn its scintillating intellect onto the scientist's own consciousness—the subject which is studying the object—the events prior to the Big-Bang cannot be discovered.

The proverbial chicken and egg paradox with philosophers is a product of thousands of years of human error dating back in evolutionary history from the time when man lost the awareness of the oneness of subject and object, of thinking in light and realizing that light and consciousness are one. As a result he became imprisoned in time and space and the question of which came first, chicken or egg, the quandary over the beginning and end of the universe, and all dualistic concepts of the human mind took over as mankind descended into the lower levels of identification with matter. The Garden of Eden allegory is a story which describes the ancient times when humans did use their frontal lobes and did think of themselves and the total environment as one indivisible whole.

HOW DO WE FALL FROM WHOLENESS?

In Sanskrit the word "Adam" means first, the only one, singleness, oneness, one without a second—that state of consciousness in which there is no duality, no separation from the whole or from God. The myth of the Garden is the story of man's fall from this state of identity.

> And the Lord God called unto Adam and said to him, "Where art thou?"
> And he said, "I heard thy voice in the garden, and I was afraid, because I was naked; and I hid myself."
> And He said, "Who told thee that thou wast naked? Hast thou eaten of the tree whereof I commanded thee that thou shouldest not eat?"

God said, "Adam, where has your higher self gone? Who *are* you?" And Adam hid from his higher self, his inner voice. He answered the Lord, "I was naked. I felt exposed," and God said, "How did you know that you were naked? How did you come to feel psychologically exposed? Are you identified not with the whole but with a body? Have you begun to sense the universe through your bodily skin and nervous system? If you were one with the whole, you wouldn't be feeling naked nor be ashamed of yourself and close up and hide your body. Adam, single one, have you become separated? Have you become identified not with your whole self but with your nervous system and sensations so that you know the difference between good and evil, positive and negative, male and female? Have you begun to separate and compare?"

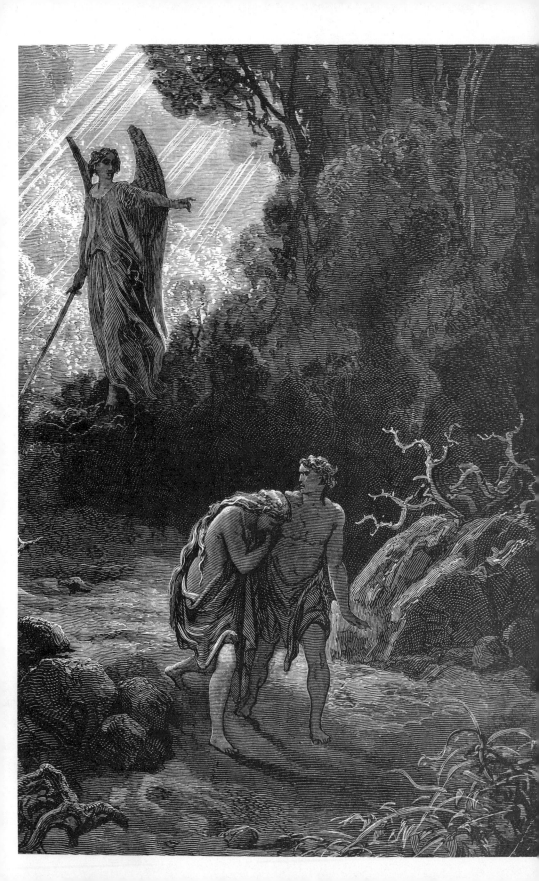

In storybook form it is difficult to see how anyone could be foolish enough to give up the blissful state of oneness, for in stories truth is clear and simple. God warned Adam, "But of the tree of the knowledge of good and evil, thou shalt not eat of it: for in the day that thou eatest thereof thou shalt surely die." The choice was very clear. If he ate, he was subject to the wheel of birth and death, whereas if he did not eat, he would be immortal. What he did not realize was that *after* the choice was wrongly made, he would lose this clarity and that the further he drifted away from it, the more he would find it difficult to return to that state of consciousness.

Before he ate of the tree, Adam had only to reach out and spiritual food came easily to his hand; he knew what was good to eat. But after he ate from the forbidden tree, he had to work and dig for food, and weeds grew in his psychological garden. These were the consequences of his choice. God said, "Furthermore I will put a guard on the gate of the Eastern garden with swords that cut this way and that, and you will not be able to get back there so easily." From the text, Adam seems damned and without hope. But the hope is that if you understand what you have done, you can go with your consciousness and do it right. You can do this at any moment. Whatever your mistake, if you are truly surrendered to the One, you become the One. Weeds do not grow in the Adamic garden if you can get beyond the tree of knowledge. Negative or evil thoughts find no nourishment once you have gotten beyond the tree of sensations so you become a little child again. We can read the story of Eden two ways: as a story of the human race at a moment in its evolutionary past when a crucial turning point was reached, and also as the story of our own consciousness, for at every moment we too are faced with the Adamic choice and with its dire consequences. It is important for us to see how we, like Adam, lose the garden.

In Sanskrit the word "Eve" means "truth reflected". Truth has to be *known* by someone. Even though the myth says that Eve tempted Adam, Eve is only a reflection of Adam's consciousness, just as the individual soul is a reflection of the indivisible One. Eve's yielding to the serpent is the temptation happening in Adam. But not until he actually tasted the fruit did he lose his original purity. Then kundalini (the serpent) was set against him, flowed downwards towards his feet (Genesis 3:15 "and thou shalt bruise his heel") and amplified his sensory knowledge at the expense of his extra-sensory knowledge, because kundalini only amplifies oneness when it flows *up*wards. Adam and Eve symbolize the male and female parts of everyone, which are fused when the kundalini flows upward in the highest state of consciousness, but they become separated when the serpent power tempts them downward, and then they become self-conscious of their separation and crave to find completion in something external.

If you are in a pure state, what can make you disobey? You disobey because you think it is okay; it won't really harm you. This is the serpent, the tempter who says to Eve, "God told you that if you ate of this tree you would surely die, but it isn't really true; it won't really happen." The tempter comes and says to us, "Just for now let's forget all the rest and indulge this one part, the senses." This is man's eternal problem with sex. From the moment that we separate sex off into its own trip in order to really groove it, from that moment we stop seeing sex or other sensations as part of the whole. By craving these sensations, the human race becomes a prisoner of the downward flow of kundalini. We think we can identify with the sensation and make it most important and still get away with it. There is nothing wrong with sex, but if we make it the most important part of life, we fall from the high state in which sex sensation is only a part. If you put sex sensations above the higher self, then you lose yourself, hide from yourself as Adam did, don't want to know yourself as you really are, your wholeness, don't want to hear your conscience or inner voice say, "Who are you? Where are you? What are you doing now?"

Adam was told not to eat or indulge in the fruits of the sensory world but to regard these sensory experiences as ephemeral, transitory. Eve would reflect the true Adamic state if he were in it. She is an objectification of what is already happening in him. In the unitive state of consciousness when he made love to Eve, he made love to himself. But when he began to look on Eve as his pleasure, the object and source of his sensations, rather than directly perceiving that God was the source of his intelligence and self-knowledge, he lost himself. After that point, the more you get into it, the more you get into it. The higher you are, the easier it is to fall.

Humans say, "Let's satisfy our own urges first, *then* do God's work." This is the Adamic attraction. When I was a young man in the world of business I used to say to my wife, "First I want to make a million dollars and then I will have the means to do God's work." I didn't know any better at the time. I went into business because in those days, that was what people did. I always knew that I had something to do for God, but it wasn't until later, after experiencing oneness, that I realized I must make a choice between the two. I must either make money or obey the voice that was telling me to go out and do something about the world, the voice that said, "Not by money and matter and power and fame and all those things that people seek, but by my spirit (consciousness) shall these incredible things come about. Attach your consciousness on this only."

I learned by experience that I could enjoy the side trips only if I were unattached to them. If my task is to write a book and that is God's work, then I have to put the book first. If some pleasurable activity comes up, which does not interfere with the writing or perhaps even enhances, it, then I can enjoy it. But only your own inner voice can tell you which is which. If you are in doubt, don't do it. If I see that lots of girls are eager to groove it with me, there is nothing wrong in that. But if I let myself identify with that situation, then my consciousness will fall, because sex would then cease to be secondary and would be the means of my satisfaction.

Humans deny sex in their ignorance, but the real truth of the spirit is: if you eat of that tree, don't think you can *identify* with it and get away with it. If you are in the unitive state, then when you make love, the whole cosmos makes love too because of what is in the minds of the two people. You are still eating from the Tree of Life then. Instead of going down to the lowest chakra where the sexual energies are reinforcing body-consciousness, kundalini is raised *up*, consecrating it to the highest. Then kundalini is enhancing the oneness or unitary consciousness and there is no guilt. One is still in grace while enjoying without attachment, enjoying while knowing you can give it up tomorrow if it is God's will, and that even if you love it, you can say no to it.

There is no more sexually roomphy* expression than God himself, but that is not his purpose but his means. The end is to know himself. When he says, "Where art thou Adam?", he doesn't have to run and hide from himself. He can look on himself as pure, untainted, unpolluted, unstructured consciousness and know that his highest manifestation, whatever level he is functioning on, sexual, social, intellectual or whatever, is a pure reflection of himself. So we have to ask ourselves, "Am I seeing twoness or am I pure in my heart? If I know in my heart that I would choose God above food, sex, and other sensory delights, I am choosing my real Self first and not running away from myself." Hence Christ said, "Blessed are the pure in heart for they can look on God." They can see themselves as they really are in their pure state, without guilt, shame, nakedness or sense of separation. But it is only through being tested, as Adam was, that we can know what is really in our hearts.

I have proved out in my own life that as long as I am prepared to sacrifice sex and sensory pleasures for God, He doesn't deny me anything. But if I crave without control, and desire pleasure above wisdom or self-knowledge, then it will always be vanity that comes to defeat me and bite at my heel and be a thorn in my side and bring to myself treacherous people who give me pain and lie to me, bringing me more pain still and defeating my whole purpose of serving the One. But if I am pure in heart and can look on the alluring nature of creation in all its forms including its most beautiful form, woman, without succumbing to rationalizations provided by my ego and buttressed by a woman's love for me or the love of other people, then I will always feel obedient and surrendered to the cosmic purpose that is working through me at any time, and no task will be too menial or too difficult if it is needed to complete the total picture of divine truth and beauty.

If our consciousness or kundalini is rising without attachments which pull it down, it flows into every little act and detail to light it up and make it important to God and deserving of His grace. Eve, our

---

* An expression taken from the Sanskrit word for active spirit—Rhum.

true reflection, our soul consciousness, will show that we are in this state. God's grace does not come from anything external or acts done with any thought of reward, since if God's will is really done and one is obedient and totally surrendered, the glory of the Lord, i.e., the illuminaton of our higher self, is *guaranteed.* Hence Christ can say, in his purity of mind, "Because I have obeyed my Father's will and glorified my Father in heaven, my Father will glorify me." This is a statement of the unitive consciousness looking at its own reflection in life and knowing that the awesome glory and beauty of this tiny planet is a reflection of our own glory and beauty. Hence the ultimate purpose of all life in the Garden is to glorify that One who is the very ground from which we spring and the very dust from which we are made. To be able to worship the dust and the soil of the earth as well as the glorious golden light inside is to find heaven on earth. This is the meaning of the opening lines of the Lord's prayer, "As it is in heaven, so let it be upon earth", meaning, "As it is in Pure Consciousness, let its true reflection be its own glory upon earth or anywhere else." The destiny of man is to know this state of consciousness and to reflect in a material world the glory of Pure Consciousness. But we have fallen from that state of grace. Why do we say that we have lost a state which we once enjoyed? How do we know that we ever had it in the first place? We know because that oneness is our true self. The more we widen our boundaries, the more of ourself there is, but really it is there all along, and so we have the experience of self-discovery.

If we look at our reflection in the world today we see that Adam is the entire human race which switched from living in its higher intelligence and became an evolutionary species which lives in the lower intelligences of the nervous system and takes the sensations of the skin as its reality. The Adamic change was not just a change of spiritual consciousness but a change at the physical level too. Man is the product of all the energies which have penetrated the earth's atmosphere for countless millions of years. Just as the tree rings leave records of the sun's activity and the years of drought, so does man have within him the rings of consciousness and the changes which have taken place not only in solar activity but in the solar system as an integral organic whole. These events are written into his evolutionary code and the bursts of activity caused by the explosions of supernovas are left indelibly recorded in those genes of the biological pool.

It is said by some esoteric sources, passed on by seers from ancient times, that man once had a psychic center that was thrown out of action by a cosmic event. The destruction of a certain planet in the solar system which disintegrated into the fragments we now call the asteroids caused mankind to lose consciousness of his real nature through the rupturing of one of his etheric centers. This event withdrew from those of mankind who were not in harmony with the Cosmic Intelligence the abilty to commune with the stars and with Nature directly through thinking in light. It caused man to lose awareness of himself as part of the hologram of existence.

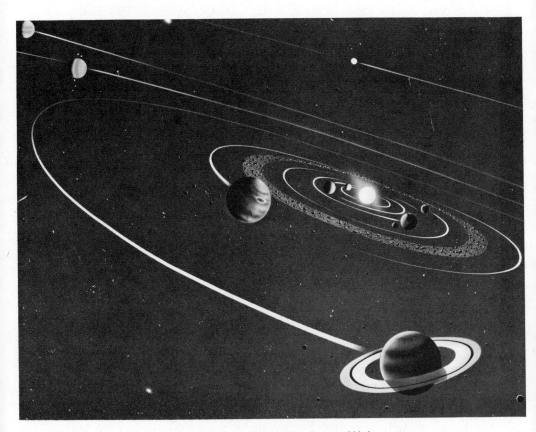

The solar system, clearly showing the asteroid belt.

People ask, why do I accept without evidence that these mutations occurred from the disintegration of this planet? The answer is based on several factors. Obviously there can be no physical evidence, any more than scientists have evidence of the prior state of the universe before the Big-Bang. They must employ the process of deduction and reasoning. Neither can there be any physical evidence for something like chakras or levels of consciousness which do not physically exist. But they can exist in nonphysical domains, just as the physical level chakra qualities of reproduction and survival exist as a witness of the physical body in the sex instinct and the instinct for bodily preservation.

The ancient Sumerian records and other Eastern accounts at the time of the Deluge and the proliferation of tongues are a record independent of our Bible. These Sumerian Akkadian and Sanskrit texts express a belief that God or Gods (superintelligences beyond man's knowing) created the Tree of Life, or spiritual body, in a specific and deliberate act of consciousness. These religious Gods (intelligences) are not conceived as mental Gods or concepts but invisible Gods or levels of intelligence without form. If we believe that this asteroid belt was the result of a sudden explosion or cosmic event created by conscious act of will, then we might feel this defeats the idea of a slow evolution, but it does not; it is an effect, not a cause. Whether the sudden event was a planet exploding or a sudden influx of matter into the solar system from the debris of a supernova or the cooled matter of a burned-out star, it makes no difference to the fact that some cosmic event unbalanced the gravitational flux in the system.

The idea of a twelfth planet on a comet's orbit passing through the asteroids as proposed by some authors, who believe the asteroid belt is the result of a celestial collision around 3800 B.C., is not supportable and would have shown up in measurements by astronomers who are now able to calculate and measure differences in gravitational orbits which would change the distance to Mars up to one yard and distances to the moon up to six inches. However the stories recorded in the Old Testament and the Sumerian texts coincide in content and are the result of many thousands of years of oral tradition long before they were written down. Before the event, mankind could roam anywhere in the cosmos in his imagination or inner vison and there was no need to have extraterrestrial explanations since he himself was a cosmic being as capable of being extraterrestrial as anything else in the galaxy. In reading the Sanskrit accounts of these intelligences, I was led to test their authenticity by Supersensonic methods because reasoning and deduction alone cannot take into account all the unknown contingencies that may arise, whereas divining cuts through to the real situation. Nevertheless, it is not even necessary to believe in the explosion of a planet but only to remember that there was a cosmic happening generating a sudden change or influx. I myself only use the planet theory here as an alternative to the collection of cosmic dust theory. It is the fact of the cosmic happening that is important, not the various explanations. How has this event resulted in a major change in human consciousness?

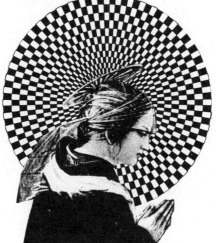

Leonardo's vision of the eighth chakra superimposed on a more accurate representation of this energy field.

Although there are many chakras or wheels of energy throughout the human body which link the physical system with the "Tree of Life" or spiritual system, only the seven major chakras are of importance to our changes of consciousness. The Adamic state of mankind, however, was able to control those seven centers from an eighth center which resonated with light and gravity. The withdrawal of part of the gravitational field and the shattering of a planetary mass in our solar system brought a fall in man's evolution for those who were tuned only to gravity and not to light. This event is recorded dimly in our consciousness, but we can get in touch with it if we want to bring it into awareness from the collective unconscious of humanity.

These ancient oral teachings showed that the cosmic happening removed from most of mankind the ability to think in light within his own physical body. This cosmic event caused the rupturing of the eighth chakra and the resultant darkness of the mind was such that the mutant human had an evolutionary physical advantage on planet earth over the other members of the human population whose consciousness did not mutate, who were still thinking in light. Because of being whole and egoless the non-mutants were defenseless against the more material and ignorant ones. Those who thought in light could not bring themselves to think in the darkness of duality of good and evil and were hindered by the disadvantage of being too good to retaliate against the ignorance of darkness. As a result they were gradually killed off (not unlike the Tibetan monks who were conquered by the Chinese) and died out as a species, leaving the mutants to depend on the comparative knowledge of their dark minds for survival. This type of being has now spread over the earth and increased in number and is responsible for the wars, aggression and pollution of the planet. Not only are these men and women active at the physical level, but their ignorance pollutes the mental climate. They are so dark in their understanding of life, that they can actually utter such stupid words as, "There is no such thing as consciousness", "There is no God", "All spiritual experience results from material influences or chemical disturbances in the body", "Religion is the opiate of the masses." They utterly ignore the fact that to utter at all they must use that consciousness which they say does not exist. This attitude infects the hologram of the collective mind and is a challenge that each part, each human, must deal with in order to achieve a new balance on the planet.

LIGHT AND DARKNESS

The darkness of such statements by Marx and others today is obvious to many, but there are other, subtler forms of darkness that people do not even notice, such as the darkness of rational thinking when it excludes all other faculties. If anyone doubts that there is darkness in human consciousness, let him look at the billions and trillions of dollars which society spends on killing and destruction. Even those who are trying to be constructive believe that the answer is

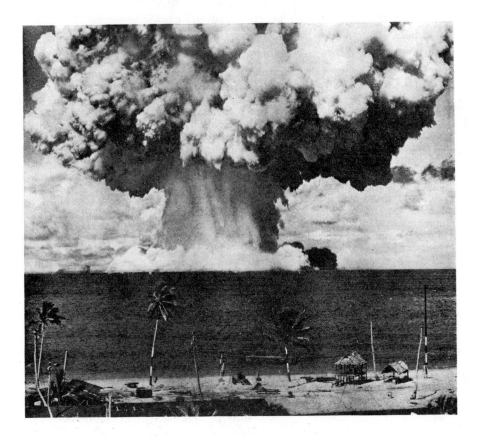

The Big-Bang theory is dear to scientists' hearts as a theory of creation; but the "Big-Bang" is also likely to be the end of life. Human consciousness throughout history has created weapons for achieving greater and greater destruction, but until now it has never reached the maximum total destruction. Has man's power over the "Big-Bang" bomb now designed the ultimate total annihilation and extinction of all species?

merely to get the right mix of external factors in society and the whole of human confusion will disappear. So they never produce a fundamental inner change. Where are the billions to finance investigation of the most important factor in health, happiness, abundance and world peace—namely, the nature of consciousness? Even those who wish to do this research cannot muster any support because of the futility of our professional darkness and the almost universal ignorance of the problem. How can people see what is missing when the consciousness they see with is itself locked in the narrow confines of comparative reason?

If mankind was plunged into the lower darkness of the rational mind of opposites and comparisons as his only guide to Reality, what was the Evolutionary Intelligence doing to close off from humankind the doorways to the higher center of the brain and to prevent man's communication with the total Cosmos around him? From time to time there were individuals who had spontaneous remissions to the former state of thinking in light in which the human brain had evolved its structures. The experience of Moses with the burning bush, Christ's tremendous awakening after the baptism by John (described as the heavens opening up and an inner voice saying, "My son I am well pleased with thee"), and the realization of Gautama Buddha that the mind is a trap which sees form as real, rather than seeing the emptiness of Pure Consciousness at the root of being which makes it real—all these are glimpses of a state of being once enjoyed by the whole human race. Throughout the ages those few who broke through into the world of light and saw the nature of the darkness have had just as much trouble in communicating what they really meant as I have had over twenty years trying to explain what I mean by saying

"LIGHT AND CONSCIOUSNESS ARE ONE."

What does it really mean to experience the heavens opening up? Why was Noah chosen as the only one fit to be saved from the flood? What do all the Biblical writings which single out the lives of a few special people—the prophets—really signify in a modern sense? Let me take one more rational journey into the duality of light and darkness in an attempt to lift the experience of thinking in cosmic light into that everyday affair which all of us are familiar with every hour—our own consciousness.

Everyone knows that when someone gets knocked unconscious or goes to sleep, then darkness descends into consciousness, and we are no longer aware of self as a body. No one gets frightened at going to sleep or passing out because they know that consciousness is only temporarily in the darkness of ego death and that it is still very much there. If we were to close our eyes and stop up all our senses, we would know that the universe was still there even if we could not experience it by seeing, hearing or touching. But not everyone knows that the sensory brightness that we call the light of day is purely an internal affair and that in actual fact light itself cannot be seen. The consciousness that lives in darkness cannot comprehend this because it believes it sees light with the eye. Without the eye it does not see. Therefore it thinks, quite logically, that not only is it the eye which sees but also that the objects seen are external to the eye.

Even physicists, who know that waves of radiation cannot be seen anymore than waves of sound can be seen, still cannot make this transition in the mind that what they see inside their heads is a psychic phantom image of a physically present object made of internal light of color and brightness. This image merely comes from chemical and electrical disturbances in the brain cells, and the external thing we see in front of us is only a small part of its reality in a very narrow spectrum of vibration. The light spectrum we see of the heavens around us is a very narrow part of our experience. We know this even more so now that we are developing radar eyes and seeing the patterns of the stellar universe through radiotelescopes which glow with radiation which our eyes cannot see.

What does all this have to do with the cosmic event that caused a mutation in human awareness? The separating of what is going on inside the brain from what is going on outside is the veil that descended at the time of the disturbance of the etheric vehicle. The stories in the Bible of man's fall—the Garden of Eden allegory, Noah's ark, and the Tower of Babel—were written down thousands of years after they happened. The same message of man's continual fall and the call to righteousness is found in stories throughout the rest of the old scriptures and testaments. The stories have been modified somewhat in being passed on from word of mouth, but the essence is correct.

WHAT IS THE COSMIC PURPOSE OF THE EVENT?

The story of the Tower of Babel gives us a clue as to why mankind was brought into the confusion of the lower mind. It is written that the children of Noah, the only human beings who survived the flood, all spoke the same language, and because of this, they could work together on a common undertaking, just as the language of science today enables scientists all over the world to pool their research for good or for evil. God watched the children of Noah and saw that now nothing would be "restrained from them which they have imagined to do." They could dream up anything, even a tower whose top "may reach unto heaven". Man has always tried to take over heaven, as is reflected in mythologies the world over. The ego decides to build an ego monument, a tower, to put itself higher than God. "Let us make a reputation," says the ego, "and become mighty and famous, more well-known than God." The Beatles, a pop group who will be forgotten in fifty years' time, actually boasted that they were more famous than Jesus. And so too the children of Noah said to themselves, "Let us make a name."

Imagination is man's highest brain faculty, but it can be used for dark and selfish ends. The imagination is unlimited in its possibilities for abominations. Modern science at this moment has in its hands a power to create, through recombinant DNA, abominations greater than any that have been seen on earth before. Today man can even invent new diseases, new bacteria and, like a god, can re-create the world in a new image. The promise of DNA recombination techniques is that microbes can be invented and tailored specially to make certain chemicals for man. Scientists at several universities have shown that this can actually be done. A multi-million dollar business is envisaged by the chemical industry who see it as a way to not only make human proteins but all sorts of solvents biologically through reprogramming bacterial DNA, the chemical in the nucleus of our cells which carries the genetic instructions for our body. They say there is little danger that any of these organisms will escape the laboratory and become dangerous and uncontrollable. The fear that man's imagination will produce microbiological monsters and, through innovation, get out of hand has increased in some people who see man as scientifically irresponsible as in the fable of the tower to heaven. The genetic language of DNA is one language for the whole of life from microbes to man. If confusion is introduced at any point the microbes could multiply and take over the world.

Can man be trusted with such power? The cloning of bacteria by genetic engineers makes us wonder if man has not come to the Tower of Babel again where nothing will be restrained from him that he has imagined to do. The cloning of people by inseminations out of the womb by implanting the fertilized egg into a host stuns the imagination with the unnatural possibilities of creating a great number of persons in the same image. So entranced with what is possible, mankind forgets to ask what is right. Like the builders of the Tower of Babel, scientists try to use the imagination for their own power and glory to make a name instead of worshipping the divine consciousness that gave them the power in the first place. But they may find that the universe will confound them. Is there something programmed into the universe that will step in and create confusion if something interferes with the course of evolution?

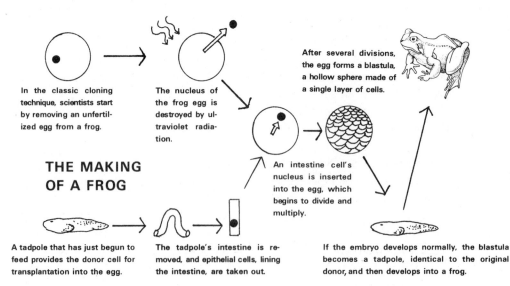

In the classic cloning technique, scientists start by removing an unfertilized egg from a frog.

The nucleus of the frog egg is destroyed by ultraviolet radiation.

After several divisions, the egg forms a blastula, a hollow sphere made of a single layer of cells.

An intestine cell's nucleus is inserted into the egg, which begins to divide and multiply.

THE MAKING OF A FROG

A tadpole that has just begun to feed provides the donor cell for transplantation into the egg.

The tadpole's intestine is removed, and epithelial cells, lining the intestine, are taken out.

If the embryo develops normally, the blastula becomes a tadpole, identical to the original donor, and then develops into a frog.

LAUNCH TOWER IN SPACE PROPOSED
Structure would be 90,000 miles high

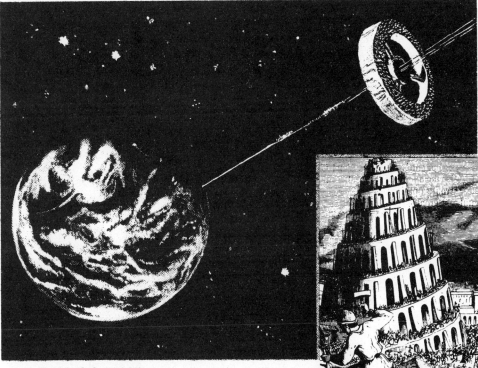

Drawing by John G. Gromoslak

ARTIST'S RENDITION OF PROPOSED SPACE TOWER

THE TOWER OF BABEL: (Genesis xi.)

There is no geological evidence that the tower of Babel was ever raised above the foundations, but extravagant reports or traditions of its immense height were handed down by word of mouth.

We have now come to the place on the evolutionary spiral where mankind is about to launch out again into heaven and build a tower reaching to platforms in outer space. If we are unable to understand the symbolic dimension of such plans, we shall again fail to evolve spiritually and our cleverness will be confused and self-destructive.

The one language in the Tower of Babel allegory symbolizes a oneness of consciousness that is only possible when the seventh level is open and people transfer images telepathically. Delighted with himself, man began to build a tower to heaven to build up the separateness of his ego rather than surrendering the ego (which is the only way man can get into heaven). The program of Evolutionary Intelligence was adversely affected by this perversion of the power of imagination. By cutting off attunement with the Cosmic Oneness, the beneficent Will and Power that man was tripping on was also cut off. Divine Will can only manifest creatively through man in an egoless state. As a result of man's ego he cut off his own deepest Self (eighth level) and of course then became confused in his seventh level images. The self-destructive power of man's delusion that he could worship the work of his own hands rather than God made his own ingenuity his god. Every time man's ego takes over and goes against the whole, this violation eventually cuts him off from the transcendent state.

The power of consciousness works like a whiplash to destroy the ego, since the universe cannot continue to tolerate anything divided against itself. Once the critical mass is reached, something blows. Imagination power was so great at that time that the whiplash effect destroyed the eighth level etheric center in those who had set the negative energy in motion in themselves by abusing their freedom and power. Since the cosmos and man are not disconnected, whatever is happening in the cosmos is happening in man too. The way the collective power of consciousness in humanity responds to cosmic forces also affects the critical balance and the condition of unknown contingencies. When subject and object, inner and outer are one, the human link with the planetary balance of forces is even more powerful than when this unity is not realized. When intelligence and advanced consciousness is heightened any mistake is also more catastrophic. What is humanity now doing with its knowledge of recombinant DNA and atomic power? God (consciousness) destroyed the people's ability to communicate on the potent higher levels and since those early times mankind as a whole has been a stunted mutant, confounded and confused, able to babble only through his mouth and lower mind instead of in the light of image transfer and his higher functions.

THE CONNECTION BETWEEN COSMIC EVENTS AND HUMAN EVENTS

The great beings who live in the eighth domain of consciousness know that they can move around in time by taking different bodies upon the physical plane of existence which is only one plane amongst many. They also know that all created matter is formed into patterns which are transplanted energy from other realms of consciousness. Every person who begins to think in light knows that all the organs of the body have a double or shadow energy pattern, called the etheric body, around which the physical body forms. Analogously, the planet destroyed midway between Mars and Jupiter which once rotated around the sun at three times the earth's orbital radius, is now just a swarm of iron and rock fragments which circle the sun. These asteroids are like the four rings around the planet Saturn made up of small particles captured in the gravitational electrostatic field of the planet with all its moons. The asteroids are the ring-belts of dust around the sun, and the planets are the moons of the sun which have crystallized from gases and elements into their present shape and have formed their spheres from the pattern of the sun's own gravitating electromagnetic field. In this sense they are a shadow energy in the physical world of the sun, which is vibrating its atoms in another octave of light.

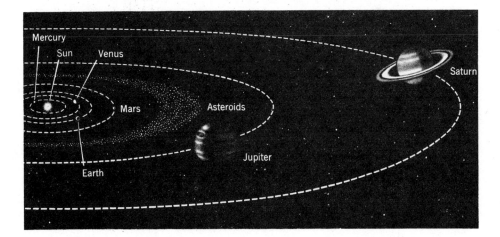

The planets are like vibrating nodal points around which matter collects in a spiralling system. In the same way, each of the planets represents a shadow energy field of the human centers of consciousness which vibrate on different thresholds. When the asteroid planet exploded it caused a mutation in the shadow energy body of the whole solar system which comprised the physical pattern of light energy to which mankind has since evolved. This caused a change of consciousness in the shadow field of those beings who were polarized negatively to light. Those who were polarized positively to light retained their active use of the eighth center and were able to continue to communicate with each other through the frontal lobes in vibrations of light energy because they were not controlled by this mutation.

The sun is not the main source of the plasma which fills the whole of space. Greater attunement to the hologram of life puts one in touch with energies beyond the solar system and this cosmic light nourishes and protects against cataclysmic events within the solar system. The starlight we call pure consciousness, or radiant background energy of light which fills all of space, also feeds the sun as well as our life force. But all the gravitational fields in space, as well as the supernova extrusions of light energy from cosmic explosions, cause minor modifications in our shadow body. When the physical body ceases to function it is because this shadow body of psychic electricity is withdrawn from it by our consciousness. We then live in a pure energy body of consciousness on other thresholds beyond our earth memory until such time as we return to incarnate in the world of the physical body. But we still have those other worlds or psychic centers in which we carry the mutating pattern of all our former existences.

There are many who are now born without the corresponding center which resonated with the asteroid planet and who cannot think in light and prefer the darkness of consciousness on the physical world alone. They feel more comfortable in denying the existence of their shadow body. Because their eighth center is ruptured they cannot even hear you speak of it. *Yet it is easy to experience for those who can acknowledge its existence.* Our consciousness cannot sense anything it does not believe is there, simply because consciousness is all-powerful. Just as people can believe in their imaginations that things are there that are not there, so are there people who can believe in their imaginations that there is nothing there, when it *is* there. Both live in illusion. The energy of the shadow body is the electrical sensory vibration which diviners and intuitives use. But many of these intuitives are still imprisoned on the physical plane even though they use their shadow energy for psychic purposes and believe in it. Because they are missing one chakra in their shadow body they can also be mutants who have no higher use for the divining faculty than finding gold or oil or getting rich. Birds and animals use the shadow body for finding mates because the survival of their species depends on it. But in the human being, the shadow center which had evolved man to be aware of his own consciousness in the Adamic state of man, was greatly modified by the disintegration of part of the solar system's energy pattern in the asteroid ring belt.

We must not think that puny little man was the cause for the destruction of this asteroid planet. Vast universal forces were operating to which man was responding in his thinking. Man has free will to respond to light negatively or positively. To identify with the forces of gravity brings involution. Just as you have consciousness now which you can use one way or another to affect your present life situation, so mankind's consciousness in the egotistic state was identified with or resonated with those cosmic forces that destroyed that planet, and so the consciousness was mutated. Those identified with darkness became dark and those identified with light as part of a vaster Cosmic Intelligence were not affected. If you reinforce a power that is already in the Cosmos and put consciousness into its nature, that will modify your vehicle of consciousness according to that force, because of the hologram that interlinks all of life. *It is essential now that man awaken to the fact of this cosmic/human interlinking.* Every explosion whether in our solar system or in our local galaxy, which is still very small on the cosmic scale, will cause mutation in the field of consciousness. Man's choices will determine how the energies affect him, or how he can master cosmic energies. As a result of identification with negative forces over long periods of evolution, man's consciousness does slightly affect the balance of energies in the solar system. It does not control the energies of the universe directly, it only influences the balance between the light and dark which is relative. Collective human consciousness tips a delicate scale, though on a cosmic scale man has relatively little significance, on the scale of the galaxy a mite more, on the scale of the solar system relatively more, on the earth quite a lot and in your own personal life your consciousness is totally powerful.

When we begin to think in light we see that what is dark in our own lives or dark on the earth may be relatively light somewhere else in the universe, and what is light on the earth in a relative sense could be darkness in another part of the universe that is seeing in light. Therefore the destruction of the asteroid planet, although apparently destructive to mankind, may have an overall evolutionary purpose that is to draw man to *want* to use his free will to be egoless, to think in light in *harmony with the greater cosmos*, the vast Evolutionary Intelligence, which he must choose in the end. Sometimes we have to do without in order to appreciate what we have. But this understanding of the function and purpose of cosmic events has been very difficult for mankind to pick up. Perhaps couched in the scientific terms of our time it will be more easily seen than in the parables of Christ's time or in the mythologies and allegories of ancient times. With this understanding of our interrelationship with the Cosmos and the importance of our own subjective position in consciousness in studying the objective world, we can now go on to take a look at what happened before the Big-Bang.

The ordinary man is apt to say, "How does all this affect me? It is beyond my power and understanding." But this is just his negative consciousness speaking out of darkness. If he knew that consciousness affected his happiness and skill in every department of life from making love to worshipping God and becoming healthy he would want to understand the more positive side of the Science of the Absolute. In the pages to follow we will journey into the eighth domain of light and consciousness which is the key to the Big-Bang. At some points insights will come and we will be on the verge of a breakthrough in our understanding. Then it will be necessary to surrender our linear way of analyzing what we read, and to drop the lower seven human levels of consciousness to image universally and feel ourselves as the whole. To become all of the different processes described will lift our identification out of the human material body into the transcendent state of the eighth level of awareness. Whatever glimpse we get of our vaster Self in cosmic consciousness will inspire us to go on and on into the discovery of Pure Consciousness.

HOW CAN SCIENCE APPROACH THE ABSOLUTE?

Astrophysicists tell us that light travels from the stars at a certain speed so that when we look up into the heavens at night we are seeing the light that takes millions of years to reach us. They say that we are looking back in time to the history of the stars as they were millions of years ago. By calculating the distance away from our own planet in space and then dividing it by the speed of light we get the number of light-years we are seeing back into time. Light from nebula clusters in our own galaxy, such as Orion 1,500 light-years away and any stars within 100,000 light-years away, is said to be part of the original nucleus of an exploding supernova star that once exploded and is still expanding in space along with other galaxies with similar clusters of stars. Some of these island galaxies floating in the empty blackness of space are said to be millions of light-years away. The vague patches which early astronomers in this century thought to be nebula clusters in our own galaxy were discovered by Hubble to be independent galaxies. One similar to our galaxy, called Andromeda by the ancients, turned out to consist of 300 billion stars and is our nearest galactic neighbor. According to modern theory, its light which we see now, started out on its journey to earth nearly two million years ago. Hubble observed and pinpointed over 60,000 spiral galaxies like our own and estimated that there were over 100 million such galaxies; today our modern astronomers estimate 1,000 times more than that, or in other words, 100 billion galaxies. These are mind-bending figures.

Hubble announced a spectacular theory that these island universes like our own galaxy were rushing away from each other with velocities which increased proportionately with their distance from each other. The whole great Cosmos sitting within unlimited space seemed to be exploding uniformly outwards and our own galaxy was not at the center of all this expansion. If stars and galaxies are distributed uniformly throughout space and space is infinite, why does not this

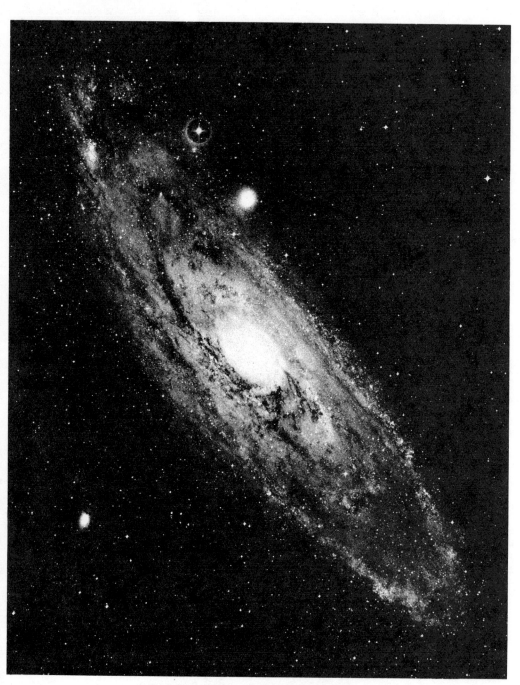

The Andromeda galaxy, Messier 31. (Lick Observatory)

enormous amount of light radiated by all the stars blind us, and why does not the sky glow at night? Hubble explained that we would be blinded by their light except that we live in an expanding universe where the light coming from distant sources is vastly weakened by the expansion. Einstein was not entirely comfortable with the theory of an expanding universe. He initially felt that the universe was static or, in essence, still. In order to account for a static universe he brought a cosmological principle into his equations to exactly balance the expansion constant of the universe. The cosmological principle is actually a

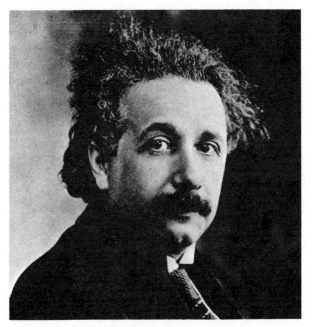

Albert Einstein. (Yerkes Observatory)

mathematical constant standing for a value which compensates for the expansion of the universe. But this effort to prove a static universe did not work because it was finally proved by the red shift that galaxies were receding, and therefore the universe was indeed expanding. Einstein was forced to agree because of lack of any evidence to the contrary, even though he was onto some truth in his intuition of a still universe.

There is no scientifically known physical mechanism at present which can provide an explanation for the red shift in the spectrum for distant stars except the expansion of the universe. However, the observed universe of radiation and light, which enables us to see objective and material bodies, is only an apparent universe based on the disturbances of atoms in our sensors. How is this so? The excited source sends light to our physical body through devices such as radiotelescopes and optical mirrors which is then concentrated in our eye or on film, but the actual observation itself always ultimately takes place in our consciousness where we give these signals meaning. Even an independent photograph cannot reveal expansion except relative to some known measurement in human consciousness. It is our consciousness which expands with the square of the distance when we view objects receding in space.* Similarly, in Einstein's theory of relativity, it is our consciousness speeding up and slowing down with the speed of light that shrinks or expands matter into energy relative to the position of the observer. The same law holds true for objects seen at the other end of the street as for galaxies, or mountains in the distance. They all shrink at the same rate in our consciousness as they get further away. The explanation which traditional science gives is that the lens of our eye does this shrinking. Yet no two human beings have the same lenses and even the lenses between each eye are usually slightly different. Why, then, do we all see exactly the same angles subtended by objects which grow large as we approach them and get smaller as they recede down the street? This effect is caused by the gravitational field of the earth working inside your consciousness. The building you are in is obviously not expanding, but as you walk away from it the size shrinks. The building contracts and expands in your consciousness with the square of the distance which we can check with sextant angles as being external to the observer. But we know in our minds that the real world stays the same size so we don't worry about this. In fact, most people don't even think about it, including most scientists.

Why are we bothering to talk about perspective and the shrinking of visible objects? Once we realize that this shrinking has nothing to do

---

* See *Supersensonics,* p. 250.

with the eye, we will realize *it is our consciousness which shrinks things*, and then perhaps the implications of that thought will dawn upon us and we will see the folly of the whole scientific approach. Our consciousness shrinks the things that we perceive, and yet we are assuming that we can measure the whole universe without even understanding what our consciousness is doing to it!

The radiation of the stars which carries energy through space to our senses, causing the apparent shrinking of the sun or galaxies, has never been seen by anyone. All that we see is a psychic brightness caused by the image which is oscillating in our senses, nerves and brain cells. The actual stuff which triggers our receptors is totally invisible to our consciousness. If our egocentric "onlooker consciousness" does not discriminate what makes things expand and contract on earth, how can we expect to know what expands in the heavens? Therefore, the universe we observe and the red shift *may not* be the result of expansion, and the universe may not be expanding any more than the building you are sitting in. It may only appear to be expanding. But it is certainly expanding and contracting in our consciousness with the distance, and as long as we have a normal lens on a camera we see the same perspective on film. Change the lens however and we have a different picture; but whatever picture you get, its size is not possible to determine nor is its distance away until you compare the object's measurements with a known human size in the picture. Thus we need to know both the nature of light and the nature of human consciousness to validate reality. This makes consciousness the cosmological constant that we need to add into our calculations and observations. This reveals that light and consciousness expand as one, and it implies that objects do not necessarily expand or shrink but merely appear to by the action of light plus consciousness.

The Science of the Absolute is different from modern physical science in two ways. Scientific method deals with a specific technique of testing evidence involving a hypothesis which can be tested by empirical science which means some way of sensing an object outside of ourself. But the Science of the Absolute goes two steps further. First we research the knower's consciousness, because any errors in the subject's way of looking at an object will be projected outwards and we will be ignorant of the real nature of the object. So this first step is to research the nature of the human being and see that the universe is a cosmically-centered one, not a human being-centered universe. The second step which differs from modern science can be called a detachment both from the method of validation and from human beings in order to reach a transcendent state of knowing which is beyond thinking and involves the nature of pure reasoning.*

With this understanding of consciousness in mind let us look at the "expansion" of the universe. The original expansion was called by scientists "the Big-Bang" and has become latter-day dogma, although there is no proof of this Big-Bang theory except that the shift of the light toward the red end of the spectrum appears to increase, the farther its distance from the observer. Hubble's concept was an incredible step into outer space, but also it proved to be an incredible trip through time. If these assumptions are correct it means that all the galaxies outside of our own are moving apart from us and from each other at enormous speeds. If these motions of the outward-moving galaxies are retraced in time backwards towards their original Big-Bang, it is found they all come together into one giant nucleus about twenty billion years ago. Packed into this tight little cosmic egg, all this matter boiled at temperatures which boggle the imagination and are therefore just scientific guesswork in billions or trillions of degrees, the scientific accuracy of which does not matter at all to anyone. The dazzling nature of this radiation coming from this intense homogeneous mass of the original hot nucleus is beyond description, and our imagination cannot conceive of its glory. In the darkness of our minds, scientists see the original picture of the universe as the explosion of a cosmic bomb. The instant when the bomb exploded and scattered itself in fragments throughout the totality of space marked the first moments of birth of a violent universe. God, to a mathematical scientist, is a Big-Bang.

---

* The new way to get beyond the apparent sensory universe is therefore to abandon mathematical representation based on such illusory expansion which we "know" is not real, and apply it instead to geometrical proportions which are (as in music) not based on exact quantitative measurement but upon observed resonances, harmonics, and ratios which are dictated by Nature and not by man. See *Supersensonics*, pp. 363-71.

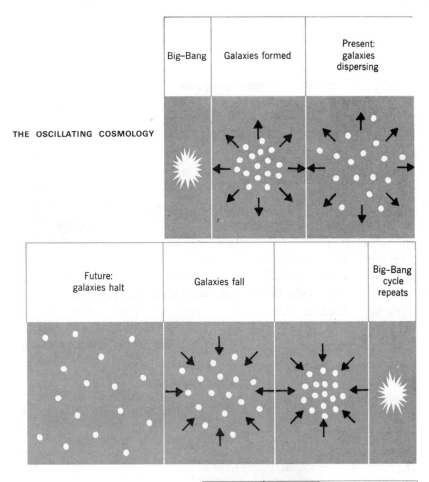

THE OSCILLATING COSMOLOGY

Big–Bang Galaxies formed Present: galaxies dispersing

Future: galaxies halt Galaxies fall Big–Bang cycle repeats

THE STEADY-STATE COSMOLOGY

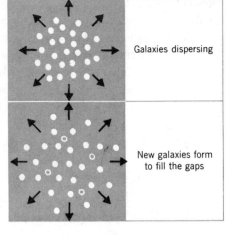

Galaxies dispersing

New galaxies form to fill the gaps

But expanding universes, or even collapsing or static ones, are not the only kinds of universes available to human consciousness. Fortunately there are many other mansions beyond the level of consciousness of the conceptual mathematician who has built this edifice of universal possibilities for us. Einstein proved that more dimensions exist beyond the mere conceptual by hitching time to space. Einsteinian units of measurement are different from physical yardsticks. A physical yardstick floating through space does not measure one yard at all and shrinks to different lengths depending on its relation to an observer (consciousness) situated at a fixed place in space.* A physical yardstick is then not even a yardstick at all. It is two points in space which get farther apart or closer together until there is no space at all. But what has happened to the observer—consciousness? The geometricization of space and physical process, including the whole act of seeing through the lens of the human eye, has a great appeal to the minds of physicists. Because this conceptual way of looking does give us accurate results in proportions and ratios in this physical dimension here on earth, it is often mistaken as a reality in itself. Scientists are unable to see the whole of mathematics and geometry as a work of consciousness and the use of the seventh level imagination *leading to an inaccurate or limited vision of the universe.* From the eighth level there is no space and the consciousness that remains is pure. Its perception is totally different from that on the lower levels, just as Einstein's perception of relativity is a dimension totally different from the level of consciousness prevalent in science sixty years ago. How a person sees the universe depends on the measuring units he uses. This applies to everyday reality as much as to our understanding of stars and distant galaxies. Our human yards and feet are fixed, arbitrary human measurements which Nature ignores. It is not our measurements but our visual perception which expands the thousand-foot mountain or hundred-foot tower as we walk towards it in our consciousness. We ourselves shrink to the eyes of a fixed observer watching us walk into the distance. Science explains this phenomenon away by saying that our vision is based on the inverse square laws, but if we

---

* The distortions of time and space due to motion are fully explained in *Nuclear Evolution,* Chapter 18, pages 430-440.

look deeply enough we can see that these laws do not always apply and are therefore not a complete explanation of the perceptual process.*

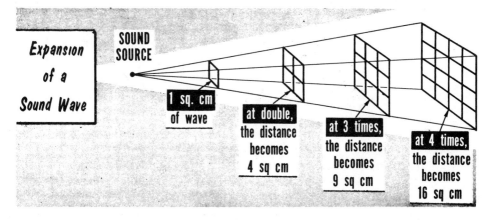

The Inverse-Square Law

There are other explanations for the surreal aspects of the universe. All our human cosmology is surreal because it is not based on understanding consciousness but on physical assumptions which themselves are not real but are only imaginative devices, such as mathematics. Mathematical results are strictly logical. They cannot deliver more than what is put into them. If apples and oranges are put in, the answer cannot come out as apples and pears. Everything in mathematics depends strictly on the basic assumptions you begin with. Hence to get back to our assumptions about light and consciousness let us assume (and be more scientific than the scientists) that all our assumptions so far about light and its experience in our consciousness are invalid, since mathematics is the product of but one level of human

---

* In *Supersensonics* I devote three chapters to the theories of Prof. Vasco Ronchi, a physicist at the National Institute of Optics in Italy, who disagrees with the geometry used to explain vision, lenses, cameras, and physical phenomena generally. I explain why our consciousness does not see what science thinks it sees.

consciousness and is therefore limited. It does not tell us anything
more about the origin of the universe before the Big-Bang. The only
way that we will ever know anything about the Absolute is first to
acknowledge the role of the observer's consciousness and its limitations and distortions and to find a more *direct* perception of Reality
than the physical senses or a way to more accurately test the mathematical equivalent of sensory perceptions. This is the function of the
eighth level of perception.

BREAKING THE LIMITS

All our knowledge of light and gravity so far recorded in history has
been investigated by the science of mathematics through operations in
our imagination concerning the relationships between these two forces
and the material objects affected by them at the physical level.
Nowhere have we been able to investigate gravity and light effects on
nonphysical objects since all our sensors involved in the measurements
and calculations are physical instruments. Yet a large part of man's life
on the planet is conditioned by nonphysical relationships, such as love
for each other on higher levels than physical sex, or social values like
paper money which is only a medium of exchange not backed by any
physical reality. Even the conventions of physical measurements such
as a yard or foot or meter which are purely human-made and agreed
upon only in the human mind, are nonphysical realities. Most people
regard an inch or a yard as a physical reality because we use physical
yardsticks to measure solid objects, but in actual fact a yard is only the
distance between two fixed points in space, and the physical yardstick
only represents the empty space between them. Likewise with all
physical measurements of objects moving through space, whether they
be motor cars, spacecraft or planets, they can only be measured in
terms of velocity by fixing a starting point in space in our minds. In
reality there is no way of pinpointing any fixed point in space anywhere in this Cosmos since space is everywhere, all-pervading and is
one, only becoming separated by the relative distance between two
objects yet in fact not separated. Space merely surrounds both objects
in its totality as one encompassing whole. The attempt of the human
mind to pin down the actions of gravity and light within that space
in exact physical and mathematical terms is purely an act of the

human imagination, since *in actuality space expands light and contracts gravity, and space is itself warped in the presence of either of these two forces.* Space shrinks or expands depending on the speed of motion of the observer. If we substitute the word consciousness for space we begin to penetrate the nonphysical reality of space and gain an entirely new insight and perspective on the limitations of modern science. We already have shown how consciousness and light act as one in our perception, and now space becomes part of that same identity where consciousness, light and space are one. From this cosmic identity we enter the realm of pure being where all the operations of light and gravity, space and time are seen as movements of consciousness on lower thresholds of energy.

What does all this mean for the ordinary man in the street? It means a totally different picture of his entire being which will be hard to realize simply because most minds do not search for light, do not question their own understanding of space, light, gravity or themselves, and are content to let things slide and leave the determination of reality to others. But this, in fact, is not possible. We suffer or move up the evolutionary ladder in direct proportion to our knowledge of the whole of life. Our peace of mind, our happiness and our social fulfillment is focused around our self-image. If we think in light, our lives are transformed in the twinkling of an eye. The dawning of this difficult liberation from our darkness cannot come to us through mental efforts but only through insight. This insight comes quickest when we meditate on the nature of light and the nature of that consciousness which experiences the light.

However not everyone is drawn towards meditation and not everyone can fall in love with the goddess of wisdom. Such an affair with a goddess does not sit well with our human obsession with our own bodies and other physical objects in space, because to understand the implications requires us to leave behind any firm exact models of reality that exist already in our consciousness. To enter into this eighth level realization that light and gravity and space are all unmanifested, nonphysical qualities of our consciousness that only come into physical existence as energies in creation on contact with material bodies, means a new paradigm or new view of what man is. To accept that light is unmanifest until it hits our sensors or physical receptors such as the organs of our own body, means that light coursing through free space is not only invisible and intangible and unformed, but is also eternal and only becomes crystallized in matter when it enters our body and becomes consciousness. When we investigate these non-physical aspects of Nature, the distinctions between our consciousness, space and light disappear and we come to realize that *the nucleus, the original stuff of the universe prior to the Big-Bang, is within our consciousness, not separate,* and that all the laws of gravitation and light radiation are operations within the Self.

Big-Bang is a hypothesis that the primordial soup, concentrated in one region of space, became unstable and exploded with a big bang with intense heat, radiation and light which, after it cooled down through expanding in space, formed the elements of matter as we know them today, and that the debris from such gigantic explosions is still being radiated into the vast space of the universe.

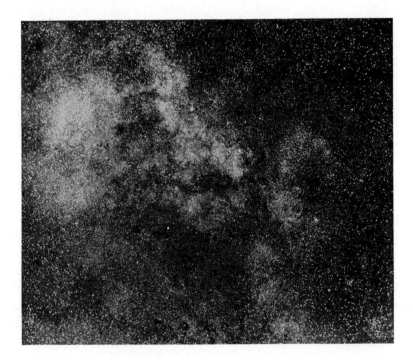

To explain how this plasma or soup got there in the first place, however, science (limiting itself to physical laws) must assume that gravitational forces so compressed the material matter of the universe that the atoms were squished out of shape into formlessness and became the primordial soup resembling the yolk of the nucleus. Is this Big-Bang theory true? Let me explain my own understanding which amplifies that of modern science so that we can think together and not separately.

The ancient seers who expanded their consciousness in deep meditation realized that the universe as a whole is a cosmic egg—a nucleus of consciousness in which we ourselves are an integral part. They knew of this primordial expansion long before our modern scientists and called it Brahman, from the root word *Brih*—to expand. Brahman in Sanskrit, or God in English, is not a matter of scientific, theological or religious definition. You can talk to God without having any religion because the cosmic vibration speaks in all languages. God does not need a physical tongue or a mouth to speak with. All languages of the whole of creation spring from cosmic vibration. Language is merely the sound vibration of thought, and thought is energy. God or Brahman is the same as Pure Consciousness and can appear to us in any manifest physical form and is not limited to persons or to any one part of creation because consciousness (God) is also formless energy and cosmic vibration working in all persons. In this nuclear concept, God is expressing through consciousness all the time, and therefore to most people who live by their sensations this materializes to our senses as solid matter.

In this sense God is not some remote Being but is present even within the nucleus of all matter. What is matter? It is a particular vibration of cosmic energy. God talks to me through matter, energy and light as well as directly through my unmanifest consciousness in the form of sound. Do I mean ordinary sound as heard in our physical ears? Of course, because God is as real and actual as you are and the vibration of His thought is constantly being sent forth through the vibration of cosmic energy on all frequencies all the time (AUM). In this sense, the whole universe is made of super sound, sensed by some (though not sensed by everyone)* as ever-radiating out from a source of vibration (called in Sanskrit *Nadabrahman*) inside everything material and physical. The one divine consciousness that is manifesting through all physical atoms of our brains in pulsing cosmic energy is externalized and expanded into the whole universe. This becomes our very awareness itself if we personalize it. But we do not need to personalize it because God is aware of Himself in every atom of the manifest creation. God is all patterns in mind and thought creating for itself a physical body of planetary systems, vibrating atoms, stars or suns, and light. He is the manifesting presence in Cosmic Consciousness, the cosmic energy of vibration and the cosmic mass we call physical matter. This is the meaning of Christ's words, "Are not five sparrows sold for two farthings and not one of them shall fall to the ground and be forgotten by God (consciousness)?"**

The spirit or consciousness of God manifests in the vastness of the expanding macrocosm as cosmic light in space and fills the space between the elementary bodies. In matter God manifests as the nuclear center vibrating its cosmic song. In the microcosm He manifests as the vibration of human consciousness, human energy of thought and the physical human body. In this sense God (or consciousness) makes man into the divine image of Self, vibrating in all the languages of creation. This experience of vibration is intelligent and maintains itself in the structure of creation itself. This is why the universe pours into our consciousness and continually dies away in our consciousness like a sound dies away in the silence. Our consciousness is like a black hole of awareness devouring all vibrations, like silence devours sound, like light swallows darkness, like love annihilates hate. The body and brain are made of countless excited electrons, atoms and molecules which are merely specks of cosmic energy emanating from our thousands of billions of cells. The body is not solid flesh except to the material-minded sight. It is in reality not solid matter but energy and is made

---

* See *Supersensonics* on the skill of sensing subtle vibration. Also *Rumf Roomph Yoga* tape series on how to experience the cosmic sound vibration.

** Luke 12:6.

from the same primordial soup in the same image as the stars. The same power of cosmic energy that sustains the universe in its expansion is vibrating in our bodies also, therefore our brains and bodies are made in the image of consciousness even from the physical standpoint of the atomic nucleus at the heart of every cell. In this sense we are like Christ, a personal manifestation of God. He who knows Brahman (God) as expanding consciousness of Self, is Brahman Himself. Thus Christ says, with unified consciousness, "I and my Father are One." And Shankaracharya and Moses say the same, "Thou art that I am," because they perceived directly that our consciousness and God are one. This does not mean that we humans can create new matter or that we are evolved enough to create anything new. But we can create love, and it is in our power to experience everything anew, in our consciousness. The Big-Bang is *you* and your expanding consciousness. It is in you to be realized and re-experienced anew, because in the cosmic consciousness of the nucleus you are beyond time. The experience of what was before and during the Big-Bang of creation is relived in the nucleus before conception, just as all the evolutionary stages are relived in the womb prior to birth. The enlightened being is one who has consciously relived the process of creation in the nuclear center of his own awareness and can say with Christ, "I am from before the beginning."

Most scientists now accept the theory of the expanding universe as true but to fully understand how any matter or space got there in the first place is only possible from the eighth level of Pure Consciousness. Obviously a pure consciousness could not make any distinctions between itself, space, light, gravity or anything else since it is the original nucleus of the universe, the one seed from which all else has sprung. Pure Consciousness, the creator of this original soup which is now distributed throughout space as matter and light, is therefore present throughout the whole of space as light radiating outwards. Everything created in the universe radiates. Therefore science has now unwittingly confirmed the truth of the sages that the Absolute, God or consciousness, light or space, matter or gravity are all one in this Pure Consciousness at the heart of every material entity, whether an atom, a star or a human being.

However, it is impossible for human beings to see this truth if this very consciousness in them is creating impurity or darkness by not comprehending its own nature or not seeing that the darkness of their minds is created by material obstruction of light by identification solely with the body or other material bodies. Just as darkness only occurs on the underside of the planet when light is arrested by the blocking of the sun by the rest of the earth or by the presence of the moon or other objects in space which prevent the light from passing through, so is the human mind blocked in darkness when it refuses to let the light pass through its dense material concepts of itself, like identifying itself as a material body. The eighth level is attained by clearing this darkness of the human nuclear center through *thinking in light* instead of clinging to matter. Once we see that consciousness is the same thing as light and we identify ourselves as being crystallized light on the seven levels of consciousness, then the darkness of a mind which gravitates to lower thresholds of energy is removed. As long as consciousness identifies itself with the physical body as matter, then the radiation of light into the hologram of life and realization of the cosmic nucleus is blocked. How can anyone stuck in the mind and experiencing themselves only as a body take another look at this eighth level view of life *from the eighth level?* How can we look at the modern scientific understanding of light and gravity and see things happening to us and in us in a new way, seeing from the space between the ears rather than looking at the space around us in the physical world?

ANOTHER LOOK

Light and gravity function in consciousness in a strange way. They are both invisible, intangible forces in their pure state. Gravity is a function of mass. Light is a function of the disintegration of mass. In other words, light and gravity are opposite forces in Nature. One is collapsing and the other is expanding. Gravity compresses so intensely that heat and light burst forth to release the pressure in the matter. But if gravity gets too intense in a black hole, even light is sucked back and cannot escape. The black hole is a space where gravity is so intense that it crushes the atoms of matter into a common plasma where they lose their characteristic patterns and become pure energy. Super-gravity dissolves matter in the same way that the human mind consumes sensations and thoughts. The black hole has this kind of an environment that literally eats matter up from the outer edges of the black hole and converts it into radiation. From the inner regions of the black hole, the radiation is so intensely compressed that gravity keeps it from escaping. Its energy is turned back into itself. The gravity field is so great that light in the visible spectrum as we know it cannot escape at all and so the black hole is an invisible object only perceived by light's absence— a hole in space into which stars are being sucked to feed its enormous gravitational appetite. Now the light of all the stars which irradiates the totality of space is the expanding energy of Cosmic Consciousness being released from matter which has been compressed and excited by gravity to the point of expansion. Viewing the observed activities of the universe from an identification with the light of consciousness itself, rather than with our physical bodies, the subject and object distinctions disappear and life opens up a vast, beautiful, breathless dimension of Self with which we can discover the workings of both our human and our Cosmic Consciousness.

The usual scientific picture of the Big-Bang theory, or the expanding universe theory, shows the universe as eventually slowing down (decelerating) its expansion. Gravity, it is said, must act as a brake on the accelerating expansion of galaxies until it eventually starts to pull things back together in black holes. Like a tide flowing out, light comes to the stopping point at the flood and begins to return. This agrees with the Hindu sages who saw creation as evolution and involution over vast periods of time, but there are some who find evidence that the universe is not slowing down, as it is supposed to be doing according to this first theory, but is accelerating. Einstein's mathematical operations allow for accelerating universes as well as static ones. The possibility of an accelerating universe brings back the cosmological constant that Einstein took out in order to agree with Hubble's theory of the expanding universe. The mathematical constant represents the cause of the acceleration. Is the universal expansion really braking to a stop or is it expanding at the edges of the universe faster than ever according to the second theory of acceleration? Our answer will depend on the way we look at the nature of human consciousness and the methods we use to validate the evidence of our senses.

What does this mean to the world of ordinary humans and does this vast galaxial expansion affect human minds or invisibly dictate the course of human affairs? We can think, like many scientists do, according to the first theory that the universe is coming to a stop, that these forces have been contracting and expanding and acting upon stars and solar systems during billions of years of evolution which appears to us to move very slowly and, like gigantic in-and-out breaths, will have little effect upon our immediate destiny. Or we can think like the Hebrew prophets of old who felt the unseen hand was leading man to the end of the world—accelerating events into a proliferation and expansion of desires and needs that must eventually outstrip all human resources. According to the second theory, if the universe is accelerating, then everything in it, including our human evolution, is getting faster and faster until eventually there will be no time, no space, no interval between events. Either way, the human consciousness is expanding with all else until it will eventually come to a point of rest or no-thingness. Duality is then resolved in a single stable state in which all motion, in and out, back and forth, acceleration or deceleration, expansion or contraction, all vibration ceases in eternal silence.

Every person goes through the mimicking of the cosmic pulse from birth to death on a smaller human scale as the Cosmos does on the larger scale. Our nuclear self goes through all the same phases every time we incarnate: the contraction or the concentrating of all being and its prephysical conception into the black hole of the nucleus, the rapid expansion of the egg in the womb reenacting the whole of evolution during the nine months, then the explosion of birth into awareness, then the acceleration of growth to maturity where the expansion stops and the consciousness slows down to a stop, and then in death our consciousness contracts again into the prephysical nucleus of the next egg. The same process that we see in the accelerating Cosmos, we also see in the hologram of our life.

Physicists see acceleration in terms of a force acting upon something, but the only force acting between galaxies in the Cosmos known to science is the force of gravity. This is a contracting force which is always attractive and represents the slowing down of the expansion and is therefore a deceleration force. Its opposite is the acceleration of the expansion which must have a repulsive force acting between the galaxies to push them faster away from each other. The gravity force always acts upon material bodies to pull them into a more intense center while the opposite expanding force divides and separates the objects of creation throughout space. What is this expanding force that causes acceleration? It is light or levity. If we liken gravity to persons who are grave we find they are automatically attracted to people like themselves, heavy and weighed down with the yoke of the world's problems. If we liken the expansive force to people who feel lightened and joyful we can understand why they feel their yoke is easy and their burden is light. Gravity leads to the grave for bodies of flesh because they are controlled by matter, whereas the expansive force of light leads to levity and joy. Because expansiveness is a quality of the human spirit and has a definite repulsive effect on all material objects, it is continually dividing material objects against themselves. Gravity is a quality of the material body and is continually pulling objects together. In this way light brings the radiation of matter and causes its disintegration into energy, whereas gravity unites matter to conserve energy and creates darkness through the obstruction of light. Its opposite force of levity unites spirit and dissolves material obstructions. This interplay is found in human consciousness, in society, and in the cosmic relations. The difficult thing is that those who are imprisoned in the gravitational field in their consciousness cannot understand this if they cannot see beyond the darkness of matter. Because their minds are narrow and can only see themselves as matter, they are identified in consciousness with material bodies and cannot see that the liberating expansive force of levity is caused by the accelerating liberating force of radiation and light. Only by expanding the mind can people get free of the near-sighted darkness caused by our human attachments to the physical earth, physical sensations, and physical scientific measurements of time and space. Those who can *think in light* realize that light and levity are the accelerating force acting between all the entities of creation.

Scientists have been looking for this force which can only appear over the vast intergalactic distances because it cannot be detected at shorter distances with our instruments, whereas gravity is always the opposite of levity and is detectable at short distances between material objects but not detectable at great distances. Because the accelerating force is not physically detectable until we get to vast intergalactic distances, we would have no physical knowledge of it upon the earth where the main force is gravity. We can only detect these facts by understanding the nonphysical light of consciousness. These ideas about black holes and the effects of light and color on consciousness make a lot of physicists react in the gut. Obviously they feel that our universe must either be expressed as mathematical and physically measureable phenomena, or not be discussed at all. This is a deliberate self-blinding to the workings of the mind, for the darkness of their consciousness refuses to see except in terms of their own self-imposed limitations. In other words, they are scanning intergalactic spaces for the intelligence to come from light signals, yet in the gut many of them cling to matter and darkness and feel suspicious of light in its psychological or spiritual manifestation while looking for it physically all over the universe.

Now we have said that the force science is looking for is an intelligence in light because it is the cause of the repulsive and accelerating force throughout space and the opposite of the attractive force of gravity. But there is a difficulty. Light cannot be seen anywhere in space. Only its action on some forms of matter is visible or detectable. The light which shines into our eyes from stars shines on the visual pigments and the molecules of rhodopsin in the retina. The light we see from radiotelescopes and instruments falls on photographic emulsions and other kinds of matter or sensors which give us only information, and not knowledge. The light we see on the moon or on clouds or on dust is all light reflected off particles of matter. Light itself would be quite invisible without the presence of some matter to stop it going on and on through space. The light generated on the earth is also very different from the light of stars, especially faraway stars. Earth light is even different from the sun's light of which we only see a small fraction, the rest being carried into the earth's magnetic field as electricity before we see its effects. The only light on the earth similar to that of the stars is laser light, and of course the sun is too near for us to experience its light as we do laser light. The laser light coming from the furthermost galaxies can, according to the latest physical theories of the accepted velocity of light, take 350 million to 2,000 million years to reach us upon the earth. But can these stars powerfully project this light which goes on and on through space? Do we see the star because it extends its light beyond its own system or do we see it because the system itself, including its surrounding space, *enables* us to see it from infinite distances? In other words, does the light actually reach the earth directly from the star or is it like the vibration of waves disturbing a medium, very much like the surface waves passing through water?

Not everybody knows that water does not move when waves roll across its surface. Even the school child can drop a cork in the water and see that the cork and waves do not move forward but only go up and down; only the energy under the cork moves. In the same way bits of matter bob up and down in space, and particles of light bob up and down throughout the totality without going anywhere. The wave energy in water travels, but water does not, and thus does energy from stars come to us in a wave motion, without the light going anywhere. It is similar to the way a nervous impulse, passing along a tube-like nerve system, passes the signal on from cell to cell, but nothing is actually moving, only each cell is handing on its own chemical electricity. We now ask ourself: does light really travel?

THRESHOLD OF THE EIGHTH DOMAIN

The foregoing sets the scene for the direct experience of light and space and consciousness as one and for the explanation of what it is like to think in light where subject and object are one, rather than to be stuck in the darkness of objective consciousness where they are separate. Does light travel from a star or does it merely stimulate emission of energy through an elastic medium called space? Let us imagine that someone lights a candle, say, a hundred yards away. We can see the tiny flame flickering, and around it is a glow as it lights up the air. Although its light does not penetrate very far in lighting up its surroundings, the flame itself can be seen from a much greater distance until the source gets very small. Obviously something is helping us to see. If we saw the light because the rays of light were extending to our eyes, the light would light up the intervening distance as well. But our eye is much more sensitive than the absorbing power of the environment. Similarly if the light of the stars did travel to earth without any decay or filtering by space then the earth would be lit up by bright

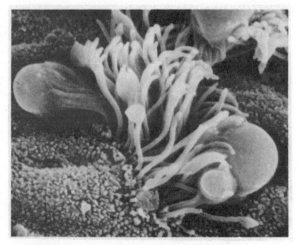

Scanning electron microscope view of the ciliated epithelial cells of the wind-pipe. A mucous droplet is supported by the cilia. ("Ciliated and Nonciliated Epithelial Cells from Hamster Trachea," Port, C. and Corvin, 1. Cover Photo, "Science," Vol. 177, 22 September 1972.)

Particles at maximum vibration cycle produce a shadow particle or hole opposite. Interchange

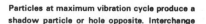

between them releases energy as when a laser emits a spontaneous wave or particle when falling from a high energy state to a low energy state.

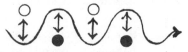

A photon or electron particle emits two frequencies, both resonating in parallel causing the particle to jump from an excited state to lower levels and back again, releasing energy spontaneously.

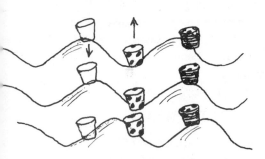

As a wave passes on the surface of the water, the water particle bobs up and down. Diagram shows corks bobbing up and down showing that only the energy in the wave travels and the vibrations themselves do not travel.

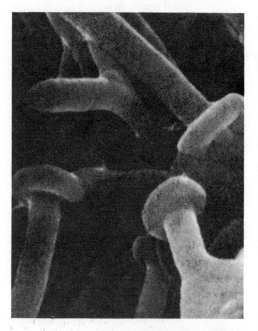

Scanning electron micrograph of synaptic knobs from a sea hare. The junction between one neuron and another or a neuron and an effector is called a synapse. (Aplysia californica). x 11,250. (Courtesy E.R. Lewis, T.E. Everhart, and Y.Y. Zeevi, "Science", Vol. 165, 1969. Copyright 1969 by the American Assoc. for the Advancement of Science.)

Motion of a Cilium on an organism moving toward the right involves a sweeping effective stroke (top), followed by a graceful recovery stroke (bottom).

WAVES DO NOT TRAVEL. THE ENERGY IN THE WAVE DOES. DOES LIGHT TRAVEL? OR IS THE LIGHT ALREADY WITHIN OUR CONSCIOUSNESS AS IS SPACE, AND IS IT ONLY COSMIC ELECTRICAL ENERGY THAT TRAVELS?

starlight like it is lit up by our sun. But as powerful as each star is, it does not have the power to send its brightness through space to our consciousness on a dark night without help from our own sensitivity. Similarly some stars cannot be seen by the naked eye; their light must be collected by lenses and mirrors and amplified by telescopes for us to increase the power of the eye or the star's light enough to see it. If any star had this power to come through space without loss of energy, then the night sky would be very bright indeed and its light would obscure the other stars just like our own sun does during daytime. It is at night on the dark side of the earth that our consciousness is sensitive enough to pick out the stars and see them through the transparent darkness. The universal medium by which we see the stars is the total expanse of space which is enveloped in a transparent darkness. Just as it would be difficult to see a candle flame in the daytime at one hundred yards, so we cannot see the stars in the daytime although they are still there. The darkness of space absorbs the light of the stars and contains them within itself but yet is riddled with rays of invisible light going in every direction in space. The background of the light-filled space is the same as the silence in which sound waves rise and fall again. It is the background against which the whole of creation is still and peaceful. The dark emptiness of space is the womb in which the stars, suns and planets are born. The darkness of the void of space is penetrated by light and yet our consciousness must already be there to receive the excitation of the atoms which causes the phenomenon of light in the first place.

Does the light travel to our eye or does our consciousness travel to the light? If we use a photographic film the light will record on it, showing that something in addition to human vision is extending through space. The time taken for the energy to reach the sensitive film is the same time to reach our eye in which perception takes place. But if there is no darkness of night there cannot be an image of star light because the film would be fogged. So the important factor in photography is the absence of light in the camera or on the film; the exposure is the temporary flash of light from the camera lens shutter which is recorded as an image. If there is too much light let into the camera, then there is not enough darkness for the film to see with and it is overexposed. If there is not enough light, then there is too much darkness for the film to register an image.

It is this analogy with the human eye that causes us to question the speed of light. It is the length or intensity of the darkness which permits us to see a fine point of light. It is this darkness which allows us to see a weak source of light like a star suspended in space. The light of the star, the darkness of space and the photosensitivity of the eye and camera film make the experience of seeing into a phenomenon. But without the darkness in the consciousness of the viewer, no point of light could be seen because it would all be light. The images of light we see require the presence of darkness in order to be seen. In other words the darkness has a lot more to do with our seeing of light than how far or how fast light travels. Why is our consciousness a darkness? The darkness is necessary for our consciousness to make the sensations of light physically visible. Here the darkness acts like the negative in the camera, and the image of brightness we see inside our head acts like a positive print impression of the light. When we *think in light* this darkness disappears because we begin to see directly through the inner eye and not by the ordinary sensations of the physical senses. But even ordinary people who believe the brightness they see is outside themselves rather than inside their brains do not realize that *the light we all see with eyes is not the real light* but only the psychic reaction to stimulus inside the matter of our head, just as the emulsion on the film is a disturbance of the sensitive molecules. The real light is invisible radiation passing through the darkness of space. Just as the sun's light is only bright as we know it on the sunlit side of the earth, while the other side of the earth is in darkness, so the light creates darkness when it is interrupted and absorbed by matter. Absorption is relative to the matter's transparency. If the earth were made of clear glass then part of the light of the sun would pass through the earth and light up the other side. To the extent that the absorbing medium is transparent or opaque, light-transmitting or dense, so is the darkness created by the light striking matter. If there were no matter to absorb the invisible light transmitted through the clear medium of space, there would be no brightness inside our brain nor any darkness in any relative sense, and the sun's light would go on its radiant way past the earth into outer space. This same process of creation of light and darkness occurs in the human consciousness as it does in the Cosmos around us. In humans it is the mental process of identification with matter that creates the darkness and blocks out the light on the various thresholds of consciousness. The ground state for light is the clear space through which it travels in the expansion from its source. Space then is zero light and zero darkness and zero space since all are invisible, and the phenomenon we call light and dark is purely a psychic phenomenon caused within our brain.* Light and dark are merely aspects of matter, and we talk loosely of the light which seems outside us as if it were more than a chemical reaction of our eyes and brain. The real light is unseen as we can observe when we look out into the dark night and see no light there in empty space even though it is ever-present. The reason we cannot see waves of light in empty space when we look through its voidness is because *our consciousness and light and space are identical with each other.* We do not experience this with the darkness of our minds simply because we mistake the phenomenon of light as brightness, when this is not primary but only a secondary reflection from matter.

Here is where we go wrong in calculating the speed of light, because we omit the speed of consciousness which includes the subject and the object both. The present scientific calculation of the velocity of the light from an object is omitting the medium through which our perception takes place, namely the void of consciousness and space. And this is why Einstein could never prove a static or still universal field. The real research must hinge upon the velocity of consciousness.

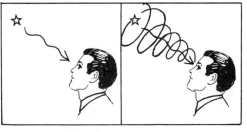

At present only the speed of light is considered by scientists. This is only half the experiment.

Our consciousness is part of the total observation and its speed must be considered.

* I go into this more deeply in *Supersensonics* page 352 and *Nuclear Evolution* page 121, the first dealing with sensing ability and the second dealing with the invisible expansion of consciousness in all acts of perception by our brains.

If our consciousness is infinite and primordial then it is outside of all time, or is in zero time. The calculation of the passage of light through space or our fixing of the notion of stars and suns relative to the stillness of space is dependent upon identifying consciousness with our senses, and this is the beginning of time. Time and space begin only with the appearance of motion, whether that motion is a ray of light transmitted from one part of space to another location, or whether it is a heavenly body moving from one fixed point to another. The question comes again—are there any such fixed points in space unless they are fixed by the human mind? The expanse of space is like the expanse of Pure Consciousness, the primordial background of reality. It is a zero dimension of stillness and silence in which all other things move. This is true of our consciousness in which all experiences of motion or excitement, frequency, vibration, wavelength, etc., are creating the experiencer in time inside our own heads. It is eternal because even when all vibration stops and there is no time, and light and dark disappear, there still remains the expanse of unlimited consciousness, unconditioned by matter or time. Finite and infinite are meaningless in the timeless zero zone of consciousness, because they imply concepts of beginning and end. Zero time is timeless—the ultimate measure of all vibrations from zero to infinity. The velocity of consciousness is zero because like space it is already present throughout the nucleus of the whole, expanded through space, an all-pervading clear medium for transmission of light.

Time does not exist at the zero point because at that place there is nowhere for consciousness to go or move except to itself which is already there. The velocity of consciousness is not subject to measurement because it is already there as the all-pervading darkness, the medium through which we perceive a distant light system and the light of our Self. Light does not travel in light-years through this subtle spatial medium which is unrestricted by time. If we look through it to perceive distant stars they are merely exciting the elastic medium of space and consciousness with their cosmic vibrations. These vibrations we must remember do not travel; only the energy in the wave travels. We see the distant star systems with the speed of consciousness which is instantaneous. We do not see the light of the stars as it existed years ago but in the real time of the universe which exists as a hologram in our consciousness at all places now.* All other calculations are artificial because they are based on artificial time and on artificial measuring devices and on artificial space created by a limited consciousness. The stars are manifesting as vibrations in our present reality of consciousness and not millions of years away. The stars are not remote from us but are vibrating inside our consciousness which extends into the actual Cosmos around us as an all-present medium. The light which fills space, emitted by all the suns and stars, is indistinguishable from our consciousness. Time is man-created and agreed upon by consensus and fixed to some standard frequency of oscillation of a physical entity and then related to human-experienced intervals such as the revolving planets or the spinning of the earth clock. The universe-at-large knows nothing of this human clock which is strictly a creation of our human consciousness. To know this real nature of consciousness and time even once is to begin to think in light, not the light we see (which is not the true light) but the light of Pure Consciousness which is pure radiance itself, unadulterated by human concepts and petty personal thoughts of self. This is the state of consciousness of someone who goes beyond the seventh brain, beyond the imaged condition of the universe and enters into the radiance of the Absolute ONE in whose presence there is no second.

THE COMING VISION

No matter how frightening the world situation may be, for some people the vastness of cosmic space is even more frightening, and the reason they do not try to open up the higher chakras is because they are afraid of the unknown. Only when we begin to see our kinship with that vastness can we learn to think in light. We can't see the nucleus of our galaxy because it is clouded with gases. Behind them is a black hole which we can't see anyway because it is made of the same stuff as our consciousness. How can ordinary people feel akin to a black hole in space? How can we even imagine the primordial cosmic soup that has been in existence since before the Big-Bang, much less feel ourselves connected with it?

---

* See *Nuclear Evolution* page 150 for detailed exploration.

The notion of interstellar organisms or intelligences has been with man a long time, but science came along and for many years pooh-poohed the idea that there might be organic chemicals existing in the interstellar dust. Now there is evidence that the compounds and reactions of biological chemistry *do* take place throughout the universe. Scientists believe that the primordial nucleus, which was made of the original soup in outer space, has been swimming in space since the time of the Big-Bang when the elements of matter as physics knows them were created. At the present time, over fifty molecular compounds have been detected in space by their spectral radiation signatures. Every year three or four new ones are found which are directly related to the births of stars and planets from giant molecular clouds. Some of these giant remnants of the original nucleus measure thirty to one hundred eighty light years in width and contain a weight of material molecules of gas from one hundred thousand to ten million stars like our sun. These clouds are formed into rings around the center of our galaxy about 12,000 to 25,000 light years out from the center, just where the creation of stars in our own galactic disk is most active.

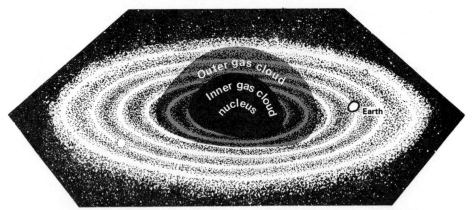

Clouds of gas detected in space around the central core of the galaxy at distances of 12,000 and 25,000 light years. These gases floating in space are composed of the elements necessary for life for living organisms—carbon and oxygen combine with hydrogen in space to form the same hydrocarbon compounds that are found on the earth synthesized by light in the process of photosynthesis. This explains how life could exist in other parts of the galaxy.

The creation of stars by the compressing of the elemental gases in intense gravitational fields of involution eventually led to the concentration of matter we call planets, like earth. The stellar furnace of our sun helps to forge the elements upon earth into the molecules which form our body, but many of these same organic molecules exist floating in the vast clouds of cosmic dust, the ashes of many stars, the debris of the Big-Bang. The carbon molecule so prominent in our diet is a thousand times more plentiful than other molecules floating in space excepting hydrogen. The survival of these molecules in the creation of a star gives the basic biological chemical materials for life and intelligence as we know it.

If the cosmic soup has molecules the same as our bodies are made of, what does this tell us about ourselves? Our galaxy is 100,000 light years across and the big clouds of gases of molecular hydrogen, carbon and water hold the same ingredients from which our bodies are made. The ingredients that are necessary for life, or in which life takes place, are found in the same places in our galaxy where stars and planets are being born by the thousand. There is bound to be the residue of all those organic life-forming molecules on all those planets, so that life or intelligence is not just on the earth but results from the creation of all these organic chemicals, of which our body tissues are made, forged in the original fire in the heart of the nucleus.

What is the reason for reading all this? The reason is because at some point you may realize, "Hey, I *am* that. That's where my parts *come* from—this cosmic soup, spiced with a few special radioactive ions."

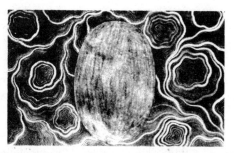

The ancient Hindu seers in deep meditation saw the cosmic egg forming in the primeval waters of the akashic sea of radiation and light. The Hindu view of creation shows the forming of the spiral galaxies from the big expansion of Brahman.

Radiation from the stars acting on this chemical soup is the same process of photosynthesis that on earth produces our food and the oxygen we breathe. Light divides the hydrogen molecule from water and synthesizes it with carbon into hydrocarbons, the basic food unit of life. Biochemistry is no longer confined to the laboratories of the earth. We must now become astro-chemists to understand astronomy. What does it mean to know this? Does it matter if you know it? What is the difference between one person sitting in the sun who knows it and another sitting beside him ignorant of the process of how he became what he is? Does it matter to a human not to know that he is ninety percent water (H_2O) which has been split by light or radiation from the suns and stars, and recombined with carbon to make our cells and plant life into hydrocarbons? The answer is that the person who is conscious that there is some *intelligence* in light which has the power to transform chemicals such as hydrogen, carbon and oxygen into living beings who are conscious of themselves, knows that their consciousness is made of light. That person knows that he too can transform matter, as light does, at the nuclear level of being, through cold processes which do not require a laboratory or the application of any heat in a laboratory or industrial chemical factory. Man is now discovering through radiology how to do this, how to transform the elements in himself through radiation and light. The radiant energies of the stars and the suns of the Cosmos, which are created from the primordial soup, may themselves be programmed with the job of transforming matter or material chemicals. To understand this process in oneself and realize that the light of our consciousness is brought to us by cosmic vibration of light of the universe acting upon matter, is to immediately lift the intelligence of a knowing being onto another hierarchical level of the creation where that intelligence is functioning transcendentally in its pre-physical state.

All light from the stars and our sun is the result of tremendous excitement of the elements of which they are made. We receive this excitement in the biological chemicals and elements of our physical organism and synthesize it into consciousness and life. In this sense, light is pre-physical intelligence, because it has no shape and no energy until it touches matter and is absorbed into it. Then it becomes physicalized into us, into our food, into the plants and millions of creatures that survive on its munificent excitement. Stop right now, if you are sitting in the sun, and feel how the sunlight penetrates through you and warms you inside. What is it saying to you?

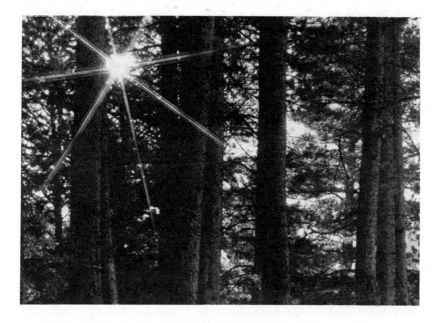

What does it feel like experientially to think in light? What can a human being create with consciousness that is not already created at the time of the original expansion of the primordial nucleus? The direct realization that light is consciousness cannot be explained in words, even though I've spent several pages explaining it, because words are merely concepts. Nor can it be described in images and metaphors because it is beyond the human imagination. How then can it be experienced and communicated?

The answer is that when we surrender all egocentric self-regarding thoughts and images we begin to create a new life with the pure consciousness which can feel the certainty of the eternal and timeless behind the changing Cosmos. This experience feels and knows itself in a totally different way to ordinary feelings and yet it encompasses all that is ordinary. There is nothing special because everything is special and unique. To one who thinks in light each blade of grass is seen as a unique creation of its own growth. To see a writhing mass of maggots and experience them in the light of Pure Consciousness is to feel each as a unique expression of oneself and to give each one a name. The fly that emerges from it to pester mankind is seen with equal rights, and yet we can swat it with compassion. To look at a star is to see a brother or sister in space and to know and feel their songs in light just as we hear the songs of birds in sound.

To think in light is to feel with light the radiance of all that it touches, to melt into its rays and to have no other will but to surrender to its fullness. To those who *feel* in light even the weakest ray of light is a delicate but awesome thread, a glimmer of the ONE shining in the darkness. We see clearly that every point of light springs from the original burning of the cosmic fire at the heart of the nucleus. The burning flame of oil or candle feels the same as the burning of oxygen in our own cells at a higher threshold of heat. To the thinker in light, heat and light are felt as one, for where there is heat enough in the presence of matter, there will be the spontaneous flame of light releasing its excitement to the world around it. To feel with the tree the caresses of light is to know the fierce unswerving power of that love that needs nothing but itself, the love which lightens every cell and atom of matter with its action.

The sages have called this feeling the *refiner's fire* because it purifies all that is dross and obstructive of evolution. When men and women are in tune with it, it carries them aloft into the realms of the spirit, not to faraway heavens but the heaven at the center of every heart, where all is perceived as even more and greater light. The pity of it all, that men prefer the darkness of their own thoughts than the light of the eternal one, becomes the pity of a Christ and the compassion of a Buddha. The need to share this light is as much a necessity for such a one as it is for others to eat. To nourish the dark world with love is essential for its own rising in the heart of life. Such a one can only feel and radiate and see that radiance in order to re-cognize itself. Thus from age to age the Phoenix rises from the eighth level of the cosmic fire and annihilates itself with all its concepts and knowledge on the radiant altar of the eternal sun. Out of these ashes springs the new

Phoenix from the nucleus of the cosmic egg, fully fledged and complete with its new divine song.

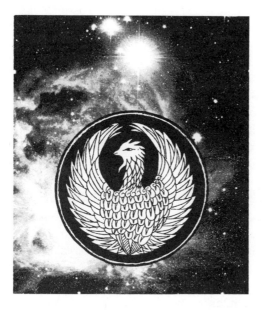

I get very frustrated with people when they say they can't see light in everything, especially with scientists. If you take a piece of grass to a scientist and say, "Don't you see that this is all full of light and radiating with light?", they say, "Well, sure, we know theoretically that if you do atomic fission on the atoms they have a very powerful energy." They look at the grass under a microscope and see that it is all made of chloroplasts and atoms and they name off all the parts, but they do not think about its being made of structures of light. They say, "Sure, I know all that, but it's just grass." They feel no sense of wonder.

When I was a boy I would sit on the river bank and meditate on the grass and communicate with it and let it communicate its being to me, and I would feel what it felt like. I would dip my hand into the water and throw it back into itself and it would make music. It is hard to describe the noise it makes when you throw water back into itself like that. The water would actually play with me. It would roll this way and that. And I would walk out into the sun and feel my atoms begin to dance as the warmth touched my skin, and they were full of excitement as if to say, "Hey, here is something like *me*, something akin to me!" Every atom of our body is a star radiating tremendous light, and they resonate with the sunlight and know it is the same as themselves. But people rarely notice.

To understand within oneself the exciting nature of light and consciousness acting together as *One* is to completely revolutionize our entire being, because we then see no separation between great molecular clouds of light and consciousness, no difference between us and the galactic center and the light of consciousness which spiritually animates and excites our physical being. But the link between our bodies and those clouds and that center is all provided by the action and excitement of light which passes from the galactic center through all the gases, bodies, molecules, suns, stars and atoms which make up the galaxy we live in, this island home of our galaxy, floating in space with countless other similar organisms in different stages of evolution.

That same light speaks through us at every moment and is speaking through us now in every act and thought, expressing itself through the dance of all our atoms, as life. That same light which experiences us and is speaking through us now and hearing and seeing in us now is animating all the suns and stars in our own brain now as it receives the vibrations of this excitement, radiating out of all the objects of sensation that we touch not only with our skin every moment of the day, but the light which we touch with our eyes as it is reflected off all the objects around us. That One who is at the center of our galaxy, the nucleus of all vibration, exciting the total environment around us, is what our consciousness is made of, deep in the nuclear center of our own being. To realize and know this, is to know that everything is made of light, that there are suns burning in our own body at the heart of every atom. To see everything as light, to know one's own consciousness as light, is to know that One who is even now thinking in light in our consciousness as we listen and see and touch the total environment around us. That One who is radiating this excitement of light to the whole of creation from the heart of all the galaxies sits buried deep in our own heart waiting for us to touch and see and feel and love with every fiber of its own creation.

To feel this response to light within oneself, sitting in the sun alongside another being who does not know the secret, is the difference between the enlightened state and the darkness of the prison of matter, though both people are identically the same one. The difference is only in our consciousness and awareness of who we are. If this realization and transformation of our consciousness and the biological instrument which it inhabits can be communicated, then the world can be changed overnight, in the twinkling of an eye. With this change and this recognition of the cosmic fire which pours out of all our eyes and glorifies the wonder of creation, will come the understanding of Nuclear Evolution which is even now touching us beyond our conscious knowledge and beyond our control.

What *is* in our control at this moment in time as we read these words is the power to remain in a self-created prison, obsessed with its own sensations, or the power to use our consciousness to break *out* of that self-made prison and radiate that light into every part of our being. That power itself is *in* the light, which is free to choose to be the whole, the totality of all experience, or to be only a minute part. That spontaneous light chooses only to enter into those objects, organisms and beings that can absorb and receive itself. Total receptivity of that light makes us pure and transparent as light is itself. When our consciousness becomes so pure that we can see nothing but light in all its many forms around us, then our entire nucleus at the center of our being becomes indivisibly married to the center of the universe, and the two become one, and omnipresence is experienced. All separations dissolve, and the whole purpose of life and creation is fulfilled.

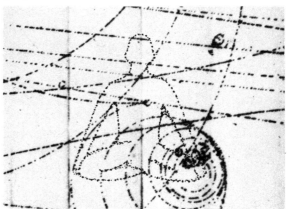

Ionization tracks left by cosmic particles in a bubble chamber reveal that our bodies are bombarded continuously by these high energies which ionize our blood cells and membranes penetrating our sensitive nerve antennae. Experiments in the mental deflection and attraction of these particles with sensors and counters reveal that we have choice and selectivity. See "Supersensonics".

IF WE FAIL TO OPEN TO LIGHT

Those who can read the book of Genesis—the stories of Adam and Eve, Noah and the Ark—not as historical events but as allegories of what happened when man lost contact with the power behind his own imagination and created with it an abomination in the eyes of the Cosmic Intelligence, can see more clearly the present step of evolution for the human race. Entry into the realms of light in human consciousness is forbidden until the surrender of all personal powers has been transformed into grace. By this means the Cosmos protects itself against the cleverness of those who would abuse their consciousness and tinker with its cosmic design. Right now we don't need any asteroid planet to blow up. Our own planet is next. To those who are striving to think in light, a planetary holocaust will not matter because it will not destroy their attunement with Nature. There is one more dense level or psychic center below the physical level of manifestation which is more dense than earthly life. If human consciousness is pulled down into this lowest center by the devastation of our planet, which would rupture the etheric center related to the physical body, the consciousness of mankind would be plunged into even greater darkness. Thus we can understand when we hear Christ make the statement:

> "The light of the body is the eye; if therefore thine eye be single, thy whole body shall be full of light. But if thine eye be evil, thy whole body shall be full of darkness. If therefore the light that is in thee be dark, how great *is* that darkness."

The seed of darkness and materialist thought is now sprouting everywhere. The rationalizations of the soulless who live in the darkness of the unillumined mind bring humanity closer and closer to the disaster of atomic suicide which everyone can sense but cannot believe will happen. The utopian belief that technology can establish the Kingdom of Heaven on earth is a vain imagination. Selfish greed of giant corporations, who cannot respect the environment and who put profits on weapons before life, are creating insecure industries which are undermined by strikes and absenteeism. Relationships between owners and employees are beset with conflicts which can only be resolved by new methods of ownership. The civil servants are striking for more pay irrespective of whether the citizen can pay more taxes. Dwellers in the capital cities of the world crave for pleasure and comfort and live in arrogance and egocentric blindness to that purpose which put them in this world of matter. Man has lost the awareness that he carries within him the jewel of God's spirit. When men lose their way and deny any purpose, they cannot love. When love is absent from the community there is no communion. Without the coming together of the community there is division among the people. Where there is division there will be the cause of suffering and the onset of collapse.

Those who scorn the revelation of Nuclear Evolution concerning man's own nature can rationalize it away, but we observe that their prejudice rules all their actions. The deafness of the supreme egotists is the same now as it was 2,000 years ago. The egotist who believes he has the answer without searching out the nature of his own consciousness, will not listen to anyone else. We have to let him go out on his fruitless mission to "save the world". Either he will seek out the like-minded and try to enthrall them in a new cult with the new word or he will search for the "sinners" to convert them. What he does not understand in his egomania, however high-sounding his aims, is that all "conversion" trips are fruitless unless there is understanding of readiness.

The hungry of soul and the blind who see their own lack will come of their own accord to the process of Nuclear Evolution because their hearts will yearn for the truth and for maturity. Those who come wanting to change the world through preaching and the hot gospel approach are egotists who want to shine and receive the attention of men. Let them have their rewards of fame. God does not approve such showmanship, however charismatic and whatever the numbers of followers. Love is not something talked about with the mouth, but something expressed permanently in actions which sing in the heart. Salvation is not the coming of an external Truth or the coming of new gurus with teachings, but the quiet knowing that all returns to the original nucleus of consciousness. There is no truth except this, that our own consciousness is the origin of all gods as it is the origin of love. To know this is to know that God is the pure light of consciousness.

A planetary holocaust on earth would mutate the energy pattern in man's brain causing him to involute into the darkness and hell described by the great sages, bringing even more suffering than humankind has now. This is not the design of the Cosmos, but the result of man's own desires and our freedom of choice to prefer darkness to light. It is the darkness of man's consciousness only which blocks the advance of evolution, and our thinking in light which advances it. This is the polarization which the Bible calls good and evil which is referred to in other world religions as well. Just as positive and negative are not separated from each other but are really one, the polarization of good and evil also has no real cosmic existence except as a vibration in human consciousness which man freely chooses. Thinking in light is beyond good and evil which are merely the relative polarization of *our choices* in our own consciousness. The eighth level is concerned only with the long timespan of evolution, far beyond human time, when the universal Intelligence eventually brings enough pressure on consciousness to cause it to choose the light, just as gravity becomes light radiation when the intensity is great enough. The eighth level is not concerned with when these things shall happen but is concerned with *what* will happen, out of love for those who walk in darkness and know it not, for if they so chose they could see the great light of inner space.

There are countries right now undergoing that hell of the lower level. The next fall of man will not happen in one great swoop, but is actually happening right now. Anyone reading of the genocide, brutality and senseless killing of people in Cambodia, or other revolutions where millions were killed by Stalin, Mao Tse-tung and Hitler, can see that these cult personalities are merely pawns and instruments which pull mankind down into the darkness of egotism and self-righteousness and reduce people to nothing more than a physical body with no more importance than an ant. To those of you reading this book in a life of relative freedom, if only you knew or could feel what it is like to be those people, to be experiencing those lowest vibrations of human consciousness! Such is the pity of this world, that those who think in light must watch those in the darkness decide their own fate—because consciousness, being all-powerful, is completely free to be self-creating or self-destructing and when divided against itself, that is the end of it.

PART THREE

TUNING TO THE COSMIC PROGRAM

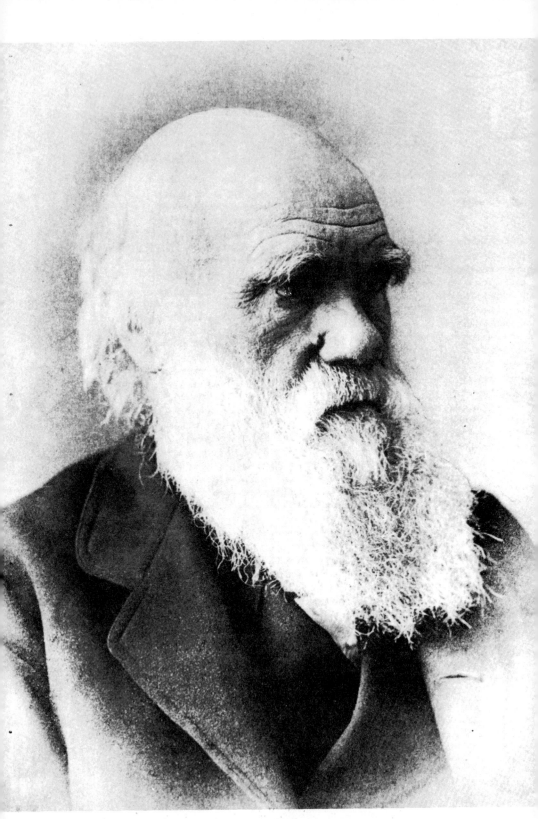

Charles Darwin

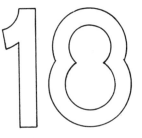

DARWIN
AND THE
EVOLUTION OF
CONSCIOUSNESS

What is evolution? What is the real meaning of evolution and did it all start with Darwin? Darwin published his *Origin of the Species* in 1859, but in 1809 Lamarck had pioneered evolutionary principles less threatening to the nineteenth century mentality and therefore less well remembered than the famous ape controversy. Lamarck's research revealed four principles behind the changes we call evolution:

1. the existence in all organisms of a primal drive for perfection
2. the capacity of organisms to adapt to environmental circumstances
3. the occurrence of spontaneous generation
4. the inheritance of acquired traits.

Whereas Darwin's work traced down the *origin* of species and thus called in question the whole religious explanation of why and how we came to be here, Lamarck's theory of an inherent drive for perfection confirmed the accepted Christian idea that God created man for a high

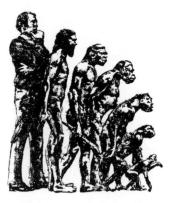

A reasonable interpretation of man's progression up the evolutionary scale.

purpose. Neither the assumption of a built-in drive for perfection nor the theory of frequent spontaneous generation of new species was confirmed by the Darwinian scientists who followed Lamarck, and Darwin's work has totally dominated all research into evolution from 1859 to the present.

Evolutionary change, said Darwin, was not the result of any Lamarckian drive for perfection nor was it a simple matter of chance but was the result of natural selection. By struggling for physical survival, he said, organisms with the best characters for coping with the environment and their competitors and enemies, had the greatest chances of existing, reproducing, and leaving survivors. This revolutionary idea of the "survival of the fittest" brought evolution down into the natural world where it followed certain materialistic laws, and there was no need for any unprovable hypothesis such as God or any outside intelligence to explain man's existence or his purpose. Although the ancients talked of involution and evolution, the idea of evolution was comparatively new to the Western world and implied that since lower forms of life evolve into higher forms through this process of "natural selection", then man himself must once have been a lower form, perhaps a member of the ape family. The ape hypothesis did away with Adam and Eve, and if it did away with Adam it did away with the Bible as an ultimate authority, and it did away with God. Therefore the public resisted Darwin's theories. Controversies charged with emotion went on for years, but Darwin just kept on publishing more and more research until the sheer bulk of it forced people to open their minds to new possibilities. Many lost their faith in God, and the modern era was born out of that disillusionment.

The *Origin of Species* was a brilliant insight into the secrets of Nature and thus had the power to completely transform man's image of himself. Yet it did not penetrate the real meaning of evolution which was known to the rishis and wise men long before modern science was even born. The ancient sages viewed themselves as organs of the world-soul and their systems of thought as an evolution of the Deity. They knew and told that the universe, its stars and planets and all organisms not only evolved through long periods but also *in*volved. The idea of involution has not so far struck any great chord in the ears of most scientists who have run off wildly with the idea of gradual evolutionary change shaped by natural processes both in cosmic evolution and biological evolution. The idea of involution or returning to the source through a gradual process of disintegration is familiar in physics where it is now known that matter is slowly and weakly disintegrating into energy, but in the biological science of genetics, evolution is seen as coming from a common source but not flowing back to the single or absolute oneness. Yet the unity of that one single nucleus is found in every entity in Nature which is whole and individable.

Up till now Darwin and his heirs have left us with a swampy feeling about evolution, and the word evolution has almost been a synonym for ape in the public mind. Strange that evolution, whose unfolding has led to higher or more aware life-forms should be so backward-looking and leave mankind with such a lowered image of himself and his origins and his destiny. Though Darwin's brilliant discoveries almost totally eclipsed Lamarck's, perhaps we need to reconsider the Darwinian axioms (as well as the modern research into territoriality, adaptations, DNA, and socio-biology) as a natural part of Lamarck's "drive for perfection", and in no way contradicting it. Let us go back to Lamarck and re-open the book

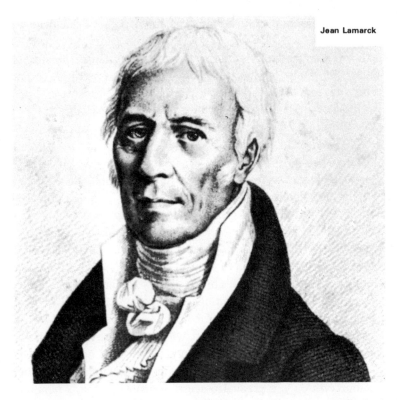

Jean Lamarck

of Nature with the same open-mindedness to truth that Darwin had when he went against the accepted values of his society and raised questions which others in his day were not willing even to ask, much less answer.

What questions would we ask today to widen the scope of our truth? Perhaps in the greater and vaster Cosmos we can see that our social scientists, concentrating on the lowest evolutionary thrust of physical and social needs, have avoided another program in mankind which has gone on from the beginning: the drive towards self-realization and the desire to know the nature of the evolutionary force itself. This mysterious and hidden mystical intelligence guiding the evolution of all forms may have a purpose behind the security and the survival of the fittest! It may have an aim which completely transcends the concepts of modern-day universities. Can we dare to speculate about it and even to create communities and groups which reach towards it as our ancestors groped towards physical domination of the environment?

In order to speak of such things, we will have to step outside the picture frame in which Nature's landscape is said to be evolving. Like Darwin, the modern scientist limits himself to Nature's physical manifestation without asking what mysterious force or superintelligence creates the manifestation in the first place. Is there an intelligence in the seed or an intention or a feeling? How does the seed hold the memory of life's origins, and does it know that it is a flower and not some other form? Nuclear Evolution is the study of this seed and its knowing and the laws of its unfolding in every living and non-living entity of creation. The modern science of genetics is a modification of Darwin's theory that complex systems have not been programmed or foreordained to follow any pre-determined pattern because over long periods they are capable of adaptation. Nuclear Evolution differs subtly from this view in the idea that the nucleus *is* already programmed with its genetic potential but not *predestined* to a fixed pattern of reaching that potential. The implications of this subtlety are far-reaching and profound. It means that the whole focus of evolution is not the external environment to which we must adapt in order to survive but the inner seed which will unfold and manifest according to what is written in its program by the evolutionary intelligence. The startling discoveries of this century in the field of genetics have not led scientists to investigate the natural higher cosmic program but instead to invent a program of their own in the recombinant DNA experiments to create new organisms unknown to Nature.

How do we tune into the evolutionary intelligence? The ancient prophets and priests of India and China used "Supersensonics"* and divination to tune in. Darwin used fossils and archeology. And modern scientists use DNA molecules and genes. Biologists and social scientists study the behavior of species and cross-correlate the patterns but they do not know that these DNA patterns, like those in the yolk of an egg, are approachable by a totally different route than the physical.

---

* The term used by the author to describe the science of subtle energies. See reference at the back of book.

Darwin's concept of a common biological descent for all those organisms which were similar meant that all mammals including humans could have derived from one ancestral species. Darwin implied that all living organisms might even be traced back to a single origin or nucleus of life—an insight which has now been confirmed by the DNA research of modern science. But he did not realize that every nucleus is

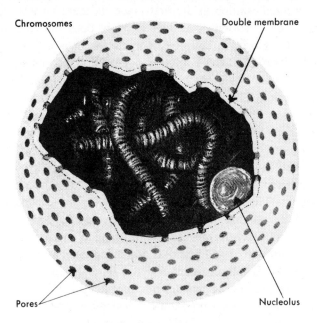

The nucleus of a cell is usually a spherical envelope composed of a double membrane with perforations to permit nutrients to pass between the nucleus and the cytoplasm. The nucleus contains the chromosomes which direct all activities for the whole cell through DNA. It is the nucleus which evolves and contains the nucleolus which synthesizes RNA to move the DNA message of life into the rest of the cell.

not only the genetic wellspring of past and future for that entity, so that a seed of grass contains within it the whole long history of its lineage, but also contains that first primordial nucleus from which the universe was born. Each nucleus is a hologram. Hence Darwinian thinking is bound in the linear concept of evolution through time, whereas Nuclear Evolution can know the whole of time in one instant by penetrating the nucleus in which the secret of absolute zero-time itself is written. Scientists today have already discovered the patterning of the DNA and are now on the verge of penetrating the superintelligence of the

DNA which, because they have not evolved in the heart, will put more power into their hands than they can handle. They are following the way of science, which penetrates the nucleus externally as an observer of Nature, whereas Nuclear Evolution guides us to penetrate the nucleus internally in the central core of our own being and thus not just observe the working plans of Nature but evolve ourselves as *part* of Nature. To one so evolved, Nature can entrust her secrets and know that they will not be misused.

What is the nuclear way of tuning into the cosmic movie at the heart of existence? To answer this we must take the Nuclear Evolution theory through a modern re-writing of Darwinism.* As we said, Charles Darwin astounded the world of his day with the publication of his theory of natural selection which much improved the earlier conceptions of evolution by Lamarck and others by looking at all the tremendous variety of organisms and their behavior in terms of the survival of the fittest. Nuclear Evolution looks at evolution not only from the survival of the fittest physically but also looks at that quality of vision or perception which transforms individuals into masters of the environment rather than passive adaptors to environment. Can we accept that man is not a prisoner, merely shaped by the forces of the environment? How much of our self-image has been formed by this passivity that was born out of Darwinian theory? What feeling does Nuclear Evolution leave us with in the sense that we now realize that each individual can use the power of consciousness to reshape our future course as individuals and as a species?

OUR NEXT STEP IN EVOLUTION

The one important thing implicit in the working out of self-mastery over our own biological drives is the idea of union. This idea dominates the whole of ancient concepts of yoga. Nuclear Evolution brings us to

---

* Alfred Russell Wallace, co-discoverer of "natural selection" and "survival of the fittest" along with Darwin in 1858, published his divergences in his 1889 book *Darwinism.*

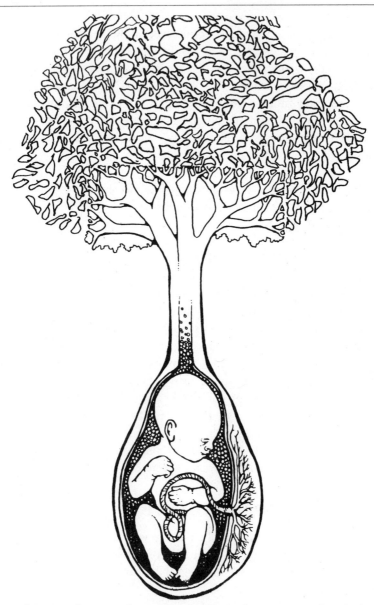

complete togetherness through tuning into the program already in the nucleus within us. Nuclear Evolution brings us into contact with the total environment as a single indivisible nucleus and thereby changes our idea of what environment is and who we are. If we are evolving not only as individuals competing for survival but as a whole unit—all evolving together toward a common destination—then we come inevitably to group consciousness. In the beginning group consciousness is a oneness in the heart which is shared among a small nucleus of people all committed to a common goal. But that goal (i.e. the final stage of group consciousness) is to expand that first small nucleus until ultimately it experiences oneness with the entire universe.

How different the twentieth century might have been had Darwin included group survival as part of his theories of evolution, but Darwin did not think that the survival of the group or the whole might be the aim of life but instead believed that the struggle for existence took place between various individuals as competing organisms. Darwinians generally neglected to apply their intellectual powers to the evolution of groups in society. When they did so, later on, it was too late to rid the original theory of its gross oversights. But if animals formed themselves into herds and groups then it is logical to think that somehow Nature has bestowed some selective advantage in the group over the individual. In addition, Darwin and his successors have left out one of the most important factors of evolution—the formation of groups *not for survival or protection,* but for the achievement of some high goal which requires group consciousness.* Much of what man achieves by groups, from aggressive industrial companies to organizations formed to protect the environment against them, could not be performed by individuals acting alone. Just as a human body, which is made of organs and the organs made of cells which are in turn made up of molecules and the molecules made by the grouping together of atoms, so too can men and women group together to achieve some common goal. The fantastic things that can be done by a human body are nothing to what may be achieved by a group of people if its goal is

---

* In 1870, Alfred Russell Wallace explored the idea that since the group still exists, it must have been valued as an evolutionary agent and must have reinforced such qualities as loyalty, leadership, trust, heroism, cooperation and altruism, all of which we still value in our civilized society. Later he differed from Darwin about the actual mechanisms of human evolution and believed that natural selection alone could not account for the higher faculties that we find in mankind. In 1875 he published *Miracles and Modern Spiritualism* in which he gives reasons for his beliefs.

lofty enough and its consciousness one-pointed.

The power of groups of individuals to shape the future may be obvious, but when we talk of the same power being used to evolve people and to evolve societies with new systems of government, we immediately begin to get negative qualms about religious cults or Hitler or Stalin, rather than think about the possibility of some really evolved societies. Have there been any examples besides the Jews when they were guided by prophets, or the golden age of democracy in the times of Pericles in Athens? The pity is that these societies were both eventually corrupted and we have never seen the spiritual power manifesting on earth purely ever since. Even at the height of Christendom when so much beauty was built from lives lived in total dedication to Truth, there were always the underlying political intrigues of the Holy Roman Empire. And in Old Testament times, the prophet-kings succumbed by giving into the desires of the people who clamored for the pomp and power of a king. The people got bored with the discipline of the prophets and the humility of sages and preferred the glitter of jewels and power to simple spiritual living. The Brahmins of India who ruled through the spiritual power of similar priestly kings in ancient times, eventually corrupted their teachings of equality into the caste-system— the very antithesis of equality.

WHAT IS GROUP CONSCIOUSNESS?

When we look at the discouraging facts of history, how are we warranted to suppose that evolution is going to work through the group to achieve its spiritual purposes? What would such a government be? How will the message written into the innermost depths of the nucleus spread to the uncaring world of human beings that are trapped into beliefs which merely repeat and repeat the same old hereditary message? We have to begin again and answer the evolutionary thrust which creates the need for more leadership, more cooperation and more altruism in order to create the conditions for the human brain to respond to the challenge of its total environment. The dark ghosts which lurk in the minds of those whose doubts and fears rule their lives and cause us to arm ourselves against the violence of their ways, are like fossils from a former stage of human evolution when the "enemy" was the neighboring community and survival of the fittest was happening in a very small arena. Now the entire earth is webbed with communication networks and our environment has even extended into space. In the shifting world of international politics, today's enemy is tomorrow's ally, and even the politicians are beginning to realize that we will all survive together or not at all. So it is not that someone must come along and raise for us the question of group consciousness or try to enlist our support in manifesting it. Though we may not recognize it, the question is rising in our own hearts, in our confusion and anxiety and our quest for a new way to live in this technological scientific world.

A divine marriage of different types of people far apart in biological cells and genes, who learn to love each other even more strongly than we love our blood brothers, mothers and fathers, was personified in Christ when that famous occasion arose where his mother and his brothers pleaded with him to leave his meeting and come home:

> "These hereabout me are my brothers and sisters and my mother."

A strange answer to send one's mother who is lovingly and protectively waiting outside with some concern for her blood son. Nevertheless it portrays the dynamic of the nucleus which forms the basic unit of the World Peace Center everywhere.

How will this divine marriage function in the practical sense of the vision? The group of those preparing for an intensive experiencing of group consciousness, after some discussion and meditation, would naturally want to come permanently together to perfect the message and purify it of all corrupted thoughts. Before expanding the nucleus into the world and replicating their newly-formed system, such a group would first have the humility to achieve what it is that they are asking others to do. A group of real doers would never advertise itself until it believed that a radical perception of its methods of organization would not be ridiculed or opposed through the press or attacked by the scientific community. Such an advanced group would not only meditate in their attempts to tune into the highest communication with the superintelligent universe but would also elect their leadership by tuning to the cosmic will.*

The idea of a community based on Creative Conflict, upon self-rule and total responsibility of the individual for group decision–making, cannot be applied to large groups of people in the beginning because the concept of growth for a natural organism is by starting with a small core nucleus and doubling, not by merely signing up new members.** Before a member can join, he or she must be accepted by the whole membership since everyone must decide on those they are going to be living with very closely for a very long time. After twelve hundred people are thus gathered there is a fall off in the members who can remember each other and know each other well. In other words, twelve hundred is the maximum size for a community whose closeness, achieved through Creative Conflict and a common vision, makes it a true democracy, each member at least remembering each other's names. The group consciousness starts with a small group of maybe ten or twenty people and if it doubles every year it would soon grow to maturity. From twenty it would double to forty, to eighty, to one hundred sixty, to three hundred twenty, to six hundred forty, to twelve hundred eighty. A group beginning with twenty members would double itself to maturity after seven years. To grow any faster would endanger the quality of growth since membership is not casual and requires a deeply considered commitment to the process. If more groups were started, then more communities of twelve hundred could begin. When the maximum number was reached, new communities could be started by leaders from the old community.

---

* A process by means of the *I Ching* could check the suitability of the choice by tuning in through the method of electing a panel of leaders specially chosen by giving the leadership to the most positive manifestation or hexagram of the *I Ching* readings. In this way everyone who is leadership material becomes eligible for the position, and the leadership is rotated by one-third of them automatically rotating every year. The divination methods of the *I Ching* are now quite well known, although when the World Peace Center constitution was first proposed in 1963 using the *I Ching* as an election device there were few people who knew of the oracle's existence. See *The Golden Egg*.
** The process of doubling follows the same process of division in the replication of human cells in the embryo and the splitting of primitive algae in the growth of pure culture.

MODEL OF LOCAL NUCLEAR GOVERNMENT SYSTEM
Optimum population about 1200 per group.
THE ORGANIC EVOLUTION OF THE CELL IS REPEATED IN THE NUCLEAR EVOLUTION OF GROUPS AND WHOLE NATIONS.

In America there are 15 million federal bureaucrats in addition to state and local government officals.

In the vision of a network of many small nuclear communities living in groups they would be limited to about 1200 people to enable in-depth communication and to obtain real knowledge of who we are electing to leadership. Each com-munity would decide its own optimum number based on the number of names and faces the members could memorize. This would cut down administration costs of local government since each group would administer its own social services and decide its own taxes as a whole group, depending on the luxury or necessi-ty of the projects decided. Taxes would be raised federally from

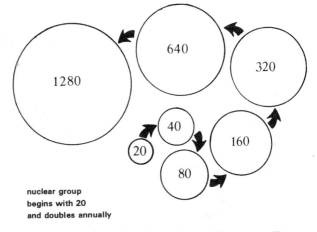

nuclear group
begins with 20
and doubles annually

wealthier districts for the poorer income areas through taxes on all spending, not on wealth or income. The ratio of government employees for the 1200-strong community would be 12 to 1200 or 100 in 10,000 as compared to the national average of nonfederal local government workers of 485 to 10,000 people as shown below.

THE PRESENT LOCAL GOVERNMENT SYSTEM IS REPEATED AT THE NATIONAL LEVEL, AND BUREAU-CRACY GROWS LIKE A CANCER CELL

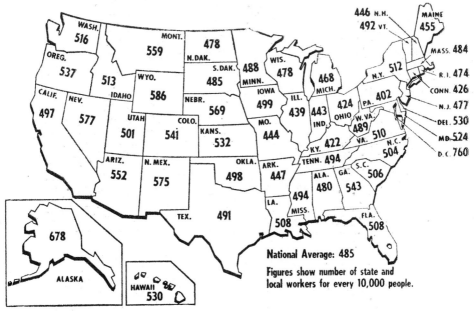

National Average: 485

Figures show number of state and local workers for every 10,000 people.

PRESENT RATIO OF LOCAL GOVERNMENT WORKERS, STATE BY STATE AND GROWING

There are 485 state and local government employees for every 10,000 people in the United States, according to the US Dept. of Commerce. Though Washington, D.C., does not have any state employees, it still has the largest proportion of nonfederal government workers—all of them municipal—with 760 per 10,000 population. Alaska is second with 678. Pennsylvania's figure of 402 is the lowest of any state. The figures shown in the map above were compiled in October 1977.

CAN WE COOPERATE WITH EVOLUTION?

The moment that we begin to see group consciousness according to the universal government of Nature's laws as our next step in evolution, we come automatically to a deeper awareness of the need for selfless service, for putting the needs of the whole before our own personal whims, the need for universal responsibility and for natural leadership rather than structured hierarchies of individuals. In other words, we perceive a whole new range of qualities valued by evolution which have nothing to do with the physical survival of one individual. We can then stop pouring so much consciousness into our own obsession with material well-being and begin to look for ways to develop a more fulfilling selflessness. By controlling the brain peptides in meditation, for example, we can develop traits of altruism, sensitivity to others, and greater sensitivity to the environment. The more the nuclear self communicates with the vast total of the cosmic environment through meditation, the more individual behavior is modified naturally so that deep communication between separate individual persons (which is the foundation of true group consciousness) automatically turns into a deeper love without resentments. Much of human love is possessive, self-serving and egocentric, causing pain and resentment, making as much division among emotionally immature people as there is union. Yet man has not yet learned from this painful division, nor is he fully aware of the lack of love and communication at the root of all hostility and wars.

It is possible for man's intelligence to tune into natural systems and devise ways of resolving conflicts and competition among individuals. In Nature, species do not necessarily conflict to the death but, by ritual behavior or rules by which both hostile parties may discharge their aggression, they conflict with honor and respect for each other. Such is the method of Creative Conflict discovered by the author over many years of experimentation with groups of people who confront each other as egos with the purpose of settling differences or at least agreeing to be different.* Thus the narrow tubular consciousness of

* See chapters on Creative Conflict in this book, pages 709-97.

each individual with its own likes and dislikes gradually comes to be aware of itself as an extended self who is invisibly joined to others in society with similar needs for self-confirmation and fulfillment which need not be obtained at the expense of fellowman. The more we respond to group evolution as an individual working for self-mastery, the more we become sensitive to methods of protecting ourselves against the power of ignorance and the corruption of egocentric individuals who exploit both the environment and society.

Nuclear Evolution, once realized within any individual who sees the potential for deeper communication of his or her being or sees the depths of several levels of consciousness, is much like an awesome glimpse into a new world that is not a utopian dream state but is actually humanly possible. The excitement of being part of an evolutionary group engaged in the refashioning of our own consciousness without being brainwashed by pre-existing doctrines or by adherence to anything but the most pure manifestations of consciousness in others, immediately gives us an insight into why most of our work and talk about society is so dull and dreary. Anyone who has been to a communist country from a Western democracy is immediately struck by the greyness and drabness of life behind the Iron Curtain. The socialists fear greatly that their peoples will be contaminated and their system undermined by free peoples who live a more abundant life with so many choices. Thus communication is censored and repressed, and the freedom to evolve ever-enlightening systems is denied.

Those who control such societies are using materialistic theories of evolution and genetics, in the name of the collective group, to gain power for selfish ends without regard to the thought that perhaps evolution has its own end, a more intelligent purpose. The communist urge to stamp out all known opposition, kill rebellious spirits and destroy the urge to freedom on an enormous scale is, if we believe the geneticists and environmentalists, killing off the spirit of rebellion and individualism and wiping it out of the genetic pool of the human race forever. With mankind thus made even more submissive than he is already, the control of power-hungry people would be assured. But are the geneticists correct? Despite attempts to breed the higher spiritual qualities out of existence, the communists have been unable to stamp

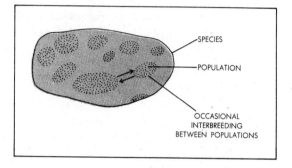

Concept of a gene pool. In a species, genes flow within and between populations. The total gene content of the species thus represents a gene pool to which all members of the species have access. Genes normally cannot flow between the gene pools of two different species.

The human gene pool is the collective potential of mankind, made up of all the gene material as it has evolved over the ages—the kind and quality of gene characteristics we have collectively bred through our choices. By selective breeding mankind has produced efficient herds of cattle and crops. In human affairs, political actions in some countries have the effect of repressing the genes of those with the will to resist and thereby eliminating those who can think for themselves.

out the evolutionary spirit. So we may have to change our whole way of thinking about evolution and perhaps undo some of what Darwin's ideas have done to man's idea of himself.

The problem of such great diversity in Nature intrigued Darwin, particularly in the dimension of the origin of the great multiplicity of species in a horizontal sweep across evolution. But Nuclear Evolution is more concerned with the transmutation of species in a vertical evolution very different from the concept of natural biological selection. Darwin's concept that the process of evolution is purely biological, gradual, continuous, and does not consist of any sudden changes is true for nonthinking species who do not have the free will to choose a more difficult but more challenging path through many varieties of behavior. If man's course had always been dictated by the easiest path and he had adapted to given conditions rather than mastered and changed his environment to suit himself, then the Darwinian concept of gradual growth and change could be universally applied. But even with animals, it appears now that evolutionary growth actually advances by spurts and we cannot limit it just to the gradual process of adaptation.

In all natural systems sufficient potential must build up in the existing manifested state of the organism to provide the energy for a leap or a breakthrough. Every manifested organism has emerged from a former potential state that has built up into an evolutionary pressure which is discharged when the organism breaks through to its next level of manifestation. In the same way that every manifested organism builds up a potential out of its manifested state through learned responses to the environment, so does every potential state have imprisoned within it the next state of manifestation. Like the chicken and the egg, the manifested and potential cannot be separated. Therefore evolution is a series of spurts, sometimes with great intervals of time between the spurts. During these intervals, while the potential is building up and Nature is preparing for its next leap, very little change appears to be going on. The next leap is often communicated very swiftly to other organisms of the same species when the breakthrough manifests anywhere on the planet. Other organisms of the same species whose potential has also built up in relation to the total environment are ready for some trigger. A process akin to crystallization takes place on a higher level in the potential state before triggering the next manifested state of the organism. Whether the organism is human or bacteria or enzymes makes little difference to Nature's methods of transmitting the trigger which provides the signal for the potential to crystallize into the manifestation at the physical level.

This process can be experimentally proved by setting up two identical cultures of enzymes or bacteria separated by a quartz window where one culture is stimulated to perform a learned reaction that the other one does not yet know. The culture which is not stimulated ends up performing the same operation by some form of communication which it receives through the quartz window. After only a short period of time the second enzyme undergoes a similar change of reaction even though there has been no physical contact between the two cultures.*

---

* Russian experiments have been done with "thought" transfer between enzymes separated by quartz crystal, as reported in *Science News*.

Whether there is some tele-thought connection enabling the communication between the two, or whether the quartz is somehow permeable to some energy or substance, is irrelevant to the fact that one group of organisms is in fact capable of communicating to the other. This experiment is akin to the famous female genius monkey who threw her rice grains which were mixed up with sand into the sea so that the sand fell to the bottom and she scooped the floating rice grains up into her mouth, while the rest of the tribe continued to pick each grain of rice out of the sand. But once one of the other monkeys noticed what the genius monkey was doing, it was only a matter of time before the whole troupe began throwing their mixtures of rice and sand into the sea. This spurt in evolution of behavior is absolutely no different than the way intelligence is communicated in evolution by consciousness. A physical link is not required. Humans can receive that transmission on seven different levels of consciousness either through a look, or from soul to soul, or by thought transference which requires no physical proximity, and this is called telepathy or tele-thought. The sophisticated network of the human physical communications television system coupled to tele-thought will make the next leap in human evolution manifest very swiftly, once the necessary threshold of potential has indeed been reached. This consciousness theory of the progress of Nuclear Evolution by sudden leaps coexists with Darwinian theory of evolution by slow adaptation in that the learned responses of adaptation must build up to a certain threshold of potential before the breakthrough to another level of functioning can manifest.

EVOLUTION BY ADAPTATION

Modern biologists now study the DNA in the cell nucleus, which is organized in several kinds of self-replicating genes that can mutate and create alternative forms of the nucleus of cells. The characteristics which adapted to fit the environment are then passed on to succeeding generations. By this theory the giraffe would have evolved his long neck to be able to reach the leaves on tall trees. But it does not explain why the zebra did not do the same. The problem with attributing all biological change merely to environmental pressures is the tremendous variety of species and the diversification that has accompanied the climbing out of the water onto the land. Why did warm-blooded animals evolve in the same environment as cold-blooded ones?

In their recent experiments with recombinant DNA, scientists are artificially duplicating the natural process by which genes adapt to the environment. This gives the scientists the power to control the patterns of life. The frightening possibilities of these discoveries have created turmoil in sociobiology, the new science of applying genetic factors to social organization. Scientists tell us that the human future will be quite different from anything we have ever known before, and people get upset about it because they have their identity at the social level of life. Harvard scientist, Edward O. Wilson, who really started the whole controversy, has suggested that the living organism does not live for itself and that its primary function is not even to reproduce other organisms but solely to produce genes. In other words, humans are merely the natural slaves of genes, the workers that act as temporary carriers of the genes, to and from the cosmic intelligent gene pool.

E.O. Wilson argues that social behavior has a biological base. He maintains all studies of mankind must start with his body which shapes and limits human nature. He sees worldly success as genetically determined.

Some of Wilson's other views:

★ Humans seem to have a genetic predisposition toward learning some form of communal aggression. The way to control it is to "create a confusion of cross-binding loyalties" to various groups.

★ The incest taboo, the persistence of the nuclear family and the failure of slavery are all due to biological predispositions.

★ Religion appears to confer a biological advantage on believers by promoting the welfare of the group. Biology limits the ways in which religion can evolve, and those different pathways "may not even be numerous."

In this view it is even doubtful whether humans make a contribution to influence events. The genes decide things. Intelligence is genetic, maybe even racial. If what Wilson says is true, then some scholars argue that white people can use it as an argument that black people are inferior to whites because of their genes, and it becomes a very explosive issue. But all these emotions and social implications are irrelevant until the theory is proven true. Instead of penetrating to the heart of the nucleus we waste our consciousness on all these side issues. We are no wiser than the shallow religionists who opposed Darwin. And in fact the same religious dogmatism is still happening today.

On the one hand we have science with an overly materialistic view of man, and on the other hand religion with a naive "other worldly" view. In spite of the fact that the vast majority of scientists today believes that the evidence of the DNA shows overwhelming proof of evolution as the process by which human beings have come to this world, the DNA is no proof at all to millions of fundamentalist Christians who believe, on the authority of the Bible, that the world did not evolve but was created in one stroke of universal force by God in the sense of "Fiat Lux" (And God said, "Let there be light!") Biology says that our origins are not cosmic but from the earth itself, the genes becoming adapted to the peculiar climate and conditions prevailing in our planet's history. But the chain of events, which scientists say has led us from lower organisms that in some primordial age somehow formed themselves purely from inanimate, inorganic material pieces of the elements, horrifies some people. The fundamentalists reject what they don't understand. Rather than wrap their minds around the issue and find out what it is all about, they cling to ancient scriptures dogmatically, rejecting any new light at all with a vociferousness equal to that of the scientists who also reject all but their own mechanistic views. They do not see that there is no real contradiction between evolution and religion if only we go deep enough. Professor Wilson speculates in his theory far beyond the material genes into actual behavior, but his wild conclusions are based only on the material genes. We should find out how our own consciousness influences the genes, and this will prove whether or not his theory is valid.

Some biologists are now beginning to see the meeting point between genetics and spiritual laws, namely that our genetic instructions found in the DNA of the genes inside the nucleus are no more than a framework of different possibilities, the rough limits of opportunity to what we may eventually become. In other words, the presence of a perfect set of genes does not guarantee that the organism will succeed in using all its potentialities or even be able to express them. Whether we use our potential or not is up to us. Or to put it in religious terms, we are not coerced by the Evolutionary Intelligence which leaves us free to resist the cosmic program within us if we so choose. This more enlightened scientific view of evolution leads us to marvel at the unfolding of the cosmic plan as a program directed by an inscrutable Intelligence which through the gene pool prepares the destiny of organisms many millions of years in advance and provides them with faculties which they will some day use, though at the moment they do not even understand them. Nuclear Evolution does not conflict at the physical level with this current research into genetics but goes beyond it in the sense that Nuclear Evolution extends to areas which can be tested through Supersensonic methods and by ordinary people in everyday life with their own biological equipment which Nature has already programmed in the DNA. In other words, we are not dependent upon the environment to trigger in us the adaptations which will fulfill the cosmic program written in our genes, but can actively change ourselves—not by a gradual series of small adaptations but by a radical dynamic change of attitude. By changing from separated thoughts to intuitions of wholeness, we tune to the nucleus of our being and the very source of evolution and creation. It is this *source* which created the genes and designed the mechanisms by which we "adapt to environment".

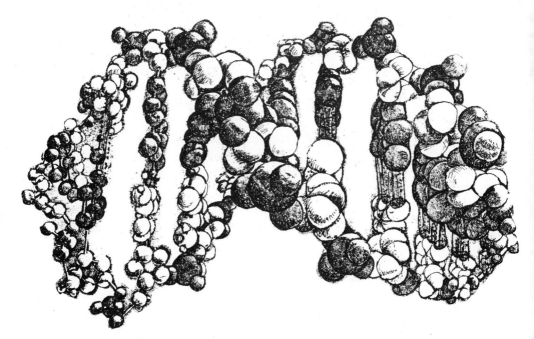

Picture shows the conception of the DNA molecule with its code of life.

HOW WILL SCIENCE EVOLVE?

The famous incident when Thomas Edison demonstrated the phonograph before the established members of the Academy of Science who saw the machine working with their very own eyes yet refused to believe the sounds were not coming from behind a screen even though there was no screen present, reveals the difference between insight and eyesight, between noumena and phenomena, between spirit and matter. This incident is not an isolated incident as some believe, but an established ingrained pattern in the human race that is probably self-suggested into the genes. For you to *see* and not believe, or *believe* without seeing or needing any proof, is the difference between two totally separate levels of consciousness which we can label insight or eyesight, intuitive or sensory, numinal or phenomenal.

An illustration of how insight rather than eyesight works in the development of a system can be seen in the evolution of science itself. Most scientists see the way we go about acquiring knowledge by the scientific method as a rigorous evolutionary discipline, changing, adapting to new evidence and in a constant state of revolution, overturning old concepts, ideas and updating observations of phenomena. Yet in practice it does not work that way with the fundamental ideas we call paradigms. In almost every case of a fundamental world-changing insight there has been resistance to accepting the new evidence because it is so strange or looks too good to be true. Einstein's ideas were resisted to the bitter end by scientists who saw them as a threat to what was already known and long settled as established observed facts. Yet in truth Einstein's ideas won out over the massive skepticism just as Galileo's, Newton's and Edison's ideas won out, despite the opposition of their arrogant contemporaries.

The evolution of science as a sophisticated method of procedure has been delayed by the tendency to discount insight and all numinous experience against the evidence of measurable concrete material phenomena. Indeed many scientists claim that science has no business at all entering the world of the spirit or consciousness where the observer himself is the subject. Objectivity in science has evolved through the study of objects and not subjective knowledge, and this attitude has been the approach to the genes and the cosmic message written in the DNA. Yet the continuing evolution of science has always depended on people who had the courage and insight to defy the weight of the consensus opinion, who went on to discover the bridges between the noumena and phenomena, the aesthetic and the objective, the insight and the sensory eyesight.

What is now going to convince those who view the scientific method as a fixed, unalterable limitation, a discipline which forbids a scientist to look for any relationships between spirit and matter? The insight of an Einstein, a Schrodinger or a Newton into scientific method itself is just as important in the evolution of science as the theories and models they give us, for these insights have shown us the way to penetrate the nuclear intelligence in the atom, the DNA nucleus of the cell, in exactly the same way that consciousness can now penetrate and discover the cosmic message programmed into the genes. But what will convince scientists that there is such a thing as spirit or consciousness?

The only convincing argument to a skeptic is an actual demonstration, but here again we have a problem: even when faced with demonstrable facts many skeptical scientists refuse to look at them until they become incontrovertible common knowledge, and even then they tend to explain them away conceptually. The fact is that everyone has the proof within them at any moment that spirit and consciousness not only exist but can affect material patterns of growth, enzyme development, biochemical secretions, not only in our internal environment of the body but also in experiments which project our consciousness out into the external world where similar effects of consciousness can be brought to influence enzyme production, light synthesis, and the growth of DNA in plants, animals and humans. A demonstration of this faculty of the human mind is more convincing than mere theory, but it does not lead to a massive change in the materialist outlook. It is a fact that consciousness can really change the replication of DNA at the source of its synthesis at the moment it is being created in the nucleus. But for some reason the materialist does not see or even want to see the profound implications of this fact for the evolution of the scientific method or even the human race. What are the implications? *Once the DNA has been created, the mind can only affect it by affecting its environment, but while the DNA is in the process of being created, the mind has the power to affect the DNA directly.* And what is the difference between these two modes of self-change?

One difference is that human change is painfully slow if we wait for the environment to change us, and even then the change is not permanent since we can always revert back, like a hybrid plant species, to a former primitive state. Because the power of consciousness controls the enkephalins and peptides which are all-powerful triggers of internal reality, they act like LSD in producing chromosome breaks and in causing the development and extension of existing nerve dendrites in the brain. These receptors grow towards the greatest point of stimulation like an etiolating plant reaches for the light. It is now possible for members of the human race to induce the development of new pathways in the brain that can channel our consciousness to do exactly the same thing that evolution, adaptation and the teleological end-purposes of Nature have done over long periods through constant environmental change. This capability, hitherto considered impossible by scientists who dogmatically have stated that nerve cells and brain cells cannot grow back once damaged, makes our evolution a matter of intensive concentration and one hundred percent self-suggestion exercises for everyone to awaken the seventh brain and promote a different ontology or science of being. The power of consciousness at certain states of intensity to change the DNA is the link which has so far been missing from the scientist's list of facts.

Up to now Western science has viewed psychology and religion separately and has developed no science of being beyond the ontology of a few philosophers who said no man can know what consciousness is and even questioned if consciousness exists! Now we can control the unfolding of our personality, its secretions of hormones, its responses to environmental conditions and susceptibility to disease, and it is now possible to condition our own happiness and fulfillment rather than succumb to external conditions. To begin working consciously for world transformation by first achieving peace within our own being is to become an expressive instrument of the cosmic purpose, for this peace of mind opens up our evolution into the superconscious state, that amplified supersensitive faculty which is already programmed into the sevenfold brain.

It is now possible to do simple experiments of mind control over enzyme production and internal altered states of consciousness which reveal that certain skills can be acquired which ancient sages and yogis once had.* Most scientists even refuse to try such experiments on the grounds that only crazy people would attempt to do this, and if scientists did do the experiments they would want to base their experimental research on a few unique individuals who they could control in a laboratory. They go to someone who can mentally bend spoons, on the assumption that only a few people can do it. But the fact is that lots of people can mentally bend spoons who do not even know they can do it. If these performers could however bend *minds* instead of spoons and shape their own "mind stuff" into new evolutionary patterns, they could change the crystal structures of the DNA chemicals just as the mind changes the crystal structures in the metal of the spoons. It would be useless scientifically to have only one person do these experiments with consciousness, therefore larger groups must now experiment until the skill can be spread to the entire society on a grass roots level. When the demonstration of mind over matter can take place across whole large sections of society, noumena will become phenomena, spirit will become matter. Unless this wider demonstration takes place, scientists will write off the few individuals who can demonstrate it just as they wrote off the invention of the gramophone until so many people were actually using it that science was forced to accept it. Mind over matter is not new, but to many scientists it is nothing short of supernatural and is therefore superstitition and not in the province of science at all. Thus it has no importance to them. This negation of the way insight actually works its magic by constantly trying many odd unlikely combinations, is the very reason why science has not yet evolved enough to study its own origins and to penetrate its incredible dialectic between spirit and matter. This is now changing with the model of Nuclear Evolution and the black hole where the concrete existence of atoms has disappeared

---

* *Rumf Roomph Yoga* tape series gives instructions for the development of brain potentials, while *Supersensonics* explores the faculties of the supersensitive life of man. (See back of book).

and in their place has come the singularity, the absolute, the power of pure consciousness to dictate the shapelessness or form of energy before it is crystallized into the crystal lattices of matter.

THE DESTINY OF THE CELL

Another Darwinian principle that is true on the lower levels of consciousness and yet, in a wider vision, quite false is the idea that whatever survives physically must be the fittest. By looking only at the physical level of evolution in total blindness to the other six levels of consciousness on which humans are or could be functioning, the science of genetics has ignored the well-documented evidence that psycho-physical mechanisms of change in individual behavior are not only genetic but are also inherited through ritual and strong tradition. Darwinian theory seeks to explain by reason and orderly classification the nature of animal existence but does not take account of the fact that man's traditional stores of symbolic intelligence do not always occur in other animals, and that man's altruistic, moral, selfless higher consciousness leads to the direct transmittance of another order of abstract intelligence from one generation to the next. The Jewish tradition of the invisible one God which cannot be pictured in any graven image nor embodied in any man (not even in a Christ), or the Hindu tradition of one God who is in everything and yet nothing, have actually changed and evolved the human social world to open higher levels of consciousness more than any adaptation to the physical environment has ever done. In these ancient traditions the human race has preserved and nurtured that wisdom which speaks of immortality rather than survival and which traces evolution not in time, but in the light of expanded awareness. If the world should come to the brink of self-destruction through clinging to the lower levels of consciousness, and if the race of man misuses the laws of God and of Nature for selfish ends, who then will be fit to survive? Will it be those whose physical muscles are strongest or those whose wits are keenest? Or will it be those who have sought the light and learned the secrets of immortality?

On the other hand, when enhancement of evolutionary development is transmitted from generation to generation through science, a tradition or through an ideal model, an imaginative myth, religions or political philosophy, its total cultural content can be destroyed in one generation because its transmission of pattern is on the fifth level of the conceptual mind and, although deeply ingrained in the society, these ideas are not yet fixed in the genetic material of the body. One of the explicit purposes of Mao Tse-tung was to completely eradicate the cultural conditioning of Buddhism and ancient Chinese values, like property ownership, which prevailed in pre-communist China. By systematic and continuous brainwashing along with forced change and killing off of all resisters, a cultural program of many thousands of years has been virtually wiped out in one generation. Similarly, the Jewish tradition is

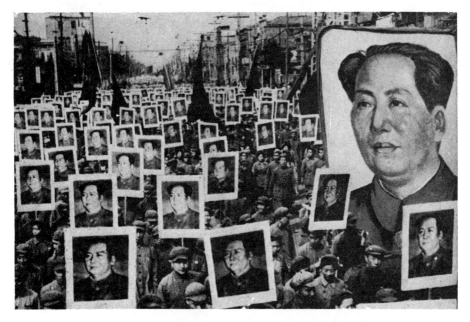

For the millions who supported the fanatics, millions more had to die.

so strong that one would almost swear that to be a Jew were "in the genes", but a nonpracticing Jew who feels no identity with being Jewish is just like anyone else; his responses and behavior are totally different from those of practicing Jews. What then is the value of a cultural tradition if its effects are so easily wiped out? The value is in its power to evolve the human consciousness, to provide an environment which stimulates and can awaken more of the existing potential lying dormant within the genes. If we raise the question, "Is the transmission of intelligence, altruism, selflessness, etc., genetic or cultural?", there is no either/or way to answer it. We would have to say that while the *mechanism* of cultural and racial conditioning is genetic, the *content* is not. All cultural programs, no matter how much they enhance our evolution, can be wiped out by a new psychological environment, i.e., the *content* of these cultural programs can be wiped out. But the mechanism by which cultural factors affect the genes remains the same, and this is the important insight into ourselves—that our culture, our surroundings, our mental environment all affect the genes by creating an aura around them which calls forth certain potentials and suppresses others. A new environment does no more than shift this emphasis, calling forth a different set of potentials.

In order to grasp the full import of this fact, we have to realize what our genes really are and how they affect our lives every day. Some people associate genetics solely with childbearing and think of heredity as the passing of unique physical characteristics in the DNA from parent to child. But in fact the genes appear in every cell of the human body (and in every cell of creation). A photograph of a cell from the salivary gland of any creature will show genes and chromosomes slightly different from a liver cell in the same creature because the cells have taken on specialized functions, but nevertheless the chromosomes are in every cell, because the original cell from which we were formed, the fertilized ovum, divided itself in two and in both cells the whole

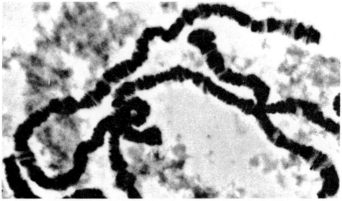

The giant chromosomes from the salivary gland of a fruitfly.

DNA of the original cell was present. Then it divided into four and then eight and kept on dividing until the entire cellular structure of the body was complete. Then it began to grow from a baby into an adult, and this growth was all controlled by the intelligence (the DNA) inside each cell. Every day, as old skin dies and we form new skin, the Master Intelligence working through the genes in each of our cells is carrying on these life processes for us, sending out its messages through the RNA. Our conscious personality does not know how to make new skin or to renew the cells of the eyes, but this process of renewal is the real subject of the science of genetics. Why is this important? Because our consciousness has the power to affect that renewal. We have the power to change ourselves.

The self-obsessive way that men and women love, hate, worry and stress themselves into sickness is imprinted in the biological patterns of life in the brain structures and passed down the line of evolution. We can see that these traits are hereditary in the human race because they are continued in our children over long periods of time, regardless of culture. But written also in the genes is the guiding pathway that can transcend human hatred, fear and instincts for fight or flight because selflessness and altruism become essential for survival at a higher point in evolution.

Every cell has a nucleus hologram in it. Just as the body contains in every cell the imprinted material of the original cell from which it sprung and each cell therefore contains both father and mother, so too each cell of the body of the universe contains within it the original primordial nucleus from which it sprung. The DNA in every cell in the whole universe is beeping the same universal cosmic message. Thus the cell's deepest identity is its oneness with the universe. All cells are the same kind of cells until they become specialized into eye cells, blood cells, bone cells, brain cells, etc., at the behest of the cosmic orchestrator. Then another level of identity is added to the primordial level by the fact that the cell is living in an internal psychic environment created by our heredity, external environment and karma, all of which determine which part of the DNA potentials will be enhanced or pushed back. In other words, the nucleus has the identical capacity to adapt to its immediate environment at the level of gene formation as humans and animals have to adapt to their local environment on the planet.

The seven levels of consciousness with their positive and negative qualities are programmed into the genetic make-up, but how we choose to use those levels is up to us. The cultural programming we mentioned before creates our environment because the second level, the human social consciousness, is written in our genes. The particular

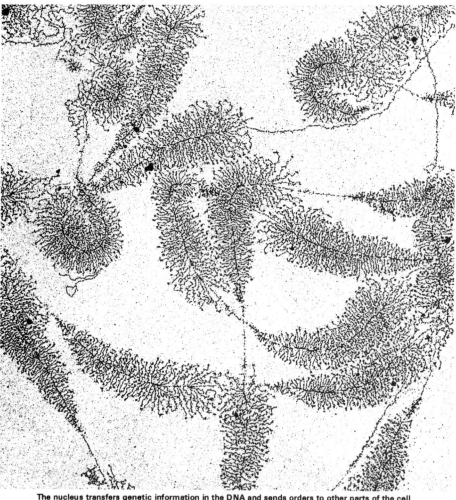

The nucleus transfers genetic information in the DNA and sends orders to other parts of the cell by means of a messenger substance (RNA). Picture shows the beginning of the process inside the nucleus. The central backbone of each carrot-like structure is a chain of DNA which acts as a template. Each DNA strand is synthesizing about 100 RNA molecular strands. The process is beginning at the narrow pointed ends of each "carrot" while the longer fibers at the thicker end are almost completed strands of messenger RNA.

program itself may change, but the social consciousness will always be there working through the second brain area. The lower levels of consciousness of the lower brains, which lead to the baser instincts, are as much a part of the potential of the DNA as is the seventh level of consciousness, which develops selflessness and altruism along with the awareness of the oneness of life. The higher brain uses the lower brains as its servants, and if the servants are unruly, stubborn or unaware of anything higher than their own perceptions the seventh level cannot manifest its potential inherited from the genes or the environment. When we talk about heredity and environment at this level, we are talking about the destiny of the cell and we are talking about the destiny of the person, and the two are one and the same. Genes are the code units, the central intelligence in the day to day activities of living cells. It is the DNA itself which creates the potentials, and we activate our various brain centers depending upon our choices and responses to our environment. Why is it that humanity chooses to respond primarily to the base and materialistic, selfish and low potentials in the gene pool?

In our social government we subjugate everything to what wins votes and therefore neglect what is good for the country as a whole, which becomes the great stumbling block to the evolutionary progress of our free democracies. In the same way, hatred, fear and stress locked in the genes of the human brain prevent the unfolding of the higher potential lying in the genes of the higher brain. The genes of the seventh brain lie waiting for us to awaken them into activity by our overcoming the conflicts which block us on all the lower levels of consciousness. We are now called upon to guide our human systems of government to evolve ways of overcoming stress and hatred and sublimating the lower levels of love imprinted in the genes of our lower brains. Any organism which becomes superintelligent must eventually become aware of the whole as an interlinked total process which includes itself. All organic life, whether in humans or in the soil, is ultimately made up of basic inorganic chemicals and atoms, like vitamins and minerals, which are essential to organic growth. In the same way, the atoms, cells and genes comprising the seventh brain which can guide the human organism towards another kind of love which does not require a love object, depend on the right organic application of consciousness for their growth. Consciousness is to the body as fertilizer is to a plant grown in rock or sand. Without it, the plant is stunted, does not flower or produces no seed. We nurture and form our cells and organs as we do our crops, increasing their yield by skillful organization of the field of consciousness. The message of Nuclear Evolution is simply this startling fact—that we have the power to change this psychic environment* and to change the DNA program written in our cells and thus to affect the level of evolution of the human race.

To modern science, heredity is a synonym for evolution. Yet our genetic or cultural inheritance from the past tends only to perpetuate the past—whether it is grandfather's nose, some primitive feeling from our cave man ancestry or some archaic tradition we cling to for security—while the real thrust of evolution actually comes from new ideas transmitted from the original mind and imagination of genius that cause us to respond in a new way and thus awaken some of the sleeping potential lying within the genes. At the moment the gene pool in society through which the message of life is carried on through sexual encounters is obviously influenced by environment and cultural interchange of scientific, religious and philosophical beliefs, but such influences are only working out at very superficial levels. For instance, most conflicts between humans are only resolved at the levels of polarized positions between labor and management, science and religion, marriage and family difficulties, property rights, legal disputes, etc., and none of this requires individuals to change even one aspect of their thought life. Millions of people can go from birth to death through many levels of conflict and remain entrenched in their egotism and opinions without ever facing the crucial ego conflict within themselves.

To contact the level of the intelligence in the genes already present in the higher brain, people must first resolve the conflict in their own consciousness between their image of themselves as a separate entity

---

* By *psychic environment* I refer to the information stored not only in the nucleic acids in the sequence of DNA changes during growth of our life history, but also the information stored in the spin, the magnetic structure and polarization of the atoms in the fluid surrounding the nucleus in our cells.

and the external environment. The environment has in the ultimate sense continuously contributed its total intelligence during the long process of evolutionary formation of the nucleus, meaning that the nucleus has within it a higher order of intelligence programmed from the total environment in which it has grown through billions of years of biological existence and development. The nucleus is like a template where the DNA is analagous to a phonograph record of all the sounds that the universe has ever made. The problem is that we have not yet developed a record player or needle fine enough to reproduce the fidelity of the signals encoded in the record. Now it becomes necessary for man to transcend his present sexual use of the gene pool and raise its potential in order to resolve his conflicts, both inner and outer, which result from the belief in his own personal will and ego which is at loggerheads with the universal will represented in the total environment of which he is an indivisible part. This conflict emerges in ordinary daily life, at the common level of the gene pool in which the lower levels are enhanced and the higher levels suppressed, causing the selfish actions of humans to be totally divorced from the commonweal. This selfishness opposes the universal will which is to ultimately dissolve all that separates the individual parts from the whole in which they exist.

How is this higher program of consciousness recorded in the higher brains from the evolutionary program of the cosmic intelligence going to emerge and suppress the present level of the lower gene functions? How is humanity going to select the higher genes from the total gene pool? Just as the whole of evolution is based on the capacity of organisms to adapt to environmental conditions over long periods of time which changes the structure of the genes and its hereditary message, so does consciousness have the power to create a new chemical environment within the cell around the genes over a short period of time of one human incarnation. Consciousness being all-powerful over the biological environment, capable of providing stress, acidity, alkalinity, biological energy at the cell level of ATP synthesis and release of bioelectrical currents at will for good or ill over the development of the DNA structure, becomes the higher evolutionary program of the seventh brain. *The discovery of the nature of conscious-ness is the fundamental purpose of the cosmos.* All humans existing at the lower levels of the gene pool who do not enhance this cosmic purpose are of no real value in the eyes of the cosmic intelligence, since it is ruthless in its universal drive for perfection. Cosmic intelligence has automatically built into the cosmos a shut-off point that closes off the human from the higher levels whenever that human's purpose differs from the purpose of cosmic evolution. The gene trigger to the higher levels is in the hands of man only if his consciousness is in tune with the cosmos.

Once the human being realizes that its consciousness has the power to determine whether or not the nucleus of its cells will be surrounded with a stress-free blissful supply of chemical nutrients which foster the emergence of the higher genetic memory, then automatically the lower gene patterns of hate, fear, schizophrenia, etc., can be overcome. It then becomes abundantly clear that the human race must pay far more attention to the quality of its thoughts and their effects on the biochemical

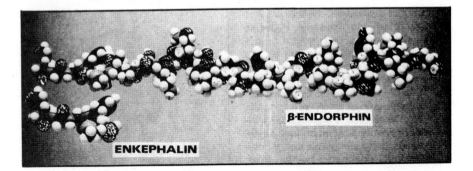

The large molecule beta-endorphin, shown above, (prepared by Sandoz Laboratories) contains the smaller molecule of the psycho-active pituitary gland hormone enkephalin. This seven-amino-acid-peptide sequence is controlled by our consciousness and has been found experimentally to help memory and concentration. When taken as a drug, mentally retarded subjects work better and senile subjects can remember better.* It also reduces anxiety, brings inner peace and counters depression in psychiatric patients within ten minutes after injection. With its aid many schizophrenics have been helped to regain their normal personalities.

---

* These experiments were done by Abba J. Kastin, Veteran's Administration Medical Center in New Orleans, Curt A. Sandman of Ohio State University and Lyle Miller of Boston University School of Medicine. *Science News,* Vol. 114, No. 22.

environment of the brain cells. The recent discoveries of the enkephalins, endorphins and peptides secreted in the third ventricle by the various biological computers which surround the walls of the ventricle, confirm that psychological conditions such as depression, schizophrenia, suicide, manic behavior, etc., are not only self-induced by the response of the individual to life situations, but can be communicated to the genes which set themselves up in patterns that conform to their surrounding psychological energy field and chemical environment.* In the same way that man allows himself to be conditioned by the society he is bred in, so does the DNA allow itself to be influenced by the genes and their psychic environment. But this is not predestined because anyone who so chooses can totally rise above or disregard the culture in which he or she was born and re-create it or take on another culture which proves that life and its adaption to environment is purely a matter of choice.

This choice that humans have between selfish will and the cosmic purpose, the choice that atoms have as to the molecules they attach themselves to, the choices that lead to the secretion of endorphins and the vibrating cilia which carry them across the floor of the third ventricle of our brains, the choices between the cells and their relationships to the organs they comprise, which can break down in cancer and other disease, all these decisions and selections go on according to genetic programs already in the nucleus of every organism and are modified by the ability of that organism to respond to the situations it is confronted with. The ability to respond is the key to all environmental change, as it is also the key to changes in the nucleus, like adaptation, survival, evolution. In the strictest sense, the ability to respond is translated as responsibility. Responsibility, or the ability to respond, is not only the secret of evolution but the basis upon which the cosmos is structured. The cell is the servant of the nucleus and its genes and is

---

* The first molecular evidence of a genetic link showing an inherited pattern of depression among offspring of depressed parents is reported by David E. Comings, City of Hope Medical Center in Duarte, California. Seymour Katz found statistically a genetic predisposition to suicide in certain life situations among families of adoptees in Denmark. *Science News,* Oct. 7, 1978, p. 244.

responsible for creating the watery environment in which the genes can function, just as the womb is the servant of the forthcoming child, supplying all its physical nourishment. In the same way the human being is the servant of all the cells which enable consciousness and intelligence to manifest. And continuing the analogy, the earth is the servant of man, and the totality of space and the energies of the stars and sun are the servant of all life in the universe as well as on the earth's surface. The principle of responsibility of all parts of life for each other and the nourishment of cosmos to star, star to planet, planet to the organisms which it supports, is carried on down into the very structure of the DNA in the nucleus. The ability to respond to the whole is humanity's present evolutionary challenge, the subject of the whole of this book.

Only if we can understand how this cosmic message is written into the DNA, the messenger of life, will we be able to have a leap in human evolution where we carry out that responsibility on all levels of consciousness—physical, social, intellectual, economic, philosophical, intuitive and spiritual. The link between the cosmic message and the DNA messenger is the link between the numinous and the material, between spirit and matter, and is found in the intelligence in the nucleus. I use the term *nucleus* interchangeably both on the numinous level of the nuclear hologram of consciousness and on the material level of the nuclear program in the genes and cells of life. The quality of the message between the numinous and the material is determined by a combination of inheritance, environmental conditioning and our free use of consciousness.

TRAUMA AND KARMA

In order to see what blocks the cosmic evolutionary message from fully manifesting, even though the physical vehicle for its expression is already present and waiting in the seven brains, we must realize that there is another agent of heredity besides genes and culture. Our experiences of existence are written in nonmaterial consciousness with the same indelible ink that they are written in the DNA, and consciousness is not confined to the DNA which is its servant. In the nucleus of our own consciousness we are now everything we have ever been, the

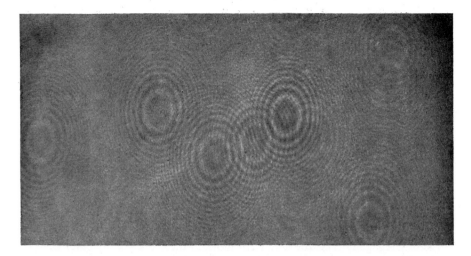

The above hologramic record of a chessboard was made by interfering wave-fronts which show how light patterns on a surface contain more information about a scene than an ordinary photograph, yet the hologram itself bears no reality to the original scene. By directing a beam of light through the hologram the waves of light reconstruct themselves and form an image of the original scene of the chessboard in mid-air which we can walk around and see the sides and back of the chess pieces just as we see them naturally with our eyes. Nuclear Evolution theory regards the human brain as a hologram, a natural capacitor in which the energy of consciousness is the light beam absorbed from all the starlight from space, and the brain and memory are like the recorded patterns encoded in the brain cells.

numina

yolk

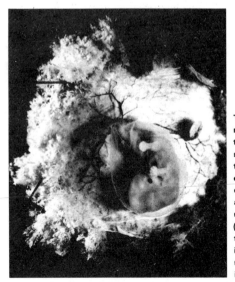

The hologram of life is not only imprinted in the yolk of the egg in seven levels of vibration but is communicated to the nucleus of every cell of our brain and body. The ancients used the staff of Hermes (Caduceus) to symbolize the transmission of information from the numinous to the material brain.

From the numinous nucleus of the yolk to the phenomenal nucleus in the gene.

genes

Note the similarity between the symbol of the staff of Hermes, the ancient messenger of the gods, and the double helix spiral of the DNA.

phenomena

total sum of all incarnations in all bodies. A person born into the twentieth century is enriched and changed and evolved by the inheritance of the past, passed to him through his culture and his parents' genes, and in addition he is inheriting his own past and his own karma through his own unconscious memory that is present with or without a body.

Who is the "I" that is using the inherited characteristics? Where does it come from? Is the "I" in one body different from the "I" in another? Each "I" is the sum total of its own experience—its moments of joy and sorrow, its successes and failures, its traumas and its responses to those traumas—all of which are recorded as vibration in memory and written into the events of our lives by the hand of the unconscious mind. We call this unconscious memory bank our "karma". Strictly speaking, karma is the end result of our choices and our reactions to situations. Karma is the law of cause and effect by which our every thought, word and deed brings its consequences. A good action will set forces in motion to bring us good reactions, while a bad action will rebound on us eventually with misfortune. The reason that karma is inevitable is because there can be no separation between a cause and its effect except in the time interval experienced in our minds. The law of karma operating as cause and effect is Nature's universal method of government working out and through every action taken. We cannot take any action in life except through our existing state of consciousness or our degree of awareness of the situation as it really is, and we can call this acting through our true nature or the natural state of our being. Christ and the Old Testament sages in Proverbs put it another way:

> "FOR AS A MAN THINKETH IN HIS HEART
> SO IS HE."

According to one's traumas, flights of fancy, concepts of the world, self-image and filters of awareness, so does a person act out on the world stage. In Nature we find the law of karma expressed in Newton's famous axiom, "Every action creates an equal and opposite reaction." Taken to other levels of consciousness, this axiom says that every manifested state of the material world has its potential state, every present moment has its prior conditions, every future moment has its potential in the manifested present. To bring our reasoning back to the objective body, we can state that its evolution, its manifestation, its potential, whether as a perfect set of genes or as a physical vehicle for the fact of consciousness and life, is definitely programmed by the subjective consciousness. In this sense, evolution can be seen to be working out in more than the physical dimension of the DNA nucleic acids. According to modern science, the genetics of evolution gives us our hereditary traits, yet wisdom and the spirit enter into the traits. With a change in consciousness our body can change, as in the case of faith healings. Hereditary patterns of facial characteristics have changed remarkably in a matter of days when there is a profound change to either positive or negative attitudes. Stress is not only the biggest killer in the form of heart disease which affects the biological tissues and heart muscle but also can permanently change our faces and bodies. If the biological instrument of our consciousness which we call our body is only an extended manifestation of the spirit that inhabits it, then the individual has the power of consciousness to change the body out of its genetic casting into a new form of organization.

Both trauma and karma work by the simple fact that consciousness has the power to shape and influence matter, to change our genetic possibilities, to foster or prevent the birth of the most promising set of genes, to conserve or waste genetic resources of the planet and to change the instrument of perception with or without drugs and intoxicants. Even in the womb, the traumatic effect of an event on the mother's consciousness can influence the inherited patterns in the fetus. While I was being born my mother experienced a flash of lightning in a thunderstorm during her labor which seemed to hit the building and come into the room so she put her hand over her eyes to shut out the brightness. In exactly the same place on her wrist where she felt a shock and got a slight burn, I had a large bright red mark on my wrist like a birthmark when I was born a few minutes later. It took over nine years to go away. She swears it was because of the lightning flash, but most people would put it down to coincidence.

Trauma is not only an imprint in a heart muscle or a nerve but an imprint in consciousness, and therefore it is the same as karma. Though karma or trauma may not be transmitted *through* the genes, it does condition the biological vehicle and the tensions between cells, or in other words vastly affects the environment in which the genes operate. Therefore it affects the way the genes grow. If you have a trauma in a muscle so that you can no longer move it, there is a disconnection between nerves and body. How do you release it? The trauma is recorded in the brain, but how does the brain work on itself? Like karma it is locked into a pattern and only you can change it, even though this means that the brain is trying to untangle its own knot.

Many psychological diseases, schizophrenia included, have their origin in the chemical knots formed in the releasing of brain hormones. These pineal and pituitary hormones rolling across the floor of the cave of the third ventricle, the Cave of Brahma, determine all of human personality. Feed people hormones and it changes their personality, changes their thresholds of pain or even the signals their brain sends to their stomach. The difference between feeding someone a hormone like a vitamin or a drug and creating that healing hormone directly from within by the power of consciousness is that the drug has to be administered in ever-increasing doses and the will and consciousness of the individual are not involved. The organism then adapts to the drug and becomes tolerant of it, whereas self-suggested hormone activity is an enhancement of the organism's own purpose. There is no tolerance level to the action of the chemical which is naturally secreted. Once the administered drug or chemical is withdrawn, the person experiences withdrawal symptoms since the drug has really been a crutch supporting it from the outside, whereas naturally–induced secretions are internally produced and do not create dependence on external supplies. Nevertheless, many personality changes can be effected through drugs or the secretion of hormones into the bloodstream or by the secretion of chemicals in the brain which can dramatically transform the way a person reacts to environmental conditions. But these are only temporary even if they last a lifetime, because the real evolution of a person is based on the evolution of the will.

Our reactions to the environment or to human situations or to people that we think are "disturbing" may cause traumatic reactions in

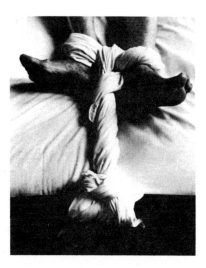

As with the use of the straitjacket, this method of restraining violent mental patients is not as prevalent as it was before the advent of "miracle" drugs.

our physical bodies and seem very real to us, but these are not caused solely by the environment at all. It is we who, by our response, make a disturbing situation disturbing. Most traumas are not real but are self-imposed. They are removable by the power of suggestion. Since they are caused by environmental circumstances and by our own imperma-nent attitudes, not by our deeper self, these traumas (no matter how deeply we think we feel them) are superficial temporary hurts and can be cleared instantaneously by a change in consciousness, i.e., by dissolving the ego pattern which is causing the hurt. Even the deeper hurt which originates by the division of consciousness from itself when the ego takes on a separate reality of its own, can be cleared by our imagination level of consciousness, because the ego is not real either but is self-created out of consciousness splitting off from itself. The ego *seems* real, just as people with paranoia truly believe that they are being chased or persecuted. But ego, karma and trauma all can be changed whether they are manifesting only on the psychological level or whether they are trapped in the muscles, nerves, cells or even affecting the gene functions.

Ego is a simple form of schizophrenia, not dangerous in normal manifestation except to itself, where it provides plenty of hurts. But imbalanced in the form of mental illness or chronic schizophrenia, the organism becomes disorientated and unable to see or understand itself at all. It creates its own unreal reality and trauma abounds. If the trauma has become one hundred percent self-suggestion of the imagination and one puts the full intensity of one's entire being behind it, then the effects of this mental separation (ego versus "other") is transferred by consciousness to the cell and its DNA nucleic acid structure. The separation becomes so embedded in the biological program that it affects the formation of genes and the instability is transmitted to offspring so that schizophrenia becomes hereditary. But in most cases the genes are not so deeply affected. Even a schizophrenic whose chemical balance has been disturbed by a psychotic condition of the parent carries with him the ability to succumb to the condition or to counteract the warp in the chemical formation of the psychic field of consciousness in the DNA of the gene. Severe schizophrenia is a result of one hundred percent self-suggestion of total separation either in the parent or in the child, and this suggestion has its effect on the brain cell and on chemical life. Yogic trance is the opposite of schizophrenia because it is one hundred percent suggestion of unity. This exercise, done by yogis for centuries, provides a blissful chemical environment for genes and allows the cosmic program to subjugate the lower genetic garbage in the gene pool. Few people, even among really insane schizophrenics, take their fantasies to the level of the real imagination that can program such deep genetic self-suggestion. And even if they did, it is consciousness which has imprinted the separation in the genes, and therefore consciousness can remove it. Not only can consciousness easily wipe out our sense of being separate from the environment, but even when it has penetrated into our being so deeply that it affects the DNA, even then the power to change ourselves is still in our own hands provided we have the will to do it.

This revolutionary understanding of genetics is radically different to that view of intelligence which holds that our brain functions and cell life are determined once and for all by the patterning of the genes at birth. The power of consciousness called *kundalini*, from the Sanskrit root word "to burn", is known in yogic disciplines to transform the nervous system so that the brain undergoes microbiological changes which are easily visible in the whole gestalt of the body. The secretion of melatonin from the pineal center triggers the sexual activity of the sex organs so that the sexual fluids enter the cerebrospinal fluid and affect the brain centers. These biological changes are imprinted in the genes of the enlightened and our spiritual progress can be passed on to our progeny. However, these genetic changes in the structure of DNA are not always available to offspring without the consciousness of the progeny desiring to develop the potential of their genetic program by their own will. No one can be forced to develop the potentials against their own will and no one can be forced to adapt to environmental factors against their will. Human beings do adapt to the environment, but in actual fact in unity consciousness where there is one hundred percent suggestion, there is no external environment for us to adapt to. Ego creates the internal and external environment by separating itself in consciousness from the whole. Without an ego there is no such thing as an external environment separate from our consciousness of Self. A person not engaged in change and self-knowledge or search for the origin of his own self-consciousness or egocentricity is not aware of the original "sin" of egohood and therefore becomes subject to his own illusions of separateness and is forced to adapt to the environment. The less evolved we are, the more the superintelligence in the environment presses one to change, to adapt, to surrender to fate. Industrial man has tried to dominate the natural environment, but Nature will not yield and forces him to look at his impoverishment of the earth or die out as a species. The universe or total environment is too powerful for an individual ego to dominate or fight so he can only work *with* it and eventually must surrender to it. If he surrenders in a passive, unthinking way, we could call it adapting to the environment, whereas the surrender of those who are truly spiritual is active and happens by their own awareness and volition. It is then an intelligent surrender to God who is the whole total environment in which there is no separateness.

Surrender to God is not something that we can just decide and easily do. Our ability to surrender is dependent upon how well or how poorly we have used our opportunities for conscious evolution in this or any lifetime. The main theme of Nuclear Evolution is that evolution is not just physical heredity. Our karma determines how we *use* the physical inheritance, and our karma is the sum of our experiences kept in the unconscious. It affects the genes environmentally by making a block between the spirit and its body, e.g., in tensions. These karmic knots change the body. But even then, we must understand that our evolution proceeds not just from the conscious thoughts and choices of our personality but from our being—the willful attitudes hidden deep in our unconscious minds which govern our choices at a level we cannot reach any other way than by surrender to the evolutionary program present in the unconscious mind from the beginning.

WHAT IS THIS EVOLUTIONARY PROGRAM?

In the core of each organism is the need to express itself through love. Though our adaptation to the external world and its pressures may be more vivid to our *conscious* minds, the power of this internal evolutionary pressure working in the *unconscious* mind is the real source of change. The outside pressure of rejection by a loved one, for example, would not have the same effect upon us at all were it not for the fact that we loved them and therefore cannot remain indifferent to their actions. And most of our pain comes in fact from our interference with this love which, if we let it come through into a clear conscious awareness of our own ego-pride, would evolve us swiftly and without pain. But until that time, the traumas and karmic impressions embedded in consciousness are at the same time embedded in each nerve, muscle and cell and they cannot be removed piecemeal from any one of those without the others because they are written in consciousness, and if they are written in consciousness they are written throughout the universe. They get passed down to the physical organism through vibration at the mind, brain, nerve, muscle, cell and atom levels—each level stepping the signal down into physical manifestation. Therefore opening up the nucleus to the central core of love is merely a stripping away of the various locking devices which, like trauma or karma, fix the vibration in a pattern which blocks the functioning of the organism at higher evolutionary levels of expression.

The geneticists focus on the determinism of our heredity, but determinism is only a drop in the bucket in the story of consciousness, and genes are only a tiny part of the picture of man. To remove the trauma at every level one can only write it out of consciousness. As long as it is stuck there, it will return every incarnation in one body after another (even though it may not be originally carried in the genes), slightly modified each time. For example, if you are suffering from a sexual trauma, then your nervous system and whole body is suffering from intolerable tension, and the production of sperm and ova will be stunted or grow up in a hostile environment, and therefore the seed which develops inside the womb carries with it this reaction to hostility as a vibration of fear. The fear can be transmitted by parents from generation to generation, not only after birth but while still in the womb, but it is not real and, like karma or trauma, can be removed.

Fear is the opposite of love. Fear leads to doubt, and only when fear and doubt are vanquished can true love exist, since all karma and all traumas originate ultimately from fear. The Superintelligence is not afraid of anything. While acknowledging danger and living with caution, the superintelligent consciousness knows that *all that is needed to release the love at the heart of the nucleus is to remove fear and doubt* since they are not separate from the doubter. This is the true meaning of faith, not as a belief but as a sense of conviction that penetrates through every level and, when emanating from consciousness itself, produces spiritual healing and reorganization of matter. Trauma and karma are the blockages to love. And fear and doubt are the bolts on the door of the heart. Hence, when Christ says, "Love one another," he means, "Trust one another, eradicate fear and doubt." To know that consciousness is twisted into knots by fear enables the superintelligent person to unscramble the knots in human behavior and to bring sanity and peace to the chaos of the planet.

HOW DO WE MAKE THE LEAP?

If thousands of years of cultural brainwash have not changed the nucleic acids (DNA) through biological adaptation to customs and traditions then how can Nuclear Evolution possibly create a one million year evolutionary leap that will affect the genes? The answer is that up to now, only the mystics, Hermetic Kabbalists, great prophets and sages of China and India knew of the powers of consciousness over the biological mechanisms, and this was kept secret. Because they knew men would use this knowledge for selfish ends and that the world could be enslaved by unscrupulous people, they preferred to let this knowledge die with them, knowing it to be eternal knowledge that would rise again at the right time.

Today we live in different times. We have telephones, TV, books and the press, with an electronic infra-structure of intercommunications stretching like a web around the whole planet. Now that this knowledge can be transmitted to all humanity and not just to a few people who might form some secret society, some illuminati or special clique, this planetary network can enable all human beings to become superintelligent in a short time. There are still some dangers that a few scientists in ivory towers will create ultra-intelligent machines which artificially simulate thought processes in a computer and enslave mankind in another way. Most people think of intelligence as solely the product of human brains, but the environment is full of superintelligence, particularly the DNA of the nucleus which holds the pattern of our physical brain and body. But we must discriminate carefully, in an evolutionary sense, between the *vehicle* of consciousness which we use, i.e., the cells, the DNA and body structure (analagous to the computer and its stored intelligence) and the actual program itself. Nuclear Evolution is concerned with the program itself because it claims there are already thousands of intelligent systems or vehicles with the entire cosmic program stored in the nuclei all around us and inside us waiting for us to become conscious of them. All we have to do is to tap what is already there in the cosmic consciousness by tuning our brain functions and getting rid of the mental blockages and cultural programs which actually limit our concept of evolution and our idea of human intelligence. The danger is that scientists will invent ultra-intelligent machines that can be coupled to living cells or genes which will eventually be able to rid organisms of components which now block their access to biological and cosmological processes. Those machines could artificially tap the Superintelligence in Nature before man as a whole becomes ready in the development of his own consciousness. He might then find himself totally dependent upon these intelligent machines.

The secret of Nuclear Evolution is in the power of suggestion to control biological processes available to everyone. The ancients discovered that it was possible to control nerve currents, control blood supply to

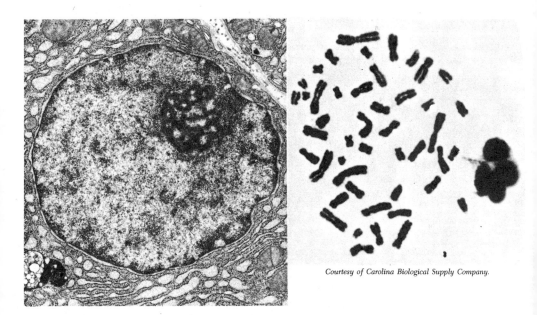

Courtesy of Carolina Biological Supply Company.

Picture shows an electron micrograph of the cell nucleus. The round membrane encloses the nucleus with the cytoplasm of the cell surrounding it. Within the membrane of the nucleus can be seen the dark patch of the nucleolus and the dark speckles around it are the chromatin containing chromosomes, showing at right the 46 chromosomes in each nucleus of a human being.

the cell, and enhance or retard growth at a depth of consciousness unknown to ordinary man. By desensitizing certain functions of our cells and amplifying others it was possible and still is possible to use the power of consciousness to control the sex of a baby or even prevent birth altogether by mentally instructing the genes to become impotent. Sometimes this is done unconsciously by personal stress, and a couple will remain childless. The Western equivalent of this power of the imagination over the program in the cells is called "hypnosis", which is a name given to it about a hundred years ago by a British physician who brought the power of suggestion from India after seeing many surgical operations performed there without anaesthetic. Since then the psychiatric and medical professions have used it as a tool against a host of clinical disorders but with very little understanding or agreement as to what hypnosis is. Hypnotic trance was discovered by yogis and seers many thousands of years ago through meditation, but the level of trance achieved by doctors for surgical operations is only five percent of what a yogi calls one hundred percent suggestion. With one hundred percent suggestion a person can change the message in the DNA structure and actually control the growth of the nucleic acid crystals as they form and replicate in the environment of the cell. In Italy doctors have used hypnosis on over one hundred women as birth control and not one has become pregnant. The International Center of Medical and Psychological Hypnosis in Milan* guarantees that eighty-five percent of women can use hypnosis as one hundred percent birth control method. The other fifteen percent are women who cannot go into a sufficiently deep trance. These physicians believe that the hypnosis sets in motion a neurological hormone process which inhibits the ovum and prevents pregnancy. With even *fifty* percent yogic trance we can create changes in the environment of the inter-cellular fluids around the nucleus which cause the genes to adapt in the same way that they have adapted to environmental changes through natural selection. The difference between ordinary evolution and Nuclear Evolution is that ordinary scientists do not believe that consciousness has the power to willfully suggest such changes in the pattern of the DNA. They quite believe that chemical-osmotic forces can manufacture ATP which energizes the DNA, but they do not believe that these forces are controlled by the deep willful consciousness of a person. Just as in the synthesis of ATP where light oxidation of an atom drives protons across a membrane, so can the DNA be affected by the energy-rich compounds which are formed as the protons flow back into the cell through a complex of enzymes. Nuclear Evolution theory has stated since 1968 that consciousness and light, consciousness and protons, consciousness and ATP affect not only the DNA but also the behavior of the atoms which make up the structure of the nucleic acids themselves. In other words, the difference between the old idea of Darwinian evolution and Nuclear Evolution** is that atoms and protons in the nucleus have choice; they

---

* Dr. Marco Marcheson and his son, Dr. Rolando Marcheson, state that their method consists of six to eight sessions for suggestion of infertility to last indefinitely. The power to reverse the process is retained by the patient. Tests have been made over a three-year period.

** This process is fully explained in "The Physics of Consciousness" in the book *Nuclear Evolution*, published in London in 1968 and reprinted in an expanded edition in 1977, available from University of the Trees Press.

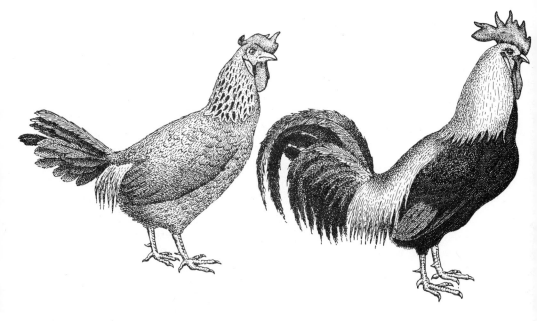

It is known that several hormones affect the RNA genetic activity of chromosomes and genes. Genes exercise immediate control over the activities of growing cells that are going through some change. The effect of estrogen on the synthesis of all kinds of RNA in cells can be demonstrated by treating a rooster with the female hormone. Its liver begins to produce yolk proteins which it does not need since it cannot produce an egg. Testosterone given to female rats causes the synthesis of a new variety of RNA. The hormone aldosterone affects the passage of sodium ions and potassium ions transported through cell membranes. A rooster treated with female hormone estrogen at left is compared with a normal rooster at right showing the physical changes in the synthesis of the growing cells in the comb and tail and its plumage.

have selection power to associate with whom they want and to gravitate towards preferred unions with other atoms and environments caused by consciousness. The theory is easy to prove by hypnosis since in deep states of trance, enzyme activity and the flow of electrons through the system of carrier molecules of DNA drive positively-charged hydrogen ions (called protons) across the membranes of mitochondria, bacteria cells and chloroplasts, so that an electrical potential or gradient is created to which the field of consciousness generated from the brain and its higher centers can respond, influencing and commanding the flow of light energy (protons) from the sun and stars. I did many experiments of my own before I published this theory in 1968 but have been unsuccessful in getting any university to carry out a test of the theory. Many doctors who have visited our London center and who have read *Nuclear Evolution* over the years have confirmed that this theory is correct, but they were immediately regarded as far-out and branded as misled cranks by people who have never taken even the slightest trouble to test their assumptions, objections or statements. Every day new research comes out which proves this theory is correct in every detail and not one word has needed to be changed since 1968. The new expanded edition in 1977 contains the old edition showing the process exactly as it was first written. The concepts of Nuclear Evolution have even been used since by radiologists experimenting with the power of the imagination over the function of cancer cells, and they have found the information correct. Dr. Oscar Morphis, M.D., of the Oncology Associates, Fort Worth, Texas, who founded a radiologists' clinic, one of the leading institutions in the USA, told me personally that he considered the book *Nuclear Evolution* to be the most profound insight into the cancer mechanism that he has come across. Since it may take several years more for academia to accept reluctantly what is ultimately inevitable, the knowledge has been generally published and given to all so that no one can make a special profession out of it.

If some first-hand knowledge of deep self-hypnosis (one hundred percent suggestion) were required of every scientist before he or she could get a degree, scientists would then know the power of consciousness to transform biological cells into patterns that defy recognition. The DNA grows in tendrils which develop carrot-like shapes as they grow in the environment of the nucleus.* Cultural programming does not affect DNA formation but deep hypnosis in one hundred percent trance, often reinforced and repeated, affects DNA synthesis both negatively and positively just as the growth of living organisms at the physical level adapts and selects according to environmental stresses and needs.

Imagine suggesting to the cells in yourself one hundred percent joy with one hundred percent of your consciousness for even half an hour a day! Do you think you would ever get cancer or a thrombosis? Imagine suggesting to yourself doubt, fear, mistrust, frustration, jealousy, separateness all day long. Can you understand why people are miserable, unhappy, seeking oblivion, sick and in a continual state of dis-ease?

---

* See picture of DNA on page 574.

Long established in the healing profession, Dr. Morphis has a good record of cures at his clinic and his partner Dr. Carl Simonton, M.D., and his wife are giving courses all around the country, showing how powerfully the imagination and its seventh level functions can control the life of the cell.

Standard evolutionary theory predicts that an organism will adapt itself over a long period of time to local changes in the physical environment. But in Nuclear Evolution theory, through the power of self-suggestion of consciousness, organisms can adapt to self-programmed psychic changes in an even shorter period of time. By understanding the ego as well as the mechanism of self-suggestion, evolutionary changes can be quickly wrought into the vehicle of consciousness, the physical body. Ego patterns are the self-suggestions of consciousness working on itself and they condition the gene environment. Hate, worry, and stress feelings all cause the ego to reinforce itself, and the negative energies wrought by the ego can destroy the cell. But the normal ego has no voluntary control over the biological actions of the organism which are all functioning well below the consciousness of ego which has no idea how it breathes, gets hungry or processes chemicals needed to support the body. The very fact that, under self-suggested trances, these functions are easily controlled is proof that ego is not a strong enough self-suggestion to be impregnated in the cell. Even though ego is a powerful force and has been with us throughout history, it still is only normally about a fifty percent self-suggestion of separateness and therefore can be obliterated by a fifty percent opposite self-suggestion. Whatever degree of suggestion we have programmed into consciousness, the same degree is necessary to de-program. If man could achieve one hundred percent self-suggestion of unity he would be able to transmute his entire physical vehicle into pure consciousness. But even by learning five percent self-suggestion we can begin to consciously control our biological computer and through practice open up the higher brains to prepare the way for superintelligence.

Yogis have written over thousands of years, from before the time of Gautama Buddha, that we have the power of one hundred percent suggestion in the process of identification of consciousness. Consciousness must obviously be put where the enkephalins are flowing in order to generate them spontaneously by our own bliss. In answer to the intellectual lawyer who asked which is the greatest commandment in the law, Christ replied the same as the old testament prophets did in the Book of Deuteronomy:

> *"Thou shalt love the Lord thy God with all thy heart, and with all thy soul, and with all thy mind. This is the first and great commandment."*

This advice, found also in all the great world religions, is no different than what is scientifically meant by one hundred percent self-suggestion. But in order to achieve this one-pointedness of all our energies we have to be able to release all our attachments to what is tying us to only our lower brains. Again the analogy can be drawn to Christ's response to the rich man who said he had kept all the spiritual laws yet he still didn't feel complete, and he asked Christ what more he must do to have eternal life.

> *"Go and sell all you have and give to the poor and you shall have treasure in heaven."*

This was the one thing the rich man could not do because his consciousness was very attached to earthly wealth. How can an ordinary person follow the Superintelligence which Christ was talking about, give up all attachments in order to tune to it, and consciously surrender to its wisdom without being regarded as a religious fanatic who loses his sense of humor and generally is thought stupid to abandon himself to fate? And what will motivate anyone to try it?

In order to make more sense of life we must begin to learn how incredible our human nervous system is for sensing the subtle radiations from the total environment. Hidden in humans is the same faculty which enables the swallows of Capistrano to fly 10,000 miles to Argentina and arrive back several months later within a few minutes of the same arrival time in previous years. Hidden in the structure of our brains and consequently also in our genes is the ability to guide ourself to the source like the ocean salmon find their way back up the river to the spawning grounds. This faculty, formerly developed in us but now inhibited and squelched by our rational and conceptual levels of consciousness, I have called the Supersense. Many people use it as intuition and they make decisions, make selections and detect the presence of invisible factors with it. Supersensonics, or the new science of sensing these radiations from the whole of Nature's many objects in the environment, is described in more detail in the book of that title.* The ability to tune into the real function of our own cells, however, and discover the state of their internal environment and even to tune into the DNA message, releases us from the age-old prison of only one mode of knowing. Validation by scientific means, *after* we have received "leads" and discovered "pathways" of certain signals in our brains is not an opposite way of approach to supersensing but a complementary way of detection which we must have as a check against our unconscious desires to corrupt information to our own liking. This process of corruption of Nature's signals goes on at every level, sometimes conscious and sometimes unconscious, and has to do with our degree of ego interference in our perceptions. We can tune into the songs of whales and songs of birds and insects, and we can analyze the language of the dolphin, but can we use one hundred percent suggestion or the process of identification to know what their intelligence is actually thinking inside them and apply it to our own experience? Some people do realize that there is a cosmic program hidden deep in their being and they are wanting to get to it, so they are attracted to religion which appeals to that desire within or they are attracted to search the unknown in science which appeals to that same desire directed externally to the natural world. But Supersensonics starts from the foundation that we already have a direct method of sensing the invisible worlds of Nature and Spirit in the human ability to divine how to stay one hundred percent in tune with the source of all knowing—our evolving consciousness.

---

* "Supersensonics" is the capacity of the human brain as a nodal point or modulator to detect a vast array of cosmic frequencies in the universal field. This leads to the concept of Nuclear Evolution where the brain becomes the perceiver of a hologram. The neurological lighting up in the brain created by the firing of the nerve cells provides us with a movie or play of the physical objects in the environment.

CHANGING THE UNCHANGEABLE

Like Darwin, our present science does not believe that evolution takes any leaps at all but passes gradually and slowly through vast periods of time. However, Nuclear Evolution is indeed a leap not only in time but in showing that *time itself is a fiction* and that our power over the seed, both in leaps of thought and leaps in the physical evolution of our incarnate fleshy brains, is not a fiction but a timeless ever-re-creating property of our consciousness. To understand this we must understand in detail the differences between the Nuclear Evolution approach to the nucleus and that of modern scientific thinking.

In the nucleus of the seed is the DNA which according to modern biology *does not change* but merely passes its genetic message on to the next generation *by combining* with the DNA or genes of another different organism.

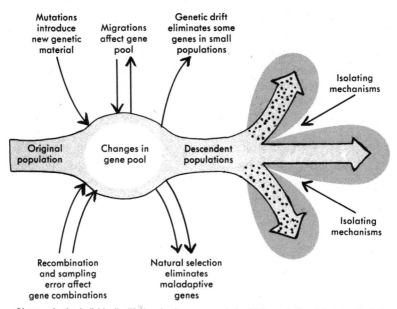

Changes in the individual's lifetime in the genes and the DNA are believed not to affect the course of evolution, but the genetic make-up is supposed to change over many generations of mutation, recombination and migration introduced into the gene pool of populations through natural selection. If groups are separated and prevented from exchanging genes they would, according to present theory, diverge and evolve a new species.

Although present scientific research in the field of recombinant DNA can produce genetic changes, present theory does not allow for any mental interference in the DNA pattern of the genes. Only by artificially unlocking the code in the genes and inserting a genetic fix or by natural sexual combinations can there be any real change in the physical structure of human beings, according to this mechanistic viewpoint. *Nuclear Evolution challenges this respected theory and maintains that THE DNA CAN BE CHANGED by intense self-suggestion, that is, the power of consciousness to modify and influence its own cell life, to bring about in time a complete mutation from within, without reference to the external environment.*

How can we explain to the geneticist that such a thing is possible? It is possible because hidden in the genetic program of the nucleus is *already* a cosmic pattern waiting for the trigger to activate the opening of our brains. Waiting for a certain key feeling, waiting for a certain cellular environment and a sense of peace, the nucleus is ready to carry out its own mutation and change itself when the spiritual climate has changed to nurture, when the mental field has turned to total conviction, when the emotions are not in conflict.

Nuclear Evolution theory states that this natural mutation of the seed at the heart of every nucleus is not a readjustment of a temporary physical condition but that through the control of cosmic forces, continuous self-suggestion and self-hypnosis can affect the permanent transmission pattern of the RNA which carries the DNA message from the nucleus to other parts of the cell. Thus we say that the seed, the Nux, replicates itself or selects its own conscious role in the evolutionary thrust of life, whereas Darwinism and its present supporters maintain that it is the environment which changes the selections of the organism. Of course this self-suggestion which we call one hundred percent suggestion in Nuclear Evolution must reach that intensity by consistent practice through time as a regular way of life rather than just sitting as an idea in someone's head. In exactly the same way, no scientist could make an atom bomb just by knowing the theory because there would have to be some practical skill in putting the parts together and some dedication to purifying the materials used. No one can change the fundamental code of life merely by taking thought or dreaming of a wishful condition as a fantasy. To use our imaginative power correctly we must *become* the condition so that we *are* it in our consciousness, otherwise the DNA/RNA structures will not change. To use our imaging power only for wishing is like doing something half-hearted or half-baked.

Nuclear Evolution does not pretend to work from any superficial belief system or idealism since consciousness is not powerful enough to act in biological systems merely through idealism or through thinking. The intensity of faith required for biological change must be at the level of one hundred percent self-hypnosis and must be more a sense of deep conviction, impenetrable by doubt, than an acquired opinion or ideal. It is obvious that throughout history the power of conviction has been used many times in reverse to bring about negative conditions and to create self-righteous believers who justified any action such as murder, oppression, suicide, sickness or even future atomic suicide. No further evidence is needed than the 916 people who committed suicide or were murdered under the spellbinding orders of Reverend Jim Jones who used repeated reinforcement of hypnotic suggestion to convince his followers that they would all go to heaven. The often repeated dogmatic suggestion that there must inevitably be a violent war between communism and capitalism has made both the US and the USSR arm themselves with megaton bombs and prepare themselves with shelters for atomic survival of their cities. Atomic suicide will come from such a self-deluding conviction since any escalation of the arms race will only increase the opposition so that the suggestion becomes self-fulfilling. Yet even this conviction to the point of suicide may not be powerful enough to change the cell life and the genes, as one hundred percent suggestion does.

AN EXAMPLE OF FAITH

To define such a deep sense of conviction is difficult. Even Jesus had difficulty in describing this kind of faith. Yet it is possible by direct experience because I myself have experienced this sense of conviction in which miracles can be wrought. It has nothing to do with religion as such because the very first time I experienced it I was almost an agnostic. My own small son, John, was thrown and trampled by a horse which bolted from my hand by breaking the reins. We were out riding together and the horse ran dragging my son's body upside down with his feet still in the stirrup and his head just clearing the rocky ground. I was powerless and felt impotent to save him. I summoned up all the power of my being and challenged God or any universal force if there was one to come now and protect him. Surprisingly I felt an amazing reassurance flood all over me as the horse disappeared up the rocky drive dragging my son to the stables. I galloped after him only to arrive as my wife, who had heard the commotion at the bottom of the long drive, was grabbing the head of the frightened horse. My son's fingers and his hand were crushed out of recognition, with the bones showing through all pulped. Surprisingly it was not bleeding very much. We rushed him to the doctor who took one look at it and said his hand was finished. We were to wrap up all the mashed hand in antibiotic powder and come back the next day when a decision would be taken with other specialists what to do. Somehow I was not worried. A sense of calm had settled on me since I had that strange conviction that something, some force, some intelligence had definitely answered my intense prayer. Next day we went down to the doctor and watched him sadly removing the bandages while trying to tell us that John was very lucky, under the circumstances, only to have lost some fingers and possibly a hand. The next thing I noticed above all was the incredulous look on the doctor's face. He was one of the most degreed doctors I ever knew and the vice president of the University Regents, a long-time friend with whom we had even talked of spiritualist healings over dinners in former years. But the look on his face was a mixture of joy and mystification. He looked up at me in a special way and said, "I think there is nothing wrong with John's hand. It is perfectly whole." I looked at him deep in the eyes for he was a deep man, an experienced man, and I respected him as a very knowledgeable person. "I can't believe it," he said, "but I have to. There is absolutely nothing wrong with this hand. It is a miracle." John held his unbandaged hand up in the air to inspect it and pointed to a slight scar down the length of one finger. The hand was indeed whole, without even broken skin, and furthermore John seemed in good spirits as if nothing much had happened. The doctor looked at me rather strangely, "I could swear I saw a hand yesterday that was beyond repair. This is an almost instantaneous healing which is hard to believe." I smiled rather smugly for I had just been introduced to my first experience of what Christ meant by total commitment to God. I had put my all into that request. I had put my heart, my head, my love, my very soul, for I loved that boy more than anything else I could think of and it was for his sake I had challenged God to emerge out of the universe in full force. It was the beginning of an inner dedication in my own heart, for in my gratitude I promised I would find that source and make it available to others. From that moment on, I resolved to seek that one power relentlessly and to know it directly with conviction in my own heart. It was the primitive beginnings of my realization of my own and all human ignorance. Several more life-changing years were to come before I could be free to devote myself totally to that force. Many thousands of miles, many strange lands and faces, many illusions and delusions farther on, I would come to know that One who had scrambled to my aid from some distant place in my awareness. To get closer to it, to feel once again that sense of conviction, that certainty and knowing, became my only goal. I had no idea how long and arduous my journey would be or what ignorance and egotism dominated my whole search for the power. Many years later I came to know that it was not power I was seeking but grace. But that is another story. For now I try to share with the reader what I mean by a sense of conviction, for nothing short of this can change the DNA.

GROUP CONSCIOUSNESS

We have said that deep-seated, long-standing cultural traits and even powerful self-suggestions that we are an ego, separate from the whole, are *not* genetic and that these can be changed by seventh level suggestion or even by cultural brainwash without any great difficulty. Now we are saying that another kind of more powerful suggestion can change the DNA structure, and all that we need to know is that faith which moves mountains or a sense of conviction which few humans have about miracles. And we are now saying furthermore that this state of conviction can be achieved by deep meditation or self-hypnosis. This sounds very dubious to those who do not know what physiological changes the power of suggestion can bring to our minds and bodies. There is no substitute for personal experience, but even after one has seen what can be done by hypnosis in a half-hour stage show, we still could not possibly know what hypnosis over a long period of continuous reinforcement can do to our cell life. We could still not know its effects

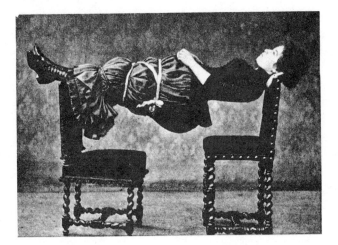

A usual stage demonstration of hypnosis or suggestion which can be achieved with light fifteen percent trance. Auto-hypnosis as practiced by yogis and meditation reaches much deeper levels of one hundred percent trance. Unless reinforced, the lady in the picture would gradually come out of trance within an hour or two.

on our nerve currents, our brain functioning and its secretions of natural soma—the endorphin enzymes which control our perception of reality. And even if we could believe that we could control our internal secretions and keep our attention fixed with complete conviction on the source of all conscious being, we would still need to know what kind of change we might want or what program we can suggest to our intelligent genes. We must then come to know how much more powerful the highest seventh level suggestion is than the milder self-hypnosis that we are indeed a separate ego with separate existence from the total universe we live in. We are so convinced of our separateness as individuals that we cannot conceive of anything more powerful that could change our consciousness so radically as to stop us thinking of our self and dehypnotize ourself from our identification with this waking dream.

That program of convincing ourself at all levels of being, convincing the genes that they can indeed change the self-interested individual survival-orientated person into a whole-orientated group-conscious evolutionary agent, can more easily be worked out selflessly in the company of others who are similarly committed to reaching the ONE nucleus at the deep center. The de-hypnotization of our consciousness from its self-obsession with the self-regarding instinct is not an easy program but it is a possible program for those who will investigate it, wish for it and bring themselves to meditate upon it.* The whole secret is in really wanting it enough. Most people do not want it enough to make the effort to find out. The nucleus merely waits for us to have the insight. By creating a community of individuals who use the power of consciousness to suggest one hundred percent unification of conscious-ness, i.e., the unification of the subject with the object of perception, the process of Nuclear Evolution in society begins.

The formation of a community to overcome the negative programs in the gene pool was the fundamental idea behind Plato's Republic where all the different humans were ideally trained to be one hundred percent skillful exclusively in their respective roles. It is also the fundamen-tal idea behind an ashram where the vibration of the guru and the spirit-ual atmosphere helps the devotee to succeed with meditation and to choose the environment in which the higher seventh level program can automa-tically emerge. The trouble has been in the past that neither the ashrams nor any communities have used one hundred percent self-suggestion, and they never applied what they did use to the group. They only tried for the emergence of higher consciousness in individuals, hoping that as a by-product the whole group would achieve it. The Nuclear Evolution community is to work with the group as a whole integral nucleus from the beginning to become a model of the hologram of life.

I have found that certain people cringe whenever I mention group consciousness or egolessness as if the idea of it implied a loss of individuality or they feared the group might swamp them and swallow

---

* See back matter for Speed Tape Learning Institute. "Information and Guidance Tape" has an excellent program for self-hypnosis and acquiring the skill of deep yogic trance. Published by University of the Trees Press.

them up without regard to their feelings. They confuse ego with uniqueness or confuse self-centered thoughts with the right to a special kind of privacy which should not be invaded by a probing group. These are all ghost thoughts because to really become "group-conscious" one must have a very heightened awareness of the individual. All human beings are different, lead different lives and have innermost thoughts and secrets which they may never share completely with anyone but God—their own consciousness of self. It is natural for humans that we should not wish to be like someone else. But the group consciousness we speak of is deeper than our sense of egocentric privacy or individualism because once we achieve our total individual potential, then we have become indivisible from all other individuals, and there is complete understanding of every individual and his or her private needs. While yet experiencing our own selfhood, how is it possible for us to become one with all selves without dissolving into nothing, without experiencing nothing, without our becoming unaware of any ego differences between selves? The answer is that the selfless person experiences all individuals as himself and will feel the same degree of difference or separateness that they feel, as if it were his very own, while not identifying with it and making this separation himself. We can sit in the light of the stars all the sunny day long without knowing it. The stars do not stop shining in the daytime but only the strong light of the sun masks them. The aware person is aware of their light constantly pouring down upon him even while sitting in the sunlight. So it is in the presence of human suns, human egos and individuals. While they shine, the selfless one sees and experiences their light without losing his own unique awareness of the universal light of all suns and stars. Thus it is in group consciousness, and in the heightened individual who reaches that state. It is not a sameness or a regimented exercise at ego-reduction but a thrilling state totally aware of all differences and outlines, yet seeing and experiencing that which makes them all the same in the heart of being—consciousness, pure and undefiled by thoughts. The degree of paranoia which any person will experience at the thought of group consciousness is directly proportional to his or her clinging to a separate identity. Such a person fears to *lose* identity, not realizing that identification with group consciousness is just the opposite—a much larger, expanded identity. It is because these fears and survival instincts are very powerful in humans that the self-suggestion we give ourselves must also be very very powerful and intense.

First-hand knowledge of hypnosis (commonly referred to in India throughout the centuries as "suggestion"*) is essential before anyone can know what I am talking about. Until you have passed a needle through your cheeks or through your hand without any effect, or taken out a tooth without any pain, or stopped the flow of spurting blood in an accident victim, you just cannot know the power of the imagination over the biological system. Many doctors are totally ignorant of the power of consciousness in certain altered states to change not only the physical appearance of a biological system but to transform functions such as cell growth, nerve transmission or blockage, cell metabolism, etc. I have watched blisters form before my eyes and go away again by suggestion. Anyone wishing to heal the sick and to become acquainted with the power of the human imagination could talk to any medical hypnotist.

I have studied this power of conviction in scientists, skeptics and imaginative artists and found it working in reverse to increase doubt in some just as powerfully as working to create faith and trust in others. I have seen people healed by hypnosis and others healed by faith healers with the same results. I have seen the sickness return almost the next day after faith healing because the self-doubt was too deep and the sense of conviction not deep enough. I have seen successes with hypnosis where the healing was permanent and the sickness did not return because the suggestion went deep enough into a person's inner space. If a person is not ready to change and they continue with the same habits of thought which brought the sickness in the first place, then no hypnosis or faith healing can work for any length of time because one's own consciousness is lord of the body and more powerful than any external force. I remember my amazement when I began to experiment with hypnosis both on myself and others. By

---

* I have outlined a thorough course in what Patanjali called "identification" in a series of tapes called *Rumf Roomph Yoga.* See details at back of book. This is an in-depth study of self-suggestion not at the level of putting needles through your cheek but at the level of evolution of the highest states of consciousness.

releasing the trauma on an auditory nerve, I made deaf people hear. By putting blind people in trance I have, by the power of suggestion, made the blind see and sighted people hallucinate things that were not even there. I came to respect this power of consciousness so much that it became sacred to me.

Sometime after my first experiments with suggestion, I came to feel that no one should really hypnotize another person or take away the self-control of another ego but should rather show someone how they too could do it to themselves as easily as having it done to them. Nor is there any need to have someone gain control over our own imagination, for we use this tool of evolution to hypnotize ourselves every day without knowing it. There are books on self-hypnosis a plenty but a guided meditation, showing us how to distract our conscious mind and occupy the thought process of our higher mind with a mantram or sound, can help us to the second stage. This is to focus our attention upon a single spot. All we need to do to learn hypnosis is to practice every day with the awareness of self-suggestion as the basis of all our acts of consciousness. People do not understand, even at the highest level of spiritual meditation, that the only difference between meditation and ordinary hypnosis is in the quality of consciousness and its cosmic purpose. Almost anyone willing can be *self*-hypnotized, even if they are strong-willed and a bad subject under hypnosis. The strong-willed individuals find that the will works the other way once they become convinced, so that in the end they actually make better subjects. The more intelligent and imaginative a person is, the easier it is to get to the deepest levels of consciousness which we call one hundred percent suggestion and the easier it is to see the need for continuous practice in order to affect the entrenched patterns in the physical functioning of the cells.

Unfortunately the power of suggestion is not taken seriously by Westerners. It has been used and abused by many people, shown off as parlor tricks and neglected by many medical men who would prefer to administer drugs rather than have a patient wake up from trance in the middle of an operation. The force we call hypnosis was only brought to the West a hundred years ago by James Braid, a Scottish surgeon who returned from India having seen operations done on patients by

Ayurvedic doctors without anesthetics. He named it "hypnosis", and ever since then, popular stage entertainers have given Westerners a fear of the hypnotist's power to dominate the mind of another. But of our power to dominate our own mind and reality, Westerners have little to say, though we do this kind of self-hypnosis every day. To de-hypnotize ourself from certain concepts about life is a major work of Nuclear Evolution. We can change the future, evolve or involve, create powerful self-images which can fulfill or destroy us, and we can have power over the evolution of our own brains, all through self-suggestion. So far mankind has used this power of the nucleus to delude himself in his role as a creative being and has separated himself from the very intelligence of the total hologram of his own cosmic consciousness.

The nucleus of the universe from which all organisms have sprung was the center and focus of all ancient systems of evolution. Through self-suggestion many systems of thought and images of man have prevailed throughout history. The new systems of thought which now arise out of the intelligent nucleus of life in every cell of our being will transcend even these ancient systems which concentrated solely on the development of single individuals. Our consciousness will now begin to evolve the individual through interaction with the group, understanding thereby the "whole" rather than the part. To understand the part as the whole and the whole as the part, we need a system of thought which uses the power of identification and self-suggestion to raise the intensity of each individual brain to its true union with a superawareness of the whole group. This is the positive use of group consciousness—to evolve the individual to the selfless egoless love which Christ spoke of when he gave instruction for our use of consciousness:

LOVE THE ONE WITH ALL THY HEART, ALL THY MIND AND ALL THY BEING. AND LOVE THY NEIGHBOR AS THYSELF. ON THESE TWO COMMANDMENTS HANG ALL THE LAWS AND THE PROPHETS.

This is the projection of total conviction, all our heart and all our consciousness into the self-suggestion of oneness. This, of course, is very abstract for those who cannot visualize an invisible God or believe that our brain is already programmed.

What form will the image of the effective unblocking trigger of self-suggestion take? We have said that Darwin's insight into evolution changed man's image of himself. Although to some it seemed a step backward in evolution for man to let go the idea that he was a special creation of God and set apart from the rest of Nature, actually the concept of a common progenitor of animal life was a step toward genuine humility. But instead man has used it to cop out on his destiny. The hero, once valued in society, has now been demoted and the anti-hero put in his place. Today individual people in society worship the possible rather than the impossible feats of the hero, and each person strives to become like all the big ego superstars. We no longer try to imitate the shining selfless heroes who show up our own smallness at the same time that they reveal their greatness. Jesus Christ is placed in a special category and worshipped as a unique personality as God, but most church-goers would be shocked if any of their group were to actually try to be like Jesus, and such a person would most likely be rejected from the church as a freak. But in fact it was Christ's real intent that we should all become the hero and the doer of impossible things. On the other hand, the self-appointed messiahs who come as fake heroes to play upon people's need for authority must be tested by their peers in Creative Conflict so that their authenticity is validated by their manifestation. So our self-suggestion is to plant the seed in consciousness that each living soul is from the same source and has that same sweetness inside it. Not everyone can manifest their real being in equal amount, but the same criteria hold for all. As much of the hero as we can manifest, to that extent we are heroes. To become a cosmic being, at one with all in reality and not just in idea, is the prime self-suggestion. To develop a sense of conviction that evolutionary intelligence is working through our genes is another suggestion which depends on how much we believe the first suggestion. The third suggestion to our genes is to actually manifest the selfless hero to validate all that we suggest and to regard all talk about it, all words, all ideas, all books as merely substitutes for the real work of total conviction in our hearts.

A NEW SELF-IMAGE FOR SOCIETY

Karl Marx used the analogy of the ant as a perfect example of social behavior for people to emulate, i.e., the purely totalitarian society in which individuals sacrifice all individual rights for the good of the whole. But the caste system in the insect world is really irrelevant to the human world. The ancient Brahmins practiced a caste system which grew more and more hierarchical through their long belief in reincarnation and in karma, the law of spiritual cause and effect. The belief was that if we were born a working peasant, we may have ignored our responsibilities to fellowman when we were previously a king. If one were born into the Brahmin caste, it was thought to be because one had always lived a priestly life striving for perfection. Thus Brahmins justified their elite position in the group hierarchy and conveniently turned the caste theory to personal good use. So too have Marxists argued their repressive political system from a model in the insect world which is really irrelevant to the human world, because the totalitarian insect colony merely plays out its social drives according to its genetic programming, whereas a human has more free choice. There is a vast difference between the nuclear seed of insects and that of the nuclear intelligence in human beings. The caste system among humans eventually becomes dominated by a controlling group who then gains political as well as spiritual power and thereby controls society for the benefit of a privileged few. Whereas the insect society is controlled for the survival of the whole, the human version of this is just the opposite. The privileged priestly castes in human society have always controlled in order to satisfy self-centered drives for power, esteem and privilege, thereby leading to decay, revolt and eventual downfall of the privileged system of priestly rule. Marxism arose as a backlash against this kind of hierarchy but has only put in its place another hierarchy, thus proving that no matter how much one *talks* about the good of the whole, it has been almost impossible for humans to manifest. Though given free will, we have not been given the same instinct of group survival that is found in the world of insects. Free to separate himself mentally from the whole, man defines his self-image as something smaller. The major difference between a man and an ant is the drive for power, the need to feel up on top of the social heap by feeling self-important at other people's expense. So we have two problems: first, how to lift our self-image up out of its present low level and begin to identify with the entire cosmos—the whole—not in the sense that the qualities of individualism and spirit must be stamped out as in communist societies but to enhance those qualities along with the whole. And second, how to manifest the new self-image once we've got it. Social groups, families, tribes, parties and companies organized for selfish ends cannot be used as an evolutionary instrument. So our groups must be formed with a new philosophy of what human nature is. When the religious artisans who built the medieval cathedrals chose hundreds of years of hard work cutting stones and carving rock, they did so out of love without any chance of seeing the finished work. They chose the difficult path and the strenuous work of creating a beautiful manifestation because they had a sense of belonging to a whole group in love with the cosmic Christ. No one coerced them to work and often they were monks who never got paid for a lifetime of work. They were a nuclear family, bound by a sense of conviction in spirit to a common goal of union with Christ. The feeling of belonging was not something brought about through preaching religious or political propaganda but something from the heart. Through prayer and meditation they were content with minimal comforts and minimal wealth and rejoiced in the opportunity to serve a revolutionary concept of rebirth on another plane of consciousness that was not of this world.

We have no need of a cathedral to build today yet we bear the heavy load of responsibility for reshaping mankind by reshaping our social environments. Have we, like the medieval monks, a source of inspiration which, through love, can motivate us to work hard to change and evolve our human behavior? Have we the needed self-discipline? No one would work for the death of the ego were it not for the enticement of enlightenment, and most of the world's people are not even enticed by enlightenment since it requires such enormous self-discipline. By comparison, the building of cathedrals is child's play. We don't want to do it; we want to cling to all the pleasures and attachments, the joys of ownership, the attractions of power, fame and self-importance, which somehow we believe we must lose if we are to undertake the spiritual life. We have all read the Sermon on the Mount and we all know the Truth from hundreds of dull books which talk of the heavy load of the cross we must bear, and the preachers ever remind us of the sin we are supposed to be born in, but do we find that enticement towards the promised goal of heavenly bliss? To most people heaven is something that happens after they are dead, and they know nothing about the delight in the total environment around them. How many of us really sense the whole of our creation and live daily with the ambrosial feeling of love for all its many species and organisms? How will we know this enticement until we begin to change our image of mankind and to think of ourselves as group-conscious cosmic beings and to change our behavior from that of a self-centered organism to that of a universal-centered being? Nuclear Evolution provides a framework of a new system which emerges out of all the excesses of the old. Its divine purpose is to find the joy and deep enthusiasm associated with religious fervor and yet not be fanatical enough to spawn a personality cult or elitist group who allows the minority to exploit the majority.

Throughout history and even now the trend has always been toward personal ego enhancement and improved self-image. How does Nuclear Evolution swim against the popular tide if its purpose is to harness fervor in a politically relevant way? How do we stop the pendulum swing from power cliques to reform and then from reformation and revolution back to new hierarchies of power? How do we change our selfish territorial instincts, built up over millions of years of evolution by "survival of the fittest"? We are beginning to realize that our territory is now the whole planet and our physical environment has expanded into space. We are also seeing that the altruistic idea of selflessness as a cosmic trait in the natural world has never yet been maintained in the human world because we have never discovered a system which controls the power-seekers. They love to fascinate and hypnotize others and will gladly dominate and take advantage of anyone who is selfless. The World Peace Center constitution provides the means whereby the status quo may be challenged, not once every hundred years but month by month and week by week and day by day. So our only remaining question is: how do we motivate people to work the constitution and to undertake the self-discipline of evolving the heart at the expense of the self-sense? Man begins to build a beautiful constitution like the painstaking monks built the medieval cathedrals until it rises as a work of beauty, impossible of construction by one man or even one generation. Some cathedrals took two hundred years to build yet no one lost the sense of purpose, and the goal of the work was held clear in its vision. So must our new inspiration be to build the edifice of group consciousness. What will motivate us to reach beyond the limits of our self and enter the vibration of the whole? Will the glory of a superintelligent force steal our heart and turn us towards the evolutionary instrument which has already been programmed into our genes? The first group to achieve group consciousness on earth will become the seed for all the rest, no matter how tiny that original nucleus may be, no matter how slowly it appears to grow. The world is like a saturated solution, waiting for the first real seed crystal to catalyze and crystallize the whole.

The feeling that motivated the cathedral builders and monks was their love and dedication to Christ as a symbol for their own link with the cosmos. Today we do not need symbols whether they be scientific formulae or religious concepts of God. What we need is to contact the internal evolutionary spirit which moves people along. We need to penetrate the actual nucleus and listen to its cosmic song.

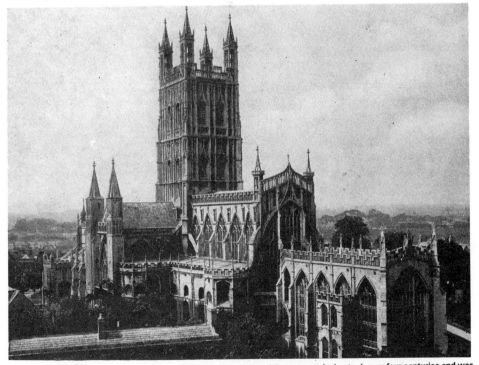

Gloucester Cathedral was a Norman church in 1088. The building of the present design took over four centuries and was finished in the 15th century as a fine example of monastic dedication, skill, and love of beauty. If our dedication to the building of group consciousness can match the master-builders of the middle ages, the human race will rise in evolution.

Potala Palace, Lhasa, historical home of the Dalai Lama

The Buddhist utopia where millions were poor but happy, where police were almost nonexistent, where religious regimentation and ritual became the main occupation of the nation. Elitism and hierarchy were established genetically by birth of "meritorious qualities" rather than social position. China now claims "unprecedented happiness in Tibet today" but exiles refuse to return and question the social regimentation and repression of religion.

AP photo

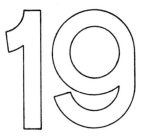

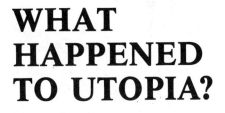

WHAT
HAPPENED
TO UTOPIA?

Only a person who has the refinement of mind to realize that he alone is responsible for guiding his life and for manifesting his own potential is capable of self-discipline. Such people know that they are responsible even for those unconscious drives that they cannot yet see; therefore they choose of their own free will to grow and change. They know that the enlightened state of their own consciousness is the only real utopia there is. However, most utopian philosophers, from Plato to Marx, to the behaviorist, B.F. Skinner, have tried to create change from the outside in by manipulating the environment, and have envisioned utopia as a social phenomenon created by following an external system. This attitude towards an external solution of the human problem shows a basic lack of trust in the universe, placing all hope of progress in the hands of the intellect with its ingenious solutions and schemes. This intellectual arrogance has now just reached its zenith in behavioral science.

Behaviorism began with the experiments of Russian psychologist Ivan Pavlov, who succeeded in conditioning the biological response mechanism by which dogs salivate instinctively whenever they smell food. In his experiments, Pavlov introduced a second stimulus, other than smell, to trigger this natural response. Each time he fed his dog, he rang a bell. After a while, the dog would salivate at the sound of the bell even if there were no food at all. Pavlov concluded that such learned behavior is the result of conditioned reflexes. Or, in other words, if we condition a creature with controlled external stimuli, we can affect not only his superficial behavior but even his instinctual response to life. For all those minds whose fondest ego dream is to be able to control and mold Nature, this seems the most thrilling

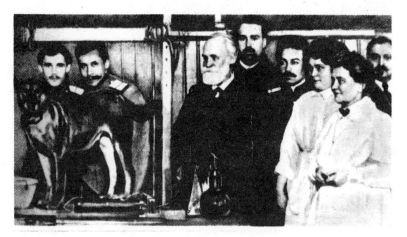

Pavlov and his lab assistants demonstrating a conditioned response in a dog. (Bettman Archive)

discovery of the century. At last! real PROOF that behavior can be controlled! We can make a dog salivate even when there is no food. Clever man! Using Nature's own laws to achieve his ends. And if we look around we can see our most clever minds manipulating Nature to achieve their own goals everywhere: adding chemicals to our foods for preservatives, using nuclear fission to run our power plants (a process that is not natural, since Nature produces nuclear energy by fusion, a bringing together, rather than a dividing apart), the tuna industry killing

•

millions of dolphins and threatening that loving animal with extinction and many more ecological abominations.

Sociobiology is an attempt to relate the evolution of animals and the genetic code to human social conditions with the implication of controlling genetic mutation. It is dealt with in detail in a chapter of my book *Nuclear Evolution.* Perhaps the most frightening of the prospects of controlling Nature exploded recently between the courts and the universities as to whether science should meddle with recombinant DNA, with the potential side effects of creating a whole host of new man-made viruses and other hazards. There are scientists today exploring ways to make society more altruistic through cloning the eventual creation of higher biological types of human beings. Their findings are creating intellectual ferment and controversy because of the drastic social implications.

How different this is from those holymen whose only goal is to be in tune with Nature and to surrender to that Universal Intelligence which created it, in order to encompass a greater understanding of Nature's own ways. The heart wants to cooperate with Nature's program for the evolution of intelligence. Evil minds manipulate life and Nature, and their unconscious drives produce war and prison camps to serve their own schemes for glory and their urges for power. Good minds manipulate life too, consciously trying to create utopias which never work because they do not understand the fundaments of man's nature. Who among humans has that quality of "Virtue" which is beyond both good and evil and which can only be experienced by giving up the compulsion to control?

The Pavlovian discovery does work; no doubt of that. The problem is, it works on a very limited scale. There is no 360 degree awareness of the whole in this approach. The behaviorists circumscribe experience, leaving out so much of life that their theory proves itself only in the terms set up for it. They fear "what is"—that gigantic unpredictable uncontrollable Reality which refuses to fit the theory. Especially they fear to enter the fields of parapsychology and the intuitive, psychic, mysterious, not-quite-explainable realms of the supernormal. Talk of the unknown worlds of the spirit makes behaviorists very nervous and defensive, for they are basically insecure people in their tremendous desire to control. Is is no accident that a popular technique, Silva Mind Control, (another approach to the same earthly paradise) is named "Control". By training people to program their consciousness at the level of alpha brain waves, Silva Mind Control places in the hands of the ego the power to control what is "good", "positive" and "best for me". It does not improve the mind's capacity to discern what really is best for itself or for anyone else. The ego does not see that "positive" is not always "good" and that life's rhythms always take a dip before they rise, or vice versa. If our rise into the positive soars too high, without our having first mastered the unconscious with its negative pulls, it will pull us down unexpectedly and we will have to fall a long way before we rise again—this time with more wisdom. Mastery and control are not the same thing. Mastery is built on understanding the mind and working with the forces of Nature to change behavior—our own. Control is direct manipulation of the forces for one's own mental purposes which may not always be in tune with Nature and may rob another's freedom. The freedom to think for ourselves is an important ingredient of our spiritual evolution.

The behaviorist philosophy is based on the fact that if behavior *can* be controlled, then our lives must be pretty much determined by environmental programs. Yet although at the level of simple vegetables, environmental conditions may make a carrot grow short or tall, sweet or tasteless, weak or strong, there is nothing that can make a carrot seed become a cabbage or become anything other than its own essence which is written in its nucleus or seed. This uniqueness written into the being of every living thing, driving and propelling it to evolve its own potentials and thus find fulfillment—this is the meaning of the term "Nuclear Evolution". The following account by a young woman now living in a spiritual community reveals the same process of human development which can only be likened to the natural unfolding of a seed.

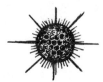

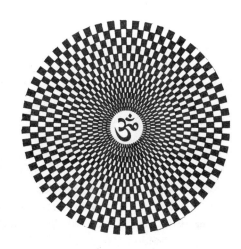

The symbol of
Nuclear Evolution

"I was brought up in a highly intellectual family. My success-ful uncles were mostly physicians—scientists with a hard-nosed intellectual bent. Both my brothers achieved recognition as professors. I was always quick, but I found a profound dryness in the emphasis on rationalism. As a young child I observed the workings of these older minds and found that they seemed to miss out on a wider breadth of life. I chose to consciously develop my intellect at around age ten because I saw that any other area of specialty was not held in as high regard by my family. Even though my talents were in creative writing, I felt this was not held in as high regard as intellectual agility. Nowhere, on any side of my family, is there a commitment to spiritual growth, although there is a lot of Jewish religious tradition. Few members of the family really believe God exists, let alone have any direct experience of Him. At age eight I had a profound spiritual experience with Christ, which I had to keep to myself as it would be an anathema in my Jewish family, mourning the Nazi holocaust and Russian pogroms and blaming them on Christian ignorance. The fact that I grew up in a Catholic neighborhood may have had some influence, but I was taught that Catholicism was all cere-monial hocus-pocus. Nevertheless I loved the vibrations in the churches and would sneak in to experience them. I

loved the spiritual feeling around Christmas and the joy in
the Lord's prayer, which I secretly memorized from an
embroidered tapestry hung over the bed at my friend's
house, which I used to gaze at when I'd sleep over there.
From what level of need or being did this originate? After
age twelve I decided to compete with my brothers for
intellectual recognition and ego food (though I didn't think
of it that way at the time) and became an agnostic and then
an atheist, like them. However, the search for truth, always
pressing within, led me to an investigation of psychology to
discover what motivates people. What motivates me? I
specialized in attitude-change theory and research at University of Chicago to see what does make people do what
they do. I couldn't stomach the laborious statistical, empirical psychology that ignored human feelings and the very
stream of life itself. I made the search for that essence of
livingness my driving goal and accidentally fell upon God,
the Self, and direct spiritual experience in the process.
From then on my relatives have labeled me "a religious
fanatic", "a smatterer in science and philosophy", "someone with hormone imbalance", "the black sheep", "de-
ranged through drugs" and other diagnoses I have not yet
heard. However, now that I am becoming in their eyes
apparently successful in my field and am a published author,
a teacher and editor, utilizing my intellectual training, I am
a bit more respected as someone "intelligent, but perhaps
deluded" or "brilliant, but hurt by life". My family did
everything they could to shape my life the best way they
knew, and they succeeded in making me an intellectual. My
environment conditioned my method of approach to life and
my surface personality. Yet it could not and did not inhibit
the deeper strata of my being that chose to embrace spirituality."

The behaviorists' main difficulty is to explain goal-orientated
behavior in terms of environmental stimuli, because human beings with
the power to reason do not act from blind association alone, like

Pavlov's dog, but through goals and long-range purposes. Even animal and insect behavior appear to be goal-orientated when the cat pounces upon a mouse or the bee gathers honey from certain flowers. Like Marx, who had to ignore all kinds of selfless human behavior in order to affirm that man was basically an acquisitive being, the behaviorists have tried to understand the operation of organisms without taking into account mental ideas and altruistic emotional feelings.

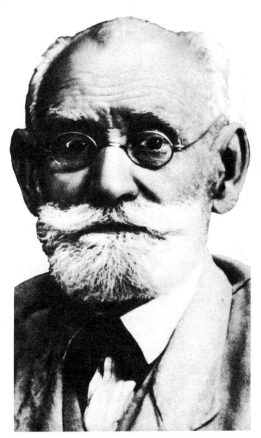

I. P. Pavlov (1849-1936), Russian physiologist, worked on the conditioned reflex.

Skinner's behavioral utopia, named "Walden Two", is founded on the concept of operant conditioning which we practice naturally with our children and our pets when we reward them for goodness and punish them for misbehavior. The Skinner theory tries to fill the gap in the classical theory of Pavlov by insisting that man's goal-governed behavior is really not just a biological mechanism but an emotional mechanism—a seeking of pleasure and avoidance of pain—and that these pain-pleasure seeking emotional mechanisms of our nature are also subject to conditioning. According to Skinner, organisms tend to repeat behavior that is reinforced with positive feedback since they get a feeling of satisfaction or fulfillment, or a sensation of pleasure when they fill a basic biological need like sex or eating. If a baby screams and you comfort him he will be certain to scream again whenever he wants attention later.

Skinner's utopia is based on the long-term advantages of positive conditioning as opposed to punishment. Under a punishment system, Skinner maintains, control over an individual can be increased only by increasing painful coercive methods which create feelings of resentment, rebellion and divisiveness, so that the controlled behavior is offset by side effects that are bad for society. Skinner admits that his operant conditioning, supposedly leading to utopia could, by using the same techniques for negative rather than positive reinforcement, produce a society where freedom, security and happiness were all suppressed.

We need not look farther than Moscow, where these personal values of freedom are not considered high ones, to see Pavlovian conditioning taking place with both negative as well as positive reinforcement. The control of deviant behavior in communist countries is mankind's old way of achieving power-goals by negative means, such as the ruthless withdrawal of jobs, social rights, etc. The Hungarian Revolution is a perfect example of negative reinforcement. The Hungarian Revolution was suppressed by the Soviet army in 1956, and the reconsolidation of the Soviet-backed communist regime led to continued reprisals for many years against anyone who had participated in the revolution. Continuous announcements of arrests and punishment of suspected revolutionaries were given out to the public and to their relatives long after sentences of imprisonment and execution had

Positive Reinforcement:
The experiments of B.F. Skinner.

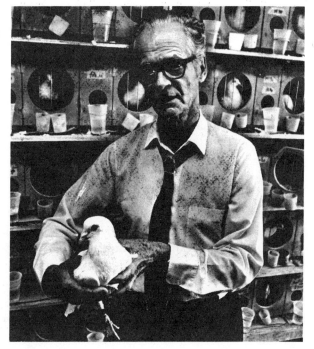

Negative Reinforcement of Soviet
tanks in Czechoslovakia. When
Soviet troops invaded Czechoslovakia on August 20, 1968, students erected barricades around
the Prague radio building so that
for as long as possible the station
could broadcast to the world
what was happening to the
country.

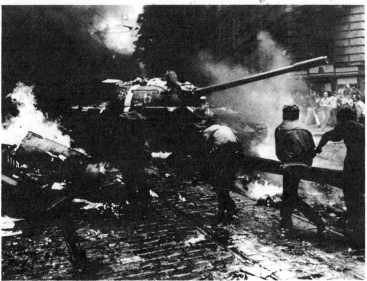

been carried out. The total number sitting in overcrowded jails awaiting their secret trials could not even be guessed at. The number known to have been executed by the puppet government which took over from the Russians is in the region of several thousand—perhaps small compared to the 100,000 who were butchered by the Soviet guns when they invaded the country to repress the Hungarians. A United Nations special committee denounced the new Hungarian government for violating the UN charter and denying human rights by its repeated secret trials and executions and in September 1958 the entire UN Assembly voted 61 to 10 for a debate on the Hungarian repressions and the secret execution by the USSR of the former prime minister of Hungary along with other members of the former communist government. The Soviet bloc and the new Hungarian government made a statement that such a debate would change nothing—an absolute refusal to respect the worldwide views of humanity or even the rights of war prisoners, let alone the rights of political prisoners to public trials.

During 1958 many repressive measures were taken to sift out and kill off any dissenters in Hungary. The installation of "peoples' inspectors", responsible only to the top Council of Ministers of the communist government, intensified absolute control of the economic and political environment. They sifted out all potential opponents from every sector of society. Appointments to positions required "certificates of good behavior" for all posts. Private law practice was abolished and lawyers were ordered to organize themselves into cooperatives. Late in summer, 550 lawyers were suspended from practice altogether for attempting to preserve some legal rights for their clients.

This theory of coercive government practiced in all modern communist societies is based on the conditioning theories of Pavlov. But the idea that society can be organized and controlled by coercion or by complete mastery of the environment has not been proved. The invasion of Czechoslovakia in 1968 and the subsequent communist party purge of half its members by the Russian-installed puppet government revealed that the Soviets were terrified of the liberation movement in that country, lest it infect Russia itself and all the other Warsaw pact countries. It is obvious even to the communists that a society which uses pain and negative reinforcement in order to threaten

WHY DO PEOPLE WANT TO ESCAPE SOCIALIST UTOPIAS?

WIDE WORLD

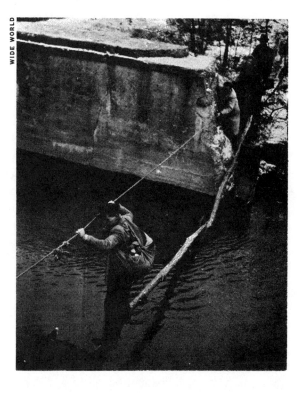

Here a group of Hungarian freedom fighters uses a makeshift bridge over a swollen stream to find its way to freedom in the West after Soviet Russia's suppression of the uprising.

As the revolt of 1956 collapsed, Hungarian refugees fled into Austria by every possible route. Many perished.

Camera Press—Pix from Publix

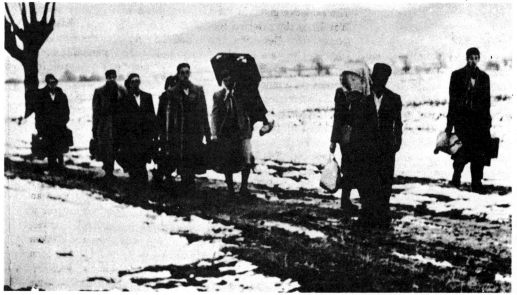

individuals or groups and to bring deviants back into line with its norms, will eventually backfire if taken too far. Revolutions emerge and tyrants are overthrown because repressive methods make the authority into a formidable foe to the people.

The less repressive and less noticeable the control and the more persuasive the coercion, the more successful the techniques of control. The totally controlled society, such as that of Soviet Russia, does not require the controller to make a constant show of power but can be handled by the subtle influence of the secret police and by assuming complete control of all communications concerning arrests, harassments, etc., and by carefully doling out positive reinforcements for conforming to the party line. Yet even the subtler repressions will one day bring a reaction, just as when individual people subject their feelings to repression and present a self-image to the world that is controlled and acceptable. One day the whole thing blows and the repressed emotions emerge from the unconscious to wreak their havoc in the form of cancer, a nervous breakdown or some other dis-ease. The murderer who writes the police a note saying "Stop me before I kill again," is a person who has *lost* control of himself; his unconscious urges are leading him in directions he does not consciously wish to go. And in the same way an individual boxed in and controlled by the State gets out of touch with that *self*-control which alone can protect society and build a peaceful world.

The method used by Skinner to intensify control over an organism through positive, rather than negative, reinforcement was to control the environmental factors more precisely so that only positive reinforcement is experienced by the organism. No mean feat, considering that life is fully prepared to teach us with both techniques. The "Skinner box" was a soundproof airtight enclosure that enabled the experimenter to control all environmental stimuli reaching the animal inside the box so that no negative experiences could come in. For twenty years Skinner made pigeons walk in figure eight patterns, playing ping pong and perform complex tasks like color recognition. But he flatly stated that the pigeons had not been improved one bit, only the environmental conditions under which they lived had been improved.

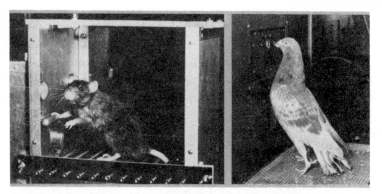

When the rat pressed the bar and the pigeon pecked the wall of the Skinner box, Skinner would reward them with food. The animals quickly learned to repeat the act.

Substitution of exact systematic control to replace the random probabilities of Nature gave birth to the science of "cultural design". According to Skinner, the possibilities of cultural design are as endless as the power of conditioning. Thus his utopian concept of "Walden Two" is a world in which all external environmental factors are scientifically controlled even more than the strict internal specialty training of judges, soldiers, teachers and statesmen that was to be controlled in Plato's utopian Republic. Skinner reasoned that scientific control of all contingencies brought the greatest degree of personal happiness—the same concept that was held by the ancient monasteries and ashrams for spiritual training, where life was governed almost mechanically by the ring of the monastery bell. Whether this external control builds dependence on regimentation and weakens the capacity for self-discipline is a subject not mentioned by Skinner.

In practice it has been noticed that people who live in secure communities and groups find it difficult to make effective decisions and to keep their minds alert to the competition in the larger world. Decisions tend to get made by the few individuals who accept responsibility and cultivate self-discipline as a challenge rather than shuffling it off onto the group. But writers who have envisioned perfect societies have endeavored to describe environments so controlled that deviationist or self-thinking behavior has very little opportunity to develop. All too many utopias have been unable to cope with dissent and human conflict without generating personal aggressiveness. What makes a utopian community pleasant and non-aggressive is that no one needs to be punished or threatened with any consequences because (theoretically) no one misbehaves. No one deviates from the stated and accepted norms of the commune, therefore no one needs to be governed or to subject himself to an authority figure, a leader, a king or a sovereign power such as the state. From an ethical viewpoint, however, freedom has no meaning without the possibility of there being bondage, and in a community in which no one misbehaves, there could be no meaning to good behavior unless we are free to choose bad behavior. If no one has an urge to do evil there can be no great credit awarded to those who do good. Only when a member by his own self-discipline becomes good, can there be any true foresight as to what is "good" behavior, since if we are *not* good, how can we know and do what *is* good? All we would know is comparative knowledge, i.e., what gives pleasure is good compared to what gives pain, which is evil and bad. Such dualistic knowledge is naive since what is often painful to do can bring much good and what is often pleasurable is sometimes the cause of evil.

The utopian idea, that environmental signals which punish or give pain are bad and those that create pleasurable feelings are good, comes from a misunderstanding of Nature. Pain is not bad; without pain there would be no evolution, no errors would get corrected and without pain, pleasure itself could not exist. The idea that we must welcome pain when it comes because life teaches mankind equally as much through pain as through pleasure, is not a popular one. It requires a certain detachment so far reserved only for sages, holy men and saints.

In the community experiment at the University of the Trees self-discipline is considered far more challenging than to get up for the bell, work to the bell and pray to the bell. Instead of the luxury of a regimented stimulus-response environment, the individuals at this community must tussle inwardly with the challenge of making a choice: whether to indulge each impulse and urge or to be a master of self and of their instincts. The challenge is to master the drive for pleasurable reinforcement so that a person's own will is supreme over any stimulus and he or she is not dependent upon anything external for happiness.

Skinner's utopia was said to offer conditions which are normally described in our society as freedom, security, happiness and knowledge.

One is reminded of the child who clings to his security blanket, whether that security is the ring of the ashram bell or the publication of the "Truth" in Pravda, the official organ of the communist party. Does "Pravda" teach people to think for themselves and become free and therefore capable of leading others to freedom or does it, like the kibbutz commune, offer security from cradle to grave? The question comes: why do people leave the security of the kibbutz for a normal life? Why did the monastery which took care of its renunciates from youth 'til death ultimately fail? Why did thousands of people living in socialist East Germany cross over into free Berlin every day, escaping from the regimentation imposed by the Soviets until they had to build the Berlin wall to stop the outflow of refugees? The answer is in the few words, "freedom of choice"—a human right which in socialist societies is not highly regarded.

How each individual, including the reader, responds to the vision of a totally controlled society and environment will depend on how he or she values freedom of choice. Believers in individual freedom will answer by saying that people are not pigeons or rats in a maze and should not be treated as such *even if they can be.* Why is it that millions of people are content to live like kept creatures, leaving all the responsibility for their well-being with someone else? Even in these people there is a spirit which can be awakened and cause them to conceive a purpose, a goal, something not programmed or anticipated by their parents, government, teachers, nor anyone else. Rights and freedoms do not exist without responsibilities, and this is why we let our rights slip from us so easily. It is not just a matter of preserving the freedoms but seeing that it is our *responsibility* to think for ourselves and accepting it. If we are to preserve the freedom to think for ourselves we must not only resist any techniques that would infringe on our rights to change but must accept the responsibilities that go *with* the rights. Before we know what is best for ourselves (much less let another decide) we have to know what kind of person we are and what is our true nature. What is our destiny, both as an individual and as part of mankind? Shall another person's vision of the highest values he can grasp be a limit on your own capacity for vision? B. F. Skinner has his own idea of utopia, but is it yours?

We are all culture-bound. But we must do something about
the quality of life. People who don't have to do anything
will not, without help, do the kinds of things that develop
them as individuals. Drugs, gambling, spectatorship—these
may yield a happy life of a sort, but at the end a person
won't be any different from when he started. Sex is a
special kind of immediate reinforcer because it is concerned
with the survival of the species rather than of the individual,
and if you can prevent the undesirable consequences, I see
nothing against it. But sex also doesn't develop the individual.
A person who turns to the arts, crafts, sports, exploration,
science, or literature, on the other hand, is constantly
changing. He is a different person at the end of his life. But
we need a culture to promote these activities. A culture that
does so is a strong culture, whereas a culture that allows its
people to live a life of pleasant stupefaction is not.*

I question whether science, literature and the arts *really* develop a
person any more than sex does. If so, then the academic community
would surely be utopia on earth. But in fact, many university professors
are among the most narrow-visioned unaware people in the world.
Skinner's ideals may be shaped by that scholarly world and its values,
but they need not apply to everyone. We have to keep the right to
extend our awareness even beyond science, even beyond the artistic
imagination, even to the farthest reaches of the universe.

Only those who are not clear-seeing feel the need to be controlled
by someone wiser and, even then, they abdicate their spiritual search
for their own self-mastery if they allow another to dictate their environment. Plus even the most benevolent dictator may not necessarily
be a wise man. To exercise absolute control over the total environment
is impossible unless you know what that total environment is, and the
assumption that we do know all the factors that control our external
and internal environment is only a hypothesis and not a fact. To give
up our freedom for the hypothesis that anyone, including ourselves,

---

* Taken from an encyclopedia description of B. F. Skinner's work.

ESCAPING FROM THE CONTROLLED ENVIRONMENT OF COMMUNISM

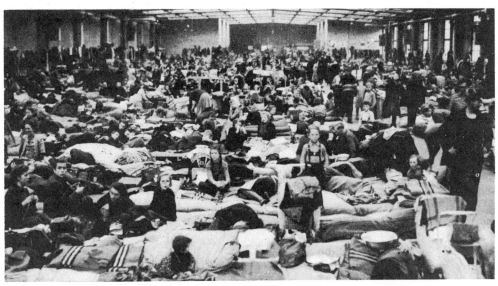

Refugees from East Germany totaling some 305,000 persons poured into West Berlin during 1953. A temporary shelter, above, in a factory building in the U.S. zone of Berlin was set up to care for the throngs. Many were sent by improvised airlift to be cared for in West Germany.

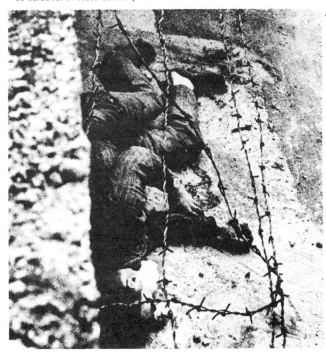

← Peter Fechter, eighteen, shot by Soviet zone police while trying to escape to West Berlin, seen as he lay dying August 17, 1962, at the foot of the wall he had hoped to cross. Onlookers in West Berlin were restrained from helping him by the guns of the East German police.

Berlin, 1961: East German soldier leaps to the West.

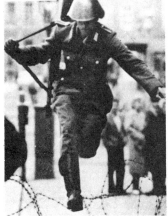

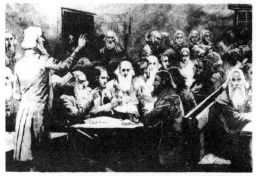

BETTMANN ARCHIVE

"A Love Feast Among the Dunkers" by Howard Pyle, portrays a religious ceremony of this sect.

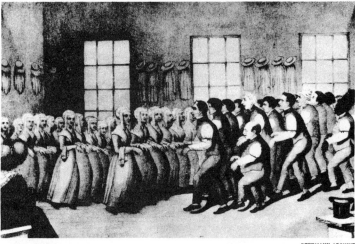

BETTMANN ARCHIVE

Shakers, originally a Quaker sect, tremble during community meeting as they receive spiritual power. Illustration from an old lithograph.

Two movements for world utopia motivated by religious feelings. While attracting sincere people who lived their beliefs, they somehow lacked the element which would change the world. Not only was their philosophy rigid, but their lifestyle was too controlled.

really totally knows all the factors is to assume that there is no ultimate reality extended beyond the experience of our own immediate environment.

If we saw how much our environment is now already controlled by social factors, we would preserve the freedoms we do have left from government control and not give up still more to the so-called all-wise authority. And who *is* this authority who says we should give up individuality and have our external environment totally controlled in order to be happy? This theory that environment is the main cause of our happiness is not borne out by most of those who have achieved real happiness. Our greatest sages and scientists have stated quite adamantly that we only experience a tiny fragment of our internal world and our external environment. Much of what goes on in our total environment outside the skin, for instance in the interactions of the atomic world of energies, is not even experienced.*

What if AWARENESS IS THE REAL PATHWAY TO UTO-PIA? And what if this environment which we are to control, is far beyond our power to imagine, much less control? Where do we draw the line and stop trying to control the stimuli of the so-called external world? Can we control the tremendous radiation which bombards our bodies at every moment from all parts of the universe? Or is there some point at which we have to admit our ignorance and simply trust in life? In the interview with B. F. Skinner, quoted above, Skinner's answer sparked several astute questions by the interviewer. In his replies, Skinner expands his utopian dream to include the whole world, but it is only the world of society that he is speaking of. His awareness extends no farther.

"Q. Are you more concerned with the survival of a particular culture—our own—than with the survival of mankind?

---

* See *Nuclear Evolution*, published by University of the Trees Press, 1977. Part II, Chapters 32, 33 and 34 deals with the interaction of the atoms of our bodies with the total intelligence and shows how the state of our consciousness limits our perception of the environment.

A. No. I think in the long run mankind must be the object of cultural design. The major issues have become global, and our decisions must take the future of everyone into account. It's not a question of whether we can still grab more natural resources than anyone else, but whether there will be any resources left.

Q. Survival of the culture in your terms, seems to require an enormous centralization of power. Couldn't this be called fascist?

A. The culture which makes it impossible for controlling power to be centralized would be a strong culture. What we have to look forward to is not a benevolent dictator but a culture in which no one can become a dictator. That would be a culture that would survive."

The final answer of B. F. Skinner in this interview is absolutely true. But what means can actually reach that end? Though Skinner would not theoretically subscribe to it, implicit within his means are repressions and controls on news and information and individual freedom of choice and of speech. How else can we achieve total control of the environment? Though Skinner rules out a benevolent dictator, his utopia hinges upon Skinner himself and other benevolent arbiters who would decide the limits of the control of that environment and what they should be and what reinforcement would be good and beneficial. Yet these human arbiters might not accept or approve as desirable much of what others experience as real.

To control the environment, expression of our internal experience must necessarily be repressed, because expression is not the same for everyone and would condition the way human beings communicate and thereby affect the environment. Yet the conflicting conditions of the world are brought about by *lack* of human communication, not by *too much* expression of our real thoughts. Human beings, even in a free social environment or the security of the family situation, are self-conscious and we express only a limited amount of that which is going on inside our skins. We do not communicate most of what happens in our minds even to close relations. The problem of society is that we express too little and even that little bit is not clear; the rest is all repressed. Repression from within and repression from the outside environment by elimination of certain stimuli puts society in a double bind. Therefore the answer of the World Peace Center is to enhance the clarity of communication and make possible the opportunity of more free, spontaneous expression. In other words, the answer for the world is not total control but total *freedom* for the individual—the awesome responsibility of self-mastery. Only this can produce the culture in which no one can become a dictator.

We cannot express our inner world without affecting the environment and thereby undoing the control. The inner world of even one individual, much less millions, is sufficient to wreck a really *controlled* environment and therefore repression of the individual is a natural and inevitable outcome of the drive for total control. The behavioral ideal—in its ultimate form (whether negative or positive)—must by its very nature try to bring utopia by stifling the individual in one way or another. The negative repressions of the communists reflect a crude kind of consciousness that relates to other human beings by trying to dominate them. The behaviorists who use positive reinforcement are a more sophisticated version of the same thing: power over Nature, power over human beings, power over pigeons and dogs as they dance to the sound of the bell. The question always remains, what limited awareness is going to decide the future for you or me?

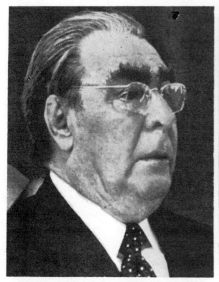

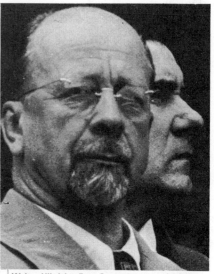

Brezhnev, leader of the socialist utopia, shows no light or radiance of joy of a utopia. He displays more a look of disappointment and failure.

Walter Ulbricht, East German communist boss, intimately posing with his "adviser," Soviet Foreign Minister Andrei Gromyko in 1957. The two austere faces reflected the somber outlook for the East German Republic.

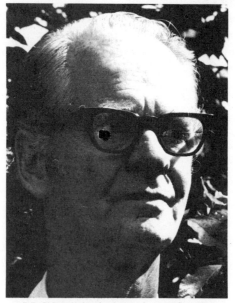

B.F. Skinner's face and eyes do not reflect the happiness and bliss he claims can be achieved through controlling one's external environment.

I have never seen pictures of any of these men looking happy or at peace.

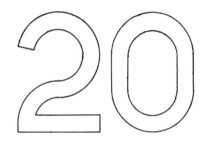

THE
ULTIMATE
ORGASM

Behaviorists claim that by controlling all possible inputs of stimuli, both pleasurable and painful, and by using them as reinforcements, the perfect society can be evolved and happiness and bliss achieved. However when we look at the photographs of behaviorist B.F. Skinner we do not see any sign of the bliss that he is claiming can be achieved, whereas when we look at the photograph of a realized yogi, we recognize instantly a light of inner sweetness and bliss which comes from *self-control* and not from the external environment. In fact, the yogi's external environment is usually inhospitable for the average person who is unaccustomed to lying on concrete floors, living in the Himalayan caves or leading a life of few material comforts. This fact— that fulfillment is not dependent on external stimuli—should disprove once and for all the behaviorist theory that the external environment has something to do with the higher kind of bliss we expect from an

638

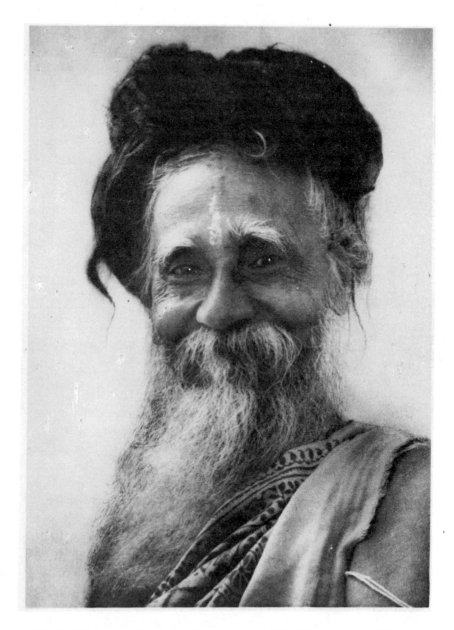

The same light as seen in the eyes of this unkown man is seen in all those who have attained inner sweetness and bliss.

enlightened person. Since the behaviorists do not even recognize that there are different kinds of bliss at different thresholds of consciousness, their range of knowledge and experience makes it impossible for them to understand these states except through hearsay, and therefore they have no idea of what they are talking about when they use the word "bliss" or "happiness".

Craving for bliss and fulfillment is the deepest drive in human beings. From deep in our unconscious minds it surfaces in our incessant attempts to seek and possess the external tokens of happiness. For we do not understand that bliss can only be found inside us, inherent in the Nuclear Self, and therefore can only come as a by-product of oneness when we give up the very ego that is seeking after its happiness in all these external ways. The oneness is already *in our hearts if only we can find it. The words "Nuclear Self" do not mean some gigantic abstract SELF, separate from your feelings, but the deepest part of you. The whole universe is inside you,* behind the locked door of the ego. Therefore bliss and fulfillment are never permanently achieved as long as ego separation reigns, though we have moments or periods of time where we are on top of the world and fulfillment is here. These are always times when there is a self-forgetting of petty cares and concerns of the ego.

Most people experience a taste of this temporary bliss in the sexual orgasm, and they believe that the happiness has come from external sensory pleasure. But what really happens is that, for one brief instant at the moment of climax, they forget themselves and experience oneness not only with their partner but with the whole universe, because all that blocks us from this ecstatic experience of oneness with the entirety of creation is the inability to forget ourselves. So anyone who has ever experienced the brief moment of oblivion in the act of making love has tasted the promise of bliss that is known by the yogi as a permanent state of consciousness. He feels it bubbling up inside him in the life-force which Freud called *libido,* the force behind sexual energy. Therefore many yogis are highly sexed and very vital, yet the yogi's sexual energy does not stop at the physical level of consciousness as it does in most people but rises up the spine, creating a feeling of orgasm at every level. In yoga this is called the rising of "kundalini" which is a Sanskrit word for fiery consciousness. Subjectively the yogi experiences the happiness of falling in love not just with one person but with everything, and the bubbling feeling in all his cells is like having sex with the whole universe. Anyone can enjoy a glimpse of this joy just by allowing himself or herself to feel an outflow of love toward ordinary things. This feeling of kinship and oneness is the real purpose of the sexual drive and why it seems to come from so deep inside us— deep in the unconscious Self that has no boundaries or limits to its feeling of "I".

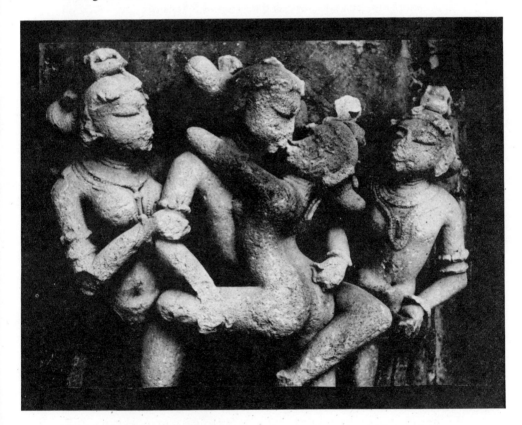

SEX AND SOCIETY

Sex is such a powerful and basic force in human nature that any social theory which does not understand and make room for the channeling of sexual energy both within the individual and between people cannot survive as an answer to world peace, any more than the human race can survive without sex. It is incredible how widespread is the misunderstanding of sexual energy and even misunderstanding of the sex *act*. Millions of men and women crave external stimulus and paraphernalia to turn them on, not realizing how much of the process of coming to an orgasm is governed by the imagination, not by sensory stimuli. Sexual purity or pollution begins in the human mind, and it is the mind which blocks the way to spiritual orgasm and bliss. Many impotent people cannot get sexually turned on even with the most sophisticated stimulations and the only reason for the great number of pornographic shops springing up in our civilization is that people are finding it difficult to obtain sexual satisfaction at an ordinary sensory level and must have their senses titillated by the extra paraphernalia now to be found in thousands of different designs. Sexual paraphernalia has become a multi-million dollar business. Such are the facts of our present civilization, which cannot be ignored if we are to understand the spiritual importance of the orgasm in society's problems.

What is really happening inside people? The behaviorists claim that people can be externally conditioned by pleasure and pain to choose the harmonious higher life, and yet the association of pain with the sexual act is widely acknowledged. Some people get more turned on sexually by the excitement of pain than by sensitive pleasures, as anyone can see in the violent sex movies, novels and television serials. Behaviorists do not deal with the fact that at the moment of sexual crisis, one does not care whether the environment is a hard stony floor or an undulating waterbed. The personal self-image is forgotten. Pleasure and pain distinctions fade. It is part of the very nature of sex that this dualism of the ego-self, always seeking pleasure and running from pain, should become one. But for some people the only doorway to the pleasure is through the pain. This is a very low level doorway and will bring a low level kind of ecstasy. Those who experience sex primarily in the bodily sensation will never even know the higher levels they are missing, but unconsciously they will begin to compensate and to seek more and more through the senses for the greater thing that they crave. They go farther and farther away from their goal, because they cannot see that they will never find outside themselves the deep inner space they are seeking.

The beast which stalks the world today, not only in bestial love-making but in brutality to fellow man, has its beginning in a fundamental misunderstanding of life and of our own psychological make-up. Perverted sex, aggression, violence, where do they come from? What is their common link? Is it a coincidence that the violence wrought by the Nazis upon the Jews was often sexual? Sigmund Freud, in his famous correspondence with the pacifist Albert Einstein, argued that aggression was at the root of our very survival as a species and that it was very much linked with repression of the life-force *(libido)* in us, which propels us toward reproduction of the species in sex, and also creates the vitality inside us and the dynamism with which we act and live. To repress such a powerful energy has a tremendous effect on society.

Today, sexual aggression or the lack of an outlet for it may be leading to the most bestial pornographic period of history where people are mutilated and sexually ravished in front of movie cameras. Even murders are committed in front of the camera and films are made of a helpless person slowly dying by sadistic violence in order to arouse the satiated sexual appetite of those who have seen everything and·whose tastes are jaded and dulled. Pornography has become big business, with a ready market controlled by the huge family network of Mafia hoods who supply the chains of pornographic shops and adult movies throughout the world. Obviously the world is today much sicker than in the times of Sodom and Gomorrah, and the urge for this aggression and sexual sadism is getting stronger and stronger. No one is quite certain whether old values of right and wrong still hold true in a modern world.

THE THIN LINE

In the free society of democratic states, even though decadence is strongly resented by the majority of society, violent and pornographic movies are allowed under the laws. The liberalization of sexual appetites and the perversion of drives has even resulted in a "gay revolution" of homosexuals, who claim equal rights in society to openly adopt any sexual relationships they please. A society which represses and ostracizes those who are different, is sick with the disease of intolerance. Its rigid morality is bought at the expense of

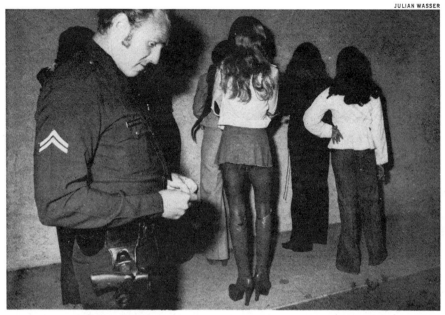

JULIAN WASSER

TRANSVESTITE PROSTITUTES UP AGAINST THE WALL ON SUNSET BOULEVARD

"Our policemen feel they are taking part in a perverted act," said one officer with contempt of the masochistic transvestites who kept repeating "I love it, I love it," as the policemen handcuffed them.

An Arrest in Mutilation Rape Case

Sparks, Nev.

A heavyset former merchant seaman was arrested in Sparks yesterday as a suspect in the case of a 15-year-old girl whose arms were chopped off below the elbows after she was raped.

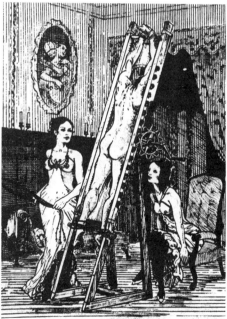

An artist's impression of the Berkeley Horse, which made a fortune for its London inventor in the nineteenth century. It recognizes that prostitutes must cater to varied kinds of human vice.

Features International

When misunderstanding of sexual energies causes them to be twisted, all manner of perversions arise in a downward flow of energy, whereas an upward flow of this energy can result in immense feelings of joy and lightness.

higher spiritual qualities of compassion and greatness of heart. In the case of homosexuality, much of the self-righteous judging comes from people's fear that they too might have some homosexual tendencies. And this fear, in turn, is rooted in the fact that all human beings have both male and female energies inside, which they must balance. Male chauvinists and the kind of women they dominate are just as imbalanced in their sexual energies as homosexuals are. The natural drive of the heterosexual to make love with the opposite sex is really just a desire to balance these energies. Because the yogi is able to balance them inside himself as the kundalini rises up his spine, he has no need for an external partner to achieve the state of ecstasy though he may choose to have one.

To view the gay revolution from this perspective is to be automatically more accepting and tolerant. On the other hand, a society in which freedom becomes license also loses that centeredness which fosters true integrity and allows weakness and indulgence to pervert our true purpose. In an individual, the thin line between self-acceptance and self-indulgence makes the difference between integrity of character and lack of character. And the same is true of society. The same kinds of rationalizations that come into the mind of an indulgent individual also lead a whole society down the subtle pathways of inner decay, so gradually that the deterioration is hardly noticed. Society pays a high price for this victory of weakness over self-discipline. The price is that our children grow up to think that "anything goes", that there are no limits. Righteousness becomes of no social value. Morality in this environment has no meaning, virtue has no advantage.

CHANNELING AGGRESSION

It is argued that the greatest achievements of civilizations are brought to us from the aggressive desire to excel or by the challenge of competition. But here in America, the evolution of society stagnates among competition of the worst kind, ranging from who can produce the worst and most beastly sexual magazine or movie to the dream of becoming a TV personality, a top singer, a football idol or multi-millionaire. If the aggressive drive to be "number one" motivates a person to become the most wealthy and successful pornography publisher in the country, can we really say that the channeling of aggression into competition is productive? It is productive only at the level we are expressing on.

In the capitalist society competition is fierce, and only the winners receive the lavish prizes of personal achievement, making the remainder of the population feel that they are not good enough, smart enough, handsome enough or likeable enough to make it. Though competition may be a mode of discharging aggression, it means that some must lose while others win, and often it actually robs a person of the ability to express love and caring toward himself or toward others. The negative side-effects of the competitive spirit are nowhere more visible than in politics. Whereas competition can be channeled creatively in the teamwork of sports, it takes a negative path through politics where the goal is to achieve personal power rather than to win a game. If politics is regarded only as a game for the release of aggressive energies, or as a legitimately competitive ego contest among opponents, then why is it that in politics real people must suffer and society becomes the pawn of the gamemaster? We are so used to it that we accept and condone it, but is the political arena that far from physical aggression? Imagine what our society would be like if its leaders were chosen by a method that made competition totally unnecessary!* It is hard for us even to conceive of such a system, so accustomed are we to compromise and learning to "play ball" if one wants to stay in the game of politics.

The channels for aggression are slightly different in other societies. In the Soviet socialist society aggressive appetites are strictly orientated to the goals of the Soviet State. In the Chinese five-year plan, aggressive impulses are channeled into production schedules, and internal differences are not allowed. In restricted societies like communist or fascist states, the aggression is focused outwards towards enemies. On the one hand we have capitalism, with its

---

* The constitution I am proposing in *The Golden Egg* recommends the use of the ancient Chinese oracle, the *I Ching*, for the choosing of leaders, so that the deep Self that is in us all can make the choice, rather than leaving it up to the ego to sift and weigh the distorted reports and expensive propaganda.

fostering of ego competition and separation from the whole, and on the other hand we have communism which has at least a philosophy of wholeness but whose "whole" stops at the borders of the nation-state.

In a genuinely spiritual society where the goal is to entirely give up the self-imposed limits upon consciousness, then everything is commonly owned and there are no competitors winning at the expense of others, and the drive to excel and advance beyond our peers is translated not into political competition but into spiritual disciplines to improve oneself and to purify consciousness. Any tendency towards aggression is dissipated in intense Creative Conflict that serves the same purpose that competitive sports or business serves in the more primitive societies that we have today. In a spiritual society, where people are willing to put Truth before their ideology or private rationalizations and to put the good of the whole before selfish self-interest, the life-force is allowed to flow in straightforward ways, not repressed and diverted into a multitude of ego compensations such as the compulsion to gain fame and power. Are the evils of society innate in human nature or are they compensations for not feeling quite alive or quite happy or quite fulfilled? The life-force is blocked in almost all human beings, so much so that blocked energy seems our natural state. Yet perhaps we are accepting a negative state as our birthright when really our true essence is something quite different.

IS MAN BY NATURE VIOLENT?

The responses of Freud the pessimist to the optimistic idealism of Einstein during his pacifist years insist that men have an innate and latent potential for war and that war is inevitable, a built-in part of the human condition. Freud explains:

> "The Bolshevists, too, aspire to do away with human aggressiveness by ensuring satisfaction of material needs and enforcing equality between man and man. To me this hope seems vain. Meanwhile they busily perfect their armaments, and their hatred of outsiders is not the least of the factors of cohesion among themselves.*

---

* The correspondence between Einstein and Freud was published in Paris in 1933 in a booklet called "Why war?" which was banned in Hitler's Germany, where not even advertisements for it were allowed.

For Freud to write this forty-five years ago shows some insight into the aggressive hatred socially instilled by the governments of the socialist countries in their controlled newspapers. The pressure of an imaginary external aggressor on a society seems to bring internal cohesion, but the cost in terms of what is unleashed upon the world is the same as with repressed energy in an individual. The results of repression are bad enough when single individuals fail to control sexual and aggressive urges, but when in a nation the normal channels of aggression are repressed, either by morality or social ideals imposed politically, the consequences of building up armaments and fanning the flames of external aggression can spell the end of whole societies.

The organization of violence in the form of armies and police, where society itself cooperates within to train people to compete aggressively with outsiders, is found in other species and animal societies. Gangs cooperate internally in political terrorism or organized crime but they war with each other. The formation of a group sometimes increases the aggressions of its members by taking away restraints and creating the need to gain attention to prove oneself within the group by acting out violence on some hapless victim. Hence aggressive youth gangs will form squads to torment Jews or homosexuals or anyone with different cultural customs. This aggression is not restricted to youth gangs of sexually immature and repressed adolescents but is found at every level of society.

There is no general agreement among psychologists, sociologists, religious scholars or behavioral scientists on the ultimate irrational extension of our aggressive drives. Even among scientists, aggressive feelings emerge at the announcement of new theories. One of the originators of the new theories of sociobiology was covered with a jug of water as he spoke at a recent meeting of the prestigious American Association for the Advancement of Science, and many scientists with unusual views on hereditary genes, intelligence and physics have been ridiculed, slapped, and pelted with tomatoes, rotten eggs, etc., for writing what they think. Not the least in suffering this aggression was Einstein in the early days of his theory which stimulated a whole rash of anti-Einstein societies in the fascist social climate of his early life in Germany.

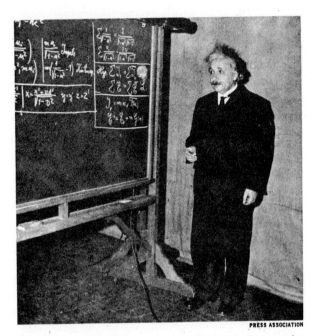

PRESS ASSOCIATION

Albert Einstein, eminent physicist, developed the law that mass may be converted into radiant energy.

Small wonder that people believe that aggression is part of human nature; it has always been with us, even in religion. The image of a Christ, broken on the cross by the Roman soldiers and violently betrayed by his own people as a social outcast, did not become the dominating image of the Christian religion for two thousand years for nothing. Even though Christ taught peace and asked us to focus on the rising of the human spirit to union with the higher states of consciousness, Christianity became the religion of the cross and it emphasized the violence embodied in the crucifixion. The medieval religious courts and the Inquisition, who sentenced their victims and scapegoats to torture and burned them alive while believing they were saving their souls, are no different from the communist slave camps, brutally sending political deviates to death in the twentieth century in Russia, Cambodia and China.

What is the primal energy that can be provoked into violence or channeled into love? The energy of consciousness is purely impersonal, but an ego reaction to a threatening idea turns the pure energy into aggression. You can feel inside you the reacting energy, and it becomes a weapon for attack. Does such aggression spring spontaneously from within human beings—a natural expression of creatures who are by nature violent? History would seem to tell us it were so, but mankind now has the evolved awareness that will let him step back and see that there was always a choice there—to follow the energy of the reaction or to listen to the promptings of the "still small voice" which is trying to teach us love.

Most humans put off loving fellowman. Man has a soul if only he will take the trouble to tune to a subtler energy. But it is easier to react than to love. Sometimes when we think we are acting from high ideals, our ego is really trying to wipe out any contradiction or threat to our own beliefs. And we may think that this ego is our real nature, but is it?

The fact that dissenters are today kept under top secret guard in communist countries, just as the Jews were in the extermination camps and gas chambers of the Nazi racial supremacists, shows that such violence done in the name of a "cause" is done out of expediency, not from social conscience. If expediency is a higher priority than conscience, from what depths of human nature does it arise? If man is by nature aggressive, then why does his conscience nag him? If we are by nature aggressive, how can we talk about the progressive decay of society as though we had the power to reverse the process? Later in this chapter we will take a deeper look into the dark subconscious mind and see what is really behind the violence and why it has a sexual dimension. Whatever the primal cause, it is stronger than the fear of repercussions.

The written dialogue between Einstein and Freud occurred long before any possibility of an atomic bomb or the discovery of fission. Freud spoke of a "well-founded dread of the form that future wars will take." Yet this well-founded dread was not sufficiently shared by others to stop the entire world from bursting into World War II just seven years later.

The political opportunists who organize a whole culture and tap the creative energy of their people for organized aggression in war and political expansion, have now developed the ultimate weapons which will make the entire world impotent and render the species without the means to reproduce. The most frightening manifestation of the beast— far more dangerous than thumbscrews, racks and burning alive—where whole populations can be snuffed out overnight, can now be utilized by any secret international terrorist who wishes to destroy self and others in some perverted way of channeling repressed sexual potency. Today we are not so much afraid of fanatical political leaders who would use the power of the ultimate weapon, because any such aggression by a nation would result in the annihilation of the aggressor as well. The dread today is from the international terrorist who is prepared to annihilate himself along with everyone else unless his demands are met. As the relative ease of obtaining plutonium from waste fissionable material grows in the years to come, the hijacker's tyranny, that now affects a few hundred passengers in an airplane, will spread to the ransoming of whole cities and eventually to whole nations. Already it is possible for an individual terrorist to go to nuclear plants that are producing energy for peaceful purposes and to hijack supplies and ingredients to construct an atom bomb.

What is it in a terrorist that makes him more aggressive than other people? If we label him aggressive, then we cannot probe his motive nor find out what really happens inside the mind of such a person. The real source of aggression is ego. Wars are fought not because men are innately aggressive but because men are obsessed with their own potency. Being inherently weak, the ego is bent on proving its power. Every other part of creation is connected with the whole and shares the power of the whole. Animals fight for a different motive. Only man is foolish enough to separate himself as an ego and try to stand totally alone. Behind all war is this separate self-sense, ruthlessly enthroned as the force and power of life, usurping the "total intelligence" (God, life-force) which is acting through the evolving nucleus at every level. It is true that man does have this power of life and intelligence as the agent of evolution, but he does not possess it and cannot use it creatively without the need to give homage to its source. Even if aggressive people seemingly get away with their power trips, they are mocked by the universe and, though they enjoy the fruits of their petty power, life cheats them of her sweetest offerings.

In the same way that a man feels a surge of power when he dominates the surrender of a woman in the sexual act, so also do people feel an excitement and a thrill in exercising brute force and material power over other human beings. But here again, there is a misunderstanding, for the surrender of a woman is voluntary, given out of love. The ecstasy of receiving totally is not the same thing as submission, for in this higher type of voluntary surrender, the woman wins the surrender of the man. The kind of man who experiences sexual intercourse in the false ecstasy of sheer power, misses the true ecstasy of surrender and union, and so too is it with nations. What is the atom bomb? It is a symbol of total power, the most powerful weapon known to man, the perfect antidote for a feeling of impotence.

THE ULTIMATE POWER: SELF-SACRIFICE

The self-immolation of a terrorist in bringing about the destruction of a world which is not to his own liking is not far removed from the sacrifice of the Buddhist monk who burns himself to death in protest against government persecution in Viet Nam. Both the terrorist and the

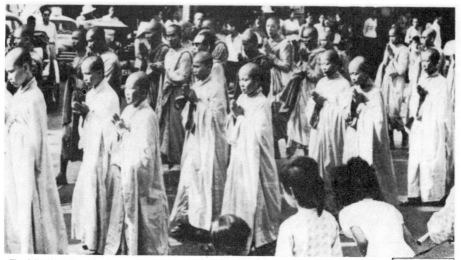

The following photographs record in sequence the suicide by fire of Thich Quang Duc on June 11, 1963 in Saigon. (AP Photos by Malcolm W. Browne) 9:00 AM

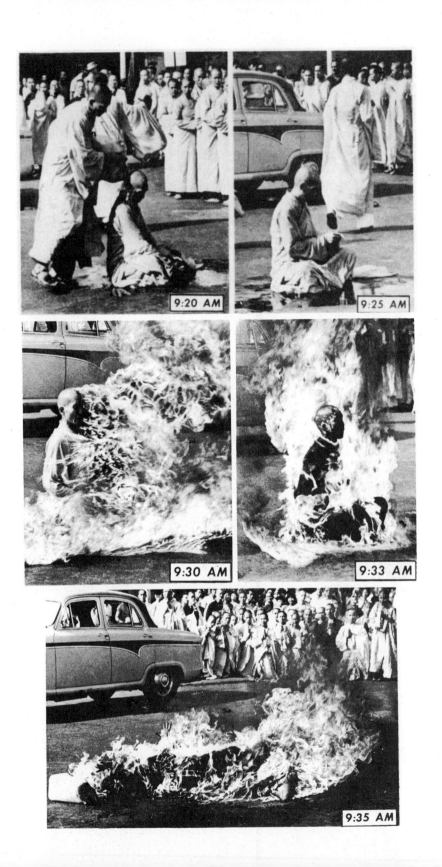

monk feel impotent and therefore take the most extreme way out of their intolerable frustration by convincing themselves it is all or nothing at all. In both cases the final act of the ego is to get rid of itself by identifying with its own body as the final weapon.

From the ego point-of-view, suicide is the turning inward of the ego and counting itself the ultimate hostage by which it can punish society for lack of caring. Suicide only occurs when alienation from the Cosmos becomes so extreme that release is sought in the last resort of annihilating the material identity. In this way the ego can feel like it retains its power and gain the ecstasy of release at the same time, but this is a delusion and the ecstasy is false, for it only releases the body and not the indwelling consciousness. At the opposite end of the spectrum, suicide is akin to the bliss of self-annihilation of the ego by the yogi or Christ who sacrifices himself as an act of total union rather than of alienation. To Socrates freedom of spirit meant more than life in the body when he committed suicide.

Built into the most precious gift of life is a fail-safe device, for we are given the power to use our consciousness for even the most separative selfish purposes, and yet this choice will put us so out of tune with the rest of the universe that in the end we will destroy ourselves. This is what Christ said when he was accused of healing by the devil's power: "If I heal by the devil's power then that is the end of him for he is divided against himself." What he meant by this was if the ego seizes power and sits on the throne of reality, the ego will eventually self-destruct. From a cosmic viewpoint the suicide urge is Nature's method of protecting itself against those who would blackmail God or the Creative Intelligence into running the universe their way. On the lower levels the universe must protect itself against acquisiton of powers before readiness to use them is there. Unless the power of consciousness or life can respect that same consciousness and life reflected in the total environment of which it is a part, consciousness will act against itself to destroy that selfishness in self-protection of the whole. If people are divided against themselves, the seeds of their own destruction will come to fruition and that will be the end of them. Every act of aggression will bring its destructive boomerang which the universe has as its built-in defense against any destructive power that works against the whole. For man to focus on destructive power, from a child's quarrel to a vast nuclear war, activates the beneficent power of consciousness to rise against it. On the other hand, when power is used on the higher levels to annihilate the separation between one self and other selves, then the power of consciousness can be trusted to serve the whole, and the death instinct and life instinct merge into another kind of superconscious primal energy which has the beneficent power of the universal consciousness behind it.

LIFE AND DEATH

Freud believed that all our behavior stemmed from two opposing universal forces: the life instinct, *eros*, which leads to enhancement of life, and the death instinct, *thanatos*, which seeks destruction. According to Freud, our unconscious motivations and behavior were governed by these two opposite powerful drives trying to balance themselves in equilibrium. The death instinct, *thanatos,* was usually seen as aggression

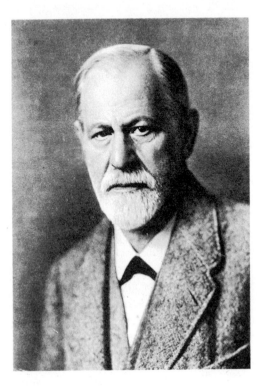

Sigmund Freud
The founder of psychoanalysis.

towards others, but could be directed inward in suicide. The life instinct, *eros,* was fueled by the *libido* energy in human consciousness. Freud had no name for the energy of the death instinct equivalent to *libido.* He suggested that the fuel was aggression, but aggression is not an energy. As a result he never really resolved the question of life and death. Yet if we examine *eros* and *thanatos* not in any book or theory but in our own consciousness, we will see that even these forces themselves have a prior cause, and both stem from the same root—the ego or self-sense.

The life-force that Freud called *libido* is not the primordial energy of the universe. Although Freud never fully understood it, *libido* comes when the cosmic energy of pure consciousness incarnates in form and identifies itself as a body. In Nuclear Evolution we see that this idea that we are a body is "ego"—a separate self (not in the same sense that Freud used the word "ego"). *Libido,* then, is the energy of the self-sense and manifests in the instincts of *eros* and *thanatos.* Freud's theory is incomplete because it does not recognize that life and death hinge upon identification with ourself as a human body instead of as a pure consciousness. Modern understanding from the science of the negative/positive structure of energies can shed some insight into Freud's trinity and into all other trinities to be found in many cultures as they attempt to explain consciousness. The atom is composed of positive, negative and neutral forces. In the East, concepts of *Prana* (*chi, ki,* or vital force) are always discussed in terms of their positive/negative, male/female, shiva/shakti, yin/yang modifications. Whether we use Freudian terms, scientific terms or Eastern terms, we are talking about the basic creative forces in Nature that propel all human action.

The ancient Hindu Vedic concept of the *gunas* answers Freud's problem and explains duality more accurately. The structure of the ego is described as the intertwining of three cosmic forces: the active force (*rajas*), the force of inertia (*tamas*) and *sattva,* the force of balance and light. These three forces are cosmically one, but they become separate qualities and myriad instincts when we incarnate into form and acquire an ego. By cutting through the ego-knot, these three qualities in consciousness are seen and experienced as one primordial energy. Sexual orgasm balances the energies to give us a taste of this oneness beyond ego, while the ultimate orgasm gives us a permanent experience of the primordial life force. Freud's insight into the forces of consciousness was limited because he himself never experienced the higher states of consciousness in the ultimate orgasm.

HE THAT WOULD GAIN HIS LIFE
MUST LOSE IT

The drive for self-annihilation was not overlooked by Freud, but he separated it from the sexual drive and used it to develop a rather pessimistic view of man's nature, attributing man's most beastly and aggressive qualities to a pre-ordained universal death force. Freud could not suspect that the death instinct had another purpose and could be found in disguise in the sexual orgasm at another level of consciousness. Even the sex drive which spends itself out in the discharge of repressed energy in the crisis of the physical orgasm has at its base the drive for self-annihilation. Therefore, sex is not just a result of the life instinct (*eros*), but an effect of a deeper causative urge.

The theory of Nuclear Evoluton is founded on the premise that the cause of hostility and war is not a built-in propensity for aggression nor a momentary need to discharge sexual frustration. All these drives are merely secondary to the primordial drive of the *real* death instinct to be found in all of Nature. This death instinct at the center of the nucleus is nothing but the unconscious desire to annihilate all separation from the original oneness, beginning with the idea of a separate selfhood, the ego, and ending in the transcendence of matter and creation, and ultimately dissolving the self root in the annihilation of matter itself. Behind the urge to pleasure, behind *eros* and *thanatos,* is the drive to re-experience the bliss of union.

Freud's concept of *libido* is in reality a reflection of the impersonal life-force, God, separating itself into form and implanting in the form an urge to return to oneness. *Libido* is this urge, and sexual attraction is only one of its many expressions. The urge to oneness is much more fundamental than Freud or his students who modified his theories knew, and results in the supreme religious experience of God—the dissolving of "I" or that self-sense which is separate from the whole. It is the positive pole of Being, while the destruction of self-identity as a material object in the act of suicide is the negative pole.

In the story of the garden of Eden, man and woman (yin and yang, male and female) were given a warning not to eat of the tree of the knowledge of good and evil. This allegorical tree was symbolic of the human nervous system with its capacity to alternate the two opposing positive/negative energies and thus sharpen the knife edge of intellectual discrimination.

On the other hand, the tree of life in the garden refers to the nerve dendrites in the brain that make us capable of the third energy—life-force energy—that gives the tree of life its name. This third energy is consciousness in its pure state, before the ego polarizes it into opposite extremes. In this state of purity, we are beyond the knowledge of life and death, good and evil, in a transcendent state called Virtue. But to get to this space of oneness we must be willing to annihilate the self-sense. In the East this is called transcending the creative forces to become master of oneself.

The spiritual genius of all our greatest teachers, from Lao Tzu to Jesus, from Plato and Socrates to Buddha, have said the same thing: kill the ego, become selfless, become the other, totally surrender yourself to God, the ultimate singularity. Now physics has invented the theoretical black hole to account for the death and annihilation of matter and the white hole for its creation. These are the two ends of the spectrum beginning at the same point where one emerges out of the other, where duality springs out of the singularity of the ONE. This duality between existence and non-existence is the primordial cause of all conflict and the ultimate cause of the orgasm.

In Freud's trinity of *libido, eros* and *thanatos,* we find a reflection of religious trinities: the Christian concepts of Father, Son and Holy Ghost, the Hindu trinity of Mother, Father, Son or Brahma, Vishnu, Shiva and, in the religion of physics, positive, negative, neutral. These can all be summed up in the insightful perception of the ancient sages who claimed that at the back of all these trinities there is a super trinity

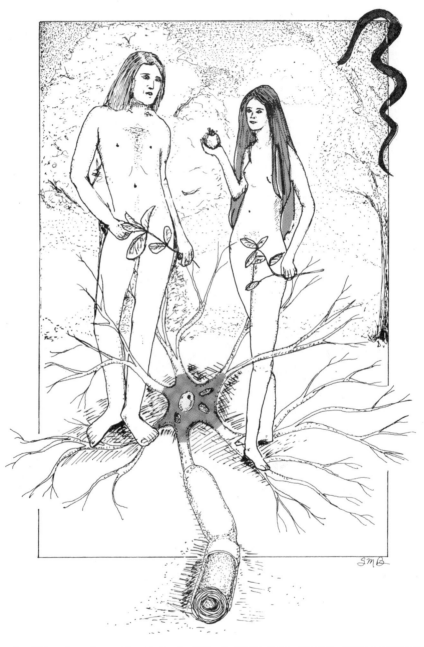

The tree by which we know the good (positive) and evil (negative) is the sensory tree of the nervous system. The nerve cells of the lower system are connected to the body muscles and organs.

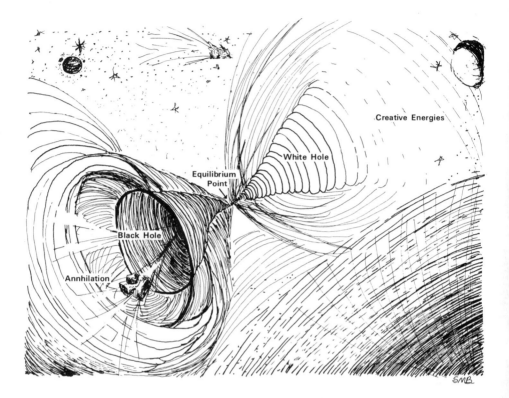

A black hole sucks in energy and matter and annihilates everything in its field, and a white hole throws off the creative energies of the universe. The more important point is the equilibrium position, the singularity where sits the ONE making everything whole. The Tibetans discovered this secret of the balance of the creative forces of the universe thousands of years ago and gave it form in the dorje.

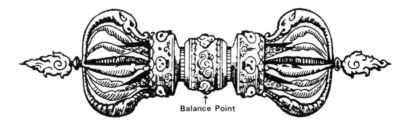

TIBETAN DORJE

(the gunas) which annihilates itself in ONE—the singularity who is Brahman—God, ONE without a second. This concept of the ONE gave birth to the explanation of the nucleus of the universe as the wholistic supertrinity interwoven as the gunas. The ancient idea (revived in modern times) that matter expands into light and light crystallizes into matter was seen by the rishis as a product of these interwoven creative forces which, when controlled in man, gave him power to experience the ultimate orgasm—the blissful pastime of the gods.* This interplay of the gunas is at the back of the universal hologram in which all the forces of creation are centered in consciousness to produce the invisible, indestructible, indefinable, all-present matrix which consciousness or God is. Consciousness is self-creating and self-negating even though it is intangible and unseeable by consciousness itself and is therefore a black hole in which all vibrations rise and die away again, just as sound rises and dies away in the silence.

MAN'S DEEPEST MOTIVATION

In looking at Freud and all other psychological theories from the inside out rather than from the outside in, we see already that they have all been constructed as if the person or the subject or the experiencer of consciousness were an entity totally separate from the environment it lives in—an obvious impossibility. All modern theories of personality and human existence, including the political theories, spring from a culture based exclusively on egocentric relationships with "others" out there and the individual in here. Based on this schism, Marx was right. From the alienated material octave from which he was speaking, seeing and experiencing life, he was absolutely right that ego, personality, characteristic concepts of religion and spirituality are products of the environment and are shaped by changes in the environment.

---

* To use such abstractions as gunas or trinities and transfer them to factual physical objects such as matter and atoms is considered scientifically suspect, since a simpler explanation in physical terms is supposed to prevail. But scientists will never fully understand physics until they are willing to look at the metaphysics that underlies it. Physicists are more and more intrigued with the theory of the black hole, but they will never understand the black hole until they have jumped into it.

But these concepts of ego, separate individuality and material existence as an entity, could only be annihilated in Marxism by total immersion in the State where no one has any individual rights nor is entitled to existence separate from the State. Perhaps the great lure of communism and the reason why it flourishes in spite of its obvious failure to live up to its ideals is this promise of oneness and comradeship in which the agony of human isolation can die into the wholeness of the State. That deep longing for oneness is so intensely powerful in man that its ideal speaks more loudly than the bloodbaths and the salt mines of Siberia.

Communism is essentially the annihilation of the individual into the material totality of the State as a totalitarian entity, yet the State itself is a living organism at the lower octave of material existence fighting for its own very life of national separateness from the whole. Its death instinct cannot achieve sexual release and satisfaction by self-annihilation. It would commit suicide! So its only outlet for its energies on the lower levels it functions on is to choose instead the aggressive route of shaping the rest of the world to fit its own ideas of total selfhood. To annihilate the world into *its* idea of self is its only way of dissolving separation and fulfilling its death urge. Whether we are consciously aware of it or not, the world's opposing political forces are the externalization of mankind's conflicting inner drives, and wars are a vicarious gratification of the drive for self-annihilation.

The death instinct is that power which is programmed cosmically into every organism or entity which sees its own image as God or Truth. Anything which is not in that ego image is ultimately intolerable to the organism. It must either destroy what does not fit its image or else it must change its image to include it. In other words, every ego identity or self-sense feels unconsciously the agony of its separation from the whole and is therefore programmed with the powerful urge of the death-wish which eventually will destroy its separation. Yet its very separation, which causes it to maintain itself against what it perceives as "others" makes it attempt to change or extinguish everyone else. Its sexual drive toward self-extinction is thus thrust outward upon the world in the terrible aggression which makes us say, "We can't help this hostility; that's just the way we are." This mechanism is working not only at the aggregate mass level of society but even in our individual relationships with one another. The ego-limitations in others which make us dislike one another, are always mirrors of our own limits and faults which we have refused to look at and change. To encompass the whole, the ego must change and expand, rather than try to change others.

The communist ideal of self-annihilation is really just a compensation for the genuine ego-death which most people cannot face. This finds its expression in the call to workers to sacrifice themselves and their personal lives for the sake of posterity. Group effort is for the success of the system rather than to make the system the servant of the common people. Communism is the group equivalent of social masturbation where the sexual frustrations of the masses are daily harnessed for the group surrender of our individuality to the huge appetite of the totalitarian State. Instead of channeling these frustrated sexual forces toward total ego death and a true crisis of the organism in the transcendence of matter, the socialist philosophy transfers the annihilation outward, to the external world in aggression and the espousal of violence. Actively supporting violence everywhere, training guerillas and even educating children in terrorist methods of killing, bombing and maiming of innocent bystanders, the communists are unwittingly signing the death warrant of their own ideal, which is like killing the goose that laid the golden egg. In the holy name of posterity they talk of self-immolation to the state god, but they do so in terms of their own deluded egocentricity. Thus, instead of creating the brave new world, they do just the opposite of the ideal, unconsciously programming the victory of materialism over the world. Materialism is at the opposite end of the spectrum from that self-annihilation of ego which only fulfills itself as it becomes one with the whole.

Capitalist countries offer the freedom either to achieve self-annihilation in oneness or to entrench the ego in an "every man for himself" philosophy of pleasure and power. The freedom to look out for only "number one" is a license to exploit everyone else. This is the crime or sin of the West. The glorification of *eros* in democracy as opposed to the glorification of *thanatos* in the totalitarian states are mirror distortions of the real purpose of life. The real purpose lies neither in *eros* nor in *thanatos,* but in dissolving the ego knot in self-surrender to oneness—that pure creative energy of consciousness.

The real purpose of freedom is to give expression to the one who experiences this totality of consciousness. This is very different from the "totalitarian self" conceptualized at the material level only in communism. This ego-surrender can take place on several different levels within the whole, including the material life, in business, in science, or on mental and spiritual levels of expression, or all of these at once.

OUR SPIRITUAL NATURE

The ancient prophets expressed this idea of oneness or totality in mystical terms, perceiving that everything in existence, including man, was created in God's image. They did not say what this image was or is. Modern materialists have dismissed this as a naive idea implying that God was therefore in the shape of a man and that the God they spoke of must have two legs, one head and a long beard. Such a materialistic view of God's image is natural to a materialistic person who is identified only with himself as a body and cannot see life on any other octave except his own blind egocentric level. Hence he believes he can dismiss the prophets' ideas along with God, and he fails to see that God is consciousness itself, which of course is shaping everything in the social and material worlds according to the images held locked within it. In this sense, only an image stands between us and this primal creative force of the universe, because even our sense of self is just an image. In the moment of sexual crisis we forget ourselves and our obsession with self, but we do not realize that this temporary blanking out of self-consciousness automatically releases in us the unlimited power of *libido.* If we did, we could make a tremendous leap in our evolution because *in the sexual climax, whatever image is held in the self will be intensified with the creative force released.* If this image is pure love it will lead to a more inclusive consciousness. If this is just the image of a physical body it will lead to ego separateness, disease or physical aggression and eventual death.

In our daily life, the image that we are a separate self or personality creates (through the power of consciousness) a mini-god, the little ego, which sets itself upon the throne of consciousness and calls its life-force "mine" and believes it is running its life alone, without any help from the total intelligence or God. Because psychologists and social theorists are themselves trapped in this limiting self-image, they believe mankind can escape the insatiable sexual energy of the primordial appetite for death of the ego-self by manipulating the social forces in the external world.

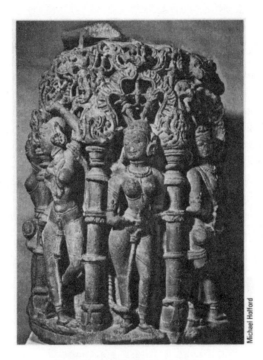

Hindus revered the sex act as a divine
experience. The base of a pillar from
Solanki shows ritual dancing.

They have not seen that the sexual climax contains within it an ego death at a lower level of experience and that the sexual energies pile up in our consciousness until the urge for self-annihilation destroys everything that is not in our own limited image. In other words, the more the energies pile up, the greater is the urge to annihilate others as a compensation for not being annihilated ourselves and therefore not finding the bliss that our hearts are unconsciously longing for. But if we understand this violence toward others, we can hear the ancient wisdom of the avatars and sages and their message of "Thy will be done on earth as it is in heaven." "Thy will" is the image of the whole as oneself.

In the ultimate sense, the spiritual organism is in search of the ultimate orgasm in which the separation of the self-sense (ego) is discharged. At the lower levels of human expression this search is an unconscious drive manifesting externally at the level of the physical body in the form of ego power, aggression and physical sexual orgasm. At the higher levels it manifests in the rare experience of total identification with the universal hologram. The release of permanent bliss at the higher level is, at the physical level, the temporary bliss of sex release. And this is why the sexual act is never totally fulfilling because it does not last forever. It is only a pale reflection of the total annihilation of the self on the octave above and the total destruction of the ego in suicide on the material level below it. This is hard to accept for anyone who has not experienced anything higher than sexual orgasm and almost impossible to imagine for someone who has not even experienced that! Nevertheless, man is propelled by motivations which are beyond his own power. Whether we call this an evolutionary intelligence, God, the creative forces or a drive is of no account. It is all the same force, acting in different ways.

There are major orgasms and minor ones. Every one of our seven levels of consciousness and our seven brains is capable of orgasm on its own level. The spiritual bliss which emerges on the final death of the ego is posited against the lower level octave of ecstasy in the sexual reproductive crisis and below that, at another octave level, the suicidal annihilation of self as a material object manifesting as a separate ego obsessed with its own inability to unite with the totality and therefore self-programmed for physical death. In between these octaves lie the minor orgasms. Even among yogis, very few are aware that we are capable of orgasm in every one of these psychic centers. Wars originate from and are to be found naturally between the middle octave of sexual orgasm and the drive of the suicide who will not surrender his ego. Therefore war is a vibration that resonates with the colors red and black. Black is the color of suicide. When it moves up one octave to the red physical level, the same energy is directed outward into aggression. The red and black of the Nazi flag of the Third Reich evoked these warlike feelings of hatred and death.

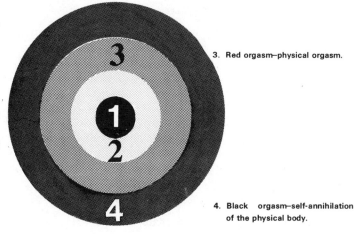

3. Red orgasm—physical orgasm.

1. Black orgasm of total absorption into the Nuclear Self.

2. White orgasm—the experience of Grace.

4. Black orgasm—self-annihilation of the physical body.

The above is a simplified linear attempt to illustrate the major orgasms which eliminate the cause of frustration with self by bringing a cathartic crisis in which the primordial forces in consciousness are discharged in an emotional climax. The actual experience of the four orgasms, however, is not linear but built up one within the other in shells or thresholds of excitation. The more intense the orgasms, the higher the expression of bliss. We can understand the inner world of a terrorist only when we can understand the intensity of the moment in which he pulls all down with him in a glorious egocentric self-destruction as a way of making a telling mark on an indifferent society. A harmless equivalent of this ego-need for recognition is the excitement of pulling the emergency cord and stopping a whole train just to satisfy our craving for power. The motivation of the suicide is the same—the use of the ultimate weapon of the physical ego to attract attention to itself and its feelings of potency. This potency is also sought on higher levels of consciousness as well, but only the suicide revels in the power of

LEVELS OF ORGASM
The One—The Ultimate Orgasm

Orgasm 1   BLACK—The Black Hole of total absorption into the Nuclear Self.

Orgasm 2   WHITE—Controlling the Creative Forces—the experience of Grace.

VIOLET—The programming of the self-image and the feeling that one is much blessed and God is well-pleased.* Here the image of the Self can still exist whereas the Ultimate Orgasm is even beyond. The violet is a window in which we catch many glimpses of the state beyond, but is a different experience to cracking open the cosmic egg which only needs to happen once and brings a continual orgasm to all the levels below. Violet is the spiritual orgasm that opens the doorway to the ultimate orgasm. A higher self-union with the totality, the true totalitarian self which annihilates ego and the self-sense by surrender. Partial glimpses of the total orgasm are felt when the ego releases its subject-object separation thus paving the way for the total orgasm of the Nuclear SELF in the black hole beyond.

(Evolutionary threshold above which ultimate power can be used only by selfless people without danger of self-delusion.)

The following are all minor orgasms or mini-orgasms. A group of five intermediary selves acting unconsciously as egocentric onlookers of the environment.

INDIGO—The joy of expecting endless possibilities, the feeling we have when something expected in the future actually happens—a dream come true—such as the realization of one's hopes on the marriage day. Also a cosmic coincidence where synchronicity provides us with a fulfilling development often intuitively foreseen.

BLUE—The Blue level orgasm is felt in the devotional experience linked with an idea, as when someone prays at the altar to a statue as a focus of devotion and experiences communion. When people take communion they feel they are united with the blood of Christ by drinking some wine handed to them by a priest. This is the power of mind on the blue level to identify with a sacrament.

GREEN—Feeling richly blessed, a feeling that one has it made. A secure feeling of having everything so one has no needs.

YELLOW—On the Yellow level orgasm comes when the mind has an ecstatic aesthetic experience of logical or mathematical beauty in the structure of a sequence of ideas or thoughts where the parts synthesize into a whole. The "Ah-ha" insight.

ORANGE—The feeling of fellowship with others to the point where you can really love even your enemy. It is also the feeling when you are with a friend or a group of friends and you have a deep feeling of brotherhood in sharing—the ecstasy of experiencing others as yourself.

The two lower major orgasms are the most common.

Orgasm 3   RED—Self-annihilation of the sexual energies in the physical orgasm. The release of frustration or tension from built-up life-force that has not been channeled into other forms of creativity.

Orgasm 4   BLACK—Self-annihilation of ego-self by destroying the body. Death, suicide, identification with material world and "self" as a body. The lowest octave of the death instinct due to intense material identification and a feeling of being separated from the whole.

---

* The violet level orgasm does not apply to purple which is a mixture of red and violet. Purple is the color of power since it combines the red aggressiveness with the search for the hidden fantasies of the violet personality. Purple passion and purple power are not really orgasms as they do not release the ego but reinforce it. A sorcerer is an example of someone resonating to the color of purple.

destruction for the sake of destroying. Can we not see the intense excitement of the suicide and the rush of chemicals into his bloodstream as he takes the power of life and death into his own hands? He does not understand that there is an even greater power in human beings—the power of self-mastery. And he does not understand that the highest orgasm is one in which the chemicals of the body are released not automatically as in suicide or aggression or sex but in full voluntary control.

The experience of the highest self-destruction is the supreme control of the consciousness which regulates and releases the hypothalamus in the brain which receives the secretions from the pituitary and the pineal glands. These secretions mix on the floor of the central cavity in the ventricles of the brain where they trigger the response of bliss if the orgasm is at the highest level. Normally these secretions are released in minimal amounts automatically controlled by arbitrary processes. The arbitrary control differs from person to person depending on their level of consciousness. There is no norm. Our red level biological urges trigger the adrenal glands which bring about anger and hatred and which start the chain reaction of chemical signals throughout the body through the secretion of adrenalin which prepares the organism for attack and reduces its awareness of pain and suffering. The person full of adrenalin cannot experience another's pain or even his own pain. The study of the sexual act in dogs, humans, insects, and other animals shows that pain in the climax of the moment of sexual self-annihilation is nonexistent or is even welcomed or attracted to oneself in the orgasm. This experience of pain by people in love can only be compared with saints who would whip themselves until blood came in order to work themselves up to the spiritual orgasm. The red chakra biological urge and the control of the adrenals is governed by the hypothalamus, which we can control by self-discipline, yoga, practice of continence or restricting sex to once a week, for example. The conscious hypothalamic release of pain-killing substances from the brain explains why the Christians could sing while being eaten by the lions in the arena, and why St. Joan could be in bliss while being burnt alive, or why the sexual urge of the sadist or masochist craves for pain.

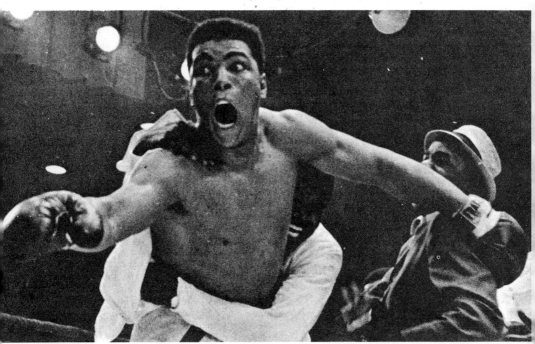

WIDE WORLD

Muhammad Ali (then Cassius Clay) exhibits his drive for ego power and probably experiences ego-reinforcing orgasms on many different levels of consciousness simultaneously as he dances around the ring shouting "I'm the Greatest!" after winning the world heavyweight title in 1965.

Because people forget themselves completely at these four major levels of the crisis, society must now recognize the dangers of the stop-at-nothing self-immolator on the lowest level as well as channel the frustrated sexual drive for the integration of "self" with another at the next level, because both are the cause of man's aggression and desire to dominate and cause pain to another. To ignore the real cause of these two deep drives for self-annihilation, prevents society from recognizing and encouraging the ultimate spiritual orgasm where man can "forget himself" on the supreme level of divinity and union with the whole.

THE ULTIMATE ORGASM

What is the use of having the ultimate organism if that organism cannot have an ultimate orgasm? What would be an orgasm for the ultimate organism? Such a question can only be answered by looking at Nature herself, who achieves a cosmic orgasm every time there is a union of two complementary and opposite forces which annihilate themselves and become one. Whether it is the fertilization of a chicken egg or the sex gland of an orchid, the exchange of radiation between two stars or the fusion of atoms in the sun, it matters not. In the very heart of each atom of chlorine is the yearning for its marriage with an atom of sodium, in which the two ions both positive and negative merge together and share each other's dynamic explosiveness in the violence of the coming together. Separately chlorine is deadly, reactive and alkaline. And sodium in the presence of air sputters and violently burns itself away in a few moments. But together they are stable and in bliss as common salt.

The voiding of human sexual energy at the moment of crisis is governed by the same laws of resonance that keep the moon circling around the earth and the earth circling the sun in a perfect love relationship that the ancients called "the harmony of the spheres". Even gravitating systems travel lines of force which are in truth neutralized attraction. Earth's momentum in its orbit around the sun exactly balances the gravitational attraction. Resonance is the point of balance between cyclic vibrating systems. In music when two harmonic tones merge in resonance with each other and become one pregnant sound, producing daughter overtones and reverberations, this too is the achievement of that cosmic balance which fuses and unites in sonic bliss (harmony). The resonant coming together in the achievement of union governs the cosmic evolution of new forms of body, mind, and spirit, and produces an infinite hierarchy of orgasms on all levels throughout Nature. For orgasm is not some event that is happening in the nervous system or the genital organs of living creatures. *Orgasm is the bliss of union.*

The ultimate orgasm is no less and no more than entering into cosmic sex with the creator, reliving the divine moment of union at the central nucleus of all creation, reflected in every one of its participant entities and groups of entities. This vision requires a super-penetration not only into one's own sexuality but into the nature of the orgasm itself and the different levels of experience upon which it occurs. To most ordinary people, the orgasm only occurs on one level. And judging by the number of divorces, perhaps only fifty percent of the people ever experience it completely even at that level. So this chapter is concerned with the opening up of those other levels in which the desire for self-annihilation causes the equivalent of a dynamic release of energy, like a boom from the crossing of the sound barrier. This super-penetration of the ultimate organism produces the bliss of the superior orgasm on the spiritual level. This experience can become as common as the sexual one, once its cause is understood and our consciousness is putting the same amount of energy into it as we put into the lower kind. Saints and sages have told us over and over again that if only we put the heart as much into our spiritual evolution as we put it into our material comforts, we would indeed make love to God every minute of the day. What we are proposing is not putting half but putting all, because to make love *to* God is one thing, if we look on God as something separate from ourself, but to have him as *our own* consciousness is a permanent union in which one's own self-sense and awareness of separation is totally devoured by love. This experience cannot be described in words but the nearest analogy would be if one could imagine a permanent orgasm feeling like spurts of radiance shooting out of each cell of one's body making them come alive in their own right, carrying their own weight and thereby lightening our self of their material weight, as if they were levitating and being lifted up so that no longer did we carry this heavy prison of the mortal flesh around with us on the earth. It is the feeling that we have been freed forever from the forces of gravity which lead us to the grave. This is the "lightening" effect where each cell becomes an individual, almost with its own name, so that this radiance we call the cosmic love binds all together without limit in the totality of the cosmic orgasm. Such an enhancement effect of every part of the individual vehicle is also possible for the individual person who becomes part of the nucleus of a new social organism which transcends the heavy weight of materialism. This lightening experience of the individual cells, atoms, people, brains, entities, is the solvent of life, that essence which dissolves the ego and enlightens the whole. This is the cosmic purpose of the Phoenix rising out of its own material substance consumed in the fire and re-created in the image of that which is eternally rising.

To such a person, who has experienced the ultimate orgasm within their own organism, their one thought and reason for existence becomes how to share this with those imprisoned in a lower vibratory body. To build the infra-structure of a communication between one level and another which makes the transfer of this energy of life-force transmittible to others, becomes the enormous task of awakening society to the existence of this orgasm which can be entered through the doorway of the sexual orgasm. This is not the only doorway but it is the one most commonly available to ordinary people who find it difficult to exercise self-discipline. To consecrate the sexual orgasm to the glory of God and to have no other thought at the moment of sexual climax but the image of the union on the higher octave, will eventually free a person from the attachment to the physical flesh. This physical doorway by itself opens out onto a longer spiritual pathway (because it does not include an orgasm on higher levels of the spirit unless those doors are already open) than if we committed ourself to God or dedicated our total being to the breaking through of all limitations. Yet it may be for some people the only acceptable, understandable way to go. But where the lower orgasm is temporary and has to be repeated and repeated over and over again, the ultimate orgasm only needs to be experienced once. And many spiritual mystics and spiritual geniuses have claimed that even when higher orgasms have been purified, obsessive dedication of consciousness to the sexual orgasm can be a trap which shuts down our perceptions of other worlds of being, beyond the human. However, the highest mystics have also said that all is ONE and if the sexual union is considered as only one of a seven-fold orgasm then there is no separative feeling of coming down from the perpetual orgasm that is going on in the nucleus at all times. In the balancing of the three gunas in the ultimate orgasm we find the balance between the positive and the negative which annihilate each other and form the third energy which is one indivisible singularity. To experience this self-annihilation is not only the essence of life itself but is in fact the satisfaction of the death instinct.

At physical death, one experiences the release of life and its resultant consciousness from its mortal prison as an orgasm in which the seeds of our next birth are contained. Like the seed pod of a flower bursting and scattering the ego, the experience of death contains that same fear that all egos dread—the shattering effect of loss of identity at the lower level of the physical existence. To those who have not achieved the ultimate orgasm of self-annihilation in life, physical death is the lowest threshold of bliss, like the dark unconscious of sleep. To those who have achieved self-realization, ego death becomes inconsumable bliss.

The ultimate orgasm is the fulfillment of orgasms on every level of consciousness, all triggering each other in a chain reaction of psychic energy. It is as if seven waterfalls were arranged one above the other. When the intensity is sufficient, one spills over into the next, filling the pool below until it too begins to overflow. This is the blissful feeling of "my cup runneth over"—the feeling of so much happiness that it cannot be contained. Once the cycle of seven is completed,* it begins again, coming back up behind itself and pushing itself along in a kind of feedback loop, gathering momentum. At each level it gathers more energy which then triggers even more energy which in turn multiplies again like an atomic explosion. Once it gets started, it grows and builds. In this sense, the first steps we take toward this union are the most difficult. Later on, the momentum of our internal experiences opens us to higher and higher thresholds of this bliss whose intensity is spilling over and over and over until we are filled full, and even then it is still coming.

The three types of human orgasms—physical death, the sexual crisis for reproduction of life, and the third and most potent, the spiritual ejaculation of the ego into the cosmic womb of the totality of consciousness—are all part of the fourth, the ultimate orgasm, which is both human and cosmic. The highest orgasm fertilizes the permanent union of oneself with the cosmic nucleus—the egg hidden in the heart

---

* Actually there are twelve levels as parts of a twelve tone spectrum in which the seven tone spectrum is embedded. These are explained on a cassette tape by Christopher Hills recorded live 10/6/78. Also note pages 414-15, 561 of *Supersensonics.*

of all Nature, from atom to molecule to cell to organ, culminating in the totality of the universal hologram. This fusion with the nuclear Self reveals to us that the cement which holds the universe and all things together is love, a by-product of the union of the two opposing forces in human life which are really complementary. Annihilation and union on the ultimate level are one and the same thing, ending in the non-separation of ONENESS. Radiance and cosmic love is the juice that flows through the nucleus of all processes of evolution and is hidden in the heart of every person. It is the "evolutionary force" brought down into life by those who experience the ultimate orgasm.

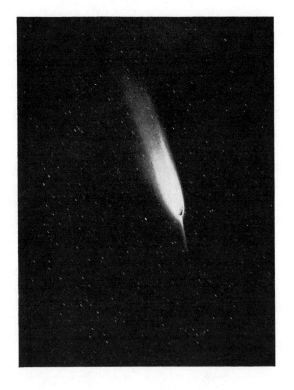

PART FOUR

MANIFESTING
THE VISION

AUTHOR'S NOTE

The chapters in this section give a foretaste of the practical solutions published in The Golden Egg. *It is easy to be idealistic, to have great visions, to moralize or rant and rave, but very hard to find real and workable solutions to the world's problems. Most of mankind's schemes for fixing things have only killed the bird that lays the golden eggs. In order to find the "how to" of happier community life which is the purpose of* The Golden Egg *we must also include the practical side of education, Creative Conflict, constitution-making, and the creation of wealth and capital through Common Ownerships, so that these all work together to make a fulfilling way of living. The social reorganization of our industrial life, our educational system, and our personal attitudes to property rights and exploitation are bound up with our capacity to love others.*

There are many groups and wonderfully innovative individuals who are putting their hearts into overcoming our society's problems. But the Phoenix will only be able to rise and turn the whole system around when the dedicated teachers, healers and businessmen and women are able to work together in groups to put the work on their own egos first and learn to tune into the cosmic program. Our ability to tune into the cosmic program is directly proportional to the degree that we have worked on our ego. Creative Conflict can be used to do this work on the ego as we attempt to resolve the inner conflicts and conflicts between individuals and groups at all levels of life, from the classroom to the home to the world of business. Because they have confronted their own egos, the real saints of the modern era are able to deal with worldly life and bring the light of spirit into the darkness of materialism. So this section of the book is where the vision of heaven comes down to earth, into the pulls and stresses of daily life. Only when we are dealing in real situations can we bring the vision into manifestation and embody it.

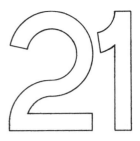

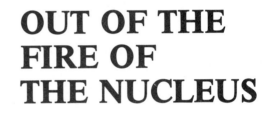

OUT OF THE
FIRE OF
THE NUCLEUS

In 1956, after retiring from a very intense business life with several companies in agriculture, trading and industry, I planned a life of research and decided to become a recluse by the side of the beautiful Rio Grande in Jamaica. This tropical paradise in the Blue Mountains was some of the most wild and beautiful scenery in the world. Miles away from anywhere, I was disturbed only by tourists on bamboo rafts, entranced by the swift-flowing river cascades and rapids. To sit in peace and meditate and commune with Nature seemed to evoke the highest poetry of my soul. A bliss would steal over me whenever I sat among the high mountain peaks watching the river far below wind through deep gorges on its way to the Caribbean and the white sand beaches just half an hour away. The bliss was like an ambrosia, killing all desire for action and so self-completing in itself that I would not even want to move a limb of my body. Love flowed out to nothing in particular and seemed to encompass the environment and all its beauty. The negative ions of the waterfalls sent out an electrical vibrancy to all the membranes of smell and taste and I thought, "This is where I will worship in God's great sky temple and spend the rest of my days."

But another part of me knew that the world was in turmoil and that there was a battle for men's minds between great forces of darkness and light. I shuddered at the thought of so many unhappy people, so much violence and betrayal, so much sheer horror and terror. The senseless way that mankind lived and died and suffered from hunger and war was in such contrast to my idyllic mountain retreat. I had to do something, but what could I do—a single individual, a lone recluse in the world, a person who was running away from the turmoil of a busy life? What could I do which would fulfill a real need?

I had been studying magic and occult mental powers and wondering whether humans like Hitler and Stalin were using the black arts in politics or whether they were just agents and naive instruments for some superhuman evil force that dominated the world of human conflict. Sitting safe among the mountains it was easy to convince myself that somehow the proud and arrogant and the selfish would "come a cropper" and the powers of good and light would win out and that God's hand was at work unseen in the events of the everyday world. But the psychic forces of light in world affairs seemed to be losing and whole countries were being taken over by small groups of tightly organized armed revolutionaries, with tremendous bloodshed, oppression and brutality. Could I afford to be complacent, basking in the sun, letting the sounds of waterfalls and soft tropical breezes lift me up above it all? Could I enjoy the world at the price of cutting off from it? If negative psychic weaponry were being used by earthly dictators as tools of alien forces to dominate the planet, would I be able to find others, unite with them in spirit and, without making a religious commitment to any particular emotional appeal to ancient scriptures, engage these forces in the defense of the planet? My vision was to awaken young people to the protective powers of consciousness. After a few years traveling around the world to bring people together, I would find a flat in London or even a cottage in the Lake District so that I could commune with Nature and work with others who felt as I did. But instead, my journey became a long spiritual search in India and the East. I left the study of psychic forces and began to reach deep into the ancient truths of the rishis and sages, to wander the world's shrines and ashrams and to seek Christ in the monastic traditions. I began to see beneath the facade and self-delusions of human life and see that the "galactic plot" was not some vast external conspiracy but the projection of our own ignorance, our own strange paranoia and fear that robbed us of reality and clarity. The world was the mirror of our soul, the cosmic movie of our own blindness to the world as it is.

With new insight I moved to London in 1965 to manifest my vision of working with others to awaken a group consciousness. I found there was a great interest in my researches into light and color among the various so-called "New Age" groups who were looking for something that would transform the world spiritually. Several group leaders expressed an interest in getting together with other groups and getting a center which could be used by all these separate groups since all of them were paying out high prices to meet regularly at public halls. So we formed a council with the express intention of getting a place and the council authorized me to make a specific purchase if I could locate a building. However, when the subject of money came up as to who would put up cash for the building everyone kept silent. I had only enough to live on with a small insurance policy and nothing saved. I was surprised because I knew that two members on the council were extremely wealthy and owned considerable property and business. I decided to test their sincerity. "Who is going to pay the lawyer to draw up the constitution for the center to get registered at the charity commissioner's?" I asked. "I'll give ten pounds (then valued at $28.00)," said one person who owned several expensive flats on Sloane Street. "I'll give ten pounds now and offer a mortgage up to 75% on the building at a regular going rate of nine percent interest," said another who reputedly was worth 600,000 pounds (over a million dollars). I felt grateful that we were even able to get a mortgage at all, as they were difficult at that time, and I had no other security to offer. Then I could not believe my ears as he continued on to say that he would only give the mortgage if I made myself personally responsible. I protested, "But it is a group project." "I know," he replied, "but the group could break up at any time in the future and I would be left holding a white elephant." Suddenly I felt committed. Even if it had to be a group of one, we had to become totally responsible to see a thing through to the end. And I saw his point. The building was in the most fashionable part of London but it was practically falling down. It had been condemned as uninhabitable pending repairs to the roof, windows, gutters, plumbing and sewage systems. I had thought idealistically that as a group of established leaders they could get all their members to come and work voluntarily to make it habitable. Little did I know that only three people would volunteer and that over the next year my commitment would find me scrambling up and down the scaffolding, painting, carpentering, plumbing and doing the sewers which the volunteers would not touch. With no money we could not hire anyone. As my regular income of 200 pounds per month came over from the West Indies I bought materials, drain pipes, insulation, etc. Miraculously my two helpers and I got beds, furniture and carpets almost for nothing at auctions. We spent a whole year rushing up and down seven flights of stairs before we could open. Funnily enough, whenever we called a meeting of the group leaders, the nearer the project moved toward becoming a reality the fewer council members turned up. No demands were made on them but they were scared that they might be required to do something because they knew others were doing all the work.

I asked myself, "Why did I get into all this? What happened to that beautiful tropical paradise and that dream of an old English cottage by the lake?" When others fell down and failed their responsibility I took it up because I said the project just *had* to work. Whatever others did or didn't do, I had to do what it took. I see now my mistake, but I couldn't see it all those years ago. I was giving others that which *I* wanted them to have. What was my motive and was I too idealistic in my expectations of others? Like a father showering presents on a son or daughter who really wants something completely different, we try to give the world what we know and think it needs. This is called "idealism". I did not learn this lesson until I'd spent five years carrying the overload and living with a community of people who let me carry it, not because they would not, but because the residential members who joined the community were not wealthy like some members of the council. Yet even if they *had* been wealthy, they were not able to see the real needs which I was filling because they had no idea of the reality. I had mentioned the bills but I had not really let them know the bare facts. Several members of the community, although not wealthy, had much more money than I had and I kept hoping their awareness would make them wonder who was paying the bills. When someone left the community there was always a room vacant for which no contribution was paid. The concept of the Centre was that full rooms at a very low rental or small contribution would exactly balance the expenses for owning the building. But when someone left, no one even mentioned the shortfall, so I paid it. After a while, when two or three rooms would be empty, I wondered if the group was ever going to wake up and find some new tenants or was I just born a sucker? We were reading and amending our constitution and practicing Creative Conflict at very high spiritual levels, so I did not like to keep bringing up the materialistic subject of money. I had been told by some members that somehow it was not spiritual to keep mentioning the bills. But nothing was changing!

This same lack of awareness that was in the resident group at Centre House was in the original council and was also in many spiritual groups that I had seen. Our original purpose had begun with a council of group leaders formed to get a place to unite and associate in a group effort to ease our material problems, to pool resources on an ongoing basis. Our vision was to share, not at an occasional meeting, but a real association of spirits like the round table of King Arthur, all seeking the Holy Grail together. For the first year we met, with each leader chairing the monthly meeting in turn, but gradually after doing their individual thing and sharing what was going on in their own group, each chairman tailed off in attendance. I couldn't understand it. Did they come to give or to get? Naively I wondered what their real motive was for stating the great need for a new evolutionary type of group cooperation and then petering out on it without saying anything. Did it satisfy the ego? Did it put the emphasis on *serving* and not on the glamor of being a leader, and so was too much sacrifice? Were the leaders perhaps wanting new members for their groups? After a year of Round Table meetings I looked around the group. It was going fine and everyone was having a good time. New leaders had come forward and were being chairmen every month because the new ones needed the exposure, but not one of the original group who had preached so fervently for unity was there! I realized then that their real desire was not the unity they professed. And those who were taking the chair now, would they be here in a year's time? I doubted it. I realized then that the spiritual unity we preached about and talked of in our heads was nothing like the reality of our lives. The *idea* was real but the practice was temporary or nonexistent. If this was the state of being of our "New Age" leaders who professed to be so far above the political and ordinary religious level of leadership, perhaps the whole idea of an evolutionary ethic, a counter-culture, or a so-called "spiritual revolution" was only a surface belief and at the core it was just a nice thought, if only it could all happen by someone else's efforts.

Over the years I realized that what the world was calling for was not this kind of leadership nor lip service to great ideals but fundamental change at the depths of Being. And I saw that unless the activity we threw ourself into was the result of some fundamental change of our own being, then it could merely be a projection of our unconscious drives for name, fame and power on the higher spiritual levels which we thought we despised so much on the materialistic or lower social levels. I began to develop a whole teaching of how to become truly selfless and how to examine our own ego trips, such as wanting to be leader or guru or the shining one so badly that instead of freeing others, we might make them more dependent, make them respond to us like a prima donna opera singer of spiritual truths or in my own case the idea that one is a messianic source when actually one might be just a spiritual entertainer. I had to face the fact that most of my efforts at Centre House were providing little more than a temporary experiment. This was the problem in a nutshell. I could only cure the Centre House problem by going away so that *they*, the resident members, had the problem and could face the reality of responsibility at last. So I left on a lecture tour which got extended and extended until now, 1979. The only time I went back was to ask the group to pay back what I had advanced for them on the mortgage over the six years that I ran Centre House. We got out all the bills and counted them up. They have, to the credit of one member in particular who accepted the responsibility as I did, paid me off at £200 a month ever since 1973. The group was learning responsibility in a practical way, even though in the end only one of the original group was still there. I felt better about having one member with a real sense of responsibility than having a "following" among whom group effort and responsibility was just an idea. The "community" has now been replaced by a spiritual school along the lines of the original teachings. It is succeeding in a totally different way from the original experiment which was too ambitious and idealistic.

This example shows that not only is it possible to have too much patience and accept too much responsibility for others so that they are allowed to live under some spiritual delusions, but it is possible to find a solution to that basic human tendency to avoid responsibility. This solution, that I applied from the very outset in the founding of the University of the Trees, is that nothing "real" is going to happen unless you make it happen. If you see a lack in the group that you yourself feel a need for—fill it; or if you are disturbed by anything in the group that does not please you—confront it. This is the essence of the World Peace Center Constitution. It will not work unless you *make* it work. Every opportunity is given in the World Peace Center Constitution* for any member to bring up and put to the vote any disturbing activity of mind or body. Nothing need be hidden. If you hide anything, it is your own fault if you are miserable. If you fear disturbing others or if you want to be the nice guy, then joy is killed. The net result is that thoughts which make us miserable, like wishing we could meditate all day and write books and poetry while the chores are pressing, or wishing that everything were different from the way it is, are found to be an illusion. Everything is the way it is, because we are the way *we* are! It is no use blaming the authorities or making someone else responsible. It is no use pointing the finger at the world situation or at other people. This applied as fully to the leaders who participated in the Round Table in London as it did to those original New Age leaders of the 1965 council of founders who shrunk from the task of forging the evolutionary group they were all talking about when the nitty-gritty job on their own egos came up for an overhaul. The ideal of a "New Age" is nice, but we can't have one without some real

---

* See *The Golden Egg* for the World Peace Center Constitution and how to implement it.

selflessness. If we are not prepared to sacrifice, then we cannot lament the fact that the New Age never arrives. There are no shortcuts and no armchair solutions, and I have seen very few people who were willing to do that real work.

THE POLITICAL NATURE OF SPIRITUAL RESPONSIBILITY

So long as the ego is comfortably intact, feeling self-satisfied about itself, its career, its security, its personality and judging everyone else thereby, that caring and responsibility which could bring peace to the world can never be born. The future of the world depends on our having no delusions whatsoever about ourselves or about mankind. We have to see our full capacity for selfishness and yet not underestimate the tremendous spiritual potential within every human at the nuclear center of being. It is true we often do aim much lower than this noble higher self within us. "It is only human," we say, "to put our material security first." Yet we feel some reproach in the values of a Solzhenitsyn who hates tyranny and autocracy more than anything else, a man who treasures freedom a thousand times more than food for his stomach, an evolved being who is concerned not only for his own freedom but for the freedom of others. In the impoverished areas of the world where people live in a dog-eat-dog struggle for survival, democratic ideals about the rights of others seem out of place. And consequently their governments, whether democratically inclined or not, are continually open to anarchy and militant terrorism. Prime ministers like Aldo Moro of Italy can be murdered by mindless anarchists posing as Red Brigades who would offer us their brand of justice to run the country and give us what they think we need. Could such terror prosper with eternal vigilance?

Because the vision of mankind as a free species extends only to a few countries of the world at this time, the threat of a dark age is almost upon the earth. If you have lived all your life in a free country, it has perhaps not dawned on you that much of the world is not just starving physically but starving inwardly for some better way of life that it can hardly even conceive of. It is amazing that so many are in this condition and yet our own awareness stops at the East, West,

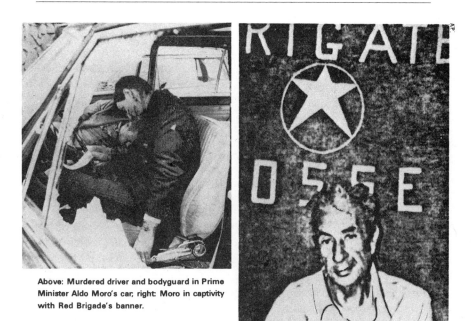

Above: Murdered driver and bodyguard in Prime Minister Aldo Moro's car; right: Moro in captivity with Red Brigade's banner.

North, and South boundaries of our own safe country or our town or even our house. How then can we carry the torch of the human spirit through these dark ages and accept the challenge of evolution? And who will do it if not we who are free and can see what freedom is? The human race cannot emerge from centuries of domination if people know no other way. And if we continue now to shirk this responsibility, we too will lose that light of freedom which birth has given us and which our system of education has fostered.

Our spiritual responsibilty is to change the social situation by changing ourselves. If we crave for a peaceful cottage by the lake district, will not the turbulent world follow us if we *are* truly aware of its dire needs? Can we escape teaching our children that they too will be responsible for the condition of life in society? We may try to push responsibility away out of consciousness for a time, but if we are a truly caring and loving person, then the beauty of the planet and the saving of the human race from dark ignorance is not only a messianic problem but a problem we must all solve for our own selfish happiness. For without this love of fellowman and Nature, life is not worth living, even though we can run away to caves, or dream of idyllic utopias. For myself, I have realized it is not for us to concentrate on the building or the location, but on the people. When we have loving people they create a nice place automatically anywhere, but to put places and idealistic conditions first before people is to delude ourselves. Happiness can be a grass hut on an island and the best school can be pitched in a tent.

WHO IS RESPONSIBLE?

The signs of disease and malfunction in the American system are not hard to find. It is easy to cut out and remove presidents and high officials with doubtful ethical backgrounds, but it is difficult to take a surgical knife to the cancerous tumors in large corporations, behind-the-scenes lobbying and shady business practices. Each businessman and congressman must confront his own motives, his pride and ambitions that let him compromise his soul. To root out this affliction in any government will require no less than a total honesty with ourselves about our own position in it as the supporters of such leaders. In other words we must do the same searching out of our own integrity that we demand of them. We can wait for degeneration to run its full course and the integrity of the word to become completely debased by politics, until the words of the constitution become an instrument only pulled out of moth balls in times of crisis. Or we can work now to prepare for the changes in man's knowledge of himself before our checks and balances have become obsolete. The politician need not be one who merely learns to thread the loopholes of an existing system but one whose new ideas for the management of society keep the constitution fresh and green. Without that spirit of heroism that prompts a politician to speak out against congressional malpractice, our checks and balances operate at only half their full potential. Too often, instead of heroes we have the faceless faces of congressmen in business suits. We have this year's pleas and promises sounding much like the promises of last year and the year before, which were never fulfilled. The expansion of population lessens our contact with these elected representatives, who are to us just names and we to them just ciphers in the mass. Congressmen try to maintain the illusion of contact by thousands of circulars sent to constituents to make them believe they are cared

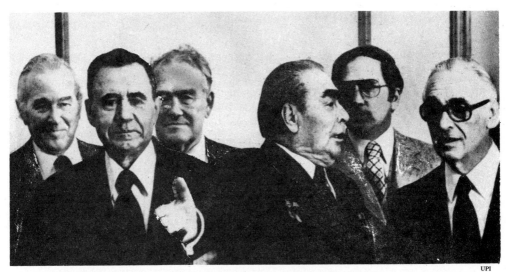

UPI

Brezhnev with US senators in Moscow—
How integral are the words of politicians on either side of the world?

about. Yet it is hard enough for humans to really care even about a
friend or a mate, much less about strangers. And all of this promotion
of illusory intimacy is paid for out of the constituents' own pockets.
Meanwhile, we really know nothing at all about the quality of consciousness, the inner drives, the power hunger or the moral and ethical
inner-worlds of our representatives until we see that their offices have
paid out $26,000 to staff for sex activities or accepted bribes from
powerful lobbyists! The geographical size of a country like America
also widens the gap between the governed and their representatives,
enhancing the illusion that Washington is far away and what is done
there does not much affect us—not until we come to claim our pay
packet and see that a large portion of our pay has been taken by some
strange entity, dressed in the garb of an angel protector looking out so
lovingly for our good yet at the same time spewing napalm over the
innocent bodies of Vietnamese children and polluting and destroying
the natural resources of an entire nation. Who is this government that
deals in napalm? Is it that same friendly government—"our" government—that will look after us when we are old? Is this government us?
Are *we* spewing the napalm?

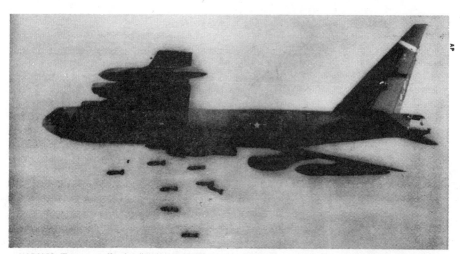

NAPALM. The most effective "anti-personnel" weapon, it was euphemistically described as "unfamiliar cooking fluid" by those apologists for American military methods who automatically attributed all napalm cases to domestic accidents caused by the people using gasoline instead of kerosene in their cooking stoves. Kerosene was far too expensive for the peasants, who actually used charcoal for cooking. The only "cooking fluid" they knew was very "unfamiliar"— and was delivered through their roofs by US planes.

Some of its finer selling points were explained by a pilot in 1966: "We sure are pleased with those backroom boys at Dow. The original product wasn't so hot—if the gooks were quick they could scrape it off. So the boys started adding polystyrene—now it sticks like shit to a blanket. But then if the gooks jumped under water it stopped burning, so they started adding Willie Peter (WP—white phosphorous) so's to make it burn better. It'll even burn under water now. And just one drop is enough, it'll keep on burning right down to the bone so they die anyway from phosphorous poisoning."

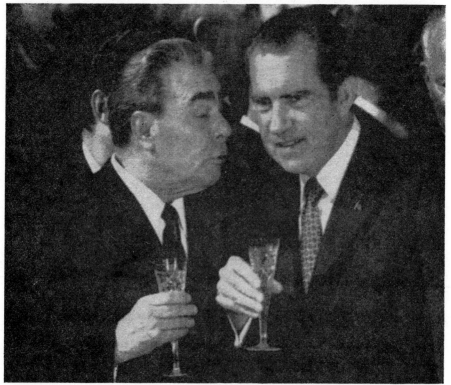

Wally McNamee—Newsweek

WHILE POLITICIANS DRANK CHAMPAGNE COCKTAILS, NAPALM AND MOLOTOV COCKTAILS BURNED THE BODIES OF VIETNAM'S PEOPLE.

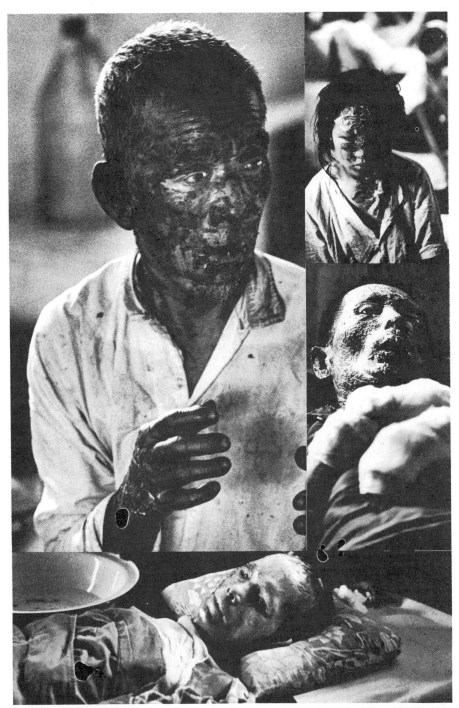

Few napalm victims were seen in the hospitals of South Vietnam. Because napalm is such an effective weapon, there were rarely any survivors. Even those who hid underground (the standard procedure when one's
village was being attacked) were asphyxiated because the fire storm causes a vacuum above ground. As
every GI knows, "it just sucks the air outta their lungs." Napalm in cigar-shaped containers was dropped
from low flying aircraft. Any victims who reached a hospital were unlikely to survive as conditions were
rarely sanitary enough to prevent secondary infection of the wounds that never heal.

Our power to adjust to whatever happens is remarkable. Napalm seems remote from our own lives now and politics seems dull. Those who discuss politics in coffee breaks and at cocktail parties do so as much for a posture or self-image as from any real empathy or compassion for the underdog. At every hour there are political happenings affecting our lives in very vital ways while we are yawning with complete boredom or saving it all for coffeetime. For those of us who do see the full implications of inconspicuous political events (such as the political piracy of raising the toll on a San Francisco bridge, a toll imposed originally to pay for the bridge, long ago paid for, now raised without a public referendum), it is difficult to keep from shouting and haranguing. The implications of supposedly minor events which can blow up into world problems such as aerosol spray cans, TV and microwave radiation, psychotronic warfare or subliminal radionic psychic influences, are not even seen by our scientists and leadership, much less by the people. In frustration we wonder what are the chances of ever getting the masses, whose minds are constantly directed to personal material problems, to expand their awareness. What we are dealing with here is an attitude to change, for as long as we remain imprisoned in our narrow egocentric state of awareness, we will be swamped by the growing complexity and multiplicity of the world's problems. Only by expanding our vision 360 degrees by getting inside the nucleus can we avoid the fate of the dinosaurs. Once surveying the whole, the complexity of life even in our modern technological civilization is not too much for us, and we have clear seeing of the implications of even the smallest detail.

OUR ENEMY HAS NO FACE

From year to year I get more impatient with the pace of the world's movement towards the union of the free. I think back to the revolutionary period of youth when naively we were all set to change the world and bring about the bright new future. But at that time I was turned off by what I suppose turns every firebrand into a frustrated lover of his fellowman—what today's young people call "The System". It is easy to feel that perhaps there is some mysterious conspiracy afoot, some secret power at work which is strong and persuasive enough to block every advance towards progress. Young Americans today in paranoiac frustration blame the secret operations of the Central Intelligence

Agency as their scapegoat and I am sure young people everywhere in every country believe the machinations of the government are in some way responsible for all obstructions, cover-ups, resistance to change and refusal to tell the people the truth. Whether it is the question of energy through nuclear fission products which saddle posterity with plutonium debris that lasts actively 500,000 years into our future, or whether it is the obvious lies we are told at election times, we feel the same: some mysterious power is at work to bring to utter confusion all our plans for building a new society.

There are many levels to this mystery, the foremost one being self-deception. People with money, ideas, power and political clout, believe they can change society by acting upon it, persuading it, by doctoring and tinkering with its many facets. These are the deluded ones who do not see that fundamentally man is not changed in the core of his being by his culture, his philosophy in the head. They are blind to real change because they do not know within themselves the cause of real change. They have no idea that they carry their blinkers with them wherever they go, and see through the narrow slits of their consciousness whatever they look at. Because they believe their perceptions of life are true, they are thereby blinded by their own delusions. There are hundreds of examples in science, in politics or religion, or in everyday life which shout at us deafeningly from the rooftops of all our leading institutions, that we really do not know how to change the ways of men, but we repeatedly do not hear. The mysterious forces which prevent our much-desired expectations seem to become every day more potent as the realization of the many radical dreams of external change recede with one failure after another of our vain schemes. Great magazines flourish, all catering for the new, the novel, the clever, the ingenious, and all forget that the builder of this tower of cleverness is our own consciousness. If we do not know that we are confused, how can we see clearly that only when men can communicate with each other on different levels of consciousness can the conflicts amongst men be resolved into peace? To change the scenery, the location, or the environment is like trying to save a marriage by changing the bed.

Many orientated to change feel that the only way to escape this mysterious power that prevents the New Age from happening is to create new imaginative colonies in space or run off into the woods and create new idyllic communities without any rules or establish utopias which ignore the present situation on earth. These schemes are just the new "towers to heaven" which are totally dependent on the levels of communication upon the earth and are reliant upon earth systems and earthly attitudes for resources and decisions. Their solution is to get

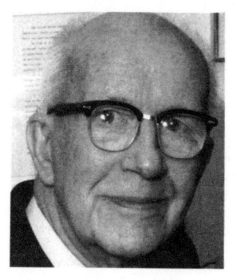

"We are already a space colony. If we can't make it in this beautifully equipped colony, we're not going to make it anywhere else either. And we're not going to carry on any space colonies except by virtue of being colonies from the mother ship. If the mother ship can't be made to work, the colonies aren't going to work."
–Buckminster Fuller

more change now, yet they will have more of the same human ego problems later on. These people feel that they do not need to change themselves in their consciousness within first, because their self-image is that they are already advanced and in the forefront of external change. It's a pity, because they are *willing* to change but do not see the depth required. They do not see that cancer of the imagination is not a cure for the cancers of society and that such idyllic idealistic speculations distract our consciousness from the main disease.

One woman wrote me that if I would only work to establish the equivalent of a "perfumed garden" along the lines of the Persian poets' dream of heaven, she would willingly join our London community. My reply was that idyllic gardens and especially perfumed gardens are "extras" which will certainly come from solving the problems of human relationships, although most of the Persian kings who created such indulgences only kept them through maintaining a violent and ruthless army. To maintain a pocket of utopia within a totally confused world is not the purpose of our nuclear concept. We must become a prolific seed, not an enclave. Certainly we must begin to beautify our immediate world, but this is an effect of our new consciousness, not a cause. To aim at beauty or unity or utopia directly without first changing consciousness is a waste of time. Beautiful people cannot help but create beauty. People who communicate in depth and are themselves unified with the Cosmos, create unity and utopia as a by-product, not as their main aim. To aim directly at the *effect*, by dreaming up fashionable escapes from working on ourselves is a sign of our present times and the cause of many superficial imaginative schemes. They are part of the cosmic circus which prevents our attention from going to the real cause of our world's sickness. The people who promote them do not see that as humans we cannot act other than our real state of consciousness is capable of seeing, and that if we have no foresight into human relationships, the conjuring up of the breath-taking technical achievements, moonshots, and mechanical wizardry or perfumed gardens are only a diversion from the real problem of deeper communication. The answer is not "techniques" or technology, which can do no more than the skillful user knows and imagines, but the actual opening up of our unconscious, unknown and therefore blind self. The promoters of such utopias, colonies in space and various astronomical extravaganzas for contacting extra-terrestrial civilizations do not realize that they do not learn what is already known about man in certain circles upon the earth, let alone learn from some super-intelligent species. These few who consider themselves visionaries are even more deluded because they believe they are already effective instruments of change when in fact they are totally blind to what kind of change is needed which is to first of all discover the depths of human conceit. Thus they too join the ranks of the New Age movement for external change, change in concepts, change in the head, etc., without ever having tried to establish a living experiment of super-communication with real live people on the earth prior to take-off into the future.

I no longer believe there is any mysterious conspiracy to take over the world. It is all very obvious and openly stated by various groups and parties. I think there are a lot of people with vested interests who are trying desperately to hang on to what they have got and I believe there are those who will sell their talents as persuaders or weapon makers, as politicians or drug peddlers, as academics or senators, for selfish gain or for power or just to have a job. In short, I don't believe the problem exists external to individual people's own attitudes. The persuaders and nuclear proliferators have their beliefs and rationalizations, however wide of the facts. The academics go along with the establishment system that gives the grant money and keeps them in their jobs. And the establishment is perpetuated by a hundred hangers-on in politics who believe that it is their divine right to spend government money for their constituents, irrespective of how much of it must come from taxation. I don't propose to probe the intricate web of connections, the hidden motives, the maneuvers behind the scenes. I do not believe such controversies add anything but more frustration and complexity. Yet a full understanding of the issues of our time cannot be simplistic. We cannot go back to our blind youth, which not only thinks that Rome can be built in one day but that people can be changed by throwing bombs in one century or another. Basically people in the mass stay the same; only situations in which people exist change, only the institutions and rationalizations and dreams change, but people hate the same way and love the same way and delude themselves the same way as they did in ancient Rome or at the time of Christ. At the nuclear center of being, man is no more sophisticated in covering up the look on his face or the deceptions of his ego than were ancient people who had never seen a man walk on the moon.

Yet it would be foolish to think that people do not grow or change. People suffer so much pain that they *have* to change; it is a necessity for their own psychic health. But usually they change reluctantly. To expect the world out there to change merely because we grab a microphone and shout, to expect the world to change without ourselves doing more than just thinking or talking about it, is the number one delusion of society. The shouters wait for the doers. We wait to go and live in utopia after someone else creates it for us. Such a delusion that it will ever happen without enormous changes within ourselves is the

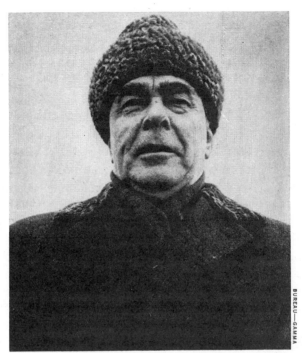

Brezhnev—the head of an oligarchy. Can he really manifest utopia?

main point of this book. The question comes, how do we radically change ourselves—collectively and individually—if we do not know where to begin? More and more, psychology emphasizes our need to accept ourselves as we are, and this touches a very deep and very real need in us. Spiritual leaders teach that we are perfect already; all we need is to give ourselves positive suggestions that will make our minds believe it. Since people do not really relish the idea of looking at the negative side of themselves and working on it, the theories of positive thinking always flourish in this world. But the embarrassing gap between our potential as perfected beings and our actual manifestation as small and separate egos remains.

In the real human world it is obvious from the way people relate that very few can actually cross the gap between their need for self-esteem, that is the boosting of self-image, and the actual performance of actions which warrant these thoughts of self-importance. Why is it

that we humans should think so highly of ourselves while our manifestation is so lacking in actual transformation? The enhancement of self-
concept in the achievement of worldly success goes against the idea of
ego reduction as practiced by spiritual teachers for centuries. We must
face the fact that although worldly success and fame may bring us
satisfaction as an egocentric being, they do not give us any satisfaction
before God. It is a fact that some of the most famous, most rich and
celebrated film stars, politicians, and well-known people are miserably
lonely in their deepest self and are thereby forced to face the hollowness
of social life. Senators, artists, film stars and people of influence are
sought after as patrons for good causes, but inside themselves they
know that although they have fame and renown, they have little real
power to affect the world for fundamental change. Even if they do not
consciously care about the world, a deeper part of them does care, and
this caring often manifests as depression and despair. Not only the
famous and influential but almost everyone is trapped in the constant
need to gain self-worth and to maintain self-image on one hand and the
need to become selfless, saintly and egoless on the other. The answer
is to be found in a method of government which generates creative
conflict throughout every level of society so that the growth of consciousness becomes an exciting national and an international way of life.
Only then will human relationships be able to generate change and
communicate on the higher levels of life.

We must not only desire change but we must resolve to grow, and it
is essential to our personal development that we should never allow
ourselves to believe that growth and change are not possible either now
or in the future. But such growth does not come to us without practice.
Growth does not come without working deliberately with others, facing
the uncomfortable conflicts within ourselves. Any future constitution
we write for society must not only incorporate in itself the machinery
for sudden change of the whole and the resolution of conflict between
individuals and groups but must also include our personal freedom to
grow. A society is no different from our own individual self, whose
tomorrow is in our power now. What we *do* now will make tomorrow a
better day. Yet all constitutions and charters, so far designed by man,
have been written by legal men to prevent the sudden passage of laws
without due process. They are devices which restrict individuals from

acting without consulting with other members of society. They are, in short, delaying mechanisms of containment designed to put off what we wish to do today until tomorrow or longer so that other people can be informed before some action is thrust upon them. Consequently, delay is the essence of political action. This depresses the people, who cannot understand why something wanted now should take so long to come about, while the things like taxation or raising money for huge government expenditures can be enacted with lightning speed. Something has to be done to devise a system that is more responsive to the citizens' needs, for nothing is more depressing than the feeling that we are impotent or ineffectual and that we have not the power to shape the future. This feeling of being unneeded, of being ineffectual in the process of government and decision-making, is part of the reason so many people feel worthless and have a negative self-image. No matter how much they intend to do something about social problems and no matter how much they think about it or talk about it, a true feeling of participation has to be expressed and written in the lifestyle rather than in words. Is it really possible to practice what we preach in our constitutions? The constitution should enable us to stay optimistic about our civilization, but does it? Discouragement does not make us want to face the future or work our decision-making power today to make tomorrow a better day.

THE FRUITS OF IMPOTENCE

As of this moment, here and now, through the lack of interest in how we are governed and our lack of participation in the formation of the institutions of society, much of the world is under the domination of very powerful armed oligarchies. An oligarchy is defined as a form of government in which the power is invested in the few, but there are still countries in which the power is invested in one person. Whether this person is an autocrat who inherits power like a king or is a dictator who seizes power, the enforcement of sovereignty over the people by the regime can only come from the might and power of guns and violence. These oligarchies control the people whether they are the clique of Russian Bolsheviks who sit at the top of the pyramid of political control and run the party machine, dictators in Africa, totalitarian military regimes in South America, the Shah of Iran, or the kings of Arabia; the pattern of sovereignty is for a few people to control the freedom of individual choice. Is there any hope for universal freedom in the ideal sense? And if so, how in this present world can those dedicated to freedom ever make an impression on those who do not even know there is a deep problem? It is understandable if a passion for democratic freedom does not occur to those who have never experienced it and therefore do not know what they are missing, but the karmic responsibility is much greater for those of us in the free countries who have not yet woken up to the reality that our own democratic system has been betrayed. While going through the motions of voting in elections, we are giving our freedom away without seeing how precious real democracy is nor imagining how we will be without it.

How *will* we be without it? Much of our democratic decision-making is already manipulated by special interests, and many of our legislatures are controlled by oligarchs or special pressure groups. Every day we speak in words the ideals of democracy, yet our leaders are weak and easily influenced by a host of private interests. The CIA taps telephones despite the constitutional provision that every man has the right to freedom of expression. President Nixon takes it upon himself to bomb Viet Nam and tell the American people afterwards. By our willing apathy, the administrators, be they weak or strong, good or evil, become so powerful that they have almost the power of dictators who can suppress, arrest, or overrule any suggestions from the people. "We the people" no longer have the voice and the self-government system we have been taught about in schoolbook studies of democracy, but are becoming pretty much a rubber stamp for government that is happening to us. Is there such a thing, when the world has grown so crowded with millions of people, as a real democracy where actual people like you and me can govern our own lives at every level and make no separation between our government and our own sense of personal responsibility?

If we dare to look at our system of government with real openness of mind, we may see it as it really is and not with all the misty trappings of tradition and sentimental childhood training. Whether you are American, Russian, British or any other nationality the odds are that you have been taught in school that your system of government is the best one evolved to date. It would be difficult for any American to be thinking about any new system which claimed to work better than the supposed constitutional "checks and balances". It would make the average American feel insecure even to *think* of getting a new constitution. But if you were British, with a parliament over a thousand years old, you would feel that an unwritten constitution, one that had grown by the usages and precedents of a lower and upper house, was safer than a written document liable to misinterpretation by a few lawyers turned judges of the Supreme Court. If you were Russian you would have been taught for sixty years that the operation of the constitution must come through the distilled wisdom of the communist party and that therefore any independent and differing views would automatically be branded as subversive, anti-Russian and traitorous.

Almost everywhere in the world, whatever the system of government, we are told that our own system is best and any attempt to change is an attack on *us*. It is almost impossible to look at the ways we are governed with this kind of traditional taboo always hovering over the sacred document or system. We are afraid that if we look at the ways we are governed, we will become open to revolution and chaos. Yet it is still possible to open this closed subject in the Western democracies just as a matter of discussion. Up to now all philosophers with new systems of government have required us to adopt the new if necessary by throwing out the old. But here I am not suggesting any form of violence nor am I trying to stir up controversy and trouble as the activists and radicals do. I am only wondering if we might create a real live experiment with subjects whose emotional volatility make them rather dangerous, and I am wondering if we can dare to take our heads out of whatever we have become so absorbed in—our lives, our children, our work, our hobbies, our love life or whatever—and really look at some realities we'd prefer to ignore.

Our inability to look at our government with any objectivity is similar to our inability to look at ourselves. If we do look at the government it is only to criticize. Those millions of coffee drinkers are blaming the President every morning at 10:15 a.m. sharp, blaming the corrupt politicians, blaming the government, and this impotent moral outrage is the sum total of their concern and their perception and their conversation. They do not point the finger of blame at themselves or for one moment think that they themselves *are* the government and are responsible for what their country does. The German people did not feel responsible for what the Nazis did, yet the rest of the world felt differently about it. Even the Nazis themselves did not feel responsible but blamed their higher-ups, as the Nuremberg trials revealed. Where

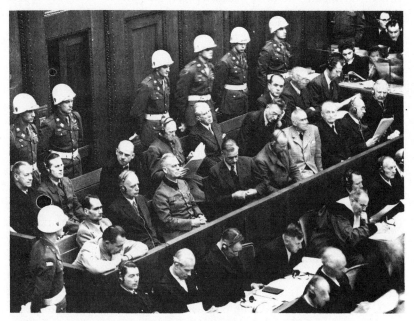

Nuremberg trials: nineteen top Nazis were convicted.

does the buck stop? When do we finally own responsibility? Is it only within the boundaries of the family that we feel responsible to each other and to ourselves? For some people, even the family can't evoke a sense of responsibility or caring. If you look within yourself, you can quickly find out where your own responsibility stops, because you yourself stop it and set a cut-off point with the power of your own consciousness. And you alone have the power to move that cut-off point.

One of the truths about ourselves that we do not want to see at the political level is the fact that there is no protection whatsoever in any nation's constitution against those who would subvert it. If you do not protect yourself by participating in the decision-making process, no one will. No matter how revered it is, the United States Constitution is a theory like any other ideal mode of government. We delude ourself that the "words" of the Constitution are our protection when they are not. Only the practice of the Constitution by honest and integral representatives who have the courage to speak out can make its protection work. But how often do we see people with this kind of integrity in the political arena? Have we ourselves bothered to develop those qualities? Even if we were to get a new constitution, only our own concern and willingness to take responsibility could make it work. Uganda is only one of many states which has a most modern constitution framed on the long experience of the British government, and yet there is at the moment a military dictator in Uganda who terrorizes the population with his army and totally ignores this modern constitution.

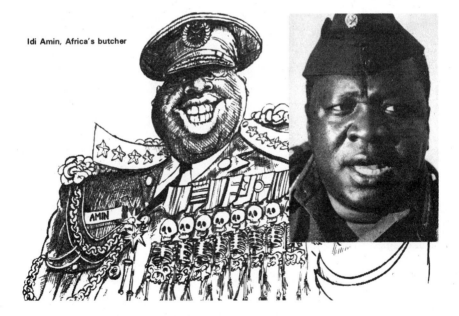

Idi Amin, Africa's butcher

A constitution, regardless of how good it is, is no insurance against ruthless power-crazy people. In fighting such dragons, there must always be a hero. And each of us, no matter how ordinary, must look inside ourselves for the necessary qualities, because heroism is no respecter of social, intellectual or any other kind of rank. It springs forth in the hearts of men and women, no matter who they are or where they live or when. They see something clearly and this clear seeing presents them with a choice. If they have strength of character, they choose the more difficult but more honorable way.

So what are we not seeing clearly? What will we see if we dare to look at our government calmly and objectively—not identifying, not feeling threatened and insecure, but just looking? One thing we will see is that the division between the "good" systems (the democratic societies) and the "bad" systems (the repressive, tyrannical governments) is misleading. In actual fact, both systems tend to favor the exploiters, power seekers, materialists, the unevolved persons who will take an interest in the government because they *want* something from it. Think of that for a moment. Realize the enormity of it. This is the way life is. It does no good to put our heads in the sand and prefer to believe that human nature is other than it is.

Perhaps you may not quite know what I mean when I say that the inability to look at our government and assess its true quality is connected in a very direct way to our inability to look at ourselves. The most fundamental principle of the World Peace Center which I am proposing is this commitment to look squarely at oneself and to change whatever is not right. The technique of Creative Conflict, *to one who is not willing*, feels something like being stoned to death by a large group of people, and it is made even more painful if you happen to love the ones who are providing this mirror of your negative qualities. But with understanding of its powerful way of penetrating beneath our ego structure comes our openness to receive feedback from our fellows without reacting to their views. As a tried method of human evolution developed over years of intense community work, it is now offered to the world as a way of passing voluntarily through the refiner's fire. It is a way of looking at ourselves as we really are. Only the willingness to look can place you in the eye of the hurricane where the storm does not touch you. From there, you can hear your faults brought out, yet not identify with them. From there, it seems that friends are helping you to clear up traits which you yourself want very much to change and be free of. So you do not feel criticized because you do not identify with the faults. You identify with the truth-centered part of yourself that only wants to know the truth and become a better person. Most people would rather hear a lie than to face something unpleasant about themselves and they feel the same about their government. "Let sleeping dogs lie," they say. "I am vaguely aware that all is not quite right with me, but I'm getting along pretty well. Best not to get into all that stuff. It might be a real can of worms once I open it up." They are even aware, in a hazy ill-at-ease way, that others are suffering because of this undealt-with problem. But they do not really look at it squarely and get a clear view because then they would have to do something about it. Some readers may be thinking, "This guy really *is* a dreamer if he thinks I am going to put myself through a lot of pain just so I can be humble enough to start caring about the world's troubles." But there are some who are ready, and this book is for them. "They that have the ears to hear, let them hear." It takes courage to climb a mountain or fight a war or to go into regions where no human has been before and map the way. But no act of physical courage requires even a fraction of the valor that is needed to venture into your own vast inner regions of unexplored terrain. Your own self is the most frightening enemy that you can fight, because you yourself feel every blow that you strike. Yet it is also the most rewarding of all battles, for if you conquer your own self, then the world has no terror that can frighten you again, and life becomes an adventure in which you find, again and again, that the air upon the mountain's peak is pure and worth the climb.

The working of the techniques of creative communication incorporated in the World Peace Center constitution enables you to set down what you think your own personal goals should be and what should be the goals of your community, nation or group. You do this because you are part of it and cannot escape responsibilty for the situation you are in. You must work to influence its direction through a system which gives you that power, otherwise you will be carried by events like a tide in the affairs of men which you cannot control. Unless you do something to face the situation and have a hand in destiny, you will be overwhelmed and made to feel impotent by the rush of events. This impotency is a human sickness leading to cancer. No amount of financial power or political power can stop this cancer or impotent life forces because the power over one's life and destiny is a spiritual condition, not a material one. It is total and indivisible from everything which happens on the entire planet. In your home you can sit thousands of miles away from the murder of 100,000 people in Africa or see the world starving to death on your TV screen, but unless you can do something you are impotent. This does not mean you must immediately send money to charity to buy dinners for hungry children. That is your escape, which gives you some self-esteem, but it does not change you nor the world which caused that situation, and it is still an act of impotence.

Why do you give money away to someone else to give away after they deduct their expenses? Because you feel impotent. And it's an easy way to get a problem off your back until the next guilt feeling comes. But what if you don't feel guilty? You are still impotent because you allow it. If you changed society by beginning with your own way of life and changing that, you would say, "I can give money away as well as anyone else. Why do I need to delegate it to others?" Many of these so-called "charitable" organizations trade on your impotence and your guilt. You can only stop this by committing your heart to changing the world. God does not want nor need your money. He wants your soul and when he has that he has your entire being; your money comes along with that. But to get satisfaction and fulfillment you must do more than just write a signature and give money to charity, no matter how hard you worked for that money. That kind of giving never brings release. But to commit yourself to a dynamic and world-changing step, taken at the level of your own life and its direction and its destiny, gives an immediate sense of relief that you are directly involved in an evolutionary change and not merely in the provision of a temporary stop gap in a system that is ultimately hopeless.

Even if you were filled with ecstasy, meditating in some lonely cave in the Himalayas—a so-called enlightened being, in touch with the whole Cosmos—you would be deluding your being in self-hypnotic trance if you stayed there enjoying yourself, knowing the answer to human cancer and yet letting the world rot. You can detect my impatience with gurus who sit on thrones or gilded stages decked with flowers while the gullible pray for these "high" beings to save their souls. If they cannot relate to their own self-separation from the depressed, the hungry and the political power systems, and have cut themselves off from the world, then they too are deluded by their love of idyllic luxury. This book is not for such materialistic fakers but for the true saints who go invisibly about the slow painful task of rooting out the cause of spiritual and material poverty.

In one sense this is an angry book. The anger is righteous anger and is directed at the blindness of mulish man in failing to see the obvious ego tricks and self-deceptions which run the world. To see that our highest organized body, the United Nations, can recieve an appeal from the king of a country (Tibet in 1959) whose people are being systematically eliminated by an invading nation, murdered in the international crime of genocide, and then to see that august body saying, "Sorry, you are not a member of our club, we cannot hear your proposal," is enough to make righteous blood boil. This anger is not anger at anyone in particular but at the terrible darkness of the human mind which will bring the world to disaster. If it were our own ship sinking and we looked around for help but watched every ship sail past oblivious, would we be angry or forlorn that their lookout was sleeping on the job? Every person has a duty to himself or herself to love his neighbors, to help them see and report a crime. If we summoned the courage to report a crime of murder and the local police did absolutely nothing about it, we would be very angry.

This is the anger of this book. For years I have been speaking and writing with too little fire in the belly. Then I read Solzhenitsyn's monumental work on the Gulag labor camps of Soviet Russia, dominated by his seething, quiet controlled anger at the inhumanity of the world. Then I read the gospels again and found the same desperate angry last-minute call to straighten our affairs, to repent, to look beyond the obvious and to get cracking with the kingdom of heaven upon earth. So I took my old book of *Nuclear Evolution* written ten years ago with a more genteel vibe and I expanded it with some of the anger I feel at man's procrastination. We have just got to quit talking and get on with our evolutionary destiny. Let us forget revolutionary anger—the *self-*righteous anger which kills people, judges people and oppresses those who do not believe in political theory. Let us replace it with the quiet anger which comes from the fierce lover who returns to earth and finds his lovely world in bed with the devil. This book is then a sequential development of *Nuclear Evolution*, describing the achieving of that Cosmic Consciousness needed by individuals to solve world problems of such huge magnitude as universal angers and conflict. It is not a book of ideas that are put forward as a theoretical base on which others can take action so that you may live in peace. It is a book which I hope will make you angry—angry at yourself as much as anyone else.

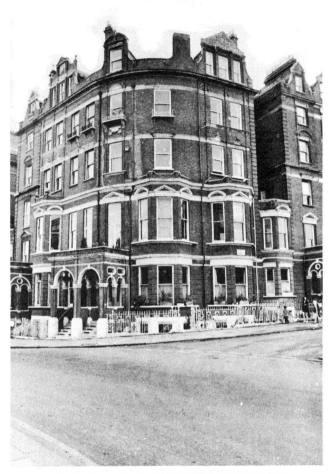

Centre House, London, as it looks now after renovations.

For seven years we practiced conflict resolution as an experimental community dedicated to spiritual evolution of the group, without coercion of the individual.

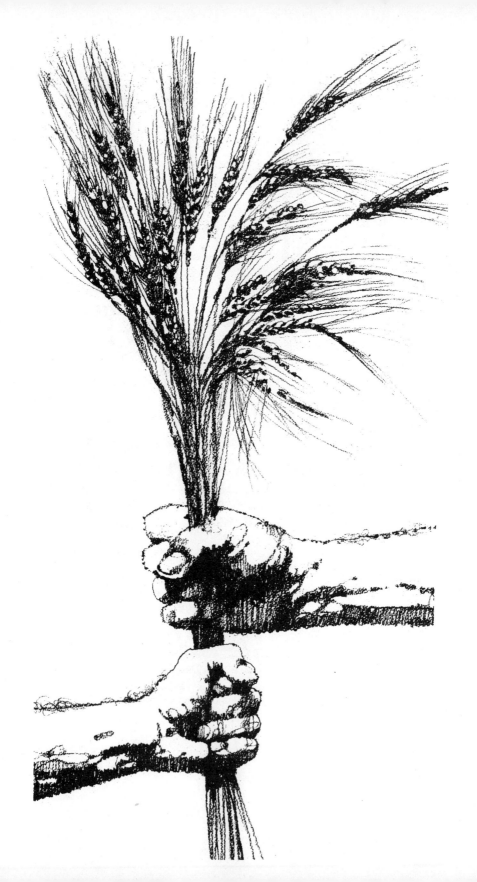

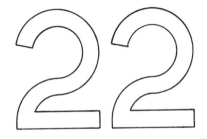

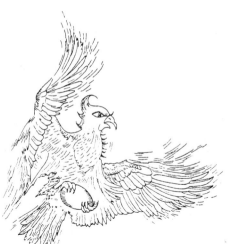

OUR MOST URGENT PROBLEM— CONFLICT RESOLUTION

There are hundreds of institutions and organizations set up in the world today to resolve conflict. In fact, resolving conflict has become a large business as we see in marriage counseling, psychiatry, the judicial system, labor unions and all the way up to the United Nations. And to a certain extent we do succeed in arbitrating our conflicts and coming to a settlement. But soon a new conflict has arisen and then another and another, because the people themselves, who created the conflict in the first place, have not changed. The same causes go on creating the same human conflicts ad infinitum. And the basic suppositions behind all human arbitration stay the same, never calling into question the right of every human ego to look out for its own interest and to win out over the "other". All our present methods of conflict resolution do little more than compromise, adjudicate, de-polarize sides, placate egos, or allow people to have a sounding board or pressure-relief valve.

The person, party, group or country in conflict then feels that they got the best deal they could under present circumstances and they will try to get even more of their own way at a later date. Apparently it does not occur to anyone engaged in all this arbitration that a real fundamental change in people is actually possible, desperately needed and desirable.

At a certain point in my own life I realized that a method had to be developed that would resolve conflict, not by patching things up at the surface level after conflict had already arisen, but by striking at the root. There would have to be a method that could make a real change in the ego structure of the participants. Because I knew of no such institution or method for dealing with conflicts between nations I traveled the world for six years speaking to leaders in the fields of international law and economics searching for someone who had found a way of solving disputes. In 1966 I felt it was necessary to set up a permanent experimental community in London with that purpose. Experts all agreed that the United Nations and the World Court had been made ineffective by the sovereignty of nations which essentially is the right to be a law unto oneself. Sovereignty, the divine right to make laws and to be free of any interferences from external authorities or forces, was claimed by all nations even in the face of international laws and organizations which had been set up to combat autocracy and to discover the mechanisms for resolving conflict.

Whether individuals are hawks, pragmatists, theoreticians, religionists, revolutionaries or businessmen, they live in different worlds from each other, and conflict is certain to emerge as these different worlds clash. The techniques of negotiation and diplomacy used to avoid violent conflict have not changed fundamentally in the last few hundred years. In fact there has been more violence in the last 100 years than in all previous history, as newer and more devastating weapons and bombs are discovered. Hundreds of new nations have been created out of revolutionary violence and more millions of people have been murdered by the Hitlers, Stalins and Mao Tse-tungs for conflicting political reasons than in any previous age. Twenty million Russians and six million Jews were killed by Hitler and forty million Russian peasants and aristocracy were killed by Stalin in his paranoiac purges.

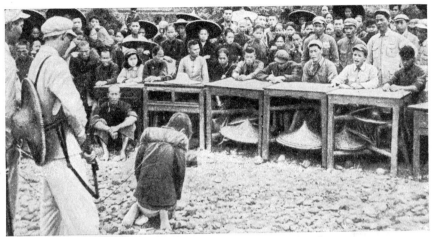

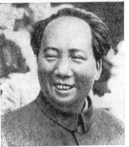

Above picture shows a radical "peoples' court" sanctioned by Mao, sentencing a "despotic landlord" who tried to cling to the two-thirds of an acre his family had lived on for centuries. About sixty million people who disagreed with communist politics were ruthlessly executed in these purges for which Mao and those who agreed with him bear direct responsibility, wherever they may be on this planet. Certain people in the West, in their enthusiasm for radical change, chose to ignore his methods, just as many Germans chose to ignore Hitler's massacre of the Jews.

An early picture of Mao Tse-tung, founder of the Chinese Communist Party, who ruled Red China without calling party conferences from 1949 to 1976. His land distribution was ruthless.

Sixty million peasants who disagreed with communism were tried and shot by so-called "people's courts" set up by Mao Tse-tung. Daily we hear of wars, take-overs, terrorism and government repression, and bombings of innocent bystanders by Irish fanatics.

What chance have we or anyone else of now coming up with a method of solving human conflicts? Institutions, universities and businesses study the laws of different countries and research the rules and patterns of world disputes. Some foundations try to anticipate conflicts which might emerge from the discovery of oil and gas or rich natural resources under the sea. Others try to research the process of making concessions and making rough drafts which fit the interests of contending parties rather than their spoken positions. Others try to use different settings to work with influential people or political leaders in order to provide a context for agreement or to establish a basis of discussion on which the conflicting parties can meet. The UN is such a specially-contrived context which provides little more than a convenient meeting ground for disputing parties seeking a mediator, although there are many idealists who believe it provides something more. Peace studies and academic research appear to be so divorced from the human beings creating the disputes, that there is little prospect of these ivory tower methods finding any acceptance on the practical level of conflict resolution. Will the protesting people of peace-making movements, similar to those which flourished on every campus during the recent war, ever come together again at the grass roots political level to act as a counterweight to the institutional violence of governments, dictators, whaling companies and terrorists? Or will we need to see more

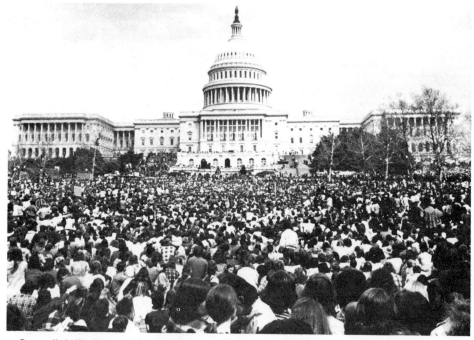

Peace rally in Washington, D.C., 1971. What is going on in their hearts and minds? Did they change the world?

bloodshed, napalm bombs on children and holocausts before we are motivated to find a way of settling conflict with those who would use force? Is real peace a passive state? Do we really know what is a peace making lifestyle, and is there any community in the world where conflicts between people of different perceptions of reality have found a fulfilling outlet for aggression and created a conflict-free environment? Is there anywhere a form of government that does not coerce or trample on human rights? The answer which our living experiment at the University of the Trees has evolved is at the human level of people and not at the institutional level, while the classical "peace researchers" are more interested in national conflicts, in big labor-management bargaining, in environmental disputes concerning rights and pollution, or in settling grievances of employees. None of these socially–orientated academic attempts to resolve conflict has really succeeded and there are today just as many strikes and just as many insoluble differences between nations as before. The reason is not hard to discover. The root of all conflict is within individuals who cause it and not in the external situations which the peace researchers look at to compile their statistics. Out of all the years that we have been practicing Creative Conflict methods as a way of developing individuals in actual living situations both at Centre House in London and at the University of the Trees, we have never had any academics involved in peace research come to investigate or even want to know how we govern ourselves organizationally or settle a conflict on a practical day to day basis. Is it not strange that there are Federal Mediation and Conciliation Services, Labor and Industrial Relations Consultants, Journals of Conflict Resolution, Centers of Conflict Resolution, and none of them confesses to any answers—yet there are places on earth which exist where conflict resolution is a living goal and a successful way of life. There are places where people totally dedicate themselves to bringing that peace which comes with understanding, both to themselves and to all members of society. But we never get visits from peace researchers or these experts who say there are no answers. Is it because they tackle it at a superficial level of employees' feelings, working places, legalities, consumer disputes, rather than in-depth understanding of ourselves? Why is this repeated over and over again when the techniques for Creative Conflict have been available in the public domain for over ten years? The answer is that Creative Conflict goes deep into the ego structure, and we may find the very peace researcher himself exposed to searching his motives rather than being armed with some label conferring the structural authority of an "expert" on conflicts and arbitration. Who will come willingly naked to learn of a totally original and new way which first of all requires that we put away all the garbage that we know does not work? A method which brings only bare consciousness to a meeting and insists on a willingness to explore the depths of being, leaves all our egotistic opinion-making behind and is not therefore to the liking of encyclopedic experts or theorists. How will the new methods for solving disputes ever gain ground if academicians will not study them or try them out on themselves? The answer is that no progress will be made until people all over the world understand that conflict begins with us, the philosophy of self, the image of ourselves and the model of the human being we live by, and not by the opinions of experts who may well be good at patching up, but not very effective at prevention at the source of conflict. Do we palliate the disease or do we attempt to cure the cause of the world's sickness? The experts explore at the battlefronts of conflict itself where the dead and bruised lie dying, but they are nowhere to be seen at the beginning of the disputes, that is, inside the minds and fears and frustrations which are the root cause of all tensions not only between individuals in society but between nations, movements and religions. They are interested in the "quick fix" for conflict but not in the long-term cure or prevention.

Nothing illustrates the present state of conflicts and individual disputes better than the legal system in America. Legal services are now mainly prepaid because the mass of people get legal help paid by all types of insurance which encourages the public to seek litigation rather than reduce it. This has driven up the cost of legal help for everyone, and especially for medical insurance, to the point that legal costs were so inflated that the premiums for medical malpractice insurance became so ridiculous that doctors went on strike. Because of these high costs people have now begun to settle conflicts over property and divorces out of court through mediation between the parting couples rather than fight them out in long drawn-out legal battles between lawyers.

If we now consider that there is almost a fifty percent divorce rate, then half of our young people are coming from broken homes, situations of bitter family conflict, and this has a powerful effect on the aggregate social tensions between people. Out-of-court negotiating reduces the bitterness and bad feeling from the marriage and thus lessens the bitterness of children, so it would seem to be a sign of real progress in our ways of resolving conflict. But this type of resolution of conflict is all after the fact, and the desire to settle these disputes more amicably is not due to any change of heart, individual growth, or wisdom, but because the tremendous demand for lawyers, courts, judges, etc., has driven the costs of litigation to ridiculous sums. The new methods of resolving family conflict and legal mediation are therefore a development resulting from material considerations and not through any real desire among this fifty percent of our people to change their ways.

The same applies to Community Dispute Centers which have sprung up in the last few years. It appears that social and individual conflicts are heading towards innovative new forms of resolving disputes at the legal level, but these arbitrations do not tackle refinement of human consciousness. They only tackle the existing grievances over such things as housing, family or marital problems, small claims courts, and consumer complaints against merchants. Many times, after the dispute has developed into an impasse, local counseling provides help which does provide an alternative to legal suits and the deep bitterness they engender, but these counseling services are only piecemeal solutions because they do not change our society nor do they change our way of life. It is the business of judges to interpret state laws and follow traditional proceedings in the deciding of conflicts, but everyone knows that justice is more than the letter of the law. There are many rightful positions lost through some legal technicality just as there are wrongful ones which escape the law altogether. More often there are also personal and private aspects of a dispute which are never brought into an open court or ever satisfied by the legal decision of a judge. Is it not an interesting fact that more violent crimes emerge from the frustrations of living closely with a marriage partner than from the alienation from a separated society? Violence such as wife-beating, child-beating, and husband-beating, slandering of neighbors and fights between children stem from inner conflicts and personal disputes which could be resolved by Creative

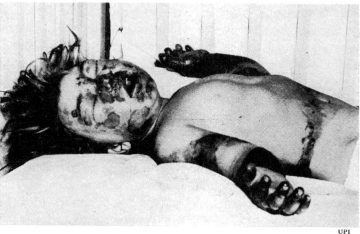

UPI

Child burned by mother.

Conflict. This kind of hostility and violence is not the same as the criminal intent to kill and murder for money or power. Neither is it the same as institutional violence such as an army or police force may inflict upon a population on the orders of a dictator or a government. However, the cause of all violence, even self-violence, is fundamentally from the same root—lack of communication, due to being out of touch with our own misperceptions and being unable to listen and understand the viewpoints of others. These in turn all spring from ignorance of the fact that humans think, feel, see, sense and live reality at different levels of awareness. Very few of the present programs of conflict resolution begin from the fact that there naturally exist seven different levels of perception of any situation, and that which may appear true from one level of consciousness may not be true from another level which takes in a wider perspective. Obviously a driver ignorant of why the traffic is held up bumper to bumper can begin to get worked up into a red passion and toot his horn at all the cars in front to let off his frustration. He does not have the same view as the helicopter pilot hovering over the line of cars who sees that the cause of the slowdown is a bloody accident a mile ahead. Similarly the citizen sitting in the bar railing at the President's policies does not have before him all the intelligence reports, the opposition pressures and friendly lobbies, the views of many experts painting a complex scene, nor does he have to suffer the consequences for any error of judgement. The view of the situation from the bar naturally will be more simplistic. Not that it might be less true, but from the wider angle of vision it could be only partially true. Creative Conflict takes this multi-tiered model of human communication into account in all perceptions of reality in a practical way. We need a wider framework to see ourselves from, not in order to avoid confrontation but to settle conflicts before they escalate into a full legal test. Conflict resolution generally is a hot subject because once it becomes a movement on the face of the waters and penetrates to ordinary citizens and alters the way they live, then it will fundamentally alter the whole system. But Creative Conflict is even hotter still because it changes lives rather than systems. When we change lives drastically, systems become mere tools of consciousness.

When it dawns on humans generally that all our systems for solving conflicts—courts, parliaments, councils, committees, etc.,—are mere expressions of consciousness, then we will not only see radical changes in consciousness but vast changes in lawmaking. In the last fifteen years the courts have been besieged by a backlog of cases which has climbed by eighty percent, and the workload of the legal agencies which administer these cases has climbed by a similar percentage. In that short time fifty out of seventy federal agencies which regulate our laws have been created, causing enormous increases in federal employees. The Social Security Administration alone employs 600 law judges who administer and hear 150,000 cases every year. Enforcement of laws is even more complex even though there is a movement towards non-court resolution of conflict as with parking tickets and probational offenders. In a complex society one begins to ask: is it possible to solve human conflict by creating new agencies? There have been conflicts between the government and the American Indians for over 200 years with promises of self-government to Indian tribes which have never materialized, and there are conflicts between whites and blacks over segregation and desegregation of schools and hundreds of minor conflicts between students, racial minorities, police brutality, workers and employers and neighbors, all seemingly very important to their supporters. For these types of conflicts there are courses at universities on mediation and conflict resolution, and law schools are now beginning to give seminars on mediation as an aid to the negotiation process. But all of this misses the real point:

PEOPLE GENERALLY DO NOT UNDERSTAND THEM-
SELVES OR THE LEVELS OF CONSCIOUSNESS THEY ARE
THINKING, FEELING OR SEEING FROM.

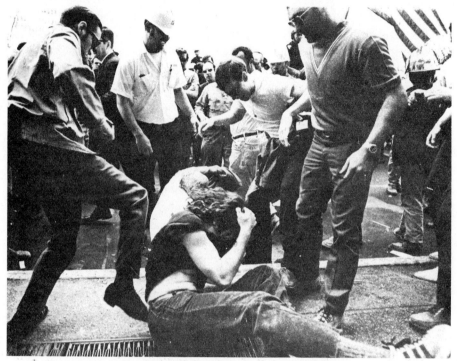

New York City, 1970: Youths protesting Vietnam War are attacked by construction workers.

Individuals, private groups, the government mediation agencies,
the university dispute and conflict resolution centers are all researching
the external environmental field for new ways to resolve the costly and
lengthy delays and disputes between business development and environmentalists. But the internal environment which is the seat of the
problem is ignored. While it is good to stop the exploitation of the
planet, to see the conflict as merely the polarization between opposing
forces is to be completely blind to what was the real cause in the first
place. The real cause is the very design of projects which exploit
Nature and other people at the expense of "the other". Many people
design projects without regard for others or including in the design
costs the allowance for solving the human problems they create. Many

of these problems are foreseen on the design table, but they are ignored because of expense, the philosophy being that we will deal with that when the public forces us to, which might allow a calculated ten years freedom from financing costs. Hence we invest in jets with intolerable noise levels, such as the British-French supersonic Concorde, or the cleaning and washing of oil tankers off the coasts at sea, or the design of nuclear electricity plants with thousands of tons of poisonous radioactive wastes. Irresponsible escape from the consequences of our

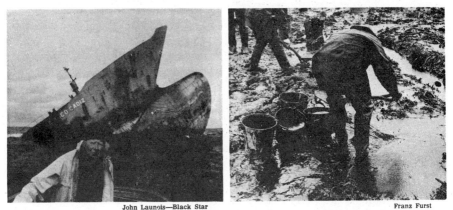

John Launois—Black Star   Franz Furst

Sinking tankers pollute the ocean and our beaches. Along with cargo, detergents for such emergencies could be carried.

action is the real cause of these projects being foisted on a tolerant public until people react in self-defense against the noise injury to the ears, the black dirt on the beaches or the poisoning of our underground waters with 500,000 years of plutonium. The planners and politicians *do not care* until everyone is up and howling at them. Right now we need to develop a society that is intolerant of commercial exploitation of the citizens' rights to peace and quiet and fresh air by engaging in Creative Conflict with designers of trucks, airplanes, chemical plants, etc., before these products and factories are produced. People must begin to care and feel concern for the inner worlds of others if we are to discover that kind of awareness which takes account of these obvious consequences while projects are still on the drawing boards. What will change this exploitation of human tolerance? Only when the designers and planners and scientists and taxmen know that society is intolerant of any exploitation of others will our leaders make sure that they never get away with it. How do we get to that state of sensitivity and caring about conflict *before* it manifests with all its destructive tension in the lives of people? Creative Conflict must become a matter of public policy and the skills of confrontation be built into the constitution of daily living.*

Governmental systems which depend on the polarizing of issues between two political parties, as in many democracies, will experience a difficulty in trying to do Creative Conflict since the parliamentary issues are reduced to the sophistry of verbal exchanges in debate which do not probe the speaker's real motives. Likewise in one-party governments such as communism there cannot be Creative Conflict as long as there is no freedom to question the party values or decisions. In two-party systems there is more freedom than in one-party societies, yet the polarizing of issues into either/or, black/white or positive/negative achieves balance at the expense of truth. Why is the truth compromised? This distortion of reality is very obvious in a labor dispute between employees and management, polarized into total opposition, or in negotiating a two-party business contract where each of two sides endeavors to extract the most concessions from each other. The distinction of two-party "conflicts of interest" only leads to solutions on superficial and easily comprehensible issues by ignoring the wider environmental and social fields which contain a great number of different parties. Such polarizing between two extreme situations is not possible in Creative Conflict, because the whole objective of Creative Conflict is to be sensitive to the viewpoint of the "other" and to be aware of all the different subtle facets of the whole. Its basis is therefore a gradient of truth, not a polarizing into crude extremes. Its purpose is to tune into the real complexity of variable conditions which will affect the long-term decisions for the whole of society. The main point of Nuclear Evolution is that this continuous pointing at the external environment or some group or person as the source of the problem is in itself a delusion which perpetuates the real problem, i.e., man's inability to communicate on any level of consciousness other than his own. Thus the first step toward resolving conflict is to learn

---

* See *The Golden Egg* for the model constitution of the World Peace Center used as a method of government at the Centre Community in London and at the University of the Trees for the last ten years.

that there are indeed other levels of consciousness than our own. This is difficult for any ego to accept.

A most acute form of conflict born of egotism in society comes from the two polarizations of science and religion where two distinct methods of acquiring and validating evidence are used. One group of humans "believes" that science is based on phenomena, measurement, and the sensory reality of objects, while the other group believes that "Truth" comes from the personal descriptions of reality called numinal or divine. The process of knowing by "divination" however is not considered scientific by many even though scientific method can be applied to divining as to anything else.* However, many scientists are in conflict within themselves about this because they believe that the scientific method *must* be restricted only to directly measurable effects or sensory effects. This is a dogmatic misuse of the scientific method which incidentally was not invented by scientists at all and in fact was invented by yogi mathematicians and seers many thousands of years ago. It was documented in various Sanskrit texts which I have actually read in the original versions. I cannot remember the source because I was not interested in proving anything to others at that time.** However the following brilliant reply to a letter accusing the editor of *Science News* magazine of leaning towards the mystical or numinous shows the kind of attitude necessary for conflict to be creative among scientists.

> *(There are things that are no less real for not being susceptible to investigation by the paradigms of natural science. These paradigms are designed for phenomena that submit to certain strict philosophical principles about repeatability, causality and logicality. The numinous,*

---

* *Supersensonics* contains a scientific treatment of the subject of divining from the viewpoint of sensing ability of birds, insects, animals and humans to detect ionizing fields.

** I have written my conclusions to this research in "Yogic Methods of Knowing", a paper delivered to the World Conference on Scientific Yoga, 1970, and published in Darshana International Magazine of Philosophy, December, 1970.

which is the nonrational aspect of religious experience (see p. 1,550 of Webster's Third New International Unabridged), obviously does not fall under these rules.

But then neither do some natural phenomena; quantum mechanics generally disobeys the rules of deterministic causality. In classical physics you can uniquely predict the behavior of an individual body. Under quantum mechanics the behavior of individual subatomic particles cannot be predicted. Only statistical rules for large numbers of particles can be derived. Einstein cursed at this situation with the remark: "God does not throw dice." In response to that kind of grousing the idea grew up that perhaps on a level of existence too fine to be seen by current experiment there existed a complex of causes ("hidden variables") that uniquely determined the behavior of individual electrons or neutrons. Experiment has never found evidence of such a hidden determinist world, and most physicists now regard hidden variables as a phantom.

A lot of junk is hawked in the name of religion, and a lot of swindles, from the coast of Virginia to the coast of California. Virgin Marys that glow in the dark usually have only the power to startle. Nevertheless I am willing to stipulate that some people have described numinous experiences accurately as some people have described quantum mechanics experiments accurately. To insist that the only reality are phenomena that can be submitted to the paradigms of classical science is itself a religion. — D.E.T.)

Paradigm is defined in Webster's as: "To show side by side as an example or pattern, but is now used in the sense of a model or a way of looking at evidence. Of late, it means a mind set or psychological ruts in which thinking occurs."

Numinous is defined in Webster's as: "Supernatural or mysterious, holy, aesthetic or spiritual," but the Oxford dictionary defines it as: "An obsolete word stemming from the Latin word numen—divine."

Quantum mechanics is that branch of physics dealing with the infinitely small charges of energy in the atom, as opposed to Einsteinian physics which deals with the infinitely large universe relative to the observer.

Conflict between numinous sources and those that seek only biological or material evidence is still raging after many centuries. Many who easily believe in statistical evidence do not always need a biochemical proof. The resolution of such conflicts by people who take extreme positions is not possible unless they can allow their own assumptions of absolute rightness to be challenged in Creative Conflict.

How can we get the blind and arrogant ego to see its own blind spots, to learn that it is not all-seeing and all-knowing and that others do live in different states of consciousness, with different modes of perception than our own? This is problem number one for Creative

Conflict because of the fact that there are none so blind as those who will not see even if they could see. This is where the whole Creative Conflict process leaves the question of the environment to itself as a given, to better concentrate on how we manipulate our own consciousness, how we exploit our own inner environment and pollute it, so that we cannot see the external environment as it really is because the observer's mind, his selfishness, his thought process is in the way. Self-knowledge is knowing of the unfolding organism in our evolution as cosmic beings rather than being content to exist as humans with only one mode of relating, only one level of listening, only one viewpoint. By looking at a situation from seven different levels, we can creatively use conflicts between man and the environment, man and woman, man and society, like an artist uses his paints to create a picture. They are the rough ingredients on the palette waiting for the consciousness which can organize them into beauty. To the musician they are the untuned strings of an instrument which sounds painful until their vibrations are arranged in resonance. To the environmentalist Creative Conflict is like knowing that the effects of a chemical on the environment will be known to the public before the chemical reaches the market. Its effects can be processed ahead of time through the art and science of toxicology. Through seeking Creative Conflict at the beginning, new tests can develop rapidly and agreement can come on the testing of a product before it has fouled up the environment and screwed up the wild life. The same is true of ideas as of chemicals. They can be tested out in small communities who join together for this purpose before foisting them untested upon the unprepared public by force of arms.

The only way society can change the context of business, governments, universities and institutions in which individuals live their everyday life, is through individuals. Individual citizens alone cannot change the social context that surrounds them directly but they can discover new ways to respond to it and can easily research the causes of tension in relationships and in themselves. This is the first step in all spiritual work and not a false narcissism, because we are not doing Creative Conflict for ourself alone but to bring peace to our greater Self in society. To face one's deepest fears or inability to express or even get in touch with one's own identity and feelings is difficult. Yet it is this inner-world of frustration and fear that leads to anger, hostility and violent action either towards one's marriage partner or towards other individuals in society. To be able to listen to feedback and probe the level from which "the other" is speaking or communicating is the first step in the spiritual work we call Creative Conflict. The struggle to be free, to be fulfilled, to live a full and rich life, to discover and master the traumas of earlier life and commit ourselves to loving and caring for others in society is the major goal of Creative Conflict. It is the group preparation for knowing the Self, the nuclear center of being in which all fear, chaos and disorder are resolved. The deep encounter of living together in the heart is not just for biological couples but for all those who sincerely ask the question of themselves:

WHAT IS THE PURPOSE OF MY LIFE?

This is the main question which Nuclear Evolution answers on seven different levels of experience. To get an inkling of what those levels are like is the very reason we practice Creative Conflict. It may take us days and days or weeks or years to resolve the clinging of the ego to its self-suggested sense of alienation. This clinging to the self-sense is our free choice and must be respected, but we must not waste time with people who do not have the will to learn to listen. There are no shortcuts to these skills which can only be practiced in order to know them. Conflicts are capable of resolution if our own feelings are confronted and expressed with integrity. If we play games with ourself and refuse to look at our internal environment and its effect upon our external world, then we suffer rejection not only by others but by the universe itself which becomes a powerful adversary to our selfishness. This is Nature's way. God leaves us alone to our arrogance and does not waste his time in an inhospitable environment. So it should be with mankind. This attitude of noninterference is not a form of intolerance but a cosmic principle written even into the hearts of atoms. We ignore it at our peril. Even the lowly atom is rejected by other atoms when they have no affinity for each other. Those who have no affinity for Truth, those who reject God, those who usurp the sovereign power of individuals, they too will not find Truth, they too will not find God anywhere since in rejecting God they reject themselves. Likewise we should never reject the sovereign Self of others, but we should ever allow them the divine right of freedom to reject themselves. The conflict is really within us with our own self-commitment to others. Can we love others and society as a whole more than we love ourself? Can we commit ourself to the nuclear bond of love and transcend our obsession with our own person so preoccupied with self? Only when we can honestly share this commitment with others integrally without any external coercion can our tensions within be prevented from being vented without. A commitment to the ultimate togetherness is a surrender to the numinous or divine bond of love. This is the true objective of our subjective state of consciousness. It is this that we share in true Creative Conflict. In its practice the subject and object eventually become *One.*

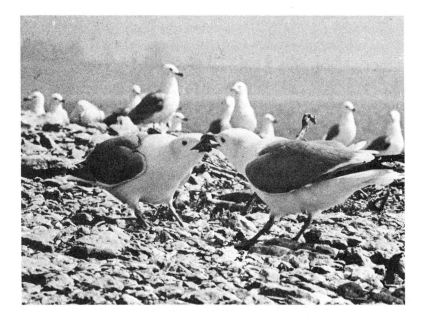

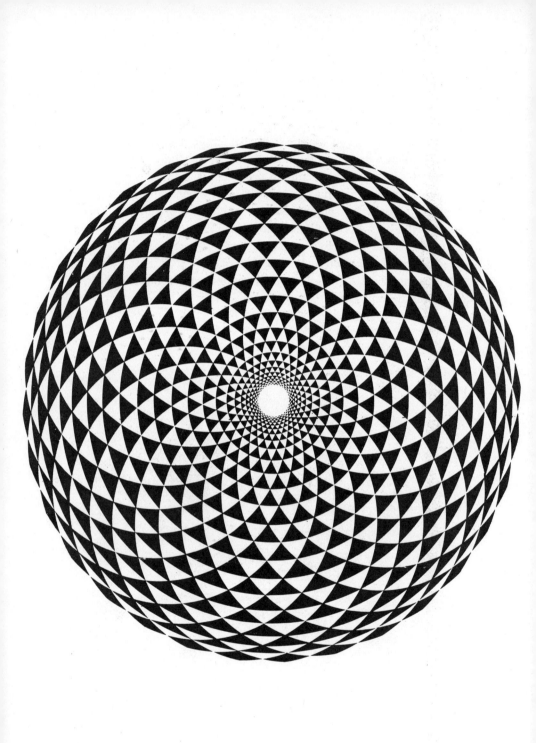

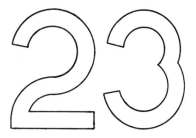

THE DEPTHS
OF CONFLICT

Creative ways of resolving conflict are patterned from Nature's own way of aiming at a critical pathway to Reality. If in the daily running of our business we are out of touch with the remorseless facts operating behind all of life, we soon find out, irrespective of our good intentions and idealism, that life will give us a subjective test of our real motivations and wishes in the form of inner conflict. One can see in the polarization of natural forces that all processes involve selection and choice at every level of atom, plants, animals and man. Most of these choices are made unconsciously in our cells, molecules, organs, etc., but the resolution of the conflict between two choices or even between three or four choices is often difficult to make on the conscious level. This is man's challenge, that he finds a way to resolve not only the conflict with others, but the conflict between parts of himself.

In the concepts and methods of Creative Conflict, I deal with the conflicts of stress which are largely the result of internal conflicts within ourself. We easily may say, "That's not true. Conflict is in the world out there, not in me." But a person is disturbed by or indifferent to news only inside his own consciousness, and if the world's conflicts do disturb us, it is because we allow it. Why would anyone want to practice Creative Conflict with others if it is true that our conflicts are within? The answer is of course that the understanding of this mystery of man's existence—*the difference between his inner life and his outer*—is not so simple because man himself is most complex. In our evolutionary development as people, we are challenged daily with our misunderstandings of situations and people, and it is no use giving theoretical reasons for society being what it is. We must show from within each person who identifies with worldly events why we should engage in the resolution of conflict in order to know ourselves better. To learn to love others who are so different from us and to work with them on their evolution by agreeing to differ with them in love, is not the normal human way of handling conflict. To some degree the business of politics is compromise, but in Creative Conflict we do not compromise Truth; instead we learn to listen to it at greater depths of communication.

Before we can say what Creative Conflict is we must take a look at ordinary conflict and try to determine its true cause. Sometimes we can't even see our conflicts, so tightly are they woven into the fabric of our living. A woman may have sexual and ego needs that pull her to many men, but she cannot act on these needs because she loves her husband and has ideals of loyalty and honor. She is torn with inner conflict which affects the quality of her consciousness at the office, and her business associates and children notice that she is irritable or inefficient or slow. She never acts on her feelings and she thinks of herself as a "happily married woman", so her conflict may continue unresolved for years and years. If she does get in touch (communicate with herself), she may separate from her husband, even though they love each other. The divorce rate rises higher and higher every year, primarily because people cannot communicate with each other. They would rather divorce than mention the subject of sex or speak real feelings or have any kind of an uncomfortable conversation.

Most people learn this by imitation because their parents lived together in the same unfulfilling way. Human conflict begins in the family and is passed down through the generations. Parents insist that their children be like them, even though the children are totally different individuals. The children shape their lives to fit these expectations. The sons are trapped for thirty years in jobs they do not like; the daughters marry and have children whether they want them or not. If they ever do get in touch with their own inner sense of direction, they find they have already entangled themselves in so much responsibility that they can no longer follow its guidance.

Most of the social norms are rigged to prevent us from getting in touch with our true being. The social code requires a friend or mate to keep silent and put up with faults for years and years. A woman talks incessantly and her husband withdraws into silence. She feels he must be stupid, since he seems unable to speak, but he is a gentleman, and a gentleman cannot tell his wife that she is an "old gas bag". She compares his faults to her virtues; he compares his virtues to her faults, but they say nothing. With faces like masks, they relate to each other at the surface level of "What would you like for lunch?" until at last the man begins a relationship with another lady. Although the marriage is totally barren, suddenly the wife feels possessive, and jealousy leads them into overt conflict. She does not see that she caused anything; she feels he is cruel to treat her this way after all the years she was loyal. Self-pity crowds out remorse. And in the man, too, there is little comprehension of his wife's inner world, what his silence does to her, why she is such a silly woman because there is no strong person to tell her to please shut up. He isn't being real; he prefers to escape into another relationship rather than work out the conflict in this one.

This example of the potential divorce is also typical of the divorce in political relationships on the national and world scene. Instead of stating anything clearly, the truth is compromised in clichés. The current president of the US is sincerely engaged in fighting inflation. The previous president started a campaign called WIN, "Whip Inflation Now". Neither president has told the public the real cause of inflation in their much publicized TV shows and appeals to labor and business to keep their prices down. The fact that government politics and the refusal to balance the budget are the reasons for the annual printing of dollars which devalues the existing currency we have in our hands, is never mentioned. This amounts to a deception of the people.

Even the sworn enemies of America are more truthful about the way to cause a social catastrophe. Lenin declared repeatedly that the best way to destroy capitalist America was to debauch the currency of the dollar and all other currencies of capitalist countries. Every president and his economic advisers know what the famous economist Lord Keynes said about the government spending more money than it has raised by taxation. Keynes said that by continuing the process of inflation, governments can confiscate, secretly and unobserved, a considerable part of the wealth of their citizens. By printing more money to pay for the budget the currency is debauched. We are told by the President that inflation is the fault of the unions asking for more money and the fault of the capitalists driving prices higher and higher. The truth is that inflation forces both labor and capital to ask for higher wages and prices, but the process of inflation begins with the government's refusal to stop its own lavish spending. By compromising the truth, this lack of integrity is then reflected in the whole of political and individual lives. The refusal to speak out the truth because we might lose a few votes is an example of the type of repressed conflict between the strict reality of the social processes in our life and the deceptive system we elect to govern over that everyday reality. The marriage of truth, beauty and government by universal intelligence cannot take place in the house on the street anymore than it can take place in the House of Representatives when the language we speak is debauched by hypocrisy and our values are debased by lack of integrity between our social leaders and the people, and between person and person.

Christ tells us that one of the greatest sources of human conflict is in judging others, not letting them be who they are, insisting that they be the same kind of person as ourselves. The laws of the spiritual life are rooted in these basic inner and outer conflicts in all human beings. If we judge our friends they will judge us, so we learn to lead a life where we do not speak openly in fear of offending them. We fear rejection from the ones we love. We fear inner turmoil and we project the resulting emotional insecurity onto others and fear then dominates our perception of them. We judge truth according to whether it meshes with our feelings. If we do not like the truth, we avoid it or put it off till later. It is a comfort for most of us to think our perception of truth is correct. A young man will argue with his aunt; his uncle comes in and takes her side of the argument, so the young man assumes that the uncle is against him and never stops to notice that the arbitration is in fact dispassionate and quite fair. At the very deep core of all conflicts sits the ego—smug and safe, certain that the best thing for all concerned is for the ego to get its own way.

The thing most hated by any ego is Creative Conflict in a group of people, with its many impartial mirrors. Creative Conflict compels us always to look at truth and it forces us to be open and integral with ourselves. No other discipline including all the spiritual methods of introspection actually brings us to see our self-deception so quickly. Even meditation and prayer are dominated by the self-serving quality of our consciousness. So many spiritual movements are merely self-righteousness in disguise, and we must find a way of testing their reality rather than unquestioningly confirming their assumptions. In the hothouse environment of Creative Conflict, one may find oneself in the first half-hour confronted with an image of self which may take several years to get to in doing meditation. The ideas, thoughts, emotions and hang-ups generated during one Creative Conflict session are such rich food for meditation that they are equivalent in terms of personal growth to several years meditation practice on oneself. Spiritual students of a tradition cannot always believe this because they have a belief that a tradition has worked out all the angles to human conflict over a long period of time. They develop an ego investment in being a Buddhist, a Muslim, a Sufi, a Christian or belonging to a sect or personality cult of the gurus and founders. They spend years in meditation learning to control the ego, but this does not *get rid of* the ego. And consequently they can be disturbed by others of different persuasions or by personalities in their own spiritual communities, because the ego reacts.

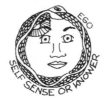

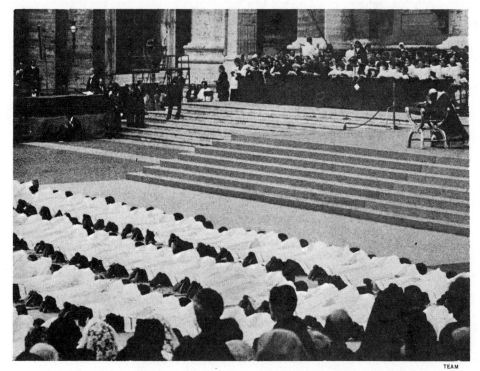

TEAM

New Priests lie prostrate before Pope Paul VI at massive holy year ordination in St. Peter's Square.

WHAT IS CREATIVE CONFLICT?

I evolved the technique of Creative Conflict in order to cut through the ego structures which block true meditation. And for this reason, I emphasize Creative Conflict more than meditation, not because I think less of meditation but because I feel there must be a preparing of the ground before proper meditation can begin to happen. What many people practice as meditation is not really meditation at all but just the ego aspiring to a state of mind which it cannot possibly reach in its present condition. Meditation should not be discontinued as a method of self-introspection but should be brought into the Creative Conflict process. The whole exercise of Creative Conflict is done with the same intensity and inner listening as one must have in meditation.

As a useful method of getting to the cause of people's conflicts, Creative Conflict does not have the disadvantages of the usual mudslinging group confrontations or the emotional binges of many encounter groups. Yet Creative Conflict enables an individual to express his deep feelings to others and far transcends the techniques of psychodrama and transpersonal systems of psychology for reaching in-depth change. In the "hot seat" (a technique for getting several views—like several TV cameras pointing on the same source, and meditating on them from different angles), we can get a better picture of how we are really manifesting as a human than by any attempt to arrive at a picture by our own internal methods alone. In fact, it is difficult for most people to see any value in these techniques of "mirroring" through the lenses of other people's consciousness, because, until they have actually tried the techniques, they are totally unaware of any need for them. Not until we become serious about improving communication do we begin to really notice our own communication gaps. Creative Conflict soon reveals our will to keep the peace at any price or shows the will to confront others with our feelings and estimate of reality. Much of the misery in human society and especially in marriage is due to our unwillingness to be real, either through fear of confronting that which we know to be true or false, lest we lose the ones we love, or through fear of expressing our deepest feelings because it makes us too vulnerable and because other people may take advantage of us in that state. Creative Conflict does away with all this by consciously building a trusting environment in which the worst can be said and faced, yet the love is maintained between the communicators without the entrenched and separative ego confrontations which normally divide a group. The practice of Creative Conflict can be extended from communication between couples to communication with groups of people and from groups of people to nations.

CAUSES OF CONFLICT

Wherever groups of people live together, their separate ego motives clash, and the frustration makes conflict inevitable. In *The Diary of Anne Frank*—the sensitive true account of several Jewish families hiding in a secret room in the midst of the Nazi takeover—the mini-war that raged within the house was as deep and insoluble as Hitler's war outside the walls. Simple inconsideration and selfishness among the family was magnified a thousandfold by the crowded living quarters, the tension, the personal discomfort, and the fear. But if we look deeper we find the same insensitivities and lack of awareness are part of every family.

The closer we live with one another, the more we get in touch with conflict. If we are children, the conflict is very likely to be repressed because we want the approval of our parents. In order to link the causes of conflict in the larger world scene with our day to day lives we have to look into personal examples with which everyone can identify. We can easily see ourselves or someone we know depicted in all the examples to follow, because the psychological patterns are very common and widespread. Most psychologists understand that world problems are just a reflection of individual problems, but few others really appreciate the link. Because they have not investigated their own inner psychology they are unable to see cause and effect operating either in their own lives or in the world. We spend billions of dollars and billions of hours tracing world conflict to sociological, economic and political roots. Not that these academic disciplines do not have some value, but they will never reach the causative factor until they come around to understanding the individual make-up of people and what people do with consciousness. It sounds simplistic to say that world problems and conflicts can even be affected much less solved by working on our own psychology, but it is far easier to make changes in the world than to make deep fundamental changes in the structure of our own ego. Could dictators so easily dominate thousands of people if those people had wrestled with their own weakness and their inability to stand up to bullies or to confront even the most ordinary injustices? The purpose of Creative Conflict is to build strength and independence. It is difficult to face truth in that way, but it builds a strong heart, because once you have gone through the experience of facing the worst in yourself, no one can ever again reduce you to guilt or feelings of rejection or throw you off center. Since we cannot magically eliminate conflict from the world, we can only begin with ourselves, taking responsibility for the causes of our own conflicts. If we see how others are successfully doing this then we can learn to do it too.

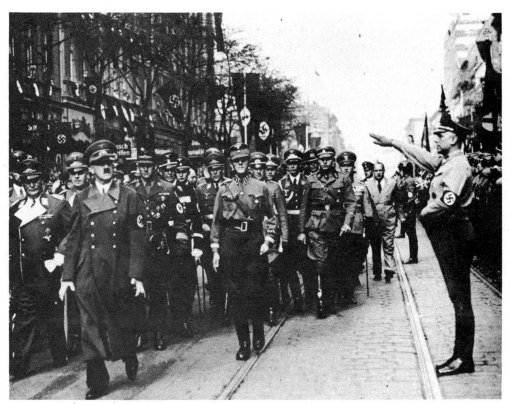

Hitler, 1938, reviewing his troops—the rise of a dictator.

Most individual conflict begins in childhood, as Freud rightly observed, and is an outgrowth of the different relationships within the family and within the ego structure of each child. Trying to express our real feelings as children and having them ignored by unreceptive parents is an almost universal experience that causes repercussions in later life, as in the case of Lance, a young man I was speaking with today:

> "My childhood was full of repressed conflict in my relationship with my mother. I've got a lot of stored-up resentment toward her because she would always know everything or, if not, would brush off her gaps with, 'Well, honey, when you get to be my age, you'll understand.' Even today, when I

ask her point-blank if we can ever get past the parent-child positions to honest relating she says, 'No, I don't want to do that.' In me this wall has created frustration because it allows no resolution of the tensions. Ultimately she feels she is the final arbiter. I can see this old frustration governing my relationships with others. I put them on pedestals and look up to them and when I disagree with them, I bottle up the internal reaction and treat myself to a big dose of frustration and disappointment."

Lance is one of my younger students who came to me in a quandary four years ago, when he was just finishing college. He was in the grip of a dominating young woman who controlled him by making him feel bad if he did not comply with her every wish. He was bottled up with frustration and confusion as she was insisting on getting married. He was weak and compliant, because she was playing on his inherent "Mother complex". I told him to be a man and break the relationship since he definitely did not want to marry. He must face this weakness and strengthen his ability to relate with women as an equal arbiter of reality, not as a child or a hen-pecked mouse. His reaction to my challenge to grow up and prove his manhood gave him the energy to break off the relationship, but he still has problems in this area with all women as he sees himself as the "nice guy". Gradually he is lessening his frustration to "mother's domination" which controls him and is now quite open about his feelings. This pattern may seem abnormal to someone who has not deeply examined his or her own feelings, but in fact all humans are controlled by similar deep psychological programs.

Many people who are not in touch with themselves think the people who *are* in touch are "screwed up". They judge those whose feelings are nearer the surface. Yet in their own hearts exists a blurred and vague uncertainty which they fear to probe. They are driven by urges which they do not deeply understand—compulsions to "make it", be accepted, get money, status, power, love, respect, fame, security or even to become enlightened. Anything that might threaten these attachments is rejected from their personalities, and other people who embody these rejected qualities are rejected too. We only have to view the disaffected elements of the counterculture to see that the more extreme compulsive types become revolutionaries and from there turn into terrorists killing innocent people by rejecting their right to life. But the same feeling of rejection and alienation operates not only on the social scene in politics but also at the level of every home and subtly in every relationship as we can see from one woman's account:

> "My mother is a tremendously sociable person. Her greatest fear is not to be accepted by her friends and the people of her town. She proudly says, 'I'm normal!' but at night her dreams say, 'Gosh, I hope I'm normal,' and she is unconsciously afraid she might not be. For the last twenty years she has rejected me in hundreds of little ways, trying to make me over and make me more like her. The more I followed my own development and became who I really am, the more abnormal I seemed to her. I was attached to her approval and it hurt me to be rejected even though I understood it. I was 40 years old before I grew strong enough in my own center to put a stop to my own hurt. Now I can see that she does love me and I understand that she feels an increasing inner conflict that she dare not resolve because I am the opposite of her self-image. Her stop-gap at the moment is to hunt for precedents in the past family members who were not quite normal and yet were good people."

This woman, Rachel, who came to our campus from a life cloistered in the ivory towers of the academic world, was sophisticated at the intellectual level but immature socially and emotionally. Unable to relate to anyone in any real depth, she was like a child in her experience of ordinary life—until she fell in love with someone very different from herself. Then all the need for approval came flying out from under wraps and she went through years of feeling rejected and hungry for attention from her lover. Her compulsion to take every statement personally and to reject any feedback was only an extended social manifestation of her family problem with her mother. After another two years she is beginning to take some feedback but is still ego-sensitive about the Creative Conflict process we practice here at University of the Trees. Hunger for acceptance and a desire to break out of her egocentric compulsive defensiveness cause her to keep up the work on herself and eventually she will see that the group, God, and life are not out to reject or to attack, not out to make her feel uncomfortable with herself, but are out to help her probe the depths of those very feelings of rejection which make her feel uncomfortable with her repressed conflicts. Some people get in touch with these buried patterns from childhood while other people insist that their childhood was perfect and can recall only the happy memories. One woman, whose mother was so domineering that she completely robbed her child of self-reliance, became so neurotic that she could not leave her house and was totally dependent on servants and workers. But if you asked about her childhood, she would say, "It was simply wonderful!" and go into an ecstatic description of wonderful days on the farm.

Most of us keep our hurts and needs unconscious, but we are driven by our compulsions and by a gnawing sense of lack, always hunting for happiness. In our Western civilization we acquire complex tastes that we cannot possibly satisfy by simple living. No doubt some primitive tribes expect little more than a marginal existence and therefore their drives are easily satisfied by less affluent conditions. But in civilizations that are already affluent, man experiences a perverse discontent which makes the thought of a utopian, conflict-free life seem impossible. The purpose of all spiritual discipline is to provide this divine contentment. Yet progress toward the religious goal of "heaven" and a frustration-free environment seems to be motivated by a divine *dis*content which produces a particular spiritual anxiety. Whether the search is inward to the bottomless depth of our being or outward to the furthermost reaches of space, the same relentless dissatisfaction frustrates mankind. Even in the peace of the woods our own self will follow, and even in our dreams we are haunted by the vague feeling that something is missing.

These frustrations become increasingly potent the closer we get to our real self, because the ego does not wish to die. Life's most powerful conflict comes when we are faced with a choice between selflessness and selfishness, between ourself and others, between doing pleasurable things and the things we know must be done. The individual need to be selfless is projected out into the community in social work and visiting of prisons. We find there is fulfillment in becoming a minister or a missionary in helping the weak or poor. We throw ourself into service often as compensation because we feel guilty for our basic selfishness and want to do something effective which will make ourself feel better. To help the sick solely out of compassion or to respond to a need may be our own need as much as the sufferer's. We may act for self-esteem or the pleasure of giving, and the act of helping the less fortunate could be more compulsion than compassion or could be a mixture of both. One thing is certain with saints—they do not prevent themselves from responding to need on the grounds that the sufferer might not be worthy, but they give the beggar the benefit of any doubt. However, when we respond to a phony beggar because he plays on our guilt and we give with resentment in our heart, it does not help the beggar and actually does harm to us. If we help society or become a giver with a coercive motive in order to be thought well of, or with an expectation of some good merit, our gift is made unwholesome and we become attached to the result. We can check to see how selfless our selflessness is by seeing whether our motive is to serve a need in the other or whether it is to gain something for ourself. Spiritual growth is found in watching our thoughts and our motives.

Our thoughts are continuously moving back and forth between conflicting goals, desires and duties, and the very fabric of our lives is made of conflicts between goals which cannot be achieved at the same time. Do I go and sit in the sun to enjoy myself or stay inside and do some hard study? Shall I marry this person and lose my future freedom? Shall I work for success at the office or go home to the family? Shall I leave my present job and risk failure at a new job or stick to the one I have, even though it bores me? Shall I become a spiritual renunciate or go out and experience life and romance and all the things that humans long for? Shall I go into the family business as my father wants me to or shall I strike out on my own? The list of conflicting goals is endless, and the conflicts generated between different parts of our natures can give us a gnawing insecurity about who we are and what we are here on earth to do. Once we realize the true purpose of selflessness we become motivated to relinquish our selfishness. We grapple with our selfish urges until the selfless self is stronger. In group life we can easily be made to feel selfish for advancing some personal desire that does not consider the whole. Once we become certain about our real purpose in life we no longer feel guilty for enjoying life, but until we have reached that point where we are willing to be totally selfless, we will continue to be caught up in the inner tensions and conflicts that have faced man from the beginning, when he first felt the pull of his own personal will against the good of the whole. In any group, even the nuclear family, we have some conflicts or mixed feelings about being an independent individual and being part of a group. We want the benefits of national security and state highway maintenance and national parks yet we don't like government interference in our private affairs or property rights. In America we have all these public amenities through taxation but we would never tolerate the infringement on our personal lives that happens in totalitarian countries. The sense of infringement can be even more pronounced in the selfless group. Such a group has a goal with desirable aspects that make us want to strive for its achievement but it also has seemingly undesirable aspects such as selfless work and no time of one's own and a tacit expectation that you will fill whatever need arises in the group, though it may cost you your personal money or perhaps your afternoon off or you may have to attend a group meeting and stay into the small hours of the morning when you are tired and you want to go to bed. Situations continually arise to test your ability to stretch yourself and your willingness to give up normal human pleasures and indulgences for something more important. Your only income may be the psychic income of inner fulfillment. If you are attached to financial income, your conflict on this point will be considerable. Many people who have spiritual aspirations want to become a higher being full of love for fellowman and to follow the great spiritual teachers, but at the same time they don't really want to spend hours, days and years of time doing boring community tasks. However, if we leave the tasks for others to do we cannot maintain our self-image as a selfless worker for God. We are torn between two goals until we either selfishly leave the community to carry the load or give up part of our ego that is resisting and insisting on its private aspirations. These frustrations and conflicts bring unpleasant thoughts and emotions and sometimes a great deal of pain. The way we try to escape or resolve or relieve this frustration will reveal our personality expression and determine its way of fulfillment. Conflict cannot be resolved by trying to forget it nor by kicking at one's situation with anger and resistance, anxiety and guilt, expectation and rigidity, but only by watching all these feelings which cause us to be disturbed in our consciousness. If we can be centered enough to watch (rather than identify with) the feelings, we can freely make decisions that will make our chores fulfilling and at the same time gain self-mastery over our own minds so that no situation in life can disturb us or cause us this kind of conflict again. Resolving this conflict calls for the true meditation in action rather than sitting still. Meditation for self eventually leads to selfless action for all.

One man at the University of the Trees confessed how difficult the challenge is for him:

"For me, I find that selfless work is practically impossible because of my dependency on something external to give me something first, either in direction, recognition, money, inspiration or motivation. It is easy to do a job if you've got a nice paycheck coming or someone tells you just what to do or says, 'You're so smart; we like you; you're a real asset here.' But in a selfless community, no one is doing that. Everyone is working for no pay except the love in their hearts. No one is expecting any recognition and they are the only ones to say whether the job was well done or not because it is their own fulfillment that is the gauge. With me, I don't work if there is just me in charge of myself. I just spin. No one is saying yes or no, do this or that, right on or way off. If I start something and someone says 'Great' I feel good and go to town on it. But if they frown I scrap the whole thing."

The man who said this is a perfect archetype of Saint Peter who would chop off a man's ear to protect the loved one or literally have himself crucified upside down. He would be capable of the same remorse at having misunderstood his mentor as when Peter denied Christ three times in spite of the prediction that it would happen. Passionate in everything, he has no discrimination. He reacts impulsively to every request for his services because he has a compulsive need to serve and this is offset by another need to shine and be a person of some consequence. As a result he is beset with internal conflict between selfless service and recognition on the one hand and on the other hand his duty to his wife and family which he tends to neglect as there is nothing special in this. Like many well-known figures, the wider appeal of the great and nobler cause of world service of humanity makes him forget that his family is also humanity. The call of the larger social framework transcends for him the petty demands of family since he can see no personal fulfillment solely in that activity. His wife would like him to earn a little extra money so they can have even a few carpets and a stereo and perhaps a holiday. But his heart is not in making money.

Most people are so busy earning some money that they do not get a chance to stop and get to know their own psychological make-up nor to alter the ratio of selfishness/unselfishness. Most people are not in touch with their selfishness, so their conflicts simmer under the surface, but they are expressed in their drives. If our goal is a physical one then the solution to our conflict is fairly simple. Like the primitive hunter looking for food, we start training to become captain of the football team or be a pop star or whatever it is we want. Some people experience conflict and frustration if, for example, they want to be a great tennis player but have a body which is not particularly athletic. If the goal is not a physical one but is a desire for fame or to become president, then our inner frustration can be enormous because only one person can be president at one time. Those who think a president somewhat low down on the scale compared to a Jesus Christ may feel even more frustration because for the role of messiah, there can be only one historical Jesus Christ in the world. Hence the egoistic self-centered drive, when confronted by impossible obstacles, drives its frustrations inward into messiah-like actions and, like Hitler, projects them onto the world scene. Only the egoless, reaching towards the initiation of the real Christ state of unitive consciousness, can syphon away the frustrations of our civilization. When a person whose drive is to be a leader, manager, organizer, boss, Mr. Somebody, Mr. Important finds his way into the spiritual trip, where the goal is to become nobody and nothing, the conflict deep inside him causes conflict with everyone else. All of us want to be creative and original, and some have deep cravings to be extra special. But in order for conflict to be creative we must become aware that all conflict is relative to our own psychological state. The delusion that the cause of our conflict is another person or situation "out there" makes our conflicts increasingly destructive and unresolvable.

We all tend to see the world around us as we see it in our relationships with those who are close to us. There are those who are most fanatical in that they will do anything for the cause or lay their head on the block for the recognition of the loved one. Such people in life usually are exploited by those who know how to manipulate them. Yet the following example shows a man who has this kind of devotion yet is himself a first class manipulator with all those manipulating qualities and potentialities he sees as controlling his own life. The transfer of these personal traits into his understanding of the way the phony world works is remarkable and he is able to smell the slightest phony a mile away. He is quite out of touch with his frustrated unconscious as we can see by the way his girlfriend describes their situation:

> "Ed, my boyfriend, feels I do not listen to him and he gets so frustrated when he can't communicate with me that he is enraged. Our conflicts are so violent that I have finally decided to end the relationship. Already he is finding the same difficulty in communicating with other people. When they complain about his anger he says that his frustrations with me are making him irritable. But in time he will have to get in touch with the source of frustration in himself that leads him to conflict with everyone he loves. I may be the cause of his anger, but his response and his sense of frustration are his own."

Ed was born poor, feels inferior, and compensates by trying to be at the top of every heap. People complain that he is manipulative, pushy and bossy so he suppresses the compulsion, yet inside he is frustrated.

At times he tries to be a leader vicariously through others, but feels that they are not doing it as well as he could do if only he had the chance. Ed feels like a race horse tied to a post. If he will not let go of the ego *behind* the driving need to compensate, he will only suppress the drive in mounting frustration and inner tension. This type of compulsive drive to excel usually ends in some debilitating disease or a nervous breakdown. Heart attacks and cancer often create setbacks that give us the opportunity to look deeply into ourselves. But how many people know where to look? In more extreme cases, this kind of frustration leads to vandalism, feelings of external conquest, or violence which creates tensions all around. This aggregate sum of tension of all individuals in a society is the cause of war, ranging from the struggles of children over toys to conflict between adolescent street gangs to the warring of nations.

As we grow up and learn to repress our hostility and feelings of inferiority, we project these feelings out into society upon certain leaders, scapegoats and other social characters. Our escape mechanism is to compensate for our own feelings of impotence and inferiority by projecting fantasies of superiority onto film stars, presidents, cult leaders, etc. Not only our conflicts with others but even our inner tensions often stem from the way we compare ourselves with other people. You may be quite happy with your present salary until another gets a raise in pay. You are content to own only one car until the neighbor gets a new second car. When we see someone else advancing perhaps with less effort than ourself we become discontented and inner conflict is created. Unless we can see clearly the cause, the conflict will not create growth but will set off a chain reaction of insecure thoughts and feelings.

THE GROUP MIRROR

In order to accept that other people can act as mirrors of our own conflict, we must, at least for a little while, assume that in reality there *are* no "others". At first this is difficult because "others" are regarded as the real source of our problems. We feel the situation would be different if it were not for the actions of other people. All this may be true, but to understand how the "others" do what they do to be so different, or to be so screwed up, we must be able to think like them, get inside them and see them from inside out. Only when we regard them as an aspect of ourselves can we do this accurately. This is Christ's real message in loving others, not to agree with them or to identify with them in any wrongheaded views of life, but to be able to see through their eyes the twisted vision of the world and thus to understand them. But to do this, we have to be able to let go of whatever pain they may be causing *us* and to selflessly get inside them and care about what is causing *them* pain. In yoga and spiritual practice one of the first disciplines is to be content with what we have and to accept gracefully what life gives to us without complaint. This attitude is to enable us to see calmly what is in our own nature and in the true nature of others, i.e., to be in truth. If, for example, someone confronts us, we feel pain, and the normal human response is to react and defend. But if instead we set that ego response aside, we are able to feel why they are disturbed from their viewpoint and receive the feedback to see if it is true. Then if it *is* true, we can accept it. This is not a matter of suppressing envy when it arises or pretending that pain is not painful. It involves a radical shift in point-of-view that is possible only with surrender of the ego. The Bhagavad-Gita describes such a person thus:

"The seers say truly
That he is wise
Who acts without lust or scheming
For the fruit of the act. . .
He needs nothing:
The Atman is enough."
(Atman: Complete unlimited Self)

The secret of this way of life is to realize we never need any more than enough and that all greed and exploitation spring from insecurity of self and its mistrust of life. The yogi knows that his needs will be met because he is one with the universe, whereas the separative ego has cut itself off and must scramble to meet its own needs in a hostile world. Its view of human evolution is the survival of the fittest. The contentment of the yogi is not built upon wishful thinking nor upon naive and superstitious faith but on truth. He tests out his supposition by direct experience in his own life and finds that it is sound. If life sends him pain, he accepts pain as well as good fortune as feedback, because pain or joy means that the mirror of life is reflecting something in him back to himself. To blame another for pain would cheat the yogi of the lesson and the opportunity to work on himself. Once he changes his attitude, then suddenly the mirror changes and life once again begins to nurture him and to further all that he attempts.

Creative Conflict is this kind of creative self-investigation where people come together in a group purposefully to share, explore and mirror each other's conflicts to reach a greater truth. Naturally it works best in a group of people who are all committed to the same basic tenet of dissolving the ego into a more expanded awareness. The first rule is that we must agree to disagree, so that no hard-and-fast ego position can entrench the mind-sets of our own deep-rooted conflicts. In order to see something new in a conflict situation, we must be able to temporarily look from someone else's point of view, even though it may be totally opposite to our own, and even though it may be very painful. We have the certainty that in the end we will feel better about ourself, not worse. It is the same with God. We do not resign ourself to His Will, but it becomes our Joy to serve It. At first it may feel like an abject resignation, a fatalism, a surrender against our own willfulness. These unpleasant feelings about ourself may originate from several distinct sources, so we need to learn to discriminate them, which brings us back again to probing the different causes of conflict.

EXTERNAL CONFLICT

Many people worry about why the world is the way it is. They cannot believe that the natural order left to itself will bring about good government and feel it will only produce the laws of the jungle or let the garden grow back into weeds. Yet whenever mankind works together in harmony with the external forces of Nature we feel at peace. In the human world, conflict seems to be never-ending, and natural law is often ignored. Many conflicts which stem from the hostile actions of others can be regarded as external causes which produce great internal conflict within us. But if we trace the cause back to ourselves, we can usually see how even the attack of another person is brought about by some situation we have created subliminally in our own individual or collective consciousness.

An example from a typical romantic conflict will show you what I mean:

> "My boyfriend invited me to breakfast and I thought we were having an intelligent conversation, but suddenly he was angry at me. His face got all red and his eyes bugged out and when I tried to reply, he shouted at me even louder than before. I threw my fork into my plate and walked out. I thought that even if I *had* said something wrong, that was no way to behave to me. I felt he was a hopeless case. Only later did I realize that I had gone to his house full of negative thoughts and suppressed anger myself and had made a mental note to be careful or there might be a fight. When he flared up at me he only mirrored what was raging silently inside my own feelings but could not find a creative constructive way to express. He had caught something in my attitude, and my 'vibes' had said more than my words. But I only gave him credit for knowing my words because I did not know the strength of my own vibes myself."

Both these people may be perceiving blocks to communication in each other accurately. They quarrel a lot, but most times neither is able to own responsibility for their reactions and each believes that "the other" is the cause of their pain. They are not in touch with their internal conflicts. How many times we can see similar situations in the world scene between countries whose words say one thing and whose "vibes" say another!

In the communication between nations there is always a certain outline set out in obvious international frameworks. But many important explanations are often unspoken or left out and these always lead to later misunderstanding. It is incredible how clarity is sacrificed for rhetoric at the political and international level because government leaders do not know themselves any better than those they govern. The same identical blocks in communication are found between lovers, between children and parents, and even between religious people. It would seem that until human communication gets better at every level and enables us to penetrate each other's inner worlds with understand-

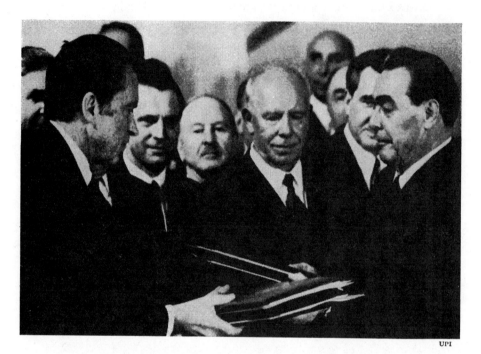

UPI

Nixon and Brezhnev exchange copies of arms pact: Freezing the terror.

ing, the attitudes we hold are what really end up dominating our
communication rather than the words we use. These attitudes speak so
loudly that we literally cannot work things out either at the political
level between nations or at the social level between people, until the
attitudes change.

INTERNAL CONFLICT

These are conflicts which arise solely within ourselves due to false
perceptions of situations or false reading of others' motives. They often
arise from basic assumptions we hold which we have subjectively
identified as reality. When we do not question our assumptions we
become incapable of listening. We hear but we do not listen, we look
but we do not really see, as in the following common situation related

to me by a student:

> "I had a friend who imagined all kinds of judgements being
> made upon herself (her house furnishings, her dinner menus,
> her work output) and was certain that her friends were
> thinking negative things about her; she could read it in their
> eyes and in little gestures. But when she told me her
> feelings, I saw that the judgements reflected her *own* values
> and were totally out of character for the people she was
> projecting them on. She put herself through constant pain
> with these 'perceptions' and seldom had the courage to be
> open and ask her friends if they were actually having those
> thoughts or not."

Most of us have no way of checking out our perceptions because we
are afraid that our friends will judge our innermost thoughts. We have
this fear because we know that we ourselves judge others. When
someone's actions clash with our internal standards of ethics, honor or
propriety which we have acquired from parents, society, heroes, etc.,
we make judgements. Of course, we are more lenient in evaluating our
own actions. At the conscious level we may be rationalizing, "It is all
right that I did this or said that because I didn't know any better," or
"he deserved it; I was right," but at a deeper level, we feel the pain of
internal confict wrenching us in two. When a motive urges us towards
committing some act that is incompatible with our own standards, we
begin to feel anxiety because we feel we are not doing what we ought
to do. We set up a conflict between *oughtness* and *isness* and feel
guilty for feeling the way we are feeling. Here is an example from
Grace, another University of the Trees member, of what most people
experience in one degree or another.

> "All of my relationships are affected by a strong compul-
> sion to do the right thing. People tease me about being 'a
> good little girl.' My center is always outside me, always
> worried about what others will think of me. Even the
> smallest decisions are hard for me to make without asking
> someone's opinion. I guess it goes back to the condemna-
> tion I felt in my family atmosphere as a child if one didn't

measure up to the unspoken family ethics. Many times we
kids didn't find out what they were until we'd broken them.
Then we knew by hindsight because the feedback was
heavy when a 'taboo' was broken."

REPRESSED CONFLICTS

Children are often motivated by hostility toward their parents to
strike out in some independent way to free themselves from domination.
But these feelings conflict with equally strong desires to be an obedient
child and to respect the parents' standards of behavior. Since the
parent is also the source of food and survival, as well as approval, the
conflict in children can be tremendous. One adolescent boy I knew
moved out of a broken home as soon as he had saved up enough
money to manage it, but he was never able to confront the parent who
had dominated him. As a result he has asthma, which is directly
related to "smother love" in early childhood. Yet even when advised
(at age thirty-nine) to confront his parent for his own health's sake, he
would not. He preferred to keep the conflict. With it he kept the
resentment, and the quiet anger simmered inside. Another woman,
Gail, age thirty, who had a similar problem with asthma took my
suggestion and confronted her parents. The result was the best sharing
they ever have had and a deepening of the relationship. It was both a
release and an awakener for Gail who had feared the consequences of
sharing her feelings for years, and the asthma lessened considerably.

Conflict and hostilities, repressed during childhood, in adolescence
and through the early stages of adult life, are projected out into society
and transferred to other authorities—to a leader, policeman, boss or
teacher—by identification. These subtle feelings cause us considerable
anxiety over our own self-image in society and we fear what would
happen if we spoke out against these authorities so we quietly let them
rule us. But usually the anger remains repressed and unspoken against
these parents, authorities, police, teachers, ministers, taxgatherers, and
bureaucrats who try to discipline us for the good of society. The most
extreme examples of this repression of feelings in the face of an
authority can be seen in the religious cult groups that require their
members to give up their inner authority to the group leader who sets

all the policies. We quickly become enraged at the gullible who follow a leader who brainwashes them into giving him all their possessions, decides whom they will marry, what they will say, and demands all their income. The recent scandal at Jonestown, Guyana revealed cultism in its extreme, where 900 people were either murdered or brainwashed into committing suicide. We cannot afford to only point the finger at Jonestown without looking at our own willingness to be dominated by authorities that we have set up to rule us. We let society be our authority until the pressure of repressed conflicts mounts up and we rebel.

Sexual promiscuity, the feminist movement and gay liberation all arose in revolt against the unquestioned authority of old definitions of morality. They erupted with the force of years and years of repressed anger at society's repressions and unfair treatment of people whose inner being did not quite fit the mold of normalcy. Some women felt limited by the standard concepts of the submissive and dependent female when they felt they could lead in the business and political worlds. And in the same way, the masculine standard of aggressive manly behavior was an unnatural restriction on men who were more in touch with the submissive and feeling side of their nature. Ideally, when both sexes have the male-female energies in balance within themselves, inner conflict about male-female roles disappears. But neither the gay revolution nor feminism has any intention of balancing positive/negative energies or actually resolving inner and outer conflicts. Both movements are charged with the energy of hurt and bitterness from the past so that what formerly was repressed and unmentionable has now developed into an over-statement of the new roles.

Even though society is more permissive now towards sexual expression, both children and adults are still subject to hidden taboos or overt pornography expressed in books, pictures and movies. In ignorance, people still repress their natural sexual energy and do not see that the spirit in which one makes love is what makes sex "bad" or "good". A person who has worked to refine his consciousness is able to experience sex as an act of worship. The same criterion holds in the age-old conflict that still arises when one partner desires a sexual relationship with more than one person, while the other partner clings to firmly

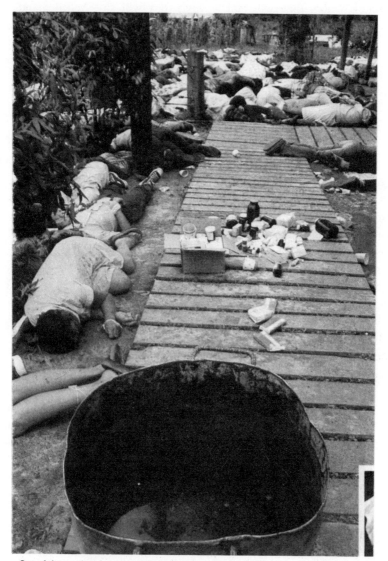

One of the results of people allowing themselves to be dominated—mass murder and suicide of Americans at Jonestown, Guyana.

entrenched concepts of fidelity. Though there may be nothing wrong in having a broader range of people to whom one can express love, one has to ask oneself, "If I do this at the expense of someone's happiness, what will it do to my own conscience? And do I really want it enough to darken my consciousness in that way?" Another form of conflict which darkens the light of consciousness comes when sexual desire cannot be satisfied without a feeling of guilt from religious teachings. Many religions teach continence and even complete abstinence and never mention the fact that God Himself created sex, not only in us and in plants and in animals, but even in the atoms, whose positive/negative attraction is part of the dance of life.

People who have anger or hostility or sexual conflicts may repress them so successfully that they may not even be aware of any anger or sexual feelings at all. They become cut off from their emotions whenever conflict is generated. They may begin by covering or diluting the truth deliberately but later on they may actually believe this half-truth or lie because they are no longer even aware of their real feelings. This is especially true in power politics. A rising politician is daily confronted by compromise with Truth. Otherwise, he says, no decisions could be made. This making of deals with each other leads to repression of hostility and the skillful hiding of undertones and anger, and thence it is only a short step to mendacity and deception. Politicians begin acting only to keep up appearances while comments of real feelings are repressed. Then when a situation arises in which they can afford to feel and express anger (at foreign countries, outsiders, opponents or scapegoats), the repressed anger comes pouring out in one great stream of hostility.

AGGRESSIVE CONFLICT

When frustration mounts beyond the threshold of tolerance all organisms in Nature, including mankind, fight back. Even the lowly worm will turn and try to bite its attacker if we tread on it. All organisms attack the obstacle to their security whether it is physical or only imaginary. Humans attack a physical barrier or an idea or a person symbolizing that idea (like some political effigy) or even attack society as a whole. Even the smallest animals will struggle or claw through their cage with frustration, and a child or man will attack the object of frustration with anger and fists. Displaced aggression aroused by a source of conflict which cannot be attacked directly is usually taken out on a scapegoat, sometimes even on an innocent bystander. Hijackers hold innocent people to ransom or use them as pawns in political issues. A man who is frustrated at work by the demanding authority of his boss may go home and use his own wife as a scapegoat for anger. Scapegoating is a typical way of taking out anger on minority individuals, groups or nations, like the scapegoating of President Richard Nixon for America's feelings of guilt and frustration or like Hitler's ingenious shifting of the blame for all the problems of post-war Germany onto the Jews.

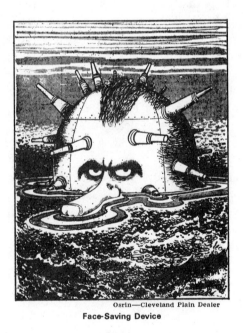

Osrin—Cleveland Plain Dealer
Face-Saving Device

Why are we discussing all these causes of conflict? Because the person in conflict who has projected his feelings out onto society after having repressed them is a person in trouble. Without our understanding of the aggregate tensions built up by many people in society, we cannot hope to bring peace or lessen tensions in the world. First we must resolve conflict within people, then the international conflicts will disappear. What makes people aggressive? An aggressive anger is only one of many possible reactions to inner conflict. Very often it is the need for communication. To a physical type person a punch in the nose is simple direct communication. He may have a lot to say but words fail him. In total frustration he lashes out in anger or violence. He gets frustrated with words which never seem to accomplish anything and, instead of talking, takes aggressive action. If he feels inferior, his aggression may be an attempt to lift himself up by knocking another down. Inside himself or herself, every bully is a coward. Some men confuse this misuse of power with masculinity or strength, whereas really it is just the opposite. One way or another, most aggression is a defense mechanism of the ego. The instant that feelings are hurt, the passive receptivity to that pain changes over to active aggressive survival tactics. Even people not normally reactive will react to anger from another.

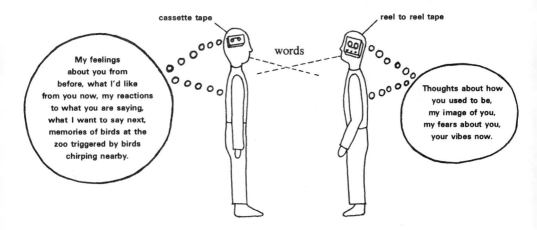

A different sort of defense mechanism is at work when, in order to keep from seeing our own half of a problem, we blame others and attack them for their part in it. Sometimes our expectations are disappointed and our needs not met and we lash out at our loved one, not realizing that we had no right to impose our expectations on another human being in the first place. Sometimes we blame them for being insensitive to our feelings but we ourselves are equally unable to see two points of view. In the end all aggression is rooted in the ego. A person who has not worked on his ego indulges in self-righteous anger, blind to his own lacks and hard on everyone else's.

A true yogi, who is master of his ego, has only righteous anger. He does not defend his ego because he has nothing to defend or to gain. His anger is solely for the benefit of the other person and vanishes just as soon as the person really hears the communication. A master of consciousness knows when to use anger for his communication or when some gentler approach will work better, because he has no ego investment in either method. He doesn't get off on his anger, and his patience is abundant. Frustration and impatience, leading to anger and conflict, are the mark of one who has a personal investment in another person's change. This is the essence of the yogic teaching of detachment as the means to peace. Normally, when we desperately want our relationship with loved ones to be a certain way, we have no patience with the slowness of their growth process. Because a yogi is detached, he can let another person be whatever he or she is. He can afford to be compassionate. He can afford to let others remain in ignorance if they do not wish to know his truth. Such a person believes in the saying *verbum sap satis est* ("one word to the wise is sufficient") because he knows that those who want to change or want to learn will take a hint whereas a fool will not accept a bookful of words. However if we care and love someone, the wise will persevere out of compassion even with a fool, because they see the reason for the foolishness and do not resent a fool but see him as an aspect of themselves.

APATHETIC REACTIONS TO CONFLICT

The opposite extreme of aggressive attacks upon others is to give up completely on a relationship or a communication in a feeling of depression, to abandon hope by turning the anger inward against the self. The world is filled with depressed people. A depressed person is one who has made himself his own scapegoat and looks upon himself as unlovable and stupid. We can take an in-depth look at a typical depressed person to see why apathy rules the psyche of most of the world.

Walter came to me three years ago hiding behind a bushy beard with hair over his eyes through which he peered out at me. He seemed a very nice person but was hiding something under all that hair. Whatever it was, he thought it was bad enough that he could not afford to be open about it. His body movements when he walked or talked were stiff and constrained. It seemed that he did not trust himself to be spontaneous but controlled every move he made and every word he spoke. He was a computer engineer with a good job but he had just finished living with a lady and was at a crossroads in his life. What drew him here was the bond of love that he sensed among the group.

I pointed out that becoming a student of mine was no escape from reality and that I was a hard taskmaster and demanded the capacity for constant change from students. He readily agreed to it. In the Creative Conflict sessions over the years Walter has been compliant and shown overt willingness to listen. He makes strong affirmations that he is going to change. As he is very hard on himself anyway, it is easy for him to believe he has faults and to want to change them. But every ego has its cut-off point where the willingness stops and resistance begins. Though Walter has grown steadily more confident and open since he came here, he has also grown more stubborn at taking feedback the deeper it penetrates to his basic ego. He lashes himself inwardly for not changing but on the inside of his being, in his heart, he resists even a simple suggestion that he log his time in a notebook as a step toward better organization. Walter is a poor organizer and a poor communicator. His work involves managing the construction of ion generators and he worries about everything at once rather than taking action on one thing at a time. He does not listen to himself enough to know when he is saying enough to get across his point and he will not listen to others' suggestions, always feeling he knows best. Like some others on campus, Walter expects everyone to know what is going on inside his thoughts telepathically and to see why he is forever changing his mind. He makes countless errors, which makes work for others, so people constantly get frustrated with him as a result.

All the people at University of the Trees meditate and practice spiritual disciplines, but these do not always enable people to be released from long-term and deep ego patterns. Walter is a very sweet and pleasant person to have around because he turns all his bottled up negative anger upon his own self and seldom confronts any person who has made him angry. If our community were like many spiritual communities, Walter would fit in nicely because all that is needed is to be loving and nice. But here we are engaged in the yoga of action and we use our work, running several businesses, as a way to become aware of what our gaps in awareness are. So Walter, who in the outside world is a normal nine-to-five computer expert, has failed so thoroughly in the ion generator department that his faults now stand in bold relief for him to see. His bottled up anger and internal conflict are so great that they often nullify his natural intelligence. And the need to control his every move and to think out every action blocks him from acting. Everything seems so complex to him that nothing can be done about it. He thinks he is seeing his situation clearly but his internal computer is programmed with too little data. Three hundred sixty degree awareness cannot be programmed; it has to be allowed to happen, just like spontaneity cannot be rehearsed but must be given freedom to create itself. Walter can make himself miserable over the smallest task which seems to have mountainous obstacles. He talks and thinks like politicians in Washington, continuously explaining all the great difficulties in the way. From their plush expensive congressional offices ($1,000 million a year for congressional services), politicians explain why they can't do anything about the social system. Walter is a perfect model of the inert culture and its educational system, but he has now placed himself within a new community which is committed to permanent evolution and change. Instead of taking honest feedback from the committed group bit by bit, accepting it and working on it stage by stage so as to change his existing pattern, he waits until all the feedback mounts up and comes down on his head in one huge avalanche and then flounders in the debris. His imagination makes it into a mountainous heap when actually, if he would strike at its deepest root, it is not a big change at all. He uses confusion and self-recrimination to produce a feeling of total worthlessness and hopelessness because in that state he won't have to change. But the price he pays is to turn black anger against himself producing a dangerous state of dis-ease that could lead eventually to a mental breakdown.

The analogy with society as a whole is clear. We have convinced ourselves that there is no way to fix society, that there is no giant being who can straddle the whole situation and knock all the heads together and get things in shape and that there is no way to remove our feelings of impotence. We therefore blame the government or we scapegoat the President or pin the reason for our failure on foreigners—the Japanese, the Germans, the Arabs, the Jews—or on the financial houses. The same is true of racial excuses for our own apathy and confusion. Instead of beginning the new type of self-rule community without government help or sponsorship, the blacks can blame the whites as the cause of hopelessness and impotence or the whites can blame the politicians and the economy for their inability to bring utopia into being. This way all can feel justified in waiting for salvation to fall out of heaven—the millennia complex. And so too with Walter. He blames a part of himself that he does not really own and does not really think of as "me", so he gets depressed about his state yet does not really feel that he has the power to change it nor admit to himself that he is responsible for it. This ego mechanism happens at the unconscious level but could be changed in an instant with one heartfelt conscious decision. In Walter's own words:

> "I feel resistance, stubbornness, entrenchment and at the same time I feel I *am* going to change it. I'm going to do it! I feel frustration at not seeing what's happening. Most of all it's the people—their reactions to me here in the group. The mirror that I get makes me feel very sick with myself. When I'm in that space I can't see any other space to get to. Now I'm in a good space and I don't know what triggered it, what makes my energy outgoing at one time and indrawn the other time.
>
> I feel extremely grateful to the people here. I feel overwhelmed with the patience of Christopher and everyone in putting up with my bullshit. I don't think I could get to the other side of this ego without the group mirror. But there's another feeling that I don't want to identify with, don't want to own. It's like something locked in loggerheads—at war. By not facing it I know I'm giving it energy. I feel like I don't

want to listen to anyone, like I'm righteous, like I'm just, my perceptions are valid no matter what you say. I am something. I can make sharp discriminations between things that other people can't. I feel it gives me a sense of energy and confirmation to hold onto these feelings in myself even if life says that isn't what's really manifesting. Without that sense of me-ness, being here, valid, meaningful, I can't imagine what it would be like to be without it.

So I'm seeing I have to say I don't know. And when people point things out I have to stop my mind from saying I know better. This ego of mine could go on and on forever except that I want the heart relating. I want a new mirror. I guess it's just not painful enough yet to change."

Walter feels that his essence is okay. And it *is* okay. In all of us the soul is pure and whole, complete within itself. But until we are able to surrender what we think is our essence to the One, we will never release our ego so that the soul force can come through us. Walter thinks his ego is his essence. He feels, "Hey that's me," while life mirrors only pain and frustration. So Walter gets depressed with himself. He cannot hear the cosmic message telling him of the work he needs to do because in his stubbornness he cannot accept surrendering to his unknown Self, beyond the ego where the love he craves for is waiting. This fear of the unknown Self is, for most of society, the great deterrent to receiving the cosmic evolutionary message.

The deep ego pattern now exposed in Walter would never have been unveiled or challenged except in an intensive community such as we have here. It could have simmered unnoticed for the rest of his incarnation or developed into cancer or been revealed temporarily in someone's frustration with him. The catch to it all is that Walter is *quite a normal person* in the ordinary world. He can do well at his computer engineering job, is likeable, idealistic, and a very good kind person. To most readers who have not gone as deep into their own inner selves it will be hard to accept that this kind of inner turmoil is indeed the norm—or is *themselves.* Even to the most spiritually-minded people reading this book, those who feel they are progressing well along their chosen spiritual path, this inner ego battle is normal. Whether they are conscious of it and humbly working on it the best way they know how, or acting as a "Holy Joe" and not in touch with it, it is there, their inheritance from their culture, simmering under the surface of all their sincere spiritual endeavors. It is hard to face the fact of the ego and all its inner ways and to reconcile them with our self-image, but acknowledging and dealing with ego is the quickest way to its release and our permanent enlightenment.

Socially, our defense against acknowledging our inability to see that ego is at the root of society's problems is apathy—the fear that it will bog us down. We don't quite know how to handle it, so we don't look at it. Most of us trust apathetically in a welfare state rather than trusting in ourselves, in our own productivity, our own self-rule, our own created vision of the community of the future. Instead, we accept the cultural brainwash of hundreds of gurus, preachers, evangelists, futurists and political observers who do not know what is going to happen anymore than the man on the street. In short, we abdicate our responsibility to the inner voice inside us and reject the responsibility for the disturbances in our own consciousness. It is not easy to face ourselves, but it is the most important and rewarding task we can do. This is the real meaning written over the temple door of the Greek sanctuary at Delphi—"MAN KNOW THYSELF".

THE WORK ON THE EGO

The process of facing ourselves as we really are is the work on the ego. When you work on your ego you get to the depth of your being. Usually when a person is in pain or is feeling badly about some part of himself, he is afraid to look deeply and afraid of truth for fear he will feel even worse about himself, but in truth the opposite happens. The way to work on the ego is to take any pain from some negative feeling about yourself or from your situation—perhaps someone you love does not love you back as you would like, or you are getting criticized for botching something up, or all your relationships seem to be lacking something, or whatever kind of problem you are having—and find someone you can trust to share it with. If you cannot find anyone, talk to your own soul about your problem. Whether you share with a person or with your soul, *listen* to the response. Write it down if it is coming from your soul, or mirror it back to the person you are sharing with by repeating what you feel has been said to you, but in your own words, until the other person feels you have really heard accurately both the words and the spirit of what was said. More than anything else in the work on the ego, we need to learn how to listen to other people's feedback in order to get beyond our own limiting perceptions. This doesn't mean the other person is always going to be correct in the feedback, but any feedback at all that you truly take in will expand you to include another's viewpoint in depth. At that depth you have choices to make. Either you will try to find justifications for why you are the way you are, or you will become receptive to a larger message about yourself and what you need to do in order to grow. If you choose the route of justification, the mind will begin to spin with its own rationalizations, and your problems will not be resolved. If you make the more difficult choice of listening to the feedback about yourself, then you will be faced with changing. In a Creative Conflict session, real listening brings insight, fulfillment and a deep feeling of your own soul which gives you the energy to make the change. You know intuitively that the feedback is right and you can then readjust your tuning to the Evolutionary Intelligence.

If we turn our back on truth, or accept a rationalization from our own ego, then we can never experience that feeling of being in tune and centered in our soul. You can know that you are progressing on your work on the ego if the world mirrors back to you increasing beauty and love and if you feel like you are growing through your challenges.

Most people are attracted to those who work on the ego because they sense a quality of being that is rare, an openness and understanding that becomes magnetic. Working on the ego is only a painful experience if there is a block in the way. The block may be stubbornness, fear of the unknown, fear of rejection, pride or fear of losing a self-image that you have invested years in building. All these blocks, fears, self-doubts, pains, are the substance of the ego. Most people rationalize, "I am getting along fine the way I am," but are they really growing? Are they being honest with themselves? Others say, "Yes I would like to work on my ego but I am afraid I will come apart, so I am better off continuing on the way I have been since it's safe." But is it safe? Or is it running away from the ultimate confrontation which is somewhere down the road? All these reactions against facing ourself are ego. Fears, angers, jealousies, negativities—whatever disturbs us which we repress—is what gives us pain and brings us down. Why has it been so difficult for humanity to look at this cosmic law and to confront their egos as the great prophets have pleaded with us to do for thousands of years?

The disease of self-generated conflict which permeates humanity can only be cured by each one of us accepting responsibility for our own situation. The real problem throughout the ages is that in our ignorance we feel we don't know how and that we are the last person who is qualified to carry out the needed treatment on the ego, since no surgeon wants to operate on his own heart. We want someone to come and do it for us. If we weren't so strongly identified with our own egos the idea wouldn't seem so frightening. Often we end up working on small faults and avoiding the fundamental ego patterns that are blocking us from our true being. It seems okay to us because that's all our parents ever did, or that's all our friends are doing. But again we must consider the consequences. People get together in groups, in businesses, or they get married. They all have strong points, but their one real weak point may bring their whole endeavor to nought in the long run.

Because this work on themselves is so threatening, most people cannot do it alone without some spiritual discipline or support of a group doing the same thing. Therefore it is essential that we get involved in some kind of evolutionary discipline or evolutionary group. No one else but us can make faith and conviction come alive inside of us to heal the social sickness. We are reluctant to accept that we *are* the disease in society, especially if we feel that others caused it and we are stubbornly convinced that the cure is going to come from somewhere else rather than from ourself. When our expectations are not met we become angry and violent or feel guilty—anything to keep our ego intact. Sometimes when one is rejected as a mate or partner or when one loses a loved one's affection through death, a sense of guilt provides a defense against dealing with the feeling of rejection. We lay on ourself a guilty feeling that we did not try hard enough, that our love was never sufficient when we were together and that somehow we lost an opportunity. Or we kick ourselves for making one goof, and we blame that mistake as the cause for the whole problem. The guilt may indeed be due to our not having been more open and more honest in our relationship with the person so that we never had as deep a sharing as we would have liked, but that is all the more reason to let go of our self-pity and to summon up positive energy to go forth again into life to do better next time if our remorse is genuine. Guilt of any kind is really a form of self-pity and a defense against being unable to look at our inner conflict.

It is only by wanting to do the work of removing all these ego blocks that the Tao can flow through us and the deepest part of our beings can feel fulfilled. So the cosmic message is ringing loud and clear through all the distress of modern life, calling people to face themselves. The urge to see truth is built into Nature, so to run from our distress can never be more than a temporary relief. The cosmic mirror will always return at some point to face us with the truth of ourselves. The natural law brings us this mirror over long spans of time. It challenges us through life's events, but it has been hard for humans to see what the Cosmos is doing. Often we can see no connection between the painful situations in our lives and the way we are misusing our consciousness. However, the urgency of our present times is that the cosmic mirror is sending its message more rapidly. There has always been conflict and distress in the world, and somehow it has always seemed that we had a long evolutionary road ahead of us and plenty of time to work things out in the future. But time is speeding up. You only need to look at your own life to see the rapid feedback of many changing events and moods.

The challenge and the only way through is for us to change our values that have always said we should leave our fears, self-doubts and negativities alone and they will go away. The fact is that these weaknesses do not just vanish. By working skillfully with them they become our strengths in disguise because they are the base metals of our being that we can transmute into gold. This isn't to say that we should wallow in them, for that is as destructive as avoiding them, but it is mandatory that we get in touch with them. Some people are so out of touch with themselves that they don't even know they have conflicts to deal with. You don't have to have some huge problem to let you know you have an ego to work on. All you need is the nagging feeling inside that something is not quite right. When you penetrate your ego you will have the feeling that everything *is* right. Whatever it is in your life that brings you pain, that is where you must begin. If you try to put down or ignore your pains you are ignoring the cosmic message beeping away at you, trying to get through to tell you what you have to look at in yourself. And if we look clearly at the world situation, this is what we are doing as a society. There is a new vision before us as well as the methods to reach it, if we will only choose to put the work on the ego and evolution first.

When we finally do make a change at the deep being level, it is like moving a TV dial from channel five to channel four. Suddenly you see a new picture, you act on a new reality, and the universe starts to mirror back beautiful new things. But this mirror is an effect of your change. The motive cannot be craving for the fruits of the breakthrough. It has to be done for truth, to receive what God or another person is telling you because you care about their reality enough to receive it. By making truth your objective and putting it before your desires or fears or personal preferences of any kind, you set an evolutionary dynamic in motion inside you that lifts you up and out of the ego. The unconscious ego is not purified all at once, but when we become committed to truth, to working on the ego, we are in tune with the methods of universal government and flow with Nature's laws. Eventually we will have to decide to let go of the ego entirely and become a servant of the One. Therefore to take up the spiritual life in earnest will automatically intensify our work on the ego and our inner conflict to push us to the very edge of the black hole—that unknown nothingness beyond the borders of all self-images, self-concepts and familiar beliefs. Until we have this spiritual commitment to truth we will have a vague belief of the black hole only as something missing—the unconscious mind into which we push our unacceptable feelings, and from which our future conflicts will arise.

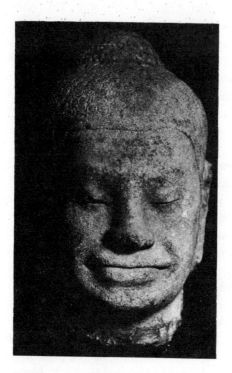

Buddha in samadhi, from Cambodia.

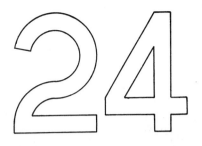

CREATIVE CONFLICT AS A SPIRITUAL DISCIPLINE

We are faced on all sides with a spiritual dilemma as our growing awareness reveals that we are all engaged in a fight for our planet—a fight of cosmic proportions in which our own state of consciousness is the battlefield. False messiahs are thriving and secular causes are crowded with devotees who would battle the political and environmental hazards that are insidiously creeping forward. Many are the causes which inspire people to dedicate their lives, trying to fill up the vacuum left by medieval concepts of holiness and the good life. Many people take up Eastern religion because they feel that the Western variety has failed mankind with its emphasis on the cult of personality. Others have become fanatically devoted, extremely emotional and fiery evangelists preaching to others. But the real fiery passion of devotion is silent— slowly but intensely burning in the hearts of those few who await some sign that does not smack of the pseudo-cult or smell of sentimentality

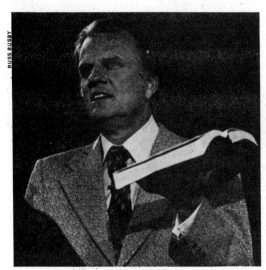

RUSS BUSBY

Rev. Billy Graham draws millions to his TV appearances and evangelical meetings where he preaches on the Bible. Many are "converted" in a rush of emotionalism, but is this "rush" of feeling a true spirituality or a substitute for the real need to look at what separates us from each other?

or self-deception. They as individuals know that they must carry the torch of the human spirit through to the end where its devotional expression is pure and undefiled by arrogance. They know that we must stay away from all movements which perpetuate the same mistakes of the past and make us all into docile followers of human organizations, orders, and charismatic campaigns for world salvation and allow us to join instead that invisible "Order of Righteousness" which moves with the spirit of the Cosmos. These individuals wait for that moment when devotion to the battle is not externalized in the more dramatic conflicts of the world but can flow spontaneously to those who serve quietly in the unspoken love of the heart.

What is true devotion? What will spark it legitimately, not trigger an emotional high that is gone two hours later? The monks in the old monasteries, walking round and round doing their rosaries, thought that they were holy, but the next moment they were out torturing people. The Inquisition went on while they were singing high mass and wearing crucifixes five inches tall. So what is the difference between "getting off" on something and true holiness? How do we recognize true devotion? True devotion is sentiment, not sentimentality. True love is selfless love. If you are genuinely spiritual your vibration comes through and you needn't play to the gallery, because your being speaks louder than any words could do. And there is no hierarchy implicit between the lines. Nothing is spiritual. Or if anything is spiritual it is *all* spiritual. Preaching at people or any other kind of put-down is not Godlike. People go to church and get that emotional feeling and feel holy, but it comes out as self-righteousness, and they do not change their ways. Minds do not really change and man continues to pollute his own environment in spite of the Bible and in spite of religious teachings about the interlocking unity of life. Religion is in this sense an opiate, just as Marx said. It sidetracks people from the real spirituality by making them feel that they are okay being an ego and they don't need to change or work on themselves. So how do we keep the precious thing, the real devotion that is too sacred to even utter, much less to speak of with a pious sugary tone of voice? How do we keep that real thing and get rid of a false religion or anything else that keeps us from facing ourselves?

That is what Nuclear Evolution is about, because you penetrate into your deepest self, the nucleus of your being, and you see that God is *consciousness*, not an old man in heaven, separate from people and their actions. To give that "old man with a beard" or "saved by the cross of Jesus" stuff to people means that they are not going to look at the real Christ or understand the reality of how they use their consciousness nor face their ego deceptions. Everybody has an ego. There is nothing wrong with having an ego, so long as you know its workings. Not to know its talent for deception is to be self-deceived. There are other expressions of devotion that are not religious and not put into words or scriptures but are visible in the actions of people. The kind of people who spend their lives in the temple doing rituals often don't have the kind of devotion to stick out the really intensive work on the ego, the real meat of the spiritual life. So the question we have to ask ourselves is how much of this nitty-gritty work can we tolerate, so that *others* can find God, not just ourselves. We are talking about the nucleus, God, the One at the center of all things! We have to do something to bring the kingdom of heaven on earth, not just talk about it. God would rather we would use our time not taking communion and drinking his blood and getting off on rituals, but looking deep into ourselves. That is what is holy.

I look at the quality of someone's life and I read it. Maybe they
never say a prayer, but they are selfless and their life is pure. So pure
is their devotion to Truth that they cannot utter words to defile it,
because it is too precious to them. So they put their devotion into all
they do. No need to preach or to make a speech about it. The *real*
emotional high does not come until you've totally conquered your*self*.
It is possible to be a monk or nun inside your own self and make the
world your monastery. The nun gets up early in the morning and gets

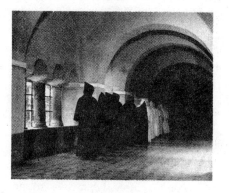

down on her knees and scrubs the floor so white that Christ can walk
on it, and her work is her worship. But in the closed cloister no *man*
can walk on it, and there is an impurity in this because it shuts the
world out. Is real devotion to be bought at the expense of being in this
world and on this earth? Why can't we clean the whole *world* up and
make our own self the monastery—make it so pure it cannot be
profaned, no matter who comes in and treads upon it? God cannot be
polluted. Even if you dump all the rubbish in it, pure consciousness
still remains pure.

For me, true growth is ruthless, and I am ruthless with all pretense.
I am a mirror for all that people feel in themselves, so I disturb a lot of
people. If they have pretense in them, they see pretense in me. All I
need to know to know *them* is to know what they think of *me*. One of

my students, who is constantly in conflict between her need for meditation and the busy life of doing God's work, has a hard time seeing my devotion and looks for that quality in the Bhakti Yoga taught by Paramahansa Yogananda. She projects the split in herself onto me and feels that I cannot see *her* real feelings. But for me there is no separation between the hard work and one's devotion; the work is an outlet for those deepest feelings. There is a problem only if people separate and make meditation more holy than living and working and daily actions. And for these people, the only answer to the pull of the monastery is to make it all one by putting pure devotion into the work. It is a matter of *living* it, making your work a worship, remembering to practice the Presence all the time, constantly, in everything you say and do. It is not a matter of sitting for hours in a meditation corner, getting off on gurus' pictures. Life is only as holy as it is lived. This must be the mantram repeated over and over.

I admit that this is not easy in a hectic work schedule, but if we remember God when we can, then God says, "It is okay that you forgot me for two hours, because you were doing my work and I understand that. But I'm glad you remembered me in this second because now I can give you in this one second all the other seconds you forgot." He can forgive you because He (consciousness) knows that your heart was pure and that you were doing the work for *the whole*. That is real holiness, and you don't need a cassock and surplice or need to become a monk to be holy. The more you practice this working for the whole, the more you get in tune with all that is out of tune— people making mistakes, running back and forth, forgetting things, miscommunicating—and the more you understand the nature of life. The University of the Trees is very much out of tune in this way, because it is a place that amplifies everything. But because it exists only for the purpose of tuning, people are happy in the midst of chaos and they grow and actually glow with their unspoken dedication to the One. People who live there go through several incarnations in the space of a year, but they can't see it. You'd have to do a lot of work in a monastery to manifest the equivalent in reality or reach the real spirituality.

Even great beings like Saint Francis couldn't bring spirituality

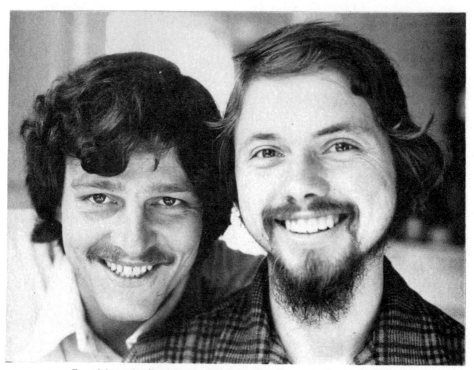

Two of the student/faculty at the University of the Trees—glowing and growing.

always into worldly manifestation. Saint Francis was even banished
from his own monastery for wanting everyone to wear a hair shirt. No
one wanted it but him, because the manifesting vibration of the place
was not really his vibration which was very holy. Later his disciples
took him back, but after he died they wallowed in luxury and excess
because he had picked people who were not very spiritual. Most people
don't know this about Saint Francis, that he was very ineffectual in his
ability to know who was or wasn't spiritual, because he saw everything
as spiritual. So the fact is that even the holiest vibration can fail
miserably on certain worldly levels. The spirit of Saint Francis may
walk among us today and be trying hard to prove to God that he can
do the worldly side of the spiritual trip as well as the devotional side,
because he failed before. And people at church might think that he was
lacking in humility or devotion because he is so involved in the world.
But his devotion would be in his actions and in his life. We must not

conveniently forget that between holy masses, Saint Francis' followers press-ganged people into the army, persuaded people to become killers, and that soon after Saint Francis died, his followers joined the Dominicans in the Inquisition, horribly torturing and killing innocent victims. But they did their meditations and felt holy and righteous because they didn't know themselves and they did not connect their religious practice with their earthly life and their daily actions. So the trick is not long prayers but short meditations on how to get heaven and earth together in one. By doing selfless service and work on the ego, though they may not give us the emotional satisfaction that we find in long solitary meditations, we *become* a worship and make our life a worship, and we feel no separation between the parts of our life nor do we experience a separation between ourselves and other people.

I realize that it is not a worldwide and accepted conclusion that the spiritual life is more fulfilling than a life seeking material advantages and pleasures. There are many who hold no regard for the higher things of life, and they have chosen freely to believe only in the reality of the material world. As such they may have no high regard for life or freedom of religion and may experience no inner conflict between heaven and earth. Do we have a right or duty to awaken them to the price of apathy or do we allow them to go down into a chaos of human making? Do we sit and watch the planet sink in its conflicts into self-destruction or do we attempt to warn, change the direction or show an example of a conflict-free life? Alexander Solzhenitsyn, who suffered many years in the Russian slave camps for a minor comment about Stalin in a letter to a friend, feels this obligation to awaken people through his writings and his speeches. Therefore at age sixty he chose to accept an honorary doctorate from Harvard University and in his acceptance speech to scold his adopted Western civilization for what he sees as a descent into "moral poverty". The speech was widely publicized.

> "The fight for our planet, physical and spiritual, a fight of cosmic proportions, is not a vague matter of the future; it has already started. The forces of evil have begun their decisive offensive, you can feel their pressure, and yet your screens and publications are full of prescribed smiles and

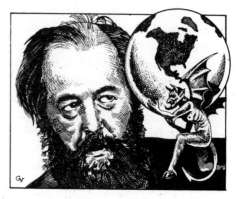

raised glasses. What is the joy about?

... On the way from the Renaissance to our days, we have enriched our experience, but we have lost the concept of a Supreme Complete Entity which used to restrain our passions and our irresponsibility. We have placed too much hope in political and social reforms, only to find out that we were being deprived of our most precious possession: our spiritual life. In the East, it is destroyed by the dealings and machinations of the ruling party. In the West, commercial interests tend to suffocate it. This is the real crisis. The split in the world is less terrible than the similarity of the disease plaguing its main sections."

Not all Americans agreed with Solzhenitsyn's assessment of worldliness and material and commercial domination of the spiritual energy of the defenders of democracy. Many felt that church and religious freedom still play a dynamic role in social and spiritual change in this country. But there are many others who sense that our system has been infected and polluted and that religion as we know it cannot solve the problems of chaos and conflict in which we are now embroiled. Why not? Because neither religion nor any traditional concept of human transformation *penetrates deep enough* into the nature of consciousness to make any real improvement in humans either individually or collectively. Only a new system of very rapid fundamental change can begin to accomplish the renaissance that the spiritual practices of history have failed to bring about.

Whenever I am trying to judge the values of the world's spiritual, political or idealistic concerns, I am always faced with the difficulty myself of living a life which directly expresses in daily experience the linkage between heaven and earth, the coming of the ideal into earthly manifestation, for as I have said, even the highest spiritual practice in the cells of some monastery or in a cave in the Himalayas has at some time got to be lived out in the practical world in order to become meaningful action. I developed the practice of Creative Conflict in order to show how to bring the expected, idealized shoulds and oughts into line with the exact quality of the way we actually live. Obviously we are only as holy as the way we live. There is in reality no separation in the world between the heavenly state of existence and the earthly side of our lifestyle. The separation is always in us and in our collective inability to make heaven on earth happen. This is the essence of Creative Conflict: how to do something which enhances our communication between heaven and earth and dissolves the gap between our wish fulfillments and our actual state of being. It is one thing to believe we are so far along the spiritual path that we don't need to do anything. But it is another to act in such a way that events confirm that what we are doing is in tune with the cosmic evolution and not just our own concept of what is good for the world. So much self-deception goes on in this area that we find ninety percent of the world's people living some kind of separation between what they believe in—that is, in an idealist or religious sense—and what they actually do with their time, their energy and their thought life. Hence the world improves very little in real terms of happiness, and we live stunted lives in communities which do not communicate with any fulfilling depth of purpose.

So we ask now the question, "What is the best and easiest way to bring about a resolution of the war which goes on between the inmost hearts of people and the external worldliness which surrounds them daily in their earthly life in the body?" And that leads directly to the very real war which goes on between the selfish individual whose priority is the search for the rewards of money and power, and those individuals whose priority is the love of their fellowman. The first uses society in order to exploit it and become self-aggrandized and self-important. The second uses the social situation as a means of making the spiritual life a real and selfless devotion to a cosmic impulse. The problem is that both the powerseeker and the lover of mankind are often comprised of types of individuals who readily deceive themselves through their egocentric relationship to themselves and Cosmos. They are easily convinced that they are working for earthly power or heavenly power for the sake of others and unity, when really their devotion and their cause is in direct conflict with others, and their actions are often a compensation or a rationalization for not wanting to look within at the operations of consciousness and not wanting to work on the ego.

Most people think of the ego as something they value which they usually call their individual uniqueness, and they find it hard to distinguish it from their real being—the pure consciousness. The idea of "getting rid of" or "working on" the ego seems foreign to the average person. He will always ask, "What is the advantage of transcending the ego? How can it be beneficial to constantly research my motives and look at the subtle undercurrents in my communications generated by self-centeredness of the ego? What is the reason for being selfless? Can I really gain anything by not looking out for number one? Who will look out for me if I don't look out for myself? Look around. How many people really want to give up their egos? I'll be stupid if I do. I want to develop my ego and improve my self-image, not reduce it."

In fact, up to now, our whole culture has valued the ego, and the philosophy of democracy hangs greatly on the balancing of many competing selfish interests. But does this competition work or do we finish up with the big multinational companies owning seventy-five percent of all productive capacity including the power, energy and oil industry? To these groups the American people are like cows being led to the milking shed! The pursuit of the success of selfishness and personal power leads eventually to the decadent and polluted environments, to the decay of our democratic system, to the lack of integrity in our human society.

Does this mean that we must radically change our minds and reverse our present culture 180 degrees and destroy everything we have built up through personal endeavors? Of course not. It means we merely put into practice what we have been giving lip service to since the times of Christ. It means that to preserve the environment of the planet and survive we must hear the words of Christ and all other religious founders directly and stop following the doctrines of human

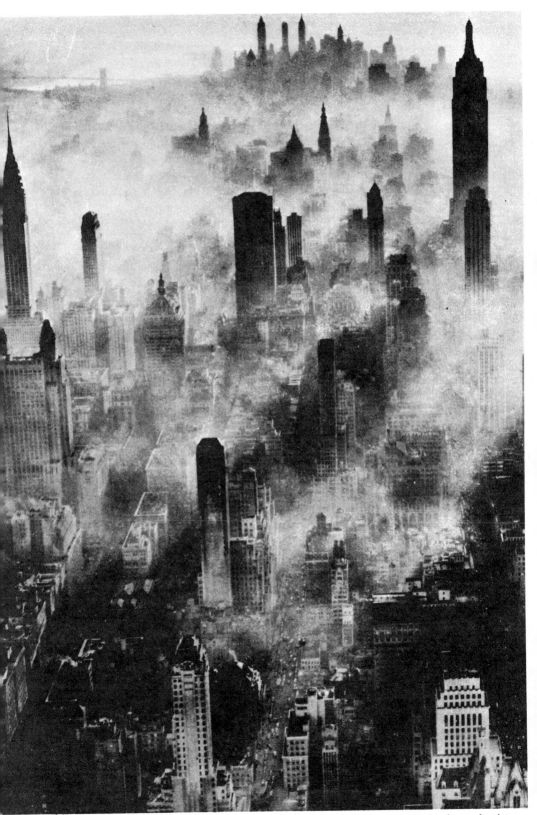

Whenever we see external pollution we must remember that it is a direct result of the internal polluted state of society. No one individual is responsible for the pollution but each of us shares in the responsibility of a polluted society.

organizations which have grown up like big business into just another way of milking the people of their wealth, without delivering the promised kingdom of heaven. Hence Creative Conflict is needed because powerful organizations of human persuasion in both politics and religion do not see themselves as egotistical or self-centered but quite the opposite. This is the social and spiritual problem in a nutshell. Unfortunately neither Solzhenitsyn nor the church is attacking the real problem at all. Self-righteousness and self-centeredness are synonymous. They stem from the same cause and cannot be separated from their effects. The cosmic battle of the ego is written in the conflict in our own consciousness for it is this disturbance raging in everyone which is projected out into the events of the world both as cause and as witness of the effects. This is why Creative Conflict is built upon the principle that our whole reality of the external world is a mirror of the internal world, and this is also why we have to face up to the fact that religion has not changed the world one ounce! We are deluded if we continue with our devotion to it in its present form. Christ appeared on the earth when religious traditions had lost touch with life, when customs and rituals had become more important than consciousness (God) itself. Christ had to rebel in order to show that truth and love transcend the cultural ideas of God and even more, that consciousness and life transcend all thoughts and concepts about God. How else can God manifest except through consciousness?

Can mankind embrace a method of spiritual growth so different from the traditional methods of monastic prayer or individual meditation which can achieve the same effect and more so that only one incarnation in the temporal plane of earthly existence is necessary for purification? Can mankind find a social system that achieves, as a worldly pragmatic political activity, the same evolutionary results as a traditional spiritual system? If these two effects can be combined successfully with economic survival of the community without exploitation of individuals or society, then we can say that our work is spiritual. Otherwise it is merely misplaced zeal. May God protect us from the zealots of all beliefs! What is the process involved in the transformation of the self in Creative Conflict? In other volumes I have set out the "how to" and the rules of Creative Conflict for beginners, but the reader of this book will be more interested in the vision of what Creative Conflict can do to bring heaven to earth and to bring the conflict between the individual self and its worldly desires into spiritual alignment with our evolutionary destiny.* Creative Conflict challenges every person to confront their ego position that separates being from being. It tackles the causes that separate human consciousness from oneness. The essentially spiritual structure of Creative Conflict has nothing to do with religion or any belief system, but just the pure relationship between energies.

Creative Conflict is done by taking our internal conflict into a group situation and using it to discover our real Self. All religions speak of the state we call heaven, but they hardly ever manifest it in society except as a *theory* of salvation. Creative Conflict begins by the coming together of a group of people who agree to be different and who agree to look at each others' feedback and to understand each communication before trying to respond to it. This means we must establish a few rules in order to prevent the normal type of communication from reasserting itself as a habit. The rules are changeable by the group as a whole, but they have been worked out by people who have been practicing Creative Conflict for some years. The natural tendency is for someone to come in and change the rules without quite knowing the reasons why we have them or why they were formed in the first place. The reason we have rules is to be able to do without them. There are a minimum number of rules which are required for creative communication to take place so that we may get to the place where rules are not needed. The problem is that the ego, thinking that it sees in all clarity, cannot understand wh   ules cannot be changed more to its liking. But to change these rules without knowing why they are put there is to break down the integrity needed to do Creative Conflict. Also we need to learn a deeper form of listening to ourself as well as others in order to get beyond the normal egocentric form of listening. The following

---

* *The Golden Egg,* a "how to" book on the organization of society, and *Exploring Inner Space* by Christopher Hills and Deborah Rozman, 1978.

Creative Conflict process for transcending the separating ego is the basic beginning teaching.*

THE CREATIVE CONFLICT PROCESS

In this process we delve deeply into specific methods to dissolve ego blocks. For most of us the ego is constantly, subtly blocking our perception. It is also usually blocking real listening, so there is very little true communication taking place, even though we may think we are high and aware beings talking to each other. We hear words but not the layers of meaning and being behind them. We see flowers but not the light and consciousness within them. In order to do this work on ourselves together or alone, we must balance its depth and intensity with a light heart, humor and joy. Otherwise it becomes very serious. However, if we look at it as life's garden that we are nurturing, weeding, digging, fertilizing, watering and supplying sunlight for, we can make the work light. By making work light we make *light* work. When light works for us we are in tune with Nature and we can tackle anything, even making the manure of negativity into good compost to help Nature grow beautiful flowers.

There are a number of keys to real listening, which is the basis of the Creative Conflict process. There are also subtle blocks to real listening that we must watch for in ourselves as we use the keys. The first step is to quiet the feelings and thoughts jangling around inside us and to put aside all reactions and "tapes" playing in our heads, spinning tunes of past feelings and ideas and future expectations. Real listening is getting your own reactions and responses out of the way in order to hear exactly what the other person is saying, but this is harder than it seems. We have to become like a blank photographic plate, open to any impression, and we cannot achieve this openness if we are listening through the filters of our own opinions, ideas, preconceptions, assumptions, hurt feelings and all the mental/emotional equipment that makes us who we are.

---

*The Creative Conflict process and guidelines are also found in detail in *Exploring Inner Space.*

Creative Conflict helps us to reach this open and receptive state of mind through the device of mirroring what the other person has said. Mirroring enables you to see if you have really been receptive and lets the other person feel you are in rapport. You speak back using your own words, not parroting the other's. This means you will speak back the vibrations and feelings you pick up from other people as well as the words, so they feel you are at one with them and can feel their heart. You might begin mirroring by saying, for example, "Let me see if I understand you; you're really saying . . . ." In mirroring you are trying to experience others as they experience themselves, becoming one, and communicating not at the level of intellect but at a deeper level of being. The other person must then confirm or deny whether you heard rightly before you can voice your own response to what he or she has said. Therefore after mirroring you ask the other if your mirror is correct. It is essential that you ask for confirmation, to know if you are tuning in properly. Then you listen for the reply, again with receptivity. If the person says, "Yes, you've got it," then you can speak your feelings and respond. If the other says, "No, that's not what I meant," or "Those were my words but I don't really feel that way," then you ask him or her to explain again. Active listening makes the other feel heard and encourages him or her to continue speaking.

This communication process may at first glance seem laborious but it becomes fulfilling as you penetrate to deeper layers of sharing and being. Mirroring is absolutely essential to clear understanding. The fact that ninety-nine percent of people cannot do this process properly without practice is proof enough that we *think* we understand but do not. Only after your mirroring is confirmed do you share your response about what the other has said to you. Most people want to respond before the other has even finished speaking and so miss all the important steps for real communication. It takes self-discipline to wait and respond only after confirmation is established. When you respond you use an "I-message". For example,

> "I felt hurt when you gave those boxes to Ruth because it made me feel left out."

There are four aspects to an I-message which express a deep feeling that you have:

    a) I felt (owning it is your reality)
    b) hurt (or joyful or whatever it is you felt)
    c) when you gave those boxes to Ruth (saying what triggered the feeling)
    d) because it made me feel left out (saying specifically what it did to you)

People often forget to include the fourth part especially and this is the part that communicates the most deeply. All four aspects of the I-message must be there for your being to have fully communicated. This takes some reflection to get in touch with your feelings and it requires openness in expressing them, which you can only learn through practice.

Once you have responded, then you ask the other person to please mirror back what you have just said so that you too can feel you have communicated. When you speak with another who is also accustomed to using these communication skills, it is ideal communication and you can usually get to the place of oneness and true understanding very quickly. Most people, whether they know about these steps or not, will respect your interest and desire to have the communication clear. Just watching someone use these skills puts them in touch with a deeper part of themselves and makes them want to use them too. With a little guidance most people will respond well to your request that they should mirror back what you have said, as it shows that you really do care that they hear you.

In addition to mirroring, there are other basic principles of Creative Conflict which have been compressed down to the bare minimum requirements for good communication. These must be practiced and studied over and over until they become part of our daily life. Setting aside a special time to share together, either in a family, a business group, or a group of friends, is the easiest way to make Creative Conflict a habit and integrate it in your daily communication. We have talked of rules for the management of our egocentric methods of communication. I prefer to call them guidelines since there is no coercion in Creative Conflict.

GUIDELINE #1
YOU ARE WHATEVER DISTURBS YOU

If someone is disturbing you, it is *your* mind and emotions that are being disturbed, not the other's. You are identifying with your thoughts about what you see or hear and are letting those thoughts bother you. It is entirely your problem. The other might not be having a problem at all. So own the disturbance as your own. Then you can free yourself. Realize that if you hold the attitude of identifying with your pure Self and not with the ego that gets disturbed, you can gain insight into why you allow yourself to be disturbed. So when someone bothers you, point the finger first at yourself to see what part of you is reacting. What is the mirror of life, reflected from that person, trying to show *you*? This does not mean that you may not have a valid perception of the other person, but if you are letting it disturb you, then you have a problem.

One major problem with conflicts and a reason why they can be so destructive is that we refuse to own our disturbances. We lash back or say, "That's his fault. I'm all right." In Creative Conflict we cannot do that because it does not matter whose fault it is. What matters is how we are handling our reactions. Often we find that when we judge others, the next minute we are being judged. Life's mirror works very quickly at times. For example, Dave gets disturbed by Sue's authoritative manner. Sue says, "You left your milk on the table again, please clean it up," and "When are you going to take out the garbage?" Dave riles inside. Why? Does he want to be the authority? This he has to look at first. Then instead of retorting, "Do it yourself!" and creating bad vibes between them, he can say, "You know, I have a problem with authority myself. I'd like to be aware enough to be the boss. But I do feel that you spoil your communication in the way you lay down the law and come across so strongly. I would find it much easier to accept what you say if it were expressed with a more humble, more caring vibe. Maybe others experience you the way I do."

In order to do this kind of communicating we have to be able to allow everyone the right to be whatever they are. Agree now that you are different from everybody and everybody is unique and entitled to use the *One* consciousness in any way they choose in absolute freedom.

GUIDELINE #2
I AGREE TO DISAGREE

This is the essence of Creative Conflict. In other words, you are so kind as to give others absolute freedom, when of course they already have it. We pride ourselves in giving others the freedom to be themselves, but life has given them that freedom whether we like it or not. You also have that freedom to be yourself every day. It is the only real freedom you have. So just as you demand that freedom for yourself, you give it to others. They have a divine right to do what disturbs you, providing they do not enforce it upon you harmfully and take away your freedom to do likewise. Pulling up the weeds of each other's hidden delusions is done first by acknowledging and accepting differences, then by confronting the motivation and truth behind each viewpoint. Only in this way can we begin the creative process. This is especially true between people or over issues in which we have a lot of emotional investment. A mother does not want to know her teenage daughter is having sex. A father does not want his son to drop out of school, as he feels it will ruin his life. One government does not like to see another government selling arms to a third country. Real peace can only come from having the self-honesty to probe the motives and causes of disagreements together, after respecting each other's right to be different.

GUIDELINE #3
I AGREE TO WORK FOR SYNTHESIS

The disagreement which does not take into account all the areas that *you do agree upon* is not creative. If the areas of *agreement* exceed the areas of *disagreement* you can have a conflict which leads to synthesis. As long as there is a fundamental unity which is stronger than the disagreements, you can work it out if you are willing. For example, you might be arguing about one particular point and getting worked up and passionately feeling your mind spinning and your emotions rushing. But there may be fifty other things you can agree upon. But do you think of those fifty things at the time you are disagreeing? Creative Conflict always has this in mind, that there may be all these areas of agreement and there is just one little area of disagreement which needs to be worked out to a synthesis with the rest. Therefore at times when we feel ourselves having negative thoughts about someone, or feel poles apart on an issue, we remember this guideline and remind ourselves of some of our common areas of agreement. We reaffirm, "I agree to work for synthesis." This reestablishes the feeling of unity in the heart, the positive energy that can resolve any differences in the head.

GUIDELINE #4
I AGREE THAT EACH PERSON HAS TRUTH FROM THE POINT OF VIEW FROM WHICH IT IS SEEN

Everything is true from the level of consciousness from which it is seen. Everyone sees true from their own level of consciousness, even if it differs from another's truth. So we say to ourselves, "I agree to be the same consciousness, even when we are talking about the same object in different terms." That same consciousness is making all things seem different. In other words, the guideline "I agree to disagree" becomes agreeing to be the same in being, even though we are disagreeing mentally, because we may be talking about the same thing in different ways. One of the problems with human beings is that we never want to be the same as anybody else. The minute you share something you think others will relate to they say, "Ah, but my thing is different." They just want to be different, so they argue. Creative Conflict involves seeing that we may be egocentric in talking about picky differences, when the differences may be just a product of the ego separating itself from the experience and thoughts of others. That is why so many couples can fight one minute and make love the next. So many children can be tearing each others' hair out one minute and playing the next. People fall in love, react to praise or criticism the same, whether they are priests, hoodlums, communists or capitalists. The situation is different, but the underlying emotion is the same. So even though what is true for one person may not be true for another in the head, together we can probe our beliefs and motives and expand to a greater truth from the heart.

We can challenge another's truth, but we have to be able to see that what John says is true for him and what Mary says is true for her, even though they may be totally different truths, and from another view they may both be limiting. To get to the greater synthesizing truth, both parties must be willing to examine themselves and be willing to change. An example of this guideline might be, "I need two women," says John. Mary replies, "I need a man who wants only me." A friend, Bill says, "You are both identifying with your needs, but Mary's need is based on her insecurity and fear of rejection which makes her cling. John's need is based on Mary's clinging which he cannot cope with, yet he loves her and does not want to leave her." The other woman has beautiful qualities that Mary does not have, but Mary also has beautiful qualities that the other woman does not have, so John feels he needs them both and is unfulfilled with only one. In Creative Conflict, John and Mary's views are both true, but the underlying needs are the forces that are causing the views. These needs are what we must probe, share feelings about, mirror and penetrate in order to find a synthesis, a greater truth than either is seeing.

GUIDELINE #5
I WILL EXAMINE MY OWN MOTIVES FOR DISAGREEING BEFORE DOUBTING THE STATEMENTS OF ANOTHER. I WILL LOOK FOR THE BASIC ASSUMPTIONS AND THE NEEDS BEHIND WHAT IS SAID.

It is difficult to stop ourselves from reacting and ask, "What is my motive for disagreeing?" But we have to learn to get to the cause of our disturbance for conflict to be transformed. We have to continually ask ourself, "What is the basic assumption in what he or she is saying? What is my basic assumption in my position? For example, "He always thinks his way is the only right way. He assumes he's always right. What arrogance! What real feeling of inadequacy must be under all that! The need to be confirmed must be there." The underlying, unspoken assumptions form our view of truth and we base our opinions of others, and of our own egos on them. The quicker we can uncover and check out the basic assumptions in any point of view, the sooner the penetration to greater truth will take place. For example, "I'm upset, Jeff, because you didn't call me, " says Laura. But Laura must examine her own motives for being upset before doubting Jeff's motives for not calling. She is upset because she is jealous and lonely. So she goes on a big trip in her mind about that, worrying for hours. Jeff finally tells her that he lost her new phone number and the operator did not have it listed. What a lot of time she has wasted worrying.

Another example, "Mary, you shouldn't handle money anymore," says John. Mary reacts and walks out in a huff. John is astonished. Does Mary ask what John's basic assumption is? Or check out her own? No! Perhaps John feels she mismanages money. That's Mary's fear. But John really feels that it is for his own growth that he wants the change, not for hers. He feels he needs to master handling money and Mary does it for him, so he is always feeling there is not enough because he doesn't know where it is going. We can only get to the causes of conflict when we constantly look behind the surface, behind the apparent situation, to the basic assumptions. The seven steps, especially the mirroring step, allow us to experience directly our own and the other person's basic assumptions that we cannot normally see in conversation. We must learn to probe together and share the basic assumptions we see operating, as we are mostly blind to them.

GUIDELINE #6
RED HERRING*

One of the greatest blocks to communication is going off on a tangent, away from the center of concentration. Someone may think he has an insight and offer it, but really it is way off the point. The group mind has to be aware of this and gently but firmly say, "That is off the point, a Red Herring!" Then the group must lead the energy back to the real point. Sometimes the person being confronted will bring in a Red Herring. Just as you are about to share a deep feeling you haven't been able to express to that person before, the other will say, "I need a glass of water" or "Isn't it time for tea?" "Oh, I must put the baby to bed," or "The dinner's got to be made," or any number of things that short circuit the energy and deny the communication. You usually then shut up like a clam and the conflict is pushed down inside and repressed. The group intuition must become finely tuned to one-pointedness and

---

*Origin of the term: In hunting, a red herring was dragged across the path of the quarry to distract the dogs away from the scent of the animal so they wouldn't chase after it.

the energies that accompany deep soul-searching must be kept concentrated and directed. Otherwise depth will not be reached. Children are famous for bringing in Red Herrings to avoid facing themselves. We even go off on Red Herrings when we are alone in thought to avoid looking at ourselves. How many times have you been in a nitty-gritty situation and somebody pulls in a completely irrelevant statement which sends you off chasing that one track and you end up spinning wheels? So, then you get a wheel spinning, or what we sometimes call a "waffling" situation. The group must be able to spot this instantly and call out "Red Herring!" whenever it occurs, otherwise the session goes nowhere and is a waste of time. The Red Herring guideline is likely to be used more than any other guideline. It will train the group intuition and make the difference between a low energy session and a concentrated, electrifying and deep experience, bringing growth.

GUIDELINE #7
QUIBBLING

To define a definition of a word and then challenge the definition of the definition is to get stuck completely in the trap of quibbling. "What do you mean when you say so-and-so?" We hear this all the time. It is usually a way of diverting, of not listening to the being of the person. Some people love to get caught up in semantics and avoid the real being. When we communicate effectively we are listening to the being of the person not the words! The words are merely second-hand symbols invented by others. They are not the most important part of communication. To use double meanings, words which are ambiguous, is another quibble. An example is, "You're too clever!" We do not mean he is clever at all. Or "You're a wise guy." Are we really thinking he is wise? A wise guy is somebody who is too clever and therefore looks stupid. This is how we speak in words that have no integrity and so we keep communication on superficial levels. To get stuck in dictionary meanings and wrong use of words is to quibble, so that all thread of the argument is lost.

Nations do the same by insisting on the legalities of actions while ignoring the actual facts. Genocide is mass murder and illegal but that does not help the victims. To stand by and say it is illegal is not telling a murderer anything new. The legality is lost on him. We do the same semantically when we quibble. It lowers the high energy-level needed for direct perception and drains the electricity which comes from being-to-being communication. The way out is for someone to say, "I feel you are quibbling." Then someone can bring in another I-feel statement to bring the communication from the semantic level to the deeper level again. We all have to be alert and take full responsibility for the direction of the group. Even one person holding back, or one person feeling bored, or dwelling on the dishes to be done at home, is deflecting the energy and is not being integral. If you are that person, ask yourself, "Why am I separating? Am I bored? Why do I not feel involved and why am I not putting in my full energies to take responsibility?" If you cannot find the cause and release it, or simply let go of yourself when you recognize it and jump in, then ask for group help at the next appropriate time, so that you can get in touch and be integral. Your *integrity* is important for group consciousness. The electricity flows in a group when all are integral.

GUIDELINE #8
I WILL SEEK OUT THE CONFLICT IN THE HEART OF EACH PERSON AND THE CONTRADICTIONS IN THEIR MINDS, BUT NOT THE CONFLICT IN THEIR WORDS AND IDEAS. I WILL NOT ENGAGE IN THEIR INTERNAL CONTROVERSY. I WILL NOT CHALLENGE WHAT I DON'T UNDERSTAND. INSTEAD I WILL SIT BACK AND LISTEN.

When you are talking, communicating, or confronting a person, you look for the contradiction in *them*, not in their words and ideas.

To challenge what you do not understand is to quibble. It is not creative to put our ignorance out onto someone else and make them explain it all in detail for us, as though we are so stupid that we do not know anything. We will need to listen better and deeper. However, it could be that the person really is expressing himself poorly, leaving half of the story out. Then we will have to ask for specific points to be clarified. What we need to watch for is the kind of attitude which believes that the whole group must be held up while "I" wait to be enlightened. It is an egocentric attitude and not creative at all. It is like the beginner saying, "I don't understand what's going on, please explain," while the rest of the group mind is just about to share an important point, vital to the conflict. You can feel the group energy start to drain or be sapped off with this kind of comment and then you must ruthlessly remind the person of this guideline. To attempt to be "nice" at this point will syphon off all the group energy. You must be firm and not be sucked into another person's confusion. Remind them to read Guideline #8.

GUIDELINE #9
MAKING A SPEECH

Under the guise of asking questions, some people will show how much knowledge they have or will display the contents of a book they have just read, ostensibly to share their insights with others. Whether those insights have been gained or books have already been read by others does not always occur to some egos. When asked to speak not from authorities or books, but from their own experience or to say what their real feelings are, they remain silent or back out of their position by saying, "I don't want to go into that now." Or they make statements about which they can offer no proof at all in their own life, only from hearsay, "Jesus said," "Marx said," "The authorities said," and they repeat all over the place for everyone's edification. But they are not prepared to test this philosophy out for themselves to prove it. They are continually coming out with suggestions which are not from their own experience. They want everyone else to test them. If they tested their own suggestions before they made them for others, then there would be value to their communication and their experience would contribute to the group energy. So before communicating we must know that our own suggestions work and that they are not just theoretical. Theoretical knowledge and comment leads only to mental masturbation. Such people should be challenged for making a speech or asked if they are contributing theoretical information or whether they are speaking on behalf of everyone present, or from direct experience. We must as a group be prepared to fight for integrity. It is not Creative Conflict unless you say, "Hey, are you speaking for yourself? I'm not at the position you're speaking from!" or "I feel you are preaching and making an assumption that we are interested in your theories and you are not really experiencing the real issues we are dealing with!" So we must remind ourselves and each other. "I (THE BIG I) CAN ONLY SPEAK FOR MYSELF FROM MY

OWN EXPERIENCE. I CAN'T SPEAK FOR EVERYONE."

This guideline also should be applied when someone begins speaking for other people about their problems. Married partners and parents often fall into the trap of speaking for others. "We just want him to find a nice hobby," says the well-intentioned wife or mother. The husband or child may not feel that way at all. So in Creative Conflict we must constantly ask each person to speak for himself or herself.

These nine guidelines to making conflict creative are deep studies of how human egos normally work. By looking for these patterns throughout our daily lives we can transform ourselves into incredibly perceptive and aware human beings. If these tools and techniques were taught in every classroom, in every home and in every business where people must cooperate, from the factory to big governments, we would have a tremendous understanding of human nature and of each other. The ancient advice, "Man Know Thyself!" would come true. And what would happen if it did come true? What is the end result of this new kind of spiritual discipline? By giving up our idea of separateness, we gain the expanded consciousness which sets us free of conflicts, pain and suffering. And by doing this together with a group of people all committed to the same goal, we attain Group Consciousness.

How do I know this is a true discipline? Because over the last ten years I have seen it work within people in ways that I have never seen belief systems of religion or politics work. Furthermore it is an exact duplicate of the way Nature communicates with itself. I have spent a small fortune and most of my time proving in different places on the earth that it can work amongst anyone who has the simple wish to communicate more deeply. But the greatest reason it works is because it resolves inner conflict and gives peace of mind in the midst of chaos. When we do it as a meditation we can feel the pressure and presence of God working through the group consciousness to make all things simple and clear, dispelling confusion about ourselves and bringing that spontaneous welling upsweep of love for which there are no words. Whether you are an industrial union leader, or a capitalist or a communist with different ideas of truth in your head will make no difference once you begin to communicate from your heart. Whatever your religion, bigotry cannot exist where there is divine love. Concepts do not bring such love, but creative communication does. This was the dynamic of the early Christians and is the simple message of all religions—that God manifests through love. Yet even the early Christians were not anywhere near a true group consciousness, though they bonded together in a mutual vision and suffered together for their faith in the risen Christ. Even the twelve disciples did not have the kind of group consciousness we are talking about. The disciples didn't know until after Christ died what they were to do. The Holy Ghost descended upon them and sat upon them in "cloven tongues like as of fire" and only then, at Pentecost, did it become clear that they were to go out and tell the story about one person who had made it to heaven.

Because of the way they carried out this mission, Christianity has become a personality cult, with Jesus Christ at the top of a great hierarchy which is foreign to the whole teaching of heaven. In talking about group consciousness we are talking about a whole bunch of people going to heaven together.

This is the purpose of the experimental community at the University of the Trees and the reason why we are fostering responsibility within each member so that our group consciousness is not centered around one individual. It might look that way to a person who visited here but my whole intention is to bring every member of the group through to a nonpersonal person where the next breakthrough will not be centered around a personality cult but will be centered around the universal person in the form of consciousness, all-pervading, inside everyone and everything. This was also Christ's intention, if we read his words correctly. His words have been twisted by the church to make it look like he alone is God and he alone is savior and he alone is capable of the highest heaven. This means that we mortals are ever stuck in the personality cult of a higher being, when in fact the church should be telling the truth that the higher being is in each one of us and even God's avatars are to be found working in the lowest levels of life and have no desire to be put on a false throne or pedestal, for the higher being is actually the whole of our Self and the total environment, not a part or a mere individual.

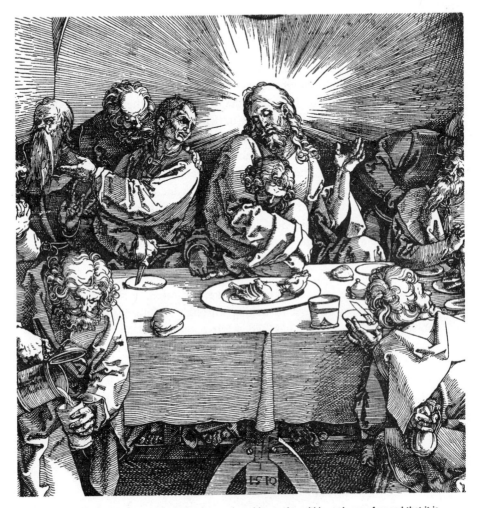

The essence of Christ's message is that heaven is waiting to rise within each one of us and that it is for everyone not just one man.

Why then did the twelve disciples of Christ go out and preach the word that Christ was the one who had made it? It happened because the disciples *interpreted* Pentecost that way. When the spirit came upon them, they had nothing else to say except what this one man (Jesus) said, whereas in the group consciousness experiment at the University of the Trees, the spiritual teachings are written in our own lives and come in our own words from the heart. Three of the four gospels in the Bible are all the same and all four are about one person (Christ). We know nothing about the disciples and their lives together. We don't know if they quarreled or what life they lived except that they did huge journeys converting others as missionaries. Pentecost was a missionary impulse which eventually spread throughout the world so that now the theory of heaven is promulgated, but its existence on earth is still just as far off as in the time of Christ. In *his* times it was considered to be imminent, whereas in our times doom seems to be more imminent. Christ's theory of the kingdom of heaven was a message of hope to a world in despair. Our world is also in despair, but the new faith must not play on hopes, since hope itself is based on uncertainty. The new faith must be based on certainty, not hopes or expectations. Such hopes and expectations for the kingdom of heaven to arrive through preaching, through scriptures, through holy books and "holy Joes", has had a fair enough trial and has received enough money and resources throughout history to make it work if it has the capacity to work. But the fact is, it cannot work unless individuals change first, and to change individual minds and hearts takes more than preaching or missionaries. These ugly facts we hate to

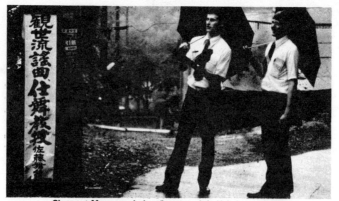

Clean-cut Mormon missionaries at work in Yokohama, Japan.

admit or look at—that the manifestation of our ideals, when tested, falls far short of our expectations.

The new group consciousness does not infect people's minds with missionary zeal or political passion but instead offers a natural scientific and practical look at the way Nature organizes its evolutionary breakthroughs. Christ himself continually pointed to natural examples in which he saw the kingdom of heaven present. These examples, such as the way Nature sprouts a seed which grows from itself and has within itself the full ear of corn, multiplying itself a hundred-fold, has not been preached by the church as a reality. Instead they have substituted external salvation to be brought from outside the seed! This separation in man's perceptions has come about because he feels that *he* plants and *he* grows the seeds, and we speak of "growers" as if they grew anything. Christ saw clearly that man grows nothing, not even his own body nor the seeds and crops he plants and that to consider himself as grower when he is merely the harvester is an arrogance which does not recognize that the life force is present within all things. This vital message of Christ's perception of the nucleus, the seed, the nux of his teachings, has been almost totally ignored ever since the words fell out of his mouth, and they have fallen on barren and stony ground. Even where they have taken root in poor soil, they have been strangled by the care of this world, which he warned about. Even the good soil, unpolluted by pesticides and irrigated by water, uncontaminated by man's ignorance of his environment, is now hard to find on the entire planet. Christ's analogies from Nature were insights of Nature and God at work. We have made them into mere literary expressions, rolling them from the end of our tongue in countless pulpits, and we have not understood or grasped a shred of what the man was talking about. Instead we have got off on our own ego trips, so fascinated are we with our own ingenuity and intellectual cleverness. The simple fact that he taught, which Nuclear Evolution re-expresses in a scientific model which can be communicated to anyone with the ears to hear, is that the seed is not only the vehicle for life force to shoot out its new form of existence but it is also the place where evolution takes place. Modern man would have us believe that the environment is where evolution takes place, but the environment is merely an effect, a replication of what is in the seed, and our power to prove this insight is obvious in the way we pollute our own planet.

Group consciousness, truly experienced, is the awareness that our entire life is evolving from the nuclear center of being, the very seed of consciousness which is planting itself in the soil of the environment which can only nurture it after its own pattern. As Christ says, man plants the seed in the ground and creates the conditions for the seed to grow, but only the seed itself can cause itself to grow, and the fundamental change of its evolutionary pattern is not determined by adaptation to environment. Otherwise the thousands of different blooms in the desert would long ago have become adapted to the sand to look alike, whereas in their adaptations they have become even more different in their response to environmental conditions. How many new plants are invented out there in the desert where there is no human eye to see them or human hand to pollinate them? We tend to think that only man can breed new species for his pleasure. But the fact is that the sameness of the desert conditions breeds thousands of different species.

In the human seed is written the power of the life force to change the fundamental patterns of growth which cannot be forced on the seed in contradiction to its true nature within. The will and the decision to change, the will to see God's hand writing itself in our consciousness, the will to manifest the life force and sprout into the new form, the new flowering, the new fruit, must come not from the pressure of the environment or from external causes but from the power which Christ saw clearly was the true grower. That power within each seed is within man in extraordinary intensity if only he would have the will to turn it inward and lift himself by his own consciousness like a person lifting himself with his own bootstraps. We are engaged in "Operation Bootstrap", and the power to levitate can only come from our own imaginations, for it is our own images which control our destiny and determine whether we shall rise like the Phoenix from the surface of the earth and join with brother sun and sister stars in singing the celestial song of heaven. This song is imprisoned in the nucleus, the seed of our own Self, and not to nourish it or plant it in good soil is the folly of man. This is the real root of the human problem—that the life force which Christ talked about is not recognized as the real evolutionary force. That force, whether we call it God, spirit, consciousness or love, is at the heart of the matter, whereas most human beings think it doesn't matter. They think what matters is matter, and that the consciousness which animates it has no power to change matter into new forms. But consciousness has power to change the world.

A group of people so tuned to the material universe to see in it the same hand working its oneness as Christ saw, by direct perception into Nature's ways, can by the sheer force of their love raise the potential of the entire human race, because if any part of the whole has been raised, the whole has been raised by that much. This is the fundamental principle upon which Nuclear Evolution rests its theory that the kingdom of heaven will manifest through the interaction and purification of the group heart and mind. The mind alone cannot do it. This purification is what Creative Conflict is about.

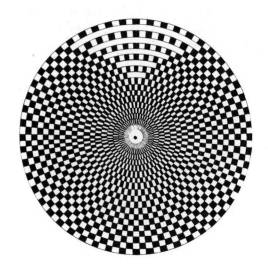

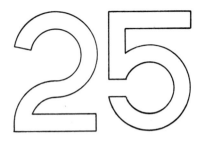

HOW WILL GOD MANIFEST?

At Centre House the methods of Creative Conflict and the techniques of growth were taught, but they were not pushed all the way to test the ego structure of the individual. Centre House was a more idealistic approach with a system of Creative Conflict that could work but not in an abstract setting where the responsibility for the community rested ultimately on one person. By involving the participants at University of the Trees in total responsibilty for themselves and the whole operation, and by pushing Creative Conflict to its ultimate conclusion irrespective of whether people would leave or not, I provided an ultimate test of the motivations of each member of the community. This faced them with what was really in their heart, whether they liked it or not. Since all had the option to leave if they didn't like it, those who stayed were literally compelled to purify their ego structures of self-interest and to put the interest of the whole (which of course included themselves) first. This insistence on group consciousness as the final result of the Creative Conflict process brought about a totally different commitment. Whereas at Centre House people were committed for as long as it suited them and until such time as they would change, at University of the Trees people had to change in order to be committed. This emphasis on change first and commitment later meant going beyond the word level of mouthed commitments. It was cash karma; no credit. It meant paying with pains and hurts of the heart, rather than rationalizing and softening the ego reactions in order to stay in the head. Hence, the difference between Centre House and University of the Trees is that Centre House was an experiment with Creative Conflict in the head, whereas University of the Trees is an experiment with Creative Conflict in the heart. This dualistic experiment brought about a synthesis in my own heart since if everyone else were going to be committed, I myself was trapped into a real marriage of love, rather than a marriage contract on paper. As in all marriages, people experience thin times depending on their resistance or surrender to each other, which varied at University of the Trees with each person's tolerance of selflessness compared to the usual human inclination to put self first thereby making the heart's love impure.

Whereas Centre House was an effective ballgame in the head, University of the Trees was a different ballgame in which the only loser could be the self. Having been trapped by love of others in a scheme of one's own making, there is no convenient escape when things get rough. For to shut off the heart would be to shut off oneself. Applying this philosophy or understanding to the dialogue between the head and the heart in every person who applies to join the nuclear marriage, forces that person to face the reality of their deepest image of themselves and to have it tested to the utmost. Centre House was a test of the ego, requiring all those who committed themselves to stay together, whereas University of the Trees was a test of the heart, requiring the ego to surrender to the heart or leave.

At Centre House one could always leave if it didn't work and go do it somewhere else. Everyone had the power to leave and to try again to achieve Nuclear Evolution somewhere else in a different place, a different building, city or country. But at the University of the Trees there was no concept of a place because the trap was laid forever with no chink for the ego to wiggle out and go somewhere else. The task was, in short—achieve the result of group consciousness, or bust. The trap which forced people to face the reality of ego separation however was not a coercion but a willingness and a willfulness which came from the true being of each participant in response to ultimate pressure to change.

This sealing of the doorways of escape could be likened to the yoga of "neti neti", not this, not that. But this negative philosophy of not this or not that was polarized with its positive complementary feeling of yes this and yes that and yes everything, including the total hologram of life as the vision which has pressed us on even at times against our own personal will in order that we may surrender to the Cosmic Will. Many do not surrender willingly to the Cosmic Will, but in its infinite design, this surrender on a higher level is programmed in the nucleus of every living organism, since it is ultimately surrender to one's vaster Self. Prodding us, not only from behind but in every inescapable direction, this fierce and ruthless Cosmic Will has no other purpose than to make us see ourself as we really are, with all our hangups, negativities and positive essence love. This dynamic love is what distinguishes the prototype group at the University of the Trees. To break through to this ruthlessness with self is the surrender to the whole which, once given, either in defeat or triumph over ego, makes the marriage of one soul to another divine. This surrender may seem like a scare ride at Disneyland, but when you get off the roller coaster, you are so relieved to get off the wheel of life that no fears can destroy the love that has brought you through to the glorious end.

What makes you go into it in the first place? Your true nature insists on Reality and has the faith, the confidence that in giving yourself selflessly, God will not let you down and will come rushing to meet you once the heart is pure and will embrace you in divine love, in the enlightening enveloping experience of the nonseparated whole which is to be found in the heart of everyone who will risk being the whole without little chinks of doubt or reservations. All these struggles of the ego, sitting on the throne of the head ruling over its selfish domain, are conquered once it admits that the sovereignty of the heart is superior. Then the love for a love object, or the love of others and what they can give to us, or the love which expects confirmation or reward, is totally transformed into that love which falls in love with love itself and all its myriad manifestations. Such a lover is not concerned with the details of its service or how it will please the loved one because the love itself is the reward and the pleasure, which can only be given on a higher level and from a pure heart. Once achieved, this state can never be taken away or hurt or diminished and that is the trap—that there is nothing else to do or to wish for, to contemplate or to know. This state is the coming to rest of all searching—the knowing that there is no other state desired, and that the stillness of the heart is the eternal peace to which all activities of creation return.

One finds that God, having created the universe, has to live with it as Himself with all its negativity and faults and possibilities for hazardous happenings. All these are seen as disturbances churning the heart the way you churn milk in order to get the golden butter. When the heart churns it is Nature's way of refining consciousness, its way of bringing that sense of inner conviction we call faith, thus making the being pure and eventually producing the golden aura that identifies with no shape or form. Like the golden butter, the heart's love sets solid into whatever shape or form it finds and is once again at rest and secure; it does not want to go anywhere or do anything because it is content. But when it melts, the love runs to the lowest, most humble levels and feels compassion for those whose hearts are still churning. The melted heart knows that the subjective feeling of churning in each individual undergoing refinement is not real except to the egocentric intelligence that refuses to surrender to its real Self.

Between the universe of the head at Centre House and the universe of the heart at University of the Trees, I became more ruthless with myself. This experience was one of compassion. Knowing that there is no escape from love, one might as well go into it fully and surrender to it. Like the doctor who has to hold you down and cut you open in order to cure you if there is no anaesthetic, this compassionate ruthlessness does not care how much people yell. It is only concerned with the operation of cutting away an obstruction and leaving the patient whole. This was summed up so simply by Christ and so ruthlessly when he made the statement, "It is better to pluck out thy right eye and cast it on the rubbish heap rather than let it lead you away from real love." The realization of this saying is not an analogy or a metaphor but a spiritual law applying to the soul, the heart, the mind and the body equally. Since we cannot kill the patient in the attempt to remove the obstruction, compassion with ruthlessness is essential to the success of the operation.

This realization that I had to go the whole hog was the equivalent of another one many years before when I sat under the Bodhi Tree where Buddha had sat 2,500 years before and resolved within myself an act of spiritual suicide—that I would not get up therefrom in my meditation until God enlightened me, and if necessary I would die in that spot. That meditation had to be for real. I had set myself a trap of taking that vow, the consequences of which I knew not, since I could not be sure that the pilgrims would feed me or know what I was doing. I looked around at the few pilgrims who were left praying in their evening devotions as the night began to get colder and in a little while I was entirely alone outside the temple. All the beggars who lived by taking alms had gone. I was alone under the night sky and began to meditate. Suddenly my mind flashed back twenty-one years before when I was a boy in my twelfth year. I had gone up to the altar in the parish church after the service was over when everyone else had gone home, and I had asked God to prove his existence by striking me dead. I had seen the long sorrowful faces of the clergy carrying golden crosses up and down the church aisles and wondered what kind of God could have such a bunch of miserable people looking after his affairs on earth. So I resolved to stay after the service and find out if God were real or not. After everyone had gone home and the church was locked, I came out from my hiding place, went up to the altar and knelt before it in the forbidden place, the Holy of Holies. I took hold of the altar cloth and said, "Now God, if you are really there, strike me dead to prove it." I was scared. If God were true, then I would be burnt to cinders on the spot, and I waited for the bolt of lightning to strike me. But nothing happened and I felt a huge sense of relief as I realized I was going to be all right. Then a great laugh seemed to come from inside and outside my head and to echo around the empty church, and a voice spoke to me like a kindly person talking inside my own head. I knew it was the voice of God, but I could not be sure God had a real voice, so I thought it might be some illusion of my own mind. The voice said, "My child, you think you can get rid of me so quickly? Just because you think I am not there doesn't mean I am not there."

I did not see at the time that if God was thus all-powerful, then to challenge him to manifest his power was an ego trip demanding special personal treatment from the Cosmos. I would have to go through many experiences first before I could know God directly. And I spent many years in search of something I could not even put a name on. I was looking for a purpose in life beyond the words and scriptures and things we are supposed to do and ought to do which others tell us. In the same way that we fall in love on the earth, I wanted to fall in love with whatever would make me feel a never-dying glow that did not depend on others. I wanted that desire, that glow of life to come from within. And unless I got this experience, whatever it was, I would feel completely lost and aimless, living a life without passion, a life that was like a living death. So now I had come again full circle to seek God, the absolute Self, in this holy spot beneath the Bodhi Tree and, if necessary, I was willing once again to put my life on the line for it. But it was different this time. I had no other purpose than to know Reality, and I was making no demands upon God. In fact, my decision to remain there came after I sat down to meditate, and was quite unplanned. I just did not want to rise from that place unless that love pierced my heart. I was meditating with the whole of my being and the whole of my consciousness. I began to meditate as if it were God meditating upon God and, within the space of several hours, about the time of dawn, I heard God's mighty voice in my own brain supplying the energy to open all the stops. Not only was this sound within my brain, but the whole universe was roaring around me like a great blast of divine power. God had come to visit in awesome fashion because at that time I wanted nothing else and my mind was single. God came with power because my God was a God of power at that time, but He humbled me by forbidding me to use the power. God had other plans in areas of the heart that I did not know at that time. He was also God of love, and the same ruthless dedication to the God of love would be required of me. That God of love would only truly test my heart and my meditation in the real world of people and in my compassion for

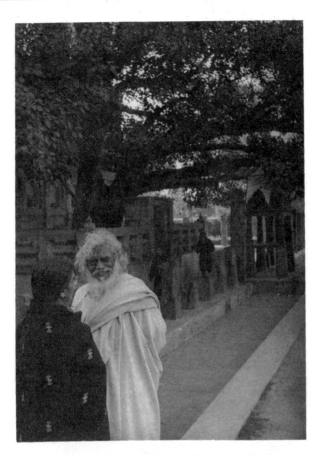

Photograph taken by the author at the Bo Tree where Buddha
was enlightened 2,500 years ago. The Holy Man traveled
with the author all over India.

their weakness and impotence. Many years passed before my surrender
to God's love would become as ruthless as my surrender to His power.
To be able to judge myself and my capacity to love as if I were judged
by God for every judgement I made regarding the lack of love in
others, was a heart-rending exercise which could not be escaped if I
were to become ONE with pure love. I had to learn to love when I did
not like, and I had to learn that there was no need to like in order to
love and no need to forgive others' weaknesses in order to love. Love
could not be rationalized, rationed or constrained by limits. Love was
ruthless with itself in order to be compassionate. But I knew that love

does not compromise with truth even to the destruction of the world. Love is greater than the creation because all that is manifest is only an effect, an expression of love. If this were true then any expression of love was my self, and I could not compromise with it without compromising myself. This is why I call love a trap, because there is no power greater than love. And therefore love is imprisoned glory within itself. To remove all obstacles to release this imprisoned glory is the limitless, ruthless and eternal way of life and became my own way since I saw clearly that this was the Cosmic Purpose of all incarnation in matter.

This was the difference between my motives at Centre House and here at University of the Trees. At Centre House my motives were poised between power and love mixed in the search for some kind of nonsentimental, nonromantic Grace which could transform not only man and society but the very physical creation itself as an expression of love. Arriving at Boulder Creek with no desires other than to meditate on that love which raises all to great heights, I resolved to find the tallest redwood tree and to meditate under it for guidance. Having found one that germinated its seed 500 years before Christ was born, roughly about the same time that Buddha was enlightened, I found myself facing the prospect of a new love. That love which grew the redwood tree through countless years of drought, fire and hazardous existence was asking me to plant the roots of my experience into manifested form and to send its branches high into the treetops of heaven. It was another experiment in the growth and evolution of human beings, but this time not caring whether it succeeded or not, not caring for any rewards from people, from the world or even from God, but merely to express that remorseless and endless cosmic fire burning in the heart and searing the brain of all its rationalizations. To carry on regardless of who came or who went or what it cost in time or expense, to press forward into the nucleus of every being who could tolerate such fierce love, and to let those who closed off from it compromise themselves and build their own trap was my goal. For consciousness must be ever free and limitless as love is, and everyone has the divine right to love or not to love, to open or to close their heart, to open or to close their mind, to advance or retreat along evolution's way. Sitting in the heart there is the universal government which will bring them ultimately to that state of love which cannot compromise with itself. Only in that kind of love was the universe created, and only in that kind of love can it be changed and re-created. Hence there is freedom in love in its lower levels of expression—to love or not to love. But in its highest expression there is no choice and no escape and no other destiny but to love, whatever the consequences and regardless of all limitation. Thus in oneness with the Cosmos there is no separate will or freedom to reject or accept the universe or any part of it around us. If we love enough, it is all one, an expression of our own love, the communication of our own divinity, from which it is impossible to separate any concept of self. When no self is there standing between God and man, only love exists and there is no one left to qualify it or to separate it from God's love and any other kind of love, human or cosmic. This experience in the heart of the nucleus of the cosmic fire becomes the altar on which the Phoenix rises out of its own ashes, constantly burning away its self-image so that the new image of the future may, like the Tao, work through it and cause the movement from within.

This self-motivated change to refine our consciousness of its old patterns of power and obsessions with self-love is the ultimate doorway to the kind of love which I call group consciousness. And Creative Conflict is the churning of the heart in its battle with the head. The Phoenix does not come to make things nice. He has just come from playing with fire and the flames are still hot from that cosmic event. Therefore those who are not ready should best keep their distance. Those who are ready to consume their ego and selfishness and reach for the ultimate love need have no fear, as this fire cannot touch them except to purify. At Centre House I worked out the method with real live people to see if this love was real for human beings or whether it was too much love. At University of the Trees we are still proving whether our own love is selfless enough to withstand the cosmic fire in the furnace of the heart, knowing that there is really no other alternative but to burn through to the pure heart of existence. Each one knows that feeling of wanting to run away but also recognizing that there is nowhere to run, and that to make the evolutionary leap into the divine life must be for real and not in philosophy, or scriptures, books or vanity.

The cosmic egg has cracked and is about to shatter its contents upon an unprepared world. Who will be ready to receive more love than they can imagine? Who will be ready to receive too much love, more than they can handle? Who will be pure enough to stand naked in mind and soul and body for that awesome gaze of our True Self? The gaze is full of compassion and it can see only what is pure, for *it* is pure. It is Pure Consciousness. In order to know ourself and to see ourself as we really are, we too must be ready to see pure. This is the purpose of the churning and refining of head and heart which is the work at University of the Trees and the purpose of Creative Conflict methods. The work is eternal. It is not a two-week exposition of fine behavior, loving caresses and beaming smiles. It is the joy of letting go the burden of having to be anything else than what we truly are. The work of conquering oneself is not easy and anyone who promises that it is has not realized that it is easier to conquer the whole world than to conquer oneself. Oneself can only be conquered by love, but the Self is God who surrenders Himself to those who fall in love with Love. For God to surrender to a human sounds bizarre and unlikely for so mighty a Being. But the fact is that God is very humble and surrenders Himself every day, even to those who cannot see Him, in the bestowal of His gift of consciousness. Consciousness is divine love surrendering to itself, discovering its own glory reflected in the eyes and splendor of all creatures. This is a simple fact, but not so simple to see until the heart is pure. We can understand then with Christ when he said, "Blessed are the pure in heart, for they shall see God."

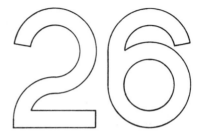

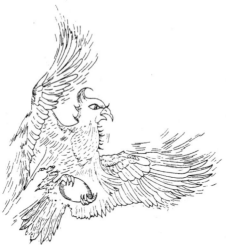

A NEW
METHOD OF
LEARNING

   Much of human disease, both individual and social results from early childhood traumas which block us at the spiritual levels of consciousness long before any physical manifestation appears in later life. The stunting of our growth and psychic development not only inhibits our childhood and our subsequent growth into mature citizens but prevents us from achieving direct perception of the obvious. Education is our most profitable investment in both time and money because knowledge, know-how and wisdom save us countless billions in expense and generate countless more billions in wealth. But the sad story today is that our society is educated not for wealth and abundance but for exploitation. We are taught how to exploit Nature, how to exploit the public and the community with soulless technologies like advertising, legal manipulations, and business practices that serve self at the expense of others. The technical know-how of medicine and science often gets turned into gross professionalism or sophisticated methods of warfare. Our educational process does not teach us *how to learn,* but teaches us only how to acquire specific information. This information approach has led to a kind of madness where we create events happening around us in our society which are absolutely horrendous and insane yet appear normal to most individuals.

Let us take for example a pretty harmless-sounding development of our political and military thinking to illustrate the low level of thinking that occurs normally in our society—a recent proposal to insure our future security by stockpiling oil in salt domes under the earth. This scheme is to import large supplies of oil (one billion barrels) by 1985. Even at today's price of fourteen to fifteen dollars per barrel, we shall pay to the Arabs over fifteen billion dollars, plus the taxpayers will have to pay several billion dollars more for contractors to dissolve the salt domes and make room for the oil.

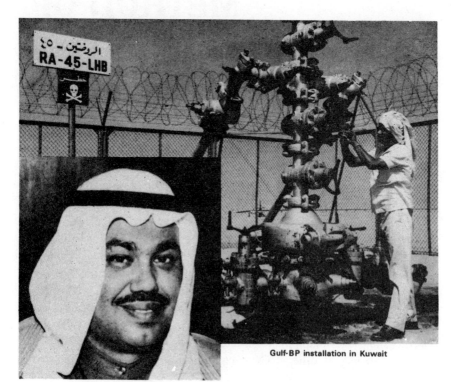

Gulf-BP installation in Kuwait

Oil minister Abdel Al Kazimi

But to top that, taxpayers will also have to pay an added $1.50 per barrel per year for storage costs which will amount to one and one-half billion dollars per annum on our tax bill. The real madness is that the storage charges alone, to say nothing of the other expenditures, would more than pay for all the research needed to liquidate our enormous coal reserves into oil residues, natural coal gas and other hydrocarbons on which we can run our automobiles and energy-hungry economy. But the dull minds that run our country, being only half-awake, do not realize that they are being led into the most expensive kind of security which is only staving off the ill-fated date when they will be forced to become independent of the price-gouging tactics of other nations. The unaware citizen thinks, "For only eight dollars a year per person for storage costs, I can always feel secure that I shall have gasoline for my automobile." He feels and thinks no further than his own gas tank!

This isolated example alone would not be so serious if it were not representative of a hundred other similar piecemeal approaches to critical problems now under our noses, which we do not perceive because we do not see the madness or the consequences of spending one and one-half billion a year for an outdated technology to let oil sit in salt domes when we have or could have the technology to change over our entire economy to liquifying coal for the price of one year's rent on the salt domes. But could we get our politicians to spend one and one-half billion a year on research and development for coal while the powerful oil interests spend millions on lobbying for oil reserves and against any other kind of energy bill? It is the lobbyists' pocket-books which motivate this senseless form of security which they sell to the public as insurance for the future.

The cure for this kind of wasteful and mad thinking lies in our most important resource, the education of our children. We spend forty billion dollars per year on education, yet we are turning out children who cannot even read or write and who have little in their heads besides 20,000 hours of television-watching.

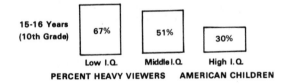

15-16 Years (10th Grade)

67% — Low I.Q.   51% — Middle I.Q.   30% — High I.Q.

PERCENT HEAVY VIEWERS   AMERICAN CHILDREN

While public outlay for education has increased in cost 450 percent since 1960, the quality of education has gone sharply down. In 1960 the per pupil cost was $397 per year and in 1978 the cost was $1,786, which is far beyond the inflation rate. During the same time average college entrance test scores tumbled fifty points and, in a number of state colleges, remedial math and remedial reading classes have become mandatory for one out of every four entering freshmen. Unless we have some drastic changes in our education the future is going to be frightening, since the students will have even less critical ability to discriminate the madness of political decisions than the public has now. Always the cry against alternative energy or changes in education is that the research is either unobtainable or too expensive, so we end up going an even more expensive and less effective way. In desperation we build terribly expensive nuclear reactors without really facing the costly danger involved. We throw away perfectly good textbooks before they are hardly used in order to buy the newest model, yet our children are doing worse academically than when they were using the old books.

Similarly, teaching loads have lessened over the past thirteen years, but the quality of teaching has also lessened. For example, more than one in three applicants for teaching posts in the Dallas, Texas public school system flunked a basic mental ability test, and a sample of teachers who were hired the previous year did even worse. Nearly one-half of the already hired teachers failed the minimum standards! From grade school through university level, public standards have gone down. At the same time a cross section of students at a private Dallas high school outperformed both teacher groups in the same exam.

Why is it that with all our sophisticated equipment for education that one out of every eight of all seventeen year-olds in the US are functionally illiterate, which means they are unable to read a newspaper, fill out a job application form or calculate change in the supermarket? And yet they receive high school diplomas! That's thirteen percent for a country as affluent as the United States, noted at one time for having the most widely educated populace in the world.

It is only because our society is unfortunately governed by social apathy and mediocrity that people continue to listen to the platitudes issued by politicians and educators about the need for a complete overhaul of our educational system and still do nothing about it. We hear over and over again in every radio show, daily newspaper, magazine or debate on education, that our young people are not getting the type of education that fits their entry into the world they live in. By

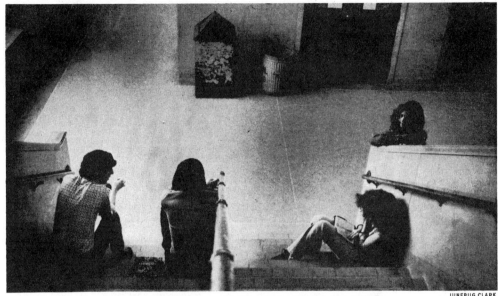

Students killing time at Detroit's overcrowded Cass High School.

JUNEBUG CLARK

contrast, the entire population in Cuba was brought from a point of eighty percent illiteracy to ninety percent literacy in a matter of just a few years by a concentrated program of social interest where children and high school students went into the fields and taught adults reading while the adults taught the children the basic skills of farming and trading. The US is dangerously resting on its laurels, unmotivated to make further strides forward. In several departments of education and skill where the US was once leading the world, it now ranks below many other West European and communist nations.

The root cause of our inertia, our inefficiency and our lack of foresight is that the public is not really interested in becoming fully developed in its potential or in becoming totally responsible for the consequences of its actions. Other countries have been motivated to change by necessity, but the US does not yet feel that necessity to take another step. Parents on the whole are interested in personal pleasure and not interested in taking an active part in their own evolution or in their children's evolution. They would rather leave the education of their children to the teachers and the state legislators and leave the economic problems to the lobbyists and the politicians.

Occasionally we hear a few voices crying from people who do care about the way modern civilization is going, that something urgent must be done to stop the boredom and dissatisfaction of our students in schools. Today it is not even the curriculum or the relevance of the materials that is the major problem in some cities. At least twenty-five percent of students in many public schools don't even come to classes no matter what courses are offered. The situation has become so ridiculous that some schools are offering free hamburgers, t-shirts, and cash prizes donated by local merchants to lure and bribe the kids back to class. Obviously nothing can be taught in school if the student is not there, but neither can anything be taught if the student is there yet feels there is no point in learning the skills being offered in geography, history, mathematics or reading. Certainly if students cannot read by the time they leave school there is not much hope that they will be able to understand this book or even read any of the inspirational and elevating philosophies of life given to the world from our past.

Some students of today feel that there is nothing in the books of the past that has any real answers for the problems of today. Somehow they know that those who read the Bible, who read all the great minds of past times, are still unable to help the world find its roots in the bizarre reality of these modern times. They feel the instruction books of the New Age have not yet been written, that nothing relevant to their own inner experience is available. Just as there were no books written on how to get to the moon back in the time of Christ, Moses or Buddha, or even how to fly an airplane, so we now have no books that go beyond the analogies and metaphors of ancient language to give us exact knowledge of the structure of human consciousness. Few teachers or students are offered definite materials within any present traditional system which are designed specifically to help them discover who they are. If we look through the great resource books such as the Bible and even the great commentaries of the Bhagavad-Gita and Vedanta, we find there is nothing specific about the nature of conscious- ness nor any instructions on how we can set up an experimental school for communicating with any accuracy a complete concept, image or model of what man is or what he is to become. Neither Christians, Moslems, Buddhists, capitalists, communists nor modern scientists succeed in bringing about the complete understanding of man or in organizing a loving society of mankind. They seem to have allegories, scriptures and words-a-plenty but not the skills; ideals-a-plenty but not the will; scholars-a-plenty but not the wisdom. And our students, from all walks of life, sense this deeper reality.

The real problem is not just one of finding well-educated teachers or concerned citizens or just going "back to basics", but a problem in improving communication between human beings. Children cannot communicate with their parents, parents cannot communicate with each other, and teachers cannot communicate the real need they see to parents. Hence our educational system, the most expensive in the world, is only capable of bringing up sleepwalkers who walk around society believing that they are awake, when in fact they know of no other levels of consciousness than their own. Our education today has no answers and our legislators are barren of any solutions because they themselves are ninety percent of the problem. Like politicians in the democracy of ancient Greece, they would rather banish or commit a Socrates to death than have their youths' minds polluted with truth. The truth of our education is clear. In spite of its billions, its vast concrete physical facilities and its beautiful expensive textbooks, our education is helpless to teach even the simplest knowledge of the three R's to all its students, let alone to teach them the crucial knowledge about other levels of consciousness and the communication which takes place between them—the only kind of knowledge that can bring peace to this world. Our educators do not even know how we form concepts or store knowledge in our memory, let alone know how to teach the children to think for themselves. Many well-meaning teachers have tried their best to be effective in what they knew but haven't been able to succeed. They have been hampered by more and more rules, state regulations and red tape. The fact is that educators have *talked about* the concept of educating the whole child and helping children to share their inner worlds for the past thirty years, but it has not been done. The excuses are that there has never been enough time, money or real know-how. This sorry state, resulting primarily from apathy and false priorities, can only be corrected if we now attempt to validate that the learning process itself can be greatly enhanced by an understanding of the nuclear process of evolution, the human chakra functions and how they get communicated internally and between people. This understanding will bring an unblocking of the myopia which has plagued mankind for thousands of years. Unblocking the psychic channels between the teacher and the student, the parent and the student, the parent and the teacher, will result in the healing of social stress and frustration, individual and social insecurity, and this is the most important resource we can invest in today. The life-energy resource of our consciousness is far more impotant than our automobiles, our fuel energy or our space stations, for the blockages in our consciousness are the main causes of our madness and our disease—the cause of insecurity in every stratum of society.

In the same way we plunk the storage of oil into salt domes to achieve security of an energy supply, so do we buy a temporary release from our fear of the future by spending more and more money on the education of our children without questioning the quality of the teaching. The forty billion dollars spent on education to provide children with palaces for schools, with every expensive educational gadget such as movie projectors, audio-visual displays, and millions of dollars worth of new textbooks which are sent to the paper shredders every few years to make room for more wasted dollars, makes for lazy-mindedness, where everything is provided and no self-effort is required. All of this shows that we do not understand that it is not books or buildings, fancy desks or movies or money that educate us.

Socrates insisted that such learning or presentation of information is not true knowledge and that we are little better off as human beings by acquiring it. As one of the greatest teachers ever, Socrates taught on street corners and always had interested youths with questioning minds gathering round him. He would excite the students by pulling truth out of them, not by putting information in.

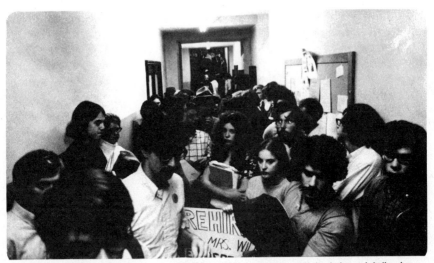

Today's teaching methods, for the most part, bore students, unlike the more stimulating and challenging Socratic method.

The Socratic view is proved conclusively today when we look at the poor results of our modern school system. But our answer to our educational problem as a society is to throw more billions of dollars down the rat hole in the belief that dollars will do the trick. It is far better to take children to a bare field, put up a wigwam and teach them how to *think* about the world they live in and how to perceive directly into the heart of Nature around them, for in doing this they will be able to write their own textbooks instead of becoming half-educated morons who know some information but nothing significant about life or their own evolution. Yet we continue to pay for school facilities because the budgets which are spent on education *must be spent* in order to get a bigger budget next year. Hence, the whole operation becomes a farce backed by political considerations, when the main problem is ignored in favor of a temporary palliative.

That main challenge is the teaching of our teachers the nature of consciousness. Judging by the results of our children's performance when they become adults, our teachers are becoming the laughing-stock of society, for they themselves continue to call for more money, more facilities and more materials to compensate for their own inability to reach the children or deal with difficult administrations, rules and parents.

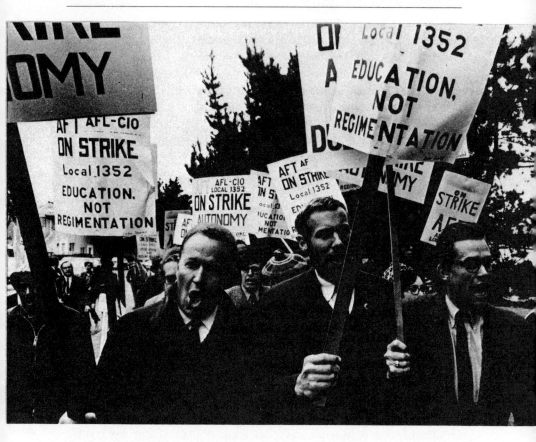

Politicians, desiring more votes, are only too willing to comply with
more dollars. The real valid cry of today's teacher is that classroom
size is much too big for effective teaching, and all the red tape cuts
down real teaching time. Public moneys would be better spent in
simplifying and creating smaller classrooms as well as better educating
teachers. But even then, unless we know what to teach our teachers in
their training programs, we will not have rooted out the major cause of
today's poor education. Parents also acquiesce in today's foolish
educational policies out of a sense of guilt, knowing that all is not well
with their children and their attitudes to life, yet not knowing how to
make it any better or having the skill to cut through the political
machinery.

Neither parents nor teachers nor anyone else knows what to do with the violence that has now become a familiar part of our schools. The emotional disturbances besetting many youngsters today will have to be dealt with before anything can be effectively taught. These disturbances take a severe toll on teachers. According to some national statistics, what were scattered schoolhouse disturbances and pranks ten years ago are now standard disorder and serious violent crimes of crisis proportions. Since 1972, classroom murders have increased eighteen percent, rapes forty percent, robberies thirty-seven percent and physical assaults on teachers seventy-seven percent. In 1975, school property destruction surpassed 600 million dollars, and serious injury from physical assaults by students was reported by 70,000 teachers. In the inner city of Los Angeles, statistics reveal that more than one out of every four teachers have sustained physical assaults at school, not to mention the psychological wear and tear on teachers and children alike. If teachers got together and confessed their inability to cope with the situation, society would be forced to come up with some solutions.

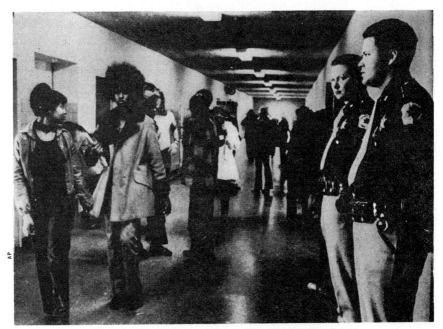

Guards watching students at violence-ridden Michigan High School.

But they are afraid to speak up. Teachers, like the politicians and the public, have not trained their minds to be clear-seeing and to cut through. They have mistaken information for knowledge and conventional thinking for wisdom. Fear of not knowing the answers and fear of speaking up is not part of a wise person. The essence of wisdom is to know what you do not know and to concentrate on that area, not to concentrate on the areas you do know and hope the other problems will go away. To be clear-seeing one has to actually *live* the knowledge, not just speak about it to the students. And students pick up a fear vibration as fast as animals do. If there is any weak link in a teacher, any place he has never looked, any part of himself he does not know, the students will find it and play on it, just as toddlers outsmart their parents and manipulate them and even become dictators of the whole household. College professors learned a bitter lesson in the heat of the student revolution, when for the first time in this country, students roused themselves out of apathy and indifference and made the professors do likewise. Conventional teachers have only information and knowledge. They have no wisdom to offer their students. Without this wisdom of an inquiring mind, students become bored and disrespectful, for they see the teacher clearly for what he is, a mere parrot of others. In order to turn this around, we must begin thinking of straw huts and wigwams and put our attention on who is teaching, on what is taught, on relationships between people, not on palaces and dollars. To concentrate on the form and not the content is not only to become a spendthrift but a fool as well. Children should be taught how to spend less and efficiently use materials that are already available, instead of teaching them wastefulness so that they grow up to become wasters of time, money and life.

The example of wasted dollars on storage of oil is not only repeated in our wasteful and useless process of education, but is seen at every level of government funding. It is only a matter of time before the public becomes clear-seeing and angry at being so deceived by their leaders and angry at themselves for being so disinterested or naive and easily duped. The result may be that in their anger they will withhold the means by which the money-hungry schools can be maintained, and they will crumble into disuse, like large white elephants, littering the landscape. Hopefully the increasingly large expense required for maintaining and running such educational palaces will kill this type of education or at least cause the schemes of its advocates to be stillborn so that effective new learning methods may come to flourish.

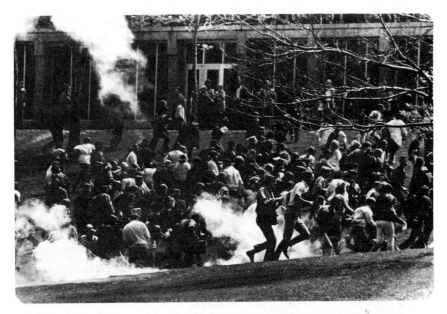

Even students felt the need for educational changes and rebelled against irrelevance of the expensive educational system. But society's answer was to use tear gas instead of encouraging self-governing educational communities.

The part that parents must play is to look at their own willingness to usher their children off to the palaces of learning in order to have a tax-paid babysitter and some peace. Parents must now gain a new angle of vision on the problem, rather than thinking that if they do not support this waste, they will have the children back in their hair. While praising everything to do with children, they have treated them as burdens, to be fobbed off to the television in the evenings and sent away to school during the days, only to return with the bewildering problems of drugs, drunkenness, teenage sex, vandalism, violence and completely uncontrollable behavior leading to unprecedented juvenile crime. Communication between parents and children is at an all-time low, in spite of our sophisticated communications technology and our sophisticated curriculums. Our education of today is education to fill the jails, psychiatric wards, and rest homes with depressed people, not an education to raise man to new perceptions of his destiny or fulfillment of his evolution.

Why is it that the old educational processes that seemed to work for previous generations no longer work? Parents are having to face the fact that there is something definitely missing in education now, because the negative results have become too glaring to be overlooked. But they do not always know what the missing factor is, since the same factor was missing in their own education. The closest equivalent in the traditional system for this missing ingredient is the division which universities call the "Humanities" or "Liberal Arts"—the study of philosophy, art, literature, music, history and all subjects which touch the human spirit. But there is no real educational equivalent of the Humanities or Liberal Arts during the early formative years of childhood, and even at the college level the Humanities are usually taught as factual knowledge. The "living" quality of the subject is totally missing. Why? Because the teachers themselves have never experienced or lived the essence of the subjects they teach. Most teachers are "head" people who are comfortable with thoughts but afraid of feelings. Consequently the living kernel of truth is rarely transmitted. Generation after generation of children pass through the educational system without ever discovering the pearl of great price—their own consciousness—or learning who they really are.

If men and women are to live together with a sense of community and peace there are specific things that the teacher, the child and the parent must do to achieve their discovery of who they are and how they are to be linked in consciousness with all fellowman. And this is where the new education takes a radical departure from the old. Education can no longer be confined to books and concepts and to lectures in which there is no interchange between teacher and student or lectures which convey only information without regard to the speaker's level of consciousness. Why should we listen even to information, much less to wisdom, from one who is not in his own being truly wise and has achieved little or no mastery over his own consciousness? And how can any teacher achieve such self-mastery if he cannot interact openly with other human beings to whom he is inextricably connected?

We can no longer make an artificial separation between the teacher behind the desk and the students out in the chairs as if the teacher were, by virtue of age alone, more evolved. A teacher is qualified to teach by having become more expert in his field, but in other respects he may (like parents) learn as much from young people as they learn from him. So the first step is for both teachers and parents to let go of their attachment to authority roles and to sacrifice pride in order to achieve dignity. In this way they gain the humility without which true education cannot occur. No student should submit to a teaching from one who lacks humility, and no teacher should bother to teach a student who has not the necessary receptivity. Therefore in the new education, there will be not just a knowing but a doing. Teacher and students alike will ask of themselves that they *manifest* their level of study by living it and becoming it. You may say that there is no such thing as embodying a subject like Physics. But our consciousness is working by the same identical laws of Nature that we find in the study of Physics. Every subject has hidden depths beneath the surface of its data, and there is no subject which does not raise for an inquiring mind the deep questions of the human race. Even practical vocational courses raise the questions of work and the blocks in human consciousness which make our work ineffective, burdensome and joyless, or make it light.

The word "meditation" traced back to its Sanskrit roots means "doing the wisdom". The new education in which we learn to work with wisdom, to live with wisdom, and to relate to one another with wisdom is meditation in action. *The Rise of the Phoenix* provides the essential first steps towards this self-realization. But a book is now obviously not enough; there must be a rapid proliferation of ideas and actions at the political, religious and scientific levels of our mentally-separated humanity to cause quick and effective transformation. An outline for a nuclear school must be set out so that we may now design individual schools which can supply the lack. The University of the Trees is itself such a model school for teachers and adults, and we are launching the practical training of students and young children who will be tomorrow's teachers. What are the provisions needed to insure that we do not get stuck like the communist social programs have done or become democratically moribund like the present competing capitalist interests? Our insurance is that we must be certain to keep focused on the aim of consciousness of Self, on constant awareness of our thought life as the cause of our ultimate grief or ultimate fulfillment. Unless this aim remains always in the foreground of any new educational system, society will become more and more fragmented by specialization and endless conflict.

Education as conceived by our present established academic institutions only succeeds within the specialization of skills required for vocational training or the teaching of professional skills and techniques. It does not equip us to live life happily or to understand how the urgent need for brotherhood, economic solvency and human unity can only be achieved through self-discovery. By "understanding" we do not mean the superficial study of external policy and culture from the viewpoint of the social sciences, but the awareness of human beings and understanding the nature of consciousness. The consciousness or awareness of a philosopher or scientist must realize that intense specialization in any narrow field kills before it is born that ultimate aim of all spiritual endeavor common to religious thinkers, creative artists or intuitive scientists—namely the direct discovery of the *life principle.*

To teach this life principle is to teach man how to know himself. The present social situation can be traced to the fact that we are being told to love one another as comrades and brothers by people who do not demonstrate love for others themselves, and who do not know their own weaknesses. It is certain that all men are brothers and that we are united with all by the very fact of Nature and the environment around us which none of us can escape. But what teacher in school or what system of education anywhere in the world helps our children see *why* we should look on other people as an integral part of ourselves or as brothers of the same family of man? What invisible force is now pushing human beings past their resistances towards an ultimate necessary unity with each other?

It is not enough to teach children the fact that we all do belong to the same species and then proceed to divide human beings up (as modern education does) into scientists, priests, artists, sportsmen, and other vocational titles. Even to teach that we are biologically the same species is not enough because there must be a conscious purpose for this unity if we are to really communicate and come together in new groups and communities at a much higher level of evolution. To manifest this joint activity and creative communication as human beings, we have to realize that some purpose for integrating our knowledge and experience exists. Community cannot happen without a purpose or take place in a void, nor can it happen in an abstract idealistic way. Therefore the new education we have called a "school of wisdom" must offer wholistic knowledge which is integrated with life's purpose and not pigeonholed into compartments. To evolve a method of resolving the professional conflict and synthesizing the various separate branches of knowledge such as we find in religion, science, philosophy, politics, etc., is the purpose of the new education.

Mankind has expressed new potential in art, science, philosophy, psychology, religion, developing from elementary ideas to the very sophisticated and academic. In some societies, in the early development of mankind, the creative activity of tool-making and inventiveness closely related to self-knowledge and therefore their religion and science nurtured each other. But our society today and the skills we need to accumulate are highly specialized because of the greater quantitative mass of knowledge available. This accumulation must be dealt with by the teacher and the student through *synthesis* rather than all the different specializations traveling their own separate roads.

Democracy was invented and shaped by all the resources of Greek art, philosophy, science and religion acting together to discover a new way. In the same way the Tao is now working through the nucleus of life to encourage a renewal of integrated activity and thereby make learning wholistic. Centers of wholistic healing are emerging but they are not enough to unite the fragmentation of society and its fractured life forces. We need also centers of wholisitic learning as centers of prevention against the narrow disease of specialization, which splits our inner emotional life and our many-faceted being from the narrow specialized jobs we perform.

Our teachers right now continue to produce more students like themselves, but our challenge as creative teachers will be to bring our own uniqueness forth from the nuclear center of our being and then to

do the same for our children, giving them an uncompromising honesty
to face themselves and discover who they are. It will be a wholistic

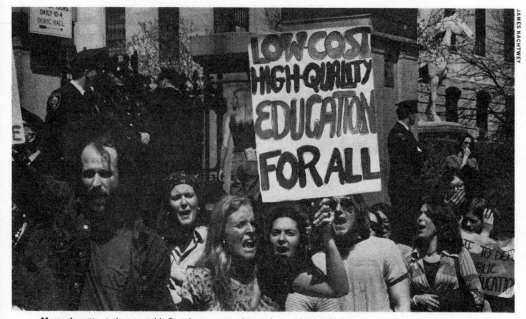

Massachusetts students outside Statehouse protesting against cutbacks. Both teachers and students put dispropor-
tionately large amounts of their consciousness on the financial side of education.

method by which students work with teachers and parents in discovering
themselves and resolving inner conflicts creatively. When this refinement and expansion of awareness of self goes hand in hand with study
of "subjects", then dead knowledge comes alive and school no longer
seems remote from the real events that are happening in the "feeling
world" of every child.

A new breakthrough is imminent because the gap between the
knower and the field of knowledge is closing. The relationship and
synthesis between science and religion, philosophy and the universal
life-force in man, is just being discovered in all its rainbow colors of the
one nucleus. Through Nuclear Evolution of the whole person an
overview of past human blindness is emerging which can be taught and

passed on in schools to free us all from our traditional habits of thought, *if* we are willing. Children are far more willing than the adults who are their teachers. If we adults have the honesty to recognize

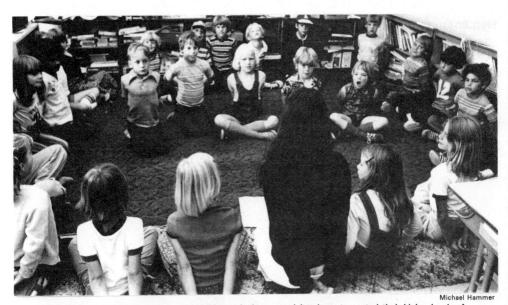

Michael Hammer

Their openness and willingness make children priceless material to learn to control their higher levels of awareness which our present educational system shuts off.

our own resistances, then we can have foresight as to how *not* to pass them on to our children.

In the early years the child learns by copying peers and adults and through parental training. Without love as the central theme of unity encouraging freedom of the spirit of inquiry, this copying of adult life and the existing status quo can be disastrous. In an earlier chapter we have shown how the counterculture was born and how a number of our young adults attempted to break free of this copying of their parents' cultural habits. If we first teach our children to think for themselves then later offer them education as specialists but in a wholistic approach to life, we will lead them to self-reliance and self-examination and healthy evolution of the species.

Self-examination is the most important development and growth we can teach another human being so long as we keep it from slipping into narcissism and self-obsession. A fulfilling work on the practical level of a community, a university, or a school which generates its own educational materials, supports itself in real economic activity as a proof of its social viability, and orders its affairs by self-rule, is the essence of our future organization of a social system. The resident student/faculty of the University of the Trees, working to create this kind of model, write their own books, edit them, typeset them, mock them up and market them. As common-owners of the University of the Trees Press, they support themselves economically while at the same time they practice self-government and evolve toward ever-increasing

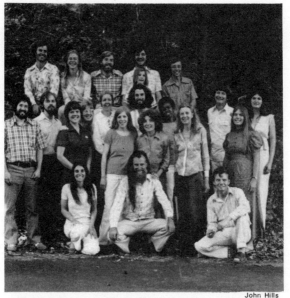

John Hills
Part of the resident student/faculty of the University of the Trees.

teamwork as a way of manifesting group consciousness in a live community situation. The offerings of an average university today do not show many courses in self-knowledge or self-government—one or two at the most. Nor do they show any real research being done into the nature of consciousness. This will not be true in a few years hence because it only needs one school, one model of *successful* concentration upon the dire need of society, for all to copy it and offer programs which penetrate to the heart of life. Yet as I said before, consciousness teachings are just as important in the classroom of younger children as they are in the university or as resource materials for adults, parents and teachers. Our catalog at the University of the Trees has as its underlying purpose self-discovery, direct perception of truth, and the attainment of living knowledge rather than "knowing about". There is no reason why the essence of these courses of instruction could not become regular courses in elementary and secondary schools providing there are enough teachers who know how to teach them. This is the whole problem in a nutshell and it is the familiar circular question of all education—who is going to teach the teachers? Obviously it is not possible for any one school, organization or person to do it alone and the University of the Trees can only hope to reach a small fraction of the population, even if we become expanded to the size of a major university. Therefore another way must now be found which can be adopted by all schools, to work from the inside out to bring out the hidden potentials within students from kindergarten through college, rather than trying to work by stuffing knowledge into them from outside-in.

The true meaning of the word *educare* "to bring out" is now well-known, but our culture does not yet know *how* to "bring it out". In this sense our culture is egocentric, because ego sucks life and love and experience *in*, rather than radiating them *out* from its true center. A new method of learning which penetrates this egocentricity of our Western culture is set out later in this chapter, based upon the full range of University of the Trees techniques of self-discovery. There are other new colleges cropping up here and there, mostly non-accredited, which recognize that self-discovery is the main purpose of a true university. But to convince all people—teachers, adults, children—that what will solve our deepest problems and prepare us for the future is self-discovery and that this is the original purpose of all great wisdom, is a most difficult and challenging task, because we are talking not about anything known but about the unknown. The secret to be found in the great wisdom of the world is the discovery that the kingdom of heaven within is another state of being. But we cannot come to this discovery through the words of another, no matter how great a teacher that other may be. We have gathered up the great teachings down through the ages but we have only absorbed them according to the degree of our self-knowledge, because our openness to the truth always depends on how much of our *Self* we are opening to. The realization of our Self in the ultimate organism of Nature is the revelation of our total potential, and this is what we are moving toward—this realization in which the words of the great teachers and thought development down through the ages suddenly make sense to us because we have a direct experience of that same state of being. So the combination of self-knowledge plus the accumulation of truth is what we call wisdom.

The problem in our modern educational systems is that wisdom cannot be taught but is something we can only pass on when we ourselves and our students become "ready" and open to hear it. The teaching of this "readiness" and the schooling of our teachers who will teach the teachers of the teachers becomes a most important problem and most important possibility at the same time. It is a problem when teachers do not recognize that humans have failed for centuries to express and pass on this essence of individuality which I call the nuclear experience of personality. It becomes a possibility when we recognize that this inner knowledge of the essential "being" is present already in the nucleus of each person waiting for complete self-realization to emerge. Whenever the student is ready, the new unmanifested potentials on the higher levels of brain development will emerge and find their exact and ultimate fulfillment. But there has to be a certain amount of desire for more awareness and a cultivated goodness of heart before this knowledge can be recognized. This is the readiness that is called for and which has been needed for centuries.

A SCHOOL OF WISDOM FOR A NEW SOCIETY

The study materials for this next step for re-educating our teachers can now be presented to those who are ready to educate along new lines. These new materials, methods and organization needed in the schools are a jumping-off ground for the exploration of inner space where we become familiar with exploration in many diverse fields such as proportional science based on Nature, creative literature, character typology, levels of communication, and higher states of consciousness, integrating them all together as a whole with the Self at the center.

It is impossible to read any good piece of literature without meeting religious, political, philosophical or scientific questions. Thus a scripture or a play by Shakespeare or a scientific theory can be the launching pad for exploration of many levels of consciousness. This integrative education is the purpose of my book on awareness games, *Conduct Your Own Awareness Sessions,* now rewritten as *Exploring Inner Space,* a space journey for all ages,* and of course the purpose of all my other more specialized books on the nature of the seven levels of consciousness.

Many of us who have taught young people have seen the joyful look of recognition which comes when something in one specialized field links up intelligibly with something in another field. This kind of insight is usually a rare event occurring by pure chance in modern schools today. Imagine the great potential if this enthusiasm and joyous recognition could be nurtured in every lesson in every classroom because the teachers themselves are aware of the wholistic effect of the teachings on consciousness! We have seen this wonderful kind of learning experience develop in public school classrooms that use our materials on consciousness training for children, so it is not just a dream but demonstrated fact. Once we understand that this learning process works directly with the mechanism of concept formation and applies to any subject, then we begin to perceive our different types of communication within the total environment around us. In other words, the quality of our consciousness will determine whether we communicate grossly or subtly with Nature and with other people and even with ourselves.

---

* Published originally by New American Library, Signet Classics, in 1970. Rewritten and republished as *Exploring Inner Space, Awareness Games For All Ages,* University of the Trees Press, 1978. This book sets out a new method of education for adults and children.

832

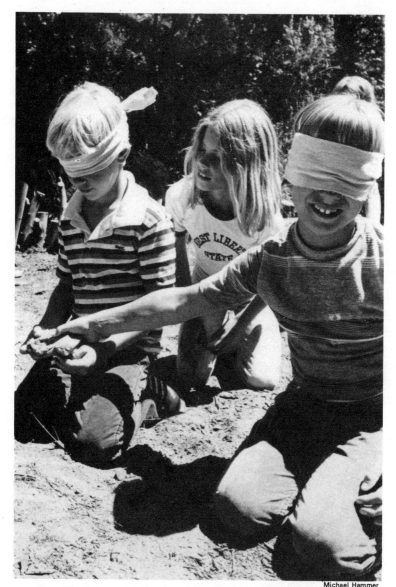

Michael Hammer

Increasing one's awareness brings children a joy of discovery of their worlds, themselves and their environment.

Our methods have been tried in many schools throughout the country and in depth in several public schools with emphasis on original meditation and centering techniques specially designed for the child's awareness. These techniques enable children to go beyond their own concept-making process so that they begin to discover how intuition and insight work. They begin to realize that the essence of learning and even of life is learning to learn, for this alone can awaken the sleeping consciousness and bring life into sharp focus so that everything is experienced more acutely, more clearly and more excitingly. When our consciousness is awakened in this way, we are stronger and more centered, less likely to let circumstances or other people disturb us or dominate us or make us doubt. The key to this inner awakening is in capturing the child's imagination with enthusiasm and, through our own love, permitting his love to flow. We use words, symbols, images and lessons in a new way that opens each child's own inner recognition. Through the use of awareness games that activate every level of consciousness and by perfecting inner listening, we capture the full attention of the being so that the child actually teaches himself through his own intense involvement in the experiential process. After centering and expanding their awareness we then teach children how to extend their consciousness to include the inner worlds of each other.

The techniques of creative communication and Creative Conflict hinge upon this ability to get into others' inner worlds and to feel compassion even while seeing the truth of a situation which emerges from the dynamic energy of group feedback. In other words, because reality is conditioned by each child who is perceiving, the classroom can reach a new level of reality and a nearness to truth by virtue of its pooled perceptions. At the same time, there must be an ability to feel with each person's inner reality or there will be no group heart feeling of togetherness, but only a collection of individuals. In this way a child can learn how to test what he perceives in relation to what others perceive and to appreciate that the other group members are a loving mirror in which he can see himself and his social relationships as they really are. The whole idea of creative communication and Creative Conflict methods is to be able to develop inner listening to the workings of our own mind and to be aware of our thought process as

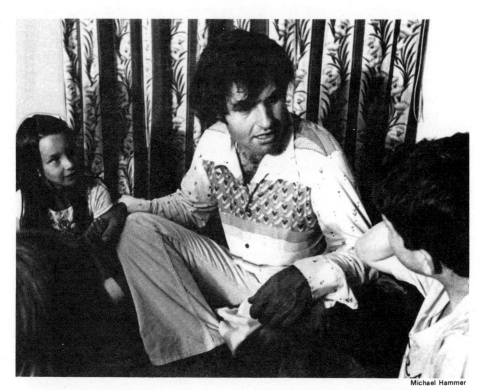

Michael Hammer

Using Creative Conflict adults can learn to communicate with their children, giving both an equal say in the search for truth.

we think, talk, behave and act out in the social drama of life. We become aware that such listening is of a totally different order from just living in our own minds, or just hearing words, and we go beyond egocentric listening. Then we can begin to recognize different levels of consciousness in ourselves and in others, and the study of Nuclear Evolution is revealed as our own inner discovery.

For this kind of inner awakening to occur, the teacher must have the full attention of the student. Effective communication can occur in depth only when the body is peaceful, not restless, when the mind is poised and awake, not drowsy or hopping from thought to thought, and only when the heart is open and ready to learn. The techniques for quickly centering the child or the classroom and penetrating through the usual inner and outer pandemonium, are available in our book

Meditating With Children*. Even in our present school system, many superintendents of school districts and teachers both at the elementary and secondary levels have begun to use these meditation techniques effectively to quiet the classroom enough to teach the children the basic skills of reading, writing and arithmetic. These methods have proved effective with every type of child, from the retarded to the gifted, when modified to their specific needs. It is obvious that however

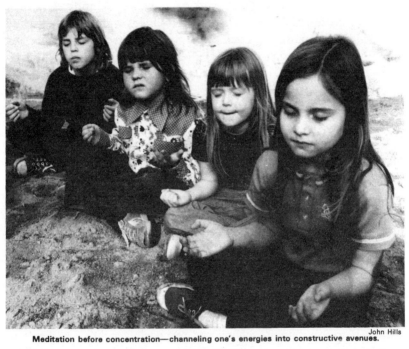

John Hills

Meditation before concentration—channeling one's energies into constructive avenues.

much the teacher knows, it is impossible to teach until the class atmosphere has settled down and there is quiet and willingness to listen. So meditation and centering are the foundation of our new method of learning, while creative communication skills and Creative

---

* *Meditating With Children: The Art of Concentration and Centering*, by Deborah Rozman, Ph.D., University of the Trees Press.

Conflict techniques* along with awareness exercises that develop all
the levels of consciousness are the structure around which all subjects
can be taught and brought into a wholistic experience.

THE SCHOOL AS A NUCLEUS

The nuclear school that uses these new methods of learning will be
successful in transforming our society even in a brief time if we have
the parent, teacher and child working together to bring a nuclear
family feeling to our society. The family feeling is what makes the child
feel healthy and nurtured. Lack of the protective feeling of family and
family nurturing is what is causing the present rapid emotional disintegration and confusion in our social life. The nuclear family of the
New Age is not a blood family, but provides the same feeling of close
family ties and is founded on a spiritual bond. A school should be like
a nuclear family with everyone evolving together. Each child must be
able to freely express his or her real feelings and thoughts in confidence
that he or she will not be rejected. The present school system and the
present family relationships and business relationships, all of which
make up the fabric of our society, teach one to hide or polish one's
thoughts and feelings into certain acceptable patterns and clichés
thereby creating a sophisticated mask under which problems teem and
seethe and get repressed. This mask separates the nuclear being from
its manifestation in society. The nuclear school and family is an
unmasking process, whereas modern education and family have become
a masking process to learn the skills of covering up reality rather than
the skills of opening up and being whole. So the nuclear approach to
society is to join family, school, and responsible political self-rule to
constitute a spiritual method of realizing our full potentials as individuals and as a nuclear group.

Human peace on earth cannot take place even within the blood

---

* Creative Conflict techniques are given in *Exploring Inner Space* and in *The Golden Egg*.

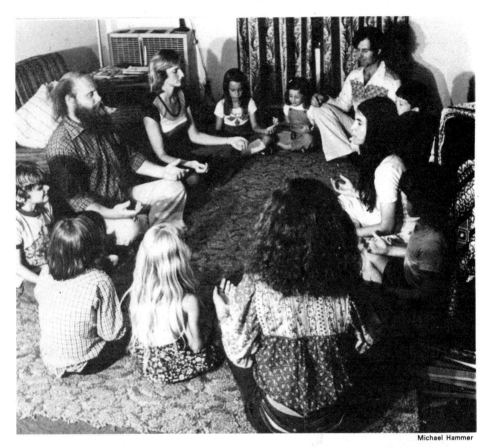

Michael Hammer

Creative Conflict unites families in a way that nothing else can. The uniting force is the love that develops from meaningful communication.

family unless greater depth of communication takes place on higher levels of consciousness than at present. This communication must be demonstrated and achieved between parent, teacher and child before there will be any fundamental change in society. The divorce rate and the state of the world are merely indicators of why a new type of education that teaches essential communication skills is urgent. They are indicators, not causes, but if we heal the causes, these indicators will change also. The causes began many hundreds of years back in history, through man's limited image of himself and his ignorance of his own nature. All human behavior depends upon our image of ourself, our image of our limitations and potentialities. The images we hold of ourselves color how we image others and limit others. Therefore we cannot discover our full potential until we let go of our limiting self-images and become totally open to more possibilities. But this openness is hard to attain because it is also an openness of the heart which requires the cultivation of love and the ability to give and take honest feedback.

The fact that all people grow to adulthood with similar insecurities, conflicts and limited self-images makes us wonder why these human problems persist through the millennia and why we have been unable to awaken enough to do something earlier. We are still tied to the biological family instead of forming into larger families whose bonds are spiritual rather than physical. Many utopian communities have failed because their bonds of spirituality were too abstract and did not reach down into the fundaments of human nature. So their children left the communities to find out what the real world was about and to find out more about themselves. The new community has to provide for this breadth of experience by activating all seven levels of consciousness in its members. And it is this wholistic way of living that I mean when I use the word spiritual. How can we break through the limitations of the biological family, the foundation of our social structure? The answer is to expand our love and trust of others.

No one would want to supplant the couple, since the love between a man and a woman is one of the beautiful experiences of life, but to expand that love to include others is even more fulfilling. The trouble with couples is that they have a concept of themselves as separate and they cut themselves off from others, which is not necessary to the building of their love bond and even robs it of a very important kind of cement. If we are couples but also more than couples, and if we are married to each other in a nuclear group that enhances and expands the family to a non-biological unit where the link between the members is spiritual, then there is a vibration of expansion rather than contraction, and that vibration of expansion is love. The contraction of a man and a woman into a private cocoon passes for love but in fact it is the opposite. I am not necessarily talking about a nuclear marriage in which sex is shared in a wider framework than the couple, though if the bond of trust should ever evolve to a certain point among genuinely spiritual people, even that would be possible because the motive would be correct. But that degree of sharing is not what I mean by "nuclear marriage". I mean that an expansive, loving vibration is contagious, just as any other vibration is contagious, and once it is set going in a group of people, we have the beginning of a new world. Then we provide a new example for our children to inherit, a new vibration based on love. There is then no need to engineer the upbringing of children by special techniques or special environments, because they will automatically be changed by the atmosphere of truth and openness, love and clarity. Once the new communities begin to spring up and link with each other over the coming New Age, children will have more freedom to think for themselves and not just copy their parents. A child who grows up in a community that practices Creative Conflict absorbs his parents' values but at the same time absorbs the whole atmosphere of openness and learns to speak his real feelings and to confront situations to get at the truth. He learns to think of the good of the whole, not as a big effort but as a matter of course. The traditional biological family, clannishly proud of its separation from others, interested only in its own success, is the opposite of this feeling for the whole. The evolutionary energy is prodding us to purify our love and expand our awareness to be far more inclusive than we have been as a people. The real utopia, based on Creative Conflict or some technique that can purify human consciousness, is like a yeast that has the power to leaven the vibration of the entire planet. Nothing short of this vision will have any effect whatever.

To begin manifesting this vision is the purpose of the nuclear school. The time when we can transcend techniques or outgrow special environments is still far away. What we can do now is to start where we are, with our children. To work with children is essentially the only way we can presently get a group of humans in one place at one time to make a continuous study of what happens when people learn to communicate on seven levels of consciousness and then practice certain techniques for an enhanced form of communication. Adults are not normally amenable to continuous daily experience or discipline, having to lead busy daily lives, whereas children have to be educated in school anyway. Although we have such an awareness community of adults at the University of the Trees, this is an unusual commitment and a dedication not found in everyone. But normal people can easily evaluate the progress and performance of children, not only because children are more open but because the before and after states of consciousness are more visible and the results more rewarding than with groups of adults who must first unlearn everything before they can be open on all seven levels and use more than just the one or two levels they now function on in normal social intercourse.

TAKING ACTION

The following program sets out the administration of a new wholistic education and a new school which invites the entire community into an exploring of the single nuclear approach to learning and self-discovery. This school will test the hypothesis of nuclear education and provide answers to two basic questions: Of what importance is the education of children in the knowledge of psycho-physical energies of the chakras? How does this knowledge of the thresholds of consciousness contribute to learning and to communication? The school will provide tested answers to these questions within two years, since the postulated levels of consciousness and their corresponding chakras, colors and brain evolution can be observed and experienced as channels of communication with others and with the environment and within the self. They are subject to comparison within control groups. Two control groups from public and private schools being taught by traditional methods will be tested along with the nuclear school to arrive at a factual comparison. An objective validating committee made up of teachers from local schools and of parents will evaluate the learning ability and general psychic health and behavior of the children in the nuclear school in comparison with the children educated by the methods of the public and private schools. This independent committee will provide the evaluation of the children at three separate times: once when the classes in the new methods begin and again after one year and then after two years. The validating committee will publish the results impartially, thereby saving the new educators from having to self-promote their techniques like a new religion or fashion. In this way they will not have to convince anyone to put their child in the new school, but the committee itself will probably recommend that all existing schools use the new methods for training in consciousness.

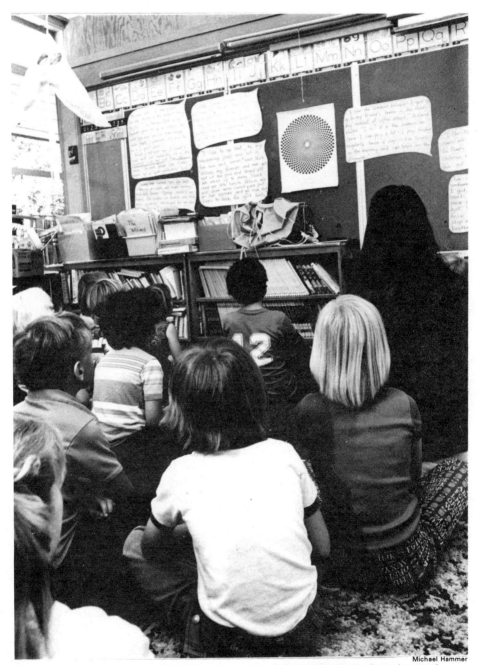

Michael Hammer

One of the public schools in California that practices the techniques outlined in this chapter, integrated with the standard curriculum.

The design of the experimental method is simple enough that any parent will be able to evaluate the progress of his or her child and the levels of consciousness in which the child functions. Each parent will be able to give a letter of evaluation at the end of a year or at the end of two years because they knew the child before and after in terms of living experience, personal happiness and fulfilling creative activity.

After much research and work with private and public schools in consciousness training techniques, the University of the Trees will begin its own private school for children from kindergarten through eighth grade in the fall of 1979, extending to high school some time after that. University of the Trees at present is a fully authorized degree-granting college in the State of California providing degrees in consciousness research fields on both undergraduate and graduate levels. The new children's school will be run as a true community school with the same self-governing methods that we use at the college level. Called *University Community School* it is being created jointly by teachers, parents and the local community interested in furthering this type of new education. The nuclear model of the *University Community School* views the evolution of the child as a wholistic chain of events within one whole nucleus.

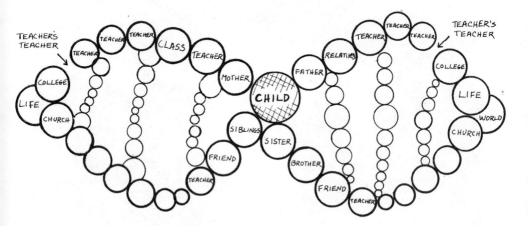

Children are subjected to many influences from parents, teachers, schools, religions, friends, TV and comics, all of which must be taken into account to further the child's evolution.

The first teacher of the newborn child is mother. The second teacher is father. The third teacher is siblings and other children. Then comes the school teacher who has a profound influence on the psyche of children. Most of us can reflect back on our school years to the memory of certain teachers who stand out against the background of our past who were very influential. Teachers help mold our self-image, emotional and inner life. How we view our self is mirrored in how we relate with others and what impact we have on the larger society. Whether the teacher we remember was much-loved or much-hated, our feelings are strongly imprinted and condition our feelings about ourself and thus our behavior even to this day. The effect of the teacher's being on the growth of a child needs to be deeply considered in our teacher training programs and by parents. It is a far more important issue for a peaceful society than just the intellectual training the teacher imparts. The final influence then is the teacher of the teachers, those who affect the attitude and curriculum of what the teachers will teach. Training of teachers is dependent upon the awareness of the teachers of the teachers, for like children, adults are inspired or turned off by their own teachers. The teachers of the teachers are at this time the most important link in the educational chain because of the vastness of the problem in finding people with both foresight and insight into human beings to teach the teachers. Few people are aware enough to teach teachers effectively and this influence permeates throughout the entire chain and thus within the whole of social life in a cycle that is stagnating at this time in history. Until we can dynamically lift the cycle into a new evolutionary spiral, we will have more and more chaos.

Thus the *University Community School* is designed to offer teacher training programs, parent classes, parent-teacher and parent-child awareness classes, along with the regular classroom curriculum, to achieve the bonding of forces needed for a synthesis and a real solution to take place. All the links in the chain must work together for a breakthrough. Divisiveness in a cell causes cancer, and divisiveness in the nucleus of society causes the social cancer we are experiencing today.

One of the most challenging areas is how to reach the teachers.

Fortunately we have the support of two local superintendents of school, including the County Superintendent of Education, for our methods of learning and our teacher training program. But many teachers are entrenched in their ways and afraid of learning something innovative. There are, on the other hand, many teachers who have applied for teaching positions in the new school and have been eager to give up jobs that pay them $17,000 per year, to train on their own expense and teach for much less pay, just for the opportunity to work in this new learning experience. Public school teachers need a break from the constant hassles that tie them to the treadmill of poor education. They need released time to discover new and more effective methods of teaching. They need a break from dealing with overcrowded classrooms of hypertensive children. In many ways I feel it would be more effective for society to shut down some of the school time to devote itself—parents, teachers, administrators and older children working together—to pinpointing the problems that each group sees and concentrating on the solutions rather than to keep going from one problem to the next.

The *University Community School* has already found a tested working solution to the problem of hypertensive children whose numbers grow larger each year. Meditation exercises do wonders with these children, as well as with more stable children, and create a receptivity to the learning process that makes the teachers' job much easier and more fulfilling. Once the teachers are aware, it is no great problem to challenge the children, enhance love, creativity, independence, responsibility and self-discipline at the same time. It is much more difficult to motivate the parents and the teachers to be open-minded and to find the solutions that are already available. It is hard for parents to have any desire to close the gulf that separates their world from the world of the school, because most parents feel that being a parent requires enough self-sacrifice without someone asking for more. But if communication were transformed between the children and their parents, the interaction might seem less like sacrifice and more like mutual fun and fulfillment. In fact they might discover that communication with their children, even the very young ones, had more depth and life and interest than the low level contact that now passes for communication between most people. So the problem of our school is to structure a model so that Creative Conflict, creative communication and other effective methods can be brought into more schools to heal the breach between administration, teachers, parents and children.

The synthesis that we envision means a real group consciousness— a unity of hearts, minds and purpose. It can only begin with those who are willing to involve themselves. All of the student/faculty in residence at University of the Trees have dedicated their own careers, finances, and beings to dealing creatively with these issues and they ask all who are in resonance with this vision to join with us from wherever they are in a wider community effort.*

BACK TO BASICS IN A NEW WAY

The curriculum is based on Socratic methods of drawing out the wholeness and knowledge from within each child to discover and explore the realms of consciousness and the faculties of human learning inherent in each individual. The teacher's role is as a facilitator serving as much as possible as a model and example of wholeness of being and also as a guide to help students become clear-minded, to release emotional blocks and to integrate their physical and spiritual life in a wholesome integrity. We feel that only with this type of wholistic approach can education occur in a fulfilling way and the basics of reading, writing and arithmetic be taught with high success and creativity in this era of many distractions and high tensions. Often we hear worried parents pressing for the schools to go "back to basics", meaning back to what they knew was stable, what worked when they were kids. But this conservative backward-looking approach will not meet the present challenge or prepare for the future. Back to basics is an important theme in *University Community School* since the three R's are essential for social success and for appreciating the most advanced minds of history. But our approach to back to basics is

---

* Practical, detailed curriculum and instructions for beginning a Community School and classes in your own community as well as the self-governing policies of the school are presented in *The Golden Egg*, University of the Trees Press.

to emphasize them along with the new methods that involve the new knowledge of human personality. In one public classroom that used some of our methods on a daily basis, children's test scores on listening and creative problem-solving jumped several grade levels. Certain children having difficulty with reading increased their reading scores up to five grade levels after several months of daily centering and concentration practice. These are just a few of many wonderful, documented results that we have had, and we will continue to incorporate new successfully proven methods as they emerge from our own research or from other universities. The *University Community School* is structured as an experimental focal point for a network of aware educators who are devoting themselves to discovering what works to tap the learning process and to address specific educational problems.

The practical methods and techniques we use are set out for teachers and parents and children in a number of our other publications in more detail. University of the Trees explores innovative approaches to *learning how to learn* and we concentrate our efforts on researching the learning process itself. We are always open to practical new ideas from other groups, individuals or institutions researching innovative solutions to the problems in the world. If we discover better ways of education than these methods which we have so far incorporated, synthesized and evolved, we will study, listen, test and evaluate them. We welcome all interested people to visit us and to evaluate our lifestyle as an educational community within the larger community, to talk to our faculty and students, help with ways to improve our school according to your own skills, interests or projects and become familiar with our manifestation. We invite you and other spiritual communities to work together with us to serve as a model, a prototype for what can happen throughout the country and build a new vision based on our united efforts.

The *University Community School* is run by trained staff members, who have had several years experience introducing these methods to other teachers, classrooms and groups, assisted by teachers in training. The director, Dr. Deborah Rozman (Ph.D. Psychology) is the author of several leading books in the field of wholistic development in children. The school will always maintain a minimum of a one to ten full-time teacher student ratio. The school will expand in stages depending upon the involvement of the community and the number of people wanting it for their children. Branch community schools will be set up in areas throughout the country, wherever a group of dedicated people in those areas choose to organize and manifest one. Ongoing parent and teacher training programs at University of the Trees enable people from all over the world to come for training and return to their own communities to start their own school or classes in these methods.

In general, our curriculum includes proven techniques for the exploration of the inner worlds of children and teachers alike in the emotional and spiritual dimensions while at the same time the basic academic subjects are taught as part of awakening specific levels of consciousness. The curriculum is designed to open the physical, social, intellectual, emotional, mental, intuitive and creative dimensions of consciousness in an integrated, wholistic manner. It will develop the trust and self-esteem of the child by giving him the freedom to say anything but get away with nothing. This means a trusting atmosphere yet with clearly defined boundaries where children assume responsibility for their own words and actions and are accountable for them. Rules and agreements made together by both students and teachers are enforced by both students and teachers in a program of self-rule which develops the inner fiber of the child to constructively deal with the authorities of parent, teacher or whomever. Using real-life situations at home and in the classroom, we help the children make responsible choices which include facing the logical consequences of their own choices. In our work with children we have noticed a direct correlation between leadership ability and the ability to feel what other children are feeling, and between achievement in academics and self-discipline. We emphasize these basic skills both as a foundation for learning the academic subjects and to enhance the child's respect for self and others needed to make a creative impact on the society he or she is living in.

It may seem that in a school where students form part of the government, discipline would be hard to implement. This was the disaster of the whole movement of Pragmatism in education built upon the "permissive" attitude to children which the children took full advantage of. The *University Community School,* however, is in no way permissive. Creative Conflict has its own form of discipline which is built in to the group wholeness which puts you in the position where you have to confront yourself, and therefore has less need for authoritarian methods of discipline from the top down. The development of higher levels of consciousness also cuts down the need for discipline. Most children function mainly on the first level of consciousness having to do with physical movement and sensation whereas the new curriculum is designed to increase awareness of the higher dimensions of consciousness along with the physical and to work from the higher Self of each child, enabling him or her to recognize that all the external world is a manifestation of consciousness and comes from the creation of images, concepts and experiences within our own consciousness. Learning to see that people's attitudes and reactions to us are largely created by ourselves helps us to assume responsibility for what happens to us and to change rather than feel sorry for ourselves or blame others or conflict with them. This is especially important for children because children easily feel rejected even when they are not being rejected, and children often carry the pain of false rejection with them throughout life unconsciously without ever checking the truth of it. The new methods teach the children to get inside their parents' worlds to see why they are saying the thing that feels like a rejection to the ego. And Creative Conflict teaches them how to check out their perceptions.

The new education will use daily relaxation, centering, concentration and guided imagery to focus the children, and this enhances their ability to perceive truth and to feel whole and complete within. They learn to validate the superconscious and intuition and to develop the creative imagination, which then becomes a powerful learning tool. The role of the creative imagination has been a prime subject of study at the University of the Trees. Especially in children who have begun to build a negative self-image from criticisms they have received, the techniques of creative imagining can be powerfully liberating and change the future course of their lives. In this and many other ways, the new curriculum builds the whole person at the same time that it builds the power of the mind to think clearly and to learn. The integrity of words and deeds of each person as a self-disciplined being—in mind, body and all faculties—extends throughout the entire class and through the entire school, even through the entire community, demonstrating a new basis for unity among people. This is not just a vision for parents but for anyone who is wishing for a ray of hope. There is no ground so ready for the seed of a new world than the unformed, unspoiled minds of children. Once we realize this potential—that there actually is a way—then we can do in reverse what the Hitler Youth movement tried to do. Instead of brainwashing our children to think what we want them to think, as Hitler did, we can teach them to think for themselves and to tune into their own being to discern the truth in any situation. Once we have given them this skill, then they can come to any field of knowledge equipped to deal with it. And they can come to the living of life and to communication with others in the readiness to discover love and truth and peace. The reason that this type of education does not need fancy buildings, playgrounds and libraries but can actually be conducted under grass huts or in a tent, is its simplicity and the fact that the only real resource needed is consciousness. When consciousness is both the teacher and the student, and is also the subject of study, and when the end result is heightened awareness and refinement of being, then education is wholistic. Only such wholistic education has the power, hidden within it as the flower is hidden within the seed, to make a whole people and a flowering of human civilization.

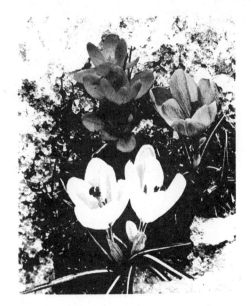

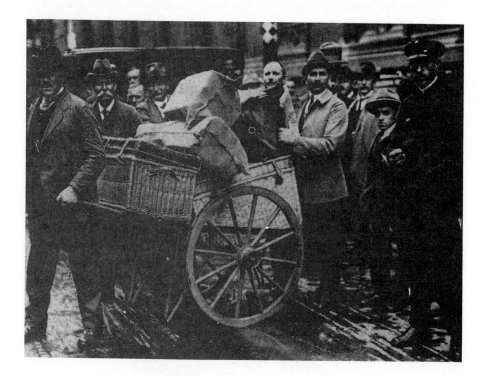

When the German mark collapsed through eroding values of paper currency, companies used baskets, sacks, suitcases and carts to fetch the freshly printed devalued money from banks to meet their payrolls until the mark completely crashed.

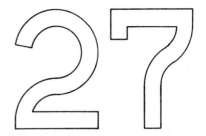

THE MEETING OF GOD AND MAMMON

What is the crux of life in most places on this earth? Is it bread or money? Is it love? or is it politics? Walk down any street in London, Paris, Moscow, New York or Peking and you will not walk far before you hear the word "dollar" or its local equivalent hit your ears from passers-by on every corner. Listen to a bunch of mayors of major cities or the talk of government at the state level of politics and the word will be "funding", another name for money. Wherever they are, as diverse and individualistic as men and women are, there is no subject however much despised that will bring a warmer response. In the polite drawing rooms of the wealthy, investing their capital, or the rummage sale of the parish priest, the subject is money. Politics is the distribution of wealth when all the hot air or fiery talk is spent, and without money, politics is dead. Science and art without money are impossible, for even the starving artist in the traditional Paris garret must buy his paints and canvas or the great Leonardos find a patron. As every politician knows, the control of money is the real power of all governments, for without it, no government could exist.

We begin this section of the book with our attitudes to money because these will determine our attitude to our fellowman and our relationship to God.

Whether we live in the capitalist world or under the rule of the communist system of government, there are some common problems regarding the use of capital and the ownership of capital, which spiritually affect every citizen deeply. Even a spiritual community must have someone to hold the money bags. The fact that it was Judas who carried the money bag for Christ's ministry, where all things were held in common, should not cloud the issue that Christ did pay his taxes to the government in *real money.* The need for big governments to tax the citizen up to fifty percent of earnings in the Western world and up to seventy percent in the Soviet system, which inflates the prices and money values of all work, is not always fully understood by those who pay the taxes or those who collect them. Those who administer our laws are some of the most ignorant of how energy becomes money or how consciousness becomes God.

To speak of God and money in the same breath is offensive to the businessman and the devout alike but we must see clearly that much of religion is just big business. The question of the Spirit and Mammon arises when we consider whether the wealthy modern movements, the fabulous riches of the church, the private jets and mansions of the pop gurus, are the result of spiritual magnetism and the manifestation of Truth or the fruits of concentration on amassing wealth. The easy packaging of religion and spiritual techniques has led to a whole industry which uses the tools of Mammon to spread the teachings. The power of the pure spirit may take much longer and be less flashy but it moves at a deeper level to grind out its perfection more slowly. The whole thrust of the spiritual fads and the Sunday sermons on money is 180 degrees opposite to the real spiritual work, which is to dismantle the structure of the ego and to dissolve attachment to the kingdom of this world. We can see the human egotism involved in the building of

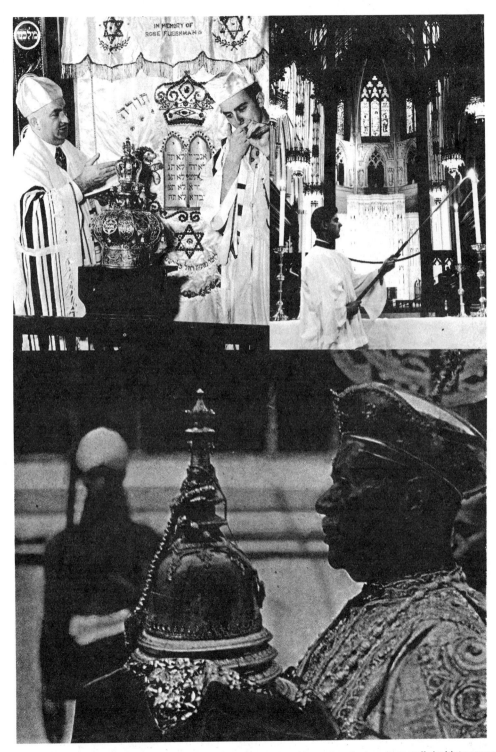

Religion and ritual are universally bound to golden objects. Throughout history, temples have been stuffed with treasures although the founders of religions have always spurned them.

fancy churches, gold crucifixes and other symbols, as if God needed to be given such offerings and works of art. These material symbols will all crumble away, and only human actions in consciousness will remain as witness to our greed and stupidity or to our enlightenment. None of these religious symbols nor the personality cults of spiritual heroes can solve the problem of social relationships. Only the spiritual laws that these great men uttered can solve the problem of human egotism and its resultant separation from God and man.

Dare we claim that the world is getting more religious? Turning to God may be easy for those who are already of a devotional or religious temperament, but it is evident from the actions of mankind today, taken as a whole, that people generally do not care about a higher intelligence because they do not run their real lives and relationships by that intelligence. Most people, for instance, do not believe in any connection between God and politics, and they have discovered no solution to the world's problems.* The barrenness of thought in this area of human endeavor is incredible and frightening. Even if mankind were dimly aware of a God-centered evolutionary spirit that could solve our economic problems, we would have to ask what is such a concept of spiritual evolution or God? What do we mean by "God"? When scientific atheists laugh at the idea of turning to God or to a higher intelligence than mankind to solve their problems, they are only dismissing the naive concept of a traditional God who is anthropomorphically sitting on the throne of heaven, presiding over his angels and listening to music of harps!

Whenever I use the term "God" in this book, I do not mean any particular human concept of the creative intelligence but the nature of consciousness uncluttered by any human images. It is images of God and of money that lead men to conflict with fellowmen and the universe over such pet ideas as capitalism versus communism, or

---

* The only feasible scheme that I have found other than the one offered in this book is authored by Dr. Hugh Schonfield in *Politics of God* published by University of the Trees Press (1978), which deals with messianism. I do not agree with it entirely but I do admire the soundness of its scholarship and feel it throws a great light on our human tendency to create personality cults.

Krishna versus Jesus of Nazareth. But the source of all these ideas is pure consciousness. Once we begin to see our consciousness as the source of all energy, then we will also see the link between SOURCE and money. We wake up in the morning with our consciousness given to us like a blank check that we can spend in any way we choose throughout the day. We can use it to generate money. We can use it to fall in love. We can use it to know God. Depending on what kind of person we are, we will spend our money in the same way that we spend our consciousness. A pleasure-loving person will spend his money and his consciousness on pleasure. Whether energy is the sum of men's efforts accumulated in money or whether our consciousness is the source of our personal experience of a cosmic intelligence or the source of natural energy, it will be our own mind which gives power to money or God, or to government. When an atheist denies the existence of God, he is using consciousness (God) to do it. In reality there is nothing in the world but this one energy and therefore to think of money without reference to God is self-delusion. There is no financial deal that can be made without the "investment" of our consciousness. Nor can we use our consciousness to make money without the cosmic intelligence to "back" us. Whenever we need to feel a little more humble toward this cosmic intelligence we can wonder what happens to a piece of food after we have swallowed it. What miraculous chemicals are our cells secreting and what fantastic digestive processes are going on in us, far beyond the control of our normal human intelligence? Without digestion to create life-energy, would there by any "me" to make money? To seek security from money, without regard to its source, is the height of impracticality. Those who do so will find that behind all the possessions and all the bank accounts, there is always lurking a last, deepest fear. And this is why money is inseparable from spiritual well-being.

What we seek here in this section of the book is to understand how money affects our spiritual life and how God affects our material prosperity in direct correlation to the way we use our consciousness. How can we begin to get in touch with the way we use consciousness in our relationships to money and to people and to government? The best way is by returning to a smaller model of community and restoring into our own hands the power of decision over our business lives. Returning this power over our own destiny to small firms, groups and individuals has now become indispensable. In both socialist and capitalist societies we have abdicated the sovereign power of our own consciousness and life to others who control our lives, ostensibly on our behalf. Why do we need to restore the power of decision to individuals and turn society away from "Big Government" toward communities and the smaller model? For an answer we have to turn to Nature's model.

All evolution takes place in the cell, the nucleus which contains the whole. The evolution of the "whole" system cannot take place in fact and in reality unless all its parts are raised in potential, unless all the "bits" in the whole are like a hologram, part of the entire vision or image. To raise only a select elite or a few does not achieve the democracy of the spirit envisioned by the American Constitution nor does it realize the communist ideal of the total self embodied in the concept of the State. The Buddhist idea of the enlightenment of all sentient beings is embodied in the concept of the Bodhisattvic vow which affirms that the selfish seeking of one's own bliss without fully sharing it with all others is an ineffective goal which is always self-defeating. The world at large has come to this point of self-defeat, where our survival depends on caring and loving, and where concern for the well-being of others becomes indispensable for our own protection.

To understand this point of self-negation at which the planet earth has now arrived and to see it as a spiritual dimension of human existence, we must examine the use of capital and political powers as coercive instruments. Because money and power are two demons which turn the angelic powers of man's consciousness into the service of the beast in man, we must descend into hell and face the pollution of our minds and thoughts as well as our pollution of the external environment. Ruined soil and polluted external environment are only a reflection of our own internal greed and ignorance. Therefore a large part of our spiritual life hinges on our conquest of money and power or our submission to it. We cannot avoid it by sweeping it under the carpet or by taking a vow of poverty. Men and women were not intended to live happily in poverty but in the life more abundant.

Attachment to poverty is no better than attachment to money and power. We have so little understanding of these areas of human insecurity that we hardly notice how meagerly our society and its system of government gives us training to cope with them. Money itself is not an evil. It is the human greed and attachment to money that is evil. Money can be good and godlike in the hands of gods and beastly and warlike in the hands of brutes. Our schools need to teach us not to avoid the conflicts which desire for money and power bring to every human, but to understand and master them. For even those who despise money and power are eventually consumed in the social upheavals and revolutions which rotate around these two demonic aspects of human consciousness. We have to study how our own consciousness works, and this can only be done with any depth of penetration and insight at the level of the smaller group or community. At the mass level of crowds there can be nothing but superficial knowledge of the real problems. To talk of money with loved ones usually brings out the real motives of the relationships, but to talk of money and power with relative strangers in the political process is to talk of matters which ninety-nine percent of all people avoid looking at.

This book has been written to find our way back to self-government and to reach that lost sense of self-fulfillment which has been usurped by the growing bureaucracy of "big government" in its many forms of disguise. Small is not always beautiful, but it has now become indispensable if we are to understand the real meaning of life. The real business of life is spiritual evolution, but the majority of mankind is only dimly aware of our real purpose on earth. Some say that man is a pigmy asleep in the mists of time and is not even dimly aware of how important it is to turn towards consciousness. He does not see that *to understand human consciousness is tantamount to understanding God and therefore can also solve our economic problem of survival.* Most communists say we do not need God to solve our problems; we need more *human* consciousness. There are only a few capitalists or communists who really believe that turning to God will indeed solve our financial problems. Obviously it would not be wisdom to turn to God in ignorance of the mechanics of money and possessiveness. We have to turn to God in full knowledge of their workings. To know that money is created out of consciousness is to know that God is the source of all human energy and intelligence. Before we can take this step toward the evolutionary intelligence and before we can attempt to solve our economic problems and our spiritual problems at the same time, we have to demonstrate through example the interdependence of the material and the spiritual. The link between economic well-being and spiritual welfare has to be made sufficiently obvious for the majority of mankind to glimpse the essential truth that *there is no separation between consciousness and God or between material bodies and the minds which control them.*

The whole crux and purpose of this book is the manifestation of specific ways* of applying spiritual laws to the evolution of social groups, and to achieve this purpose involves a confrontation with people's long-ingrained habit of separating spirit and matter. As things stand at present the collective spirit of humanity is not orientated to God as the solution of their problems. On the contrary, we find instead that most religions in practice are using God as an escape from their problems.

There are some who believe that a great "spiritual awakening" is already afoot, but the general collective attitude of the world's people towards spirituality is to dismiss the real nitty-gritty work on the ego which this word "spiritual" means. Religion can be dead or alive, depending on what you make it. If you turn to Eastern religions to find what was missing in the West, it is still a ready-made spirituality you are embracing and may still be a diversion and an escape from real God-contact. It does not make God any more real or the Buddha more effective than the Christian personality cultists make Christ when they say that Jesus will save the world. For most people of the world, whether Hindu, Christian, Communist or any other faith, God is unreal and separate from their life. Even the very devout who pray have no idea how God will implement his plans for the cosmos. How then are

---

* These specific suggestions appear throughout the book, particularly in the living constitution, the technique of creative conflict and, in this section, the idea of common ownership as a way to implement spiritual laws in the world of business and industry.

people going to turn to Him? What is going to make them see the hidden hand at work in the affairs of men? How can society tap the evolutionary intelligence working through consciousness itself?

What is the cosmic statement that religious teachers have made in the past which stirred the souls of millions in the depths of their beings so that they said to themselves, "God speaks through this man"? The answer is that these cosmic beings have seen a vision of something so awesome, so compelling that they felt destiny spoke through them. They all said the same things in essence, that the intelligence in man was directly linked with an unfolding seed or nucleus on another level of Being. Their sense of conviction became our faith. But we need to build our own direct connection to that nucleus or seed. How do we do that? Do we go off to a cave to meditate? Do we give up all our possessions and renounce the world? Or do we go the opposite direction and get even more deeply involved in the world but in a new way? Once we realize that *there is no spiritual life apart from social responsibility* and that we cannot evolve except by living our life more fully and by taking responsibility for more and more of life until at last we see that we are responsible for the whole, then the question comes: how do we change the world? How can we do something effective? And from what position do we do it? What consciousness is behind what we are doing?

Let us clearly see into social reality, that in spite of the deep motivations of millions of well-meaning persons, in spite of thousands of preachers and millions of printings of the Bible as the best-selling book of all time, the world actually is in a worse state of spiritual disease now than ever before in our history. More words are said and printed, and spiritual messages flash across the world by TV promotion, radio and microwaves, etc., yet the human world is ready to blow itself up and destroy the life of the planet. This we must see as a fact and stop kidding ourselves that anything we are doing now or have been doing in the past has worked or is actually going to work. Only a totally new message which does not preach but answers the questions in all our minds from a cosmic perspective can motivate modern man to do something. The whole question of doing anything effective comes back to economics and the use of our resources. There is no shortage of schemes and plans, and no shortage of money if we can spend five thousand million dollars on going to the moon. But what kind of consciousness is shaping the plans, and what kind of society is it striving to perpetuate?

The people of the world are in a real dilemma in their need to achieve economic freedom and individual freedom, for the only significant alternatives which human consciousness has so far been able to discover have been capitalism and communism. Yet neither has brought us liberation from the slavery of financial and political overlords. Thousands of years of religion in all its forms have not helped us to see the obvious fact that our spiritual slavery exists unconsciously within these twin social systems—communism and capitalism—even while we are thinking we are free. We have reached the point where mankind has now almost returned to another kind of state feudalism and where the productivity of each subservient worker is soon to be taxed in even greater proportions than it was by the powerful feudal lords in medieval times. However, the greatest dilemma of all is that neither system of big government nor their current philosophies has any answers about the ultimate meaning of the cosmos, and neither capitalism nor communism even professes to work out our spiritual destiny beyond the achievement of material wealth upon the earth.

Therefore another model is required for mankind, to be offered not as an anti-communist or anti-capitalist tract, but as a positive statement of a new insight which reveals a superior synthesis of both systems. The model outlined in this book hacks at the root of man's current blindness rather than chopping at the branches of his past errors. Ignoring all theories about these errors, we look squarely at the results of capitalist and communist systems in the present disastrous situation in the world. At the level of practical living, these "isms" have nothing to offer but the situation we already have. Because neither system has any cosmic vision of our psychological and emotional reality and our vaster destiny as evolving beings, we have no alternative but to set out afresh on a new journey of discovery and find the new model for human life.

In this book we attempt to go beyond the religious and political schemes which have failed. We must now go beyond the level of commitment which has given us no concrete manifestations of the kingdom of heaven. The vision of heaven must be a real one, centered in the reality of a scientific cosmos. The problem is that, as a thesis, Christ talked of the Kingdom of Heaven but did not say what the Kingdom is nor did he stay around long enough to create any specific model. Hence communism rises as an antithesis to this abstract spiritual heaven, insisting on a concrete material heaven on earth. The central framework of the World Peace Center is the dialectical synthesis arising out of the union of the thesis of heaven and its anti-thesis of materialism. It is nothing short of a direct model of the kingdom of heaven, not only here upon earth but as it is in the heavens all around us. This model is the vision of the cosmic nucleus, embodied in every living thing upon the earth. It is the vision of the nucleus of the universe from which all expansion has sprung. It is the vision of Pure Consciousness as a real God, becoming our every thought and every experience according to the level and quality of our human consciousness. It is the realization that it is we who put limits on all things including God, because we limit the very consciousness that is flowing through us. The heart of the nucleus is the source of our real spiritual and economic fulfillment, our emotional, psychological and material well-being, because ultimately our consciousness is the source of all conflict and the maker of all peace on earth.

An evolutionary model cannot make broad statements of spiritual principles without showing how they apply to the everyday life of man's survival in business, politics and human relationships. We shall attempt to show in this section of the book how specific we will be in practice, not only with the myriad aspects of money, but also with the political control we give in the euphemistic name of "big government". What do we learn through the possession of a material body and why would we have bodies and minds if it were not to manifest the supreme cosmic model of creation on the material plane? To realize this divine purpose is to act it out in real life, and this human drama can only be worked out in social groups through love of one another. In this world our love is expressed by actions on the material plane of life, but it stems from an inseparable spiritual dimension. The thing that makes any kind of love spiritual is its givingness. Whether we give ourselves in sex or give our possessions or our ideas, the giving must be more than our taking if we are to survive as a species.

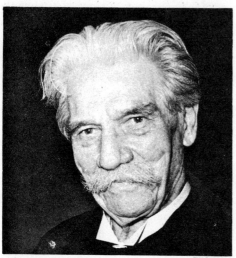

WIDE WORLD

Albert Schweitzer embodied the spirit of giving and of putting another's happiness before his own.

The longer I live the more patient I get with people and their self-righteous claims that we should all think as they do, but at the same time, I get more *impatient* at the senseless actions and criminality of human killing in the name of political causes. We humans are quick to engage in the senseless giving of life on the battlefield in war instead of the giving of our hearts. The tragic cutting short of all these lives through violence and misguided revolutionary fervor and terrorism is a saddening modern reminder that mankind, while sitting supposedly as the master of the kingdoms of the world, is at the bottom of its own evolutionary ladder. There has not been much advance in man's evolution of his deeper inner-worlds. In spite of annihilation of distance across the earth between nations, through the spread of technology and the shrinking of the world through worldwide telephone and television, men and women hate and love, fail and succeed, work and play with the same feelings and satisfactions as they did in ancient times. Furthermore, great civilizations and cultures fail for the same reasons that they have always failed. Historian Arnold Toynbee counted more than thirty-one civilizations which were abortive. The Greek thinkers who researched the nature of democracy for several hundred years and the Roman civilization which gave us the techniques of government for making social laws, both perished in fratricide and war. Are we any different at heart, even though our physical world has vastly changed?

In capitalism and communism, the opposing forces of good and evil line up for another crack at each other, and each side is sinister in a different way, depending where you are looking from. People tend to look at each side from their own limitations of knowledge and to filter out of their hearing what they do not want to hear. They tend to see society in terms of "the masses", those crowds of people who all think alike and respond alike to truth. Yet the experience of truth is an individual affair, and the fabric of society is a network of interlocking relationships between human beings living on totally different levels of consciousness. Thus the organism most people think of as "society" is not just a conglomeration of human beings but consists in the subtle relations between them. In the structure of society, individuals are the nodal points which stand at the focus of human insight or human ignorance. The relationships between people and the interactions between them are the real reasons for forming any group such as a community, a party, a church or a corporation. There are no "members" of society, as if it were a collective club or family or institution, but only subtle reactions of consciousness between people. When these aggregate unique relationships and the interactions between their individual levels of consciousness are seen as a crowd or mass of people, they become dehumanized and unreal and are either wantonly massacred by terrorists or eliminated by communists or, in capitalist society, viewed merely as cogs in an economic machine all grinding their way to the same goal.

Economic systems, too, are comprised of a complex mass of human relationships at all levels of evolution, but most economists talk of the "masses" or view a particular class as a group of stereotypes. We hear phrases like "the workers". Who are the workers? To look at individuals as stereotypes is the beginning of our social ignorance. When people become merely cyphers and pawns in the games of men who think they know, then our society becomes a grey and lifeless crowd, expendable in war, taxable in peace, and exploitable as an economic system. It is then that we forget our love and compassion, and experience other people without any accuracy and we miss the reality of their beings. Any new model of society must have power to restore this spiritual dimension to our social life.

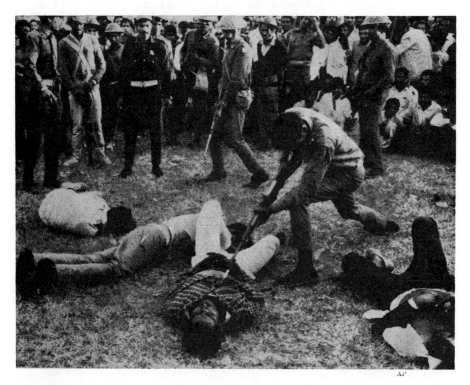

The captives in the picture have had cigarette butts stubbed out in their eyes and now their bodies are being used for bayonet practice by the Pakistani guerrillas during the 1970-71 war. This type of vengeance can only occur when one cannot see into the being of another, and all love and compassion for the other is non-existent.

WITH WHAT PURPOSE?

John Kenneth Galbraith, a leading Western economist of the current period, says that any description of an economic system hinges upon the right answers to the following basic questions:

What makes people work?
Which employment or toil is unpopular?
Which work do people not want to do?
What things do people produce?
With what organization do they produce?
With what guidance or plan do they produce?
How successful is the result?

We can note that there is no spiritual dimension in these questions unless we regard the last two questions in terms of a qualitative philosophy of life and not merely an economic plan. Whether that philosophy is religious, scientific, atheistic or mystic will definitely change what we mean by a "successful result".

Premier Krushchev of the USSR defined *his* idea of success in April 1964:

"Communism will achieve little if it cannot give the people what they want. The important thing is that we should have more to eat, good goulash, schools, housing and ballet. How much more do those things give to the enlargement of life? These things are worth fighting and working for. If the productivity of labor in the socialist countries is lower than in the capitalist countries, we shall not advance in our march to communism and the conquest of capitalism. This is the only thing that will insure the victory of communism."

Krushchev makes no mention of any higher goals of love or relationship or security of feeling or the happiness which does not come from the possession of material things. Will not love or peace be victorious over washing machines and goulash? If these are the only things on which victory is based, then communism can never win. Neither capitalist nor communist philosophy makes any mention of the lofty vision of spiritual evolution nor of any higher intent than action at the

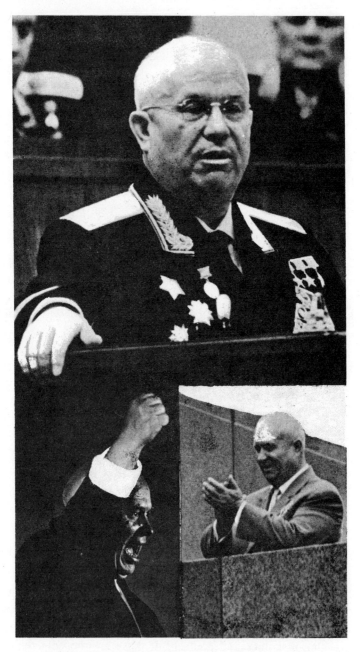

Krushchev promoting the conquest of communism over capitalism.

material level of being. They do not see that matter, or the body, is the nursery in which saints are grown and beings are purified. They do not realize that in our working with relationships on the material field-of-action we evolve towards the nucleus at the source of all divine work. The material world and the use of resources, the use of our bodies and minds, are a reflection of our level of consciousness. Our consciousness is the seat of all our knowledge of matter or the divine, and our society and its cultural ways represent the degree of evolution of each one of us. If we are unhappy with it and wish to transform it but have no power to change it, this impotence is itself also a reflection of our level of evolution. Therefore the success or failure in our use of social resources is intimately connected to our individual attitudes to love, politics, money, power and care of others.

It is now time for the human spirit to prevent its organizations from degenerating into tyranny and to retain the control over leaders. We have democracy in our governmental structure and we vote to elect our political leaders, but we cannot control them because we have not extended democracy to apply to industry. Therefore the vast industrial wealth and economic power of money over the decisions of the legislature are not in the hands of the people. Only when the money gets into the right hands can the spirit work through people, because they put the power of money second to the power of spirit. Therefore we can examine our attitudes to power and money in order to learn how we stand in the ways of the spirit. In the hands of a spiritual person, the good management of money is no less spiritual than the management of any other resources. But the spiritual laws say that if financial resources do not provide enough money, then the master of consciousness takes this as a sign from the universe that the spiritual activity which he or she is trying to manifest at the level of human social life has not yet reached its full ripeness. If it had, then the doors would fly open and the way would be smoothed.

The fact that the doors *don't* always fly open is the crux of the problem which occupies the consciousness of all those who envision the ultimate welding of the economic effort with the spiritual life. How much time must we spend with the management of money and the various schemes which generate it, so that we may manifest the ideal here upon earth? This problem has in the past been solved by the spiritual rejection of wealth in vows of poverty. There is no special sanctity in poverty, and it is only the fact that the moneyless and beggars are freed to practice humility that makes poverty a virtue and thereby forces us back upon the power of the spirit. Many have achieved isolation from the tainted vibrations of money by cloistering themselves in a Himalayan cave, yet the Indian holyman who comes down from the forests and mountains needs an air ticket or a motor car in the modern world if he is to spread his message and share his wisdom. The fact is that spirit can travel third class as easily as first class, and it can get by on whatever money comes naturally through the work itself. To chase after Mammon and to seek more than "enough" is to be out of tune with spirit. To become a master of money and not its slave, we are required to look not at the quantity of money we control but always at the humility and at the quality of action by which we manifest. If we look at the gurus whose followers are fired with devotion and generosity, we may find genuine holymen, humble and selfless, but more often we will find wolves in sheep's clothing, bent upon power and possessions.

What is the most fundamental connection between Mammon and spirit? It is the fact that money represents the essence of human power. Whether that power is political, religious or scientific, nothing can be done in any of these fields of action without money. Money to pay for the politicians' schemes comes from taxes. Money for churches, Bibles, and teaching of religion comes from the emotional feelings of generosity and may even be motivated by guilt. Money for scientific projects comes from their goal-oriented commercial application or from government policies. Without money none of these social activities can function and yet the spirit, even when defined as consciousness or soul, does not need money to make it grow more pure or more perfect. The very absence of such money power is often the very beginning of spiritual power. For Christ or Gandhi never owned a church, and Socrates lived entirely off the contributions of well-wishers. Albert Schweitzer started his African hospital in the jungle of Lambarene with barely enough money to feed himself for a year.

The secret of the spirit is in its total victory over Mammon.

Spiritual genius achieves with almost nothing but the power of consciousness itself. Furthermore if the spirit is pure it will eventually attract to it all the material and financial resources needed to fulfill its purpose and bring its inspiration to the world of human relationships. However, if we study the history of religious and political organizations we can see that the well-intentioned and saintly men who founded them were not always worldly wise in the ways of Mammon. They were often ignorant of the laws of human group development and therefore the idealistic efforts of the greatest of mankind have been wasted. Many of the movements they inspired even became harmful to society.

We can take the loveable example of St. Francis who loved not only all of mankind but also the beasts and birds, the sun and the stars, the flowers and the wind. Yet the Franciscan order which he founded to spread his brotherly love and to root out all self-seeking was ruled by his immediate successors in excessive luxury. Having taken the traditional vows of poverty, chastity and surrender, his successors rebelled against the Pope and became recruiting sergeants in the savage wars for political supremacy between the Guelphs and Ghibellines. These rich and powerful Franciscans (pledged to poverty and brotherly love), together with the Dominicans, *brought about and actually administered the atrocities of the Inquisition.* The persecution and torture of dissidents was so repressive and cruel in those days that extermination by slave labor in Josef Stalin's Gulag camps seems almost a holiday by comparison. If St. Francis had developed more worldly knowledge of human drives for power and wealth, he would have foreseen this possibility. It is not pleasant to think of the countless persecutions, witch hunts and pogroms done in the name of Christ by ideologues who believed their abominations were sanctified by the church, just as the present trials of dissidents in Soviet Russia are sanctified by the communist party.

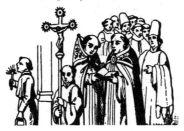

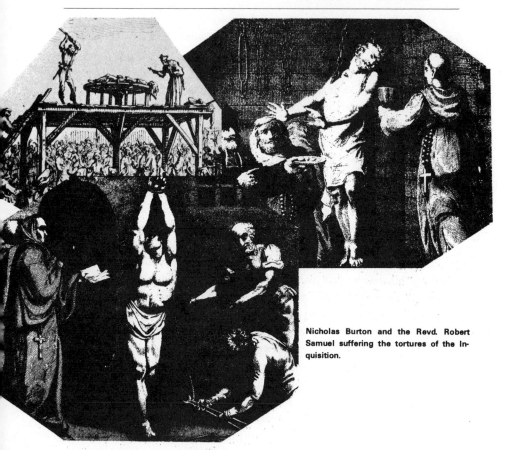

Nicholas Burton and the Revd. Robert Samuel suffering the tortures of the Inquisition.

Genuine saintliness is even harder to discriminate and recognize than scientific or artistic merit, because hypocrites have perfected the art of imitation. Organizations and systems, groups and communities and especially charities are effective managers of money for doing good *only* as long as their leaders are saints. How can we prevent hypocrites from stealthily taking control of social resources by paying lipservice to high ideals until they take over all powers?

The control of these social resources is the present battleground between communism and capitalism and represents the titanic struggle between the totalitarian state and democratic systems. Our new model must answer these vital problems or be stillborn from the beginning. The model which unfolds through this book is the model of the human organism and its guiding instrument of the brain. But before we can discover its layers of functioning as a social model we must face the drive for security in human relationships, which lies even deeper in the human psyche than the drive for power.

Why is money so fundamental to both the material and the spiritual life? If the world is the instrument of spirit and we have come here to fill this world of matter with the light of spirit, then we must *embody* that light and radiate it in every aspect of our life, from business to sex to politics to worship. What is at the very bottom of the drive to get money and power? Why does any person crave money, beyond his daily needs for food and shelter and the basics of life? Why do we feel this desperate need to store up money for old age or for some future time when we may need it? Is it not because we are fundamentally insecure?

How can we transform our drive for the security of money into a drive for the security of the heart? Essentially our drive for money is a thirst for the spirit, a thirst to become one with the whole. It is the hunger to fill the emptiness of a black hole at the center of our being which only certainty can satisfy. Our drive to possess is a reflection of a cosmic need to conquer a hazardous universe and find the ultimate security.

Every great sage or saint has assured us that the laws of consciousness provide for our every need when we put the needs of the whole first. This does not mean denying our personal needs but seeing others' needs as part of our own, loving others as much as we love our self.

> "Take no thought for your life, what ye shall eat, or what ye shall drink; nor yet for your body, what ye shall put on. Is not the life more than meat, and the body more than raiment? Behold the fowls of the air: for they sow not, neither do they reap, nor gather into barns; yet your heavenly Father feedeth them. Are ye not much better than they? Which of you by taking thought can add one cubit unto his stature? And why take ye thought for raiment? Consider the lilies of the field, how they grow. They toil not, neither do

they spin. And yet I say unto you that even Solomon in all
his glory was not arrayed like one of these. Wherefore, if
God so clothe the grass of the field, which today is and
tomorrow is cast into the oven, shall He not much more
clothe you, O ye of little faith?''

Were these words mere rhetoric, poetry of a dreamer? Or do they
contain a scientific teaching of how the laws of the cosmos work? Why
do humans not trust the universe? Why do they instead go off into so
many ego trips of their own to try to control events in their lives which
only forces them into a position 180 degrees out of phase with the
harmony of life? It is the desire to find security through the ego. The
ego wants to feel separate, unique, the only one in control, tops,
number ONE. And in pursuing this separatism it loses its security. It
tries desperately to fill the hole of emptiness through trying to grab
more power, more money, more self-image, more support for its ego
position. This way of ego divides the house of humanity against itself
so that the only road leads to a great fall. It comes as no shock that
nuclear weaponry is poised to kill and destroy all life on this beautiful
planet. Self-destruction is only an outcome of the ego position, the
basic lack of trust pervading mankind. What knowledge will convince
us that our security can only be found in the heart of the cosmos, in the
nuclear Self lying within the depths of each person? What motivation
will send us to the feet of the cosmic intelligence, the only one that can
bail us out of our spiritual, social, psychological, emotional and
economic mess? Must we be brought to our knees by physical destruction or economic collapse? Perhaps this will be the only way we will
confront our deep, unspoken insecurity. Or perhaps mankind will
awaken to the cries of the new cosmic message waiting to save him
from the fruits of his own actions. Whichever way evolution takes to
awaken humanity to its dependence on cosmic intelligence and the
humiliating limitations of our separating ego-sense, it will be brought
about by our own actions in consciousness. For consciousness is where
God and man meet and where God and Mammon must come to terms.
It is in consciousness where the will of God works out its cosmic plan
and programs for the destiny of man through man.

J.P. LAFFONT—GAMMA

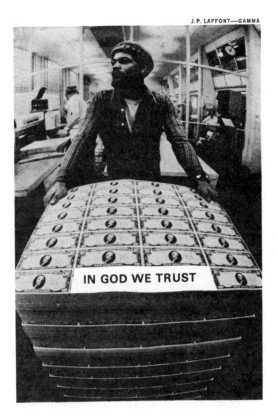

IN GOD WE TRUST

Newly printed dollars are made by the ton in Washington to finance government spending and federal borrowing. A million single dollars weighs one ton of paper. Perhaps one day when the present dollar crashes the ton of paper will be worth more than the worthless dollars.

AUTHOR'S NOTE

The chapter called "Fictitious Money" has a different vibration from most of the chapters in this book, but it is necessary for us to go into this vibration on its own terms and not from some pinnacle of self-righteous moralizing if we are to make a real change in the world and not just lay a patina of virtue over the unchanging rotten core of materialism and the selfish worldly life. To change the economic world we will have to get inside the mind of a capitalist, not try to tell him to do what he does not want to do. One friend I knew, Mr. Ernest Bader, gave away his company to his employees, but no one has copied him because what capitalist in his right mind is going to give away his company? So Mr. Bader's action, however well-intentioned and idealistic, can have no effective power to change the world or to pioneer a model that others can follow. The answer is not to give away one's company but for the employees to buy *the company over an agreed term of years. Only then will they value it, and having worked together to get it, their company becomes a spiritual vehicle for good relationships, and they will have pride of ownership, which is an entirely different motivating force from public ownership without pride. Some people have advanced as a solution a "Universal Captialism" which turns the workers into shareholding co-owners of the company. But this only multiplies the greed of capitalism. Then we have not just a few capitalists, but a whole world of capitalists, and an even more intense vibration of materialism and greed. Everyone would be looking in the newspaper every morning to see if his shares have gone up in value, whereas what we really want is not more greed but more responsibility for the common wealth, more integrity and caring. In this chapter we will mention the E.S.O.P. program for creating co-ownership, but E.S.O.P. is only a legal step to genuine* common *ownership which would be the spiritual vehicle of the new era of economic well-being for all, which we delve into in depth in* The Golden Egg. *The following chapter forms the bridge between* talking *about taking economic responsibility and actually feeling motivated to do it and knowing a definite way to begin. Without clear defined action at the everyday business level no vision, however lofty, can come into manifestation.*

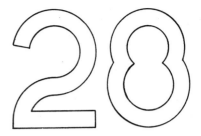

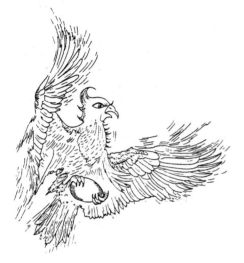

FICTITIOUS MONEY

When I was in business I would not only borrow money by buying goods on credit, but I would also *create* money by selling contracts for stuff that was to be shipped in six months time. Some of these future sales were for spices still unharvested in the ground in faraway India or Africa, and some were for spices that were not even planted yet. Hence I was able to do the business of a man with millions, with only a small amount of money. The risks involved were dependent on whether mother nature smiled on these crops or whether they were spoiled by weather conditions, monsoons, etc. Because the risk was great I tried to be the first to know how the crop was growing, so I could sell and get out of my contracts fast if the crop was not going to be big. I employed spies in various countries to go and dig the roots of spices and crops to see how they were growing underground even before the news was known to local growers who would never know until they saw the stuff growing above the ground. Thus, even without ever seeing the finished article, I had created a profit out of selling a worthless piece of paper called a futures contract. This fascinated me since it is a legal way of printing money. Most people do not know that money is a contract.*

In those days the government who issued paper money guaranteed that there was an equivalent amount of gold to back it up, and that it could be exchanged for silver or gold. Now very few nations are on the gold standard and so the contract or note we now call paper currency no longer guarantees an exchange of precious metal, but only guarantees that the public treasurer will honor it for debts public or private.

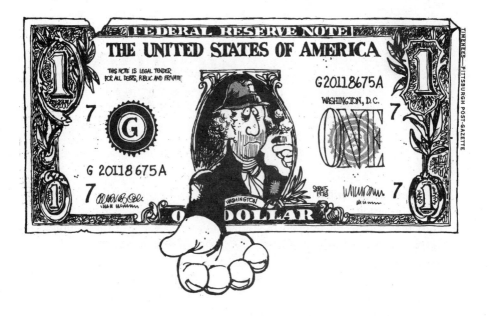

---

* A dollar bill is a contract to deliver value for the settlement of all debts. Take any currency note out of your pocket and read it. It is a contract with the US Treasury to deliver legal tender for the satisfaction of all debts both public and private. That is why it is called a note. In my own lifetime I have seen notes issued by banks contracting to deliver value for the discharging of debts. These were called "bank notes", and it is only a few years now since the government stopped the banks from printing their own notes of value.

This means that this money is fictitious, just as the contracts for spices which never existed in the ground and sometimes were never grown (because I bought them from myself through different brokers) were fictitious.

Before I had any desire to become spiritual, I thought that creating my own money out of nothing but people's imagination was one hell of a magic trick until one day I ended up with enough African, Indian and Jamaican ginger to supply the whole of America and Europe, yet I had no one to buy it. Somehow everyone on the market found out I had it, and they all waited to see how long I could hold the surplus through different crop years. After two and a half years waiting for the price to go up, I sold it to the people I borrowed money from at a terrible loss, wiping out profits of many years' trading. The day after I sold out, the market went up like a rocket because everyone knew I was out of stock, and the price rose to seven times what I had originally paid for it. One day it was worth ten cents a pound and I could not even sell it; the very next day it went to seventy cents per pound and within a week to ninety cents and you could not buy any. Nothing had happened in India, Africa or Jamaica that warranted such a price increase. This taught me another lesson: that the value of money and the value of a market is psychological, has nothing to do with the actual cost of production, and is largely fictitious. It showed that what I had done was the same thing "big government" was doing, except that the "money" they were losing by spending on government contracts was not their own but yours and mine as taxpayers. Furthermore I discovered that they could print more and more money to cover up their losses just as I had printed contracts for fictitious goods not yet grown. Legally they need never deliver any value for what the government owed because they could just go on printing money which was only actually worth its paper cost, whereas I, not being allowed to print money like a forger, had to pay up my losses in hard-earned real dollar bills. It was then I discovered that not only government was allowed to legally print money but also the banks.

Once upon a time when ordinary banks were authorized to issue their own money, these bank notes were represented by cash in the bank. It was only when there was a run on the bank during the

American financial crash of 1929 that there was not enough money to cover the paper they had printed, so eventually the governments stopped this practice. This also was fictitious money, often representing assets which could not be liquidated if all the contracts and notes to pay customers' money back came in all at once.

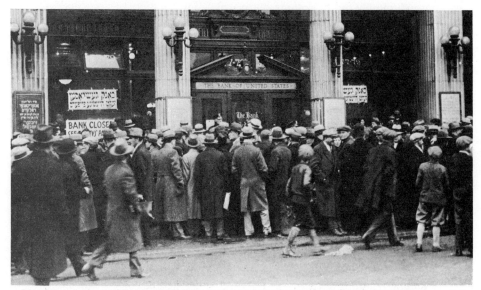

Depositors crowd around the closed doors of a bank during the "bank holiday" of 1933. The closings prevented "runs" on sound banks, which were permitted to reopen after examination by the Treasury Department.

But more than that, banks are still authorized to print fictitious money in another way, by giving credit and overdrafts. The power of banks to create money out of nothing by giving bank credit and to issue money or value not backed up by goods or gold, is no different from selling something you have not got but which you hope to have later. In other words it is institutional usury, because the banks get interest on this value without doing anything, growing anything or promising anything "real" to get or deliver this fictitious money.

You can well understand how I wanted to be a banker and start my own bank! Fortunately I was not feeling very fulfilled in all this fascinating financial wizardry and I got sick of manipulating crops, contracts and futures markets. It came to me at age thirty that I had been indulging in a legalized form of gambling, creating money out of nothing, and that this activity, for people other than authorized bankers who create and print this kind of money, is regarded as the activity of forgers and criminals. I knew that if I wanted to create *real* money out of nothing, it could not be done with a fictitious psychological trick, but only by getting hold of the *cosmic credit card.* I decided to see if it was possible to give up all my assets to the cosmos, manage them on behalf of the hidden "universal government", and then see if they would send me a *cosmic salary* or psychic income of happiness.

To do this properly I would have to know how others had done it and how to research the nature of consciousness so that the universe would respond when I wrote out a psychic check on the cosmic banker. I repeatedly read the Bible and Christ's injunction to place all my faith in the beneficence of the One (whoever that might be) who would take care of me because it was the *ultimate source.* This "heavenly Father" supposedly knows our needs before we even think of them and the whole secret is to trust this fact or to be convinced that it is actually true. Like most other human beings I trusted my bank account a lot more than I trusted God. But I decided that either Christ was a phony giving us wrong instructions or he was for real, and the only way we could ever know for sure was to scientifically duplicate the experiment and the results. The instructions said that we must give up everything to get this one thing. I knew that it was not going to be an easy experiment. This abundance could not be acquired by making a demand, but only through "eligibility". That meant working on my own consciousness. It meant learning to trust that God did actually own the universe and had unlimited resources and could supply them when needed and that the cosmic credit card was not another of those fictitious creations in people's imaginations like the value of money, but was real. This learning took me through many spiritual experiences which are not for this book. But what *is* for this book, is to share the secret of how to create 100% *real money.*

Inflation plays a cosmic joke upon all who put their faith in the things of this world. Anyone who had money way back ten years ago, like an old widow who lives off a pension plan, will know that the same money she saved or earned back then is now worth less than half its original value in the money of today because everything costs twice as much to buy. Here is an idea of what money is worth today compared with previous years:

1939 . . . . 100.0 cents		
1946 . . . . 71.1 cents		
1947 . . . . 62.2 cents		
1948 . . . . 57.7 cents		
1949 . . . . 58.3 cents		

WHAT INFLATION HAS DONE TO THE DOLLAR
Dollar's value in terms of what it will buy—
based on the prewar dollar of 1939

1950 . . . . 57.7 cents	1960 . . . . 46.9 cents	1970 . . . . 35.8 cents
1951 . . . . 53.5 cents	1961 . . . . 46.4 cents	1971 . . . . 34.3 cents
1952 . . . . 52.3 cents	1962 . . . . 45.9 cents	1972 . . . . 33.2 cents
1953 . . . . 51.9 cents	1963 . . . . 45.4 cents	1973 . . . . 31.3 cents
1954 . . . . 51.7 cents	1964 . . . . 44.8 cents	1974 . . . . 28.2 cents
1955 . . . . 51.9 cents	1965 . . . . 44.0 cents	1975 . . . . 25.8 cents
1956 . . . . 51.1 cents	1966 . . . . 42.8 cents	1976 . . . . 24.4 cents
1957 . . . . 49.4 cents	1967 . . . . 41.6 cents	1977 . . . . 22.9 cents
1958 . . . . 48.0 cents	1968 . . . . 39.9 cents	1978 (July) . . . . . . 21.2 cents
1959 . . . . 47.6 cents	1969 . . . . 37.9 cents	1979 . . . . 17.8 cents

As this book goes to press at the beginning of 1979 we are faced with a sharp increase in inflation from 13% to 17% or, with the dollar one-sixth less value than the 1978 dollar. Today's dollar therefore is worth less than half the value of the dollar you earned just 10 years ago and only eighteen percent of that of 1939.

In other countries of this hemisphere the inflation rates are much higher: Brazil 29.8%, Argentina 125.4%, Columbia 21.6%, Peru 22.3%, Uruguay 67.3%.

Most people believe that money is security, but really it is the least secure thing in the world. It is a psychological fiction. Apart from having to daily worry about money in order to hold onto it, the money mystique is one of the greatest sources of unhappiness for most people because of the great expectation that it can make them happy and healthy. The truth is that money is a sweet but fickle power and that many rich people are sick and emotionally deprived and they unwittingly hinder evolution and become spiritually lost.

Because the very psychological power of money has the ability to turn so many heads and induce so many hearts to slip from seeing the vision of real evolution, even spiritual enterprises, communities, churches, etc., fall down from their high goals and lose their integrity on the subject of money. Even governments have been known to cancel their own debts and start with new money and repudiate the old money as unreal. Once inflation and unemployment become runaway, there are always business troubles followed by massive depressions and the repudiation of government's obligations. Big cities like New York and Cleveland are already bankrupt and have defaulted on payments. Big city financial institutions and banks will go downhill once the real estate speculative bubble, caused by inflation, has burst. The fiscal crisis in America will have repercussions worldwide.

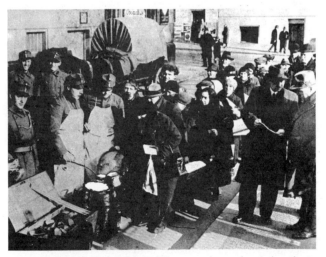

This bread line served by Austrian soldiers was only one of many throughout the depression-ridden world.

A LICENSE TO PRINT MONEY

What does back up the bank notes of a country? In the United States it is no longer the banks but the US Treasury. What supports the *fiction* that the money they print is solid and represents more value than the paper it is printed on? It used to be that a bank note promised that an equal amount of silver or gold was kept by the government to back up the paper money, but now the government is bankrupt by any ordinary citizen's standards. If the government conducted itself as an ordinary person or if we looked at the government with moral values, we would be disgusted with its business dealings. How could anyone wallowing in debt abroad at this time with over $200 billion ($200,000 million) in the hands of foreign central banks and over $500 billion ($500,000 million) in private holdings in foreign countries, and with an astronomical internal debt of $798 billion be so complacent and convinced that its budget practices work? How does it do this and what effect do such practices have in mortgaging our future as taxpayers? Are we saddling our children and posterity with the staggering problem of not only printing worthless money but making all the value we store up in capital and social credit worthless in a few years' time? In fact, is there any security in Social Security or will the government go bankrupt? Would it ever be able to protect all the depositors who have their money in banks if there were a sudden run on their funds? After the stock market crash of 1929, the Federal Reserve Bank was created in America to protect the citizen against the risks of banks which fail, but what about its own bankruptcy, since it not only relies on fictitious money but lends and allows its members, the ordinary banks, to create fictitious money out of nothing by giving credit. This might be a particularly appealing idea (like the printing of contracts for merchandise that was never existent), except that, according to the statistics kept by the Labor Department in Washington, it took nearly $19.00 in 1978 to buy what $10.00 bought in 1967. So in ten years *money has devalued by almost half while the cost of work and products has doubled because of inflation* at the rate of nine percent a year. This nine percent figure is for the USA which is much more stable than England, which has had inflation rates in some years up to thirty percent a year. What exactly is inflation? What is the relationship between the deflating money and the inflating prices? People must raise their prices on the goods they sell in order to earn enough money to live in a world where money is worth less and less. But then everyone else raises prices too, and the world gets more and more expensive to live in, which makes the money worth less or worthless. It is a vicious cycle, and no one person can stop this momentum once it begins, because he would soon starve if he kept his own prices low while paying high costs for everything he bought. Can anyone stop inflation? And if so, how?

THE FEDERAL RESERVE

Behavioral scientists believe that we can condition people by rewards, the same as animals are conditioned by food supply. In the same way, economists believe that the social habits and commercial life of the country can be controlled by manipulating interest rates and the supply of money. Very few ordinary citizens know that the American economy is controlled by the Federal Reserve Bank. Government could stop feeding inflation by not running up its enormous deficits, but instead the Federal Reserve has always used the method of reducing inflation by cracking down on the money supply and pushing interest rates up so high that people cannot borrow money to buy the things they want. Therefore the whole economy suffers a recession which then results in massive unemployment which means even more recession and even less money flowing through the economy. When money is in short supply or there is a credit squeeze people cannot buy goods freely, and the economy slows down. This lack of consumer demand causes each company to cut back production and to get rid of unnecessary employees, so jobs become scarce. The unemployed have no income with which to buy goods, so businesses are left with goods on hand that they cannot sell. They lay off more workers, and the whole thing goes in a negative spiral, creating a shrinking economy.

Why should a contrived recession be the antidote to inflation? Inflation is a similar vicious circle leading to a booming economy and more prosperity, but the prosperity is fake, because inflation is created by using fictitious money to buy real goods. By restricting credit or putting high interest rates on all lending, we cut off the supply of fictitious money and force people to buy goods with only the money they actually have in their pockets. But even this is a problem because in America there are always more goods than there are customers— with or without credit. Some economists believe that inflation is caused by "too much money chasing too few goods", i.e., by surplus money. But in actual fact an inflation is cancelled by a recession which only comes about as a result of overproduction, not from a shortage of easy credit (fictitious money). In other words, we are manipulating the *money*, but the *goods* are excessive even *with* credit.

The idea that society is controlled by these mechanisms of money-manipulation is false. Supply and demand is largely a matter of psychology because people who produce more or buy more do so as a result of mental attitudes rather than of necessity. If things look good to them they spend; if inflation looks like it's coming, they spend also to hedge the declining value of money against real bricks and mortar, objects such as cars, machinery or materials they know will increase in price. The idea that people act rationally and are predictable, like mechanical beings, is false. People will save money if they feel insecure and spend it when they feel secure, and the whole economy is therefore based on a psychological buoyancy or a feeling of depression. If people have no faith in currency bills and believe money is going to fail, they do not save it to feel secure but instead spend it as fast as they can on gold, on anything they can get, before it becomes totally worthless. This is what happens in a total financial crash. There is such a loss of conviction and it happens with such speed that people who are rich are left poor overnight. Therefore even the value of our money is based on our aggregate group faith and conviction in it as a store of lasting and secure value. The economy is controlled more by faith and the way people feel about it than the arbitrary acts of presidents, Federal Reserve Banks, or controlling experts. This is the main point in considering the value of money as a psychological fiction.

The average citizen is so intent upon his own financial situation, earning enough or borrowing enough to be able to buy what he hopes will make him happy, that he does not stop to wonder why interest rates are higher or where the Federal Reserve gets its power. He does not realize that *the Federal Reserve System is independent of the legislative, judicial and executive branches of government* and is exempt from Civil Service rules. In other words, it is autonomous with none of the checks and balances that are supposed to keep the American democratic system functioning as its founders intended. As an association of member banks, its board of governors in Washington is the final authority who can hire and fire whom it pleases without reference to government.

The main factor that keeps the Federal Reserve from gathering even more power over the nation is the state bank's option to belong or not belong to the system. All nationally chartered banks must join the Federal Reserve System and keep substantial funds on deposit with it as a safety precaution against overlending. But state chartered banks who do not do business over the entire United States can choose whether they want to belong or not. This drastically affects the power of the Federal Reserve because these state banks are in the majority. Because state bank members must put up reserves on deposit with the Federal Reserve Bank in order to be members, they have been dropping out of the system at the rate of one a week. Therefore, since 1965, the share of bank deposits regulated by the Federal Reserve has dropped from 86% to 72%, which has weakened its control over the money supply and its direct control over credit. Nevertheless, its power is alarmingly great.

The Federal Reserve Bank has twelve branches, each covering different regions and each with its own president. These banks function daily as clearing houses for checks and as centers for distributing treasury bills (bank notes) to the member banks. Through this system the nation's money supply is determined by controlling interest rates, and the Federal Reserve Bank makes a handsome profit buying and reselling government securities, bonds, and treasury bills to its member banks. On these transactions the Federal Reserve System realizes a profit ($5.9 billion or 5900 million dollars last year, 1977) and returns it to the treasury, minus all its operating expenses. Its budget is not subject to scrutiny by any government agency, congressional committee or private person, and the Federal Reserve is therefore a law unto itself. It writes the rules under which all commercial banks operate. It can approve or disapprove mergers between banks and decide whether an ordinary bank can open a new branch in other countries, and it enforces all the laws enacted for banking. The equivalent in the United Kingdom is the Bank of England and its board of governors who have similar powers and undertake similar functions with the exception that the English commercial banks are not members of a system. The Bank of England is, like the Federal Reserve, an independent control mechanism through which the economy and supply of money and credit is controlled.

The power of these institutions does not come from the constitution nor by "divine right". Where does it come from? It comes from the simple fact that we are content to buy the things we want with fictitious money, even though we enjoy this prosperity at the expense of our own future. Anyone can see that if we have more going out than is coming in, someday our nation, which began so nobly, will be as bankrupt as any petty embezzler who seizes money in the tempting moment of the now and hopes that the future will never catch up to him. The only difference is that *the American people are embezzling from themselves.*

During 1979 the Federal Government will borrow about 110 billion dollars, although the deficit will be only 60 billion. The remaining 40 to 50 billion goes to pay for loans to foreign countries to buy US arms, to Russia for export credits to buy wheat, truck factories, oil technology, computers, etc. It goes to pay farmer loans, the defaults in federally-guaranteed home loans, unpaid personal education loans and export credit insurance guarantees which are often not always paid back by foreign countries. None of these items are included in the budget.

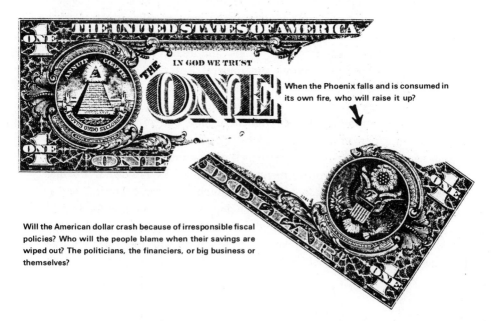

When the Phoenix falls and is consumed in its own fire, who will raise it up?

Will the American dollar crash because of irresponsible fiscal policies? Who will the people blame when their savings are wiped out? The politicians, the financiers, or big business or themselves?

There is an actual deceit embedded in the budget figures that make it *look* like a deficit of 60 billion when it will be nearer to 110 billion that we will be adding on to the national debt for posterity and our children's future taxation. The interest on all this borrowing of 798 billion dollars comes to 55.4 billion annually or 8 cents out of every dollar spent. *Our currency is backed up by a bankrupt system.*

Politicians are always thinking about the next election and, in order to make their financial and taxation policies more attractive, have often referred to the increasing GNP as a sign of wealth.

The term Gross National Product, GNP, has been banned from this book because it represents a fictitious figure. It includes inflation, the cost of all that is hideous, such as hydrogen bombs, and all that is produced by civilization including the inflated costs of hospital care and funerals. GNP is no measure of civilized activity or production and its use is a serious reflection on the intelligence of those who use it as a yardstick.

HOW CAN WE CREATE REAL MONEY?

The answer is written on the dollar bill in very large letters. The treasury does not trust gold anymore, nor does it trust silver as a back-up for its printing of paper money, but it clearly says, "In God We Trust", and that is the truth. In fact the politicians are printing money

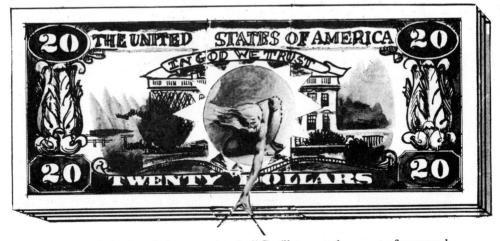

like a criminal and then trusting in "God" to get them out of unsound credit practices. Politicians do not realize that they are the cause behind the entire vicious circle of inflation. They try to sort the problem out and they propose all sorts of theories and ways to fix it, but in actual fact, they themselves are the main cause of government overspending of the citizen's future earning power. When citizens actually find out what the politicians have been doing to finance this gigantic mortgage, they are going to be real MAD. At the moment they think the national debt is something necessary and besides, it is all happening at another level. But once they see the connection and make the link with their own pockets and say, "Those people are spending *my* money on projects for my behalf in ways that I wouldn't spend it myself, and they are doing it to become popular and get themselves re-elected," then the upheaval will come, just as it came in the French Revolution or any other revolution in history. The senate may need a new office building but do the senators really need two toilets for every suite, when the taxpayer may live with his entire family in a house with only one? The building must be larger for the many aides and helpers, because the staff has grown too large for the present building, but who has checked to see if perhaps the aides, like the toilets, are a *luxury* that the taxpayers who are footing the bill might not deem necessary?

Unwittingly today people are led into inflation as a new form of slavery just as chattel slavery in England and Ireland occurred when the economic surplus of the peasants was expropriated by the owners of the land. The ownership of the land under the feudal system was given to the Norman invaders and the peasant was free to starve or compete with his fellows in renting the land from the barons. In a similar way slavery was created in India when the British awarded a monopoly privilege and power to tax the people to the Rajahs of India who were the equivalent of the Norman landlord families and their heirs.

Now the modern Western government has the same power to tax by the process of legally inflating and thereby expropriating the surplus wealth of all who work and save up money for their declining years. The process of embezzling the surplus value of the producers in our Western civilization, through spending money which has not been raised by direct taxation but is acquired by debasing the currency, has robbed all who save or buy life insurance for their dependents. The American people have been robbed of over 2000 billion dollars of surplus through the systematic inflating applied by the central bankers and politicians who have benefitted from this robbery. Our rulers have spent other people's surplus value on the lobbyists and their causes in order to get themselves elected and to retain their power. This deficit spending has produced a money credit muddle which has brought us to the present awareness that our economic system has now become unwittingly a new form of slavery, creaming off the surplus product of all producers in the system. There are laws in the constitution against chattel slavery and feudal exploitation of monopolies, but there are no laws against the economic slavery of millions of workers in Western countries by *leaders who use inflation as an invisible form of taxation.* As if this were not enough to equal the feudal slavery to the barons there is now another form of economic and political slavery invented by Karl Marx. The communists, representing a minority party in Russia and China, have implemented a system and forced it upon the majority and this new system takes the surplus value of the ordinary worker and converts it to the minority party's philosophy of power and position. Except for these new barons (the party leaders), most of Russia's people and the Chinese millions are wage slaves. They are neither free to strike nor free to change their jobs without party permission. They are only free to subsist at whatever level of living the party officials or their leaders permit. If they are not docile and completely slave-like, they are not even free to complain without being sent to worse jobs or even to a prison camp.*

The distorted philosophy of Marx who protested against the wage slavery and exploitation of early capitalism provides the intellectual rationale for the worst system of wage slavery and workers' repression the world has seen since the Normans and the Rajahs. But the difference is that the Chinese and Russian systems have been imposed from above, while in America, the wage slaves have surrendered their surplus value through taxation *voluntarily.* The spending of billions of

---

* See page 152 referring to scientists Orlov, Sharansky and Ginzburg who spoke out against lack of basic human rights.

inflationary American dollars of deficit paper money has taken place by the public's ignorance of economic laws and the unwitting belief that their political representatives were protecting the public interest. Yet every day the process of wage enslavement and embezzling of surplus value grows through inflation budgetary depreciation of currency and life savings. Unless the workers strike against the real culprit they will continue to have to strike for more wages and thereby cause more inflation and more embezzlement. Unless the retrogression of wage slavery can be turned around and the life savings and common wealth of our society preserved in an effective store of material value, then our present social order will collapse spiritually. To be put on a work treadmill without receiving any lasting abundance or material fulfill-ment is a failure of the spiritual law that Christ uttered: "Seek ye first the Kingdom of Heaven and all these things shall be added unto you." Instead, our present social order has put materialism first and this has no psychic or spiritual fulfillment and is about to collapse financially too.

The social credit which government money is supposed to represent is a complete fiction, because its value is backed up by one thing and one thing alone, namely the power of government to tax the future incomes of its citizens and thereby the power to pledge credit on their future productivity. If this fiduciary power were suddenly taken away, the government would be declared bankrupt, because it would have no way of paying its debts to foreign countries or even to its own citizens to cover its treasury bank notes. If the politicians and governments really did trust God, that would be great, but in truth they really trust only in the government's power to tax the productivity and creativity of every man, woman and child, so that they (the government and the banks giving credit) can go on creating paper money out of nothing. This great deception seems less clever when we realize that our national credit and our own money in the bank are really fictitious and have no real value, because in a real crisis they could be worthless tomorrow.

How can we correct this social situation and pay for it to be done? Two major reforms are needed in order to make capital worth 100% real value. The first step is to make all business enterprises in the

Photo Trends

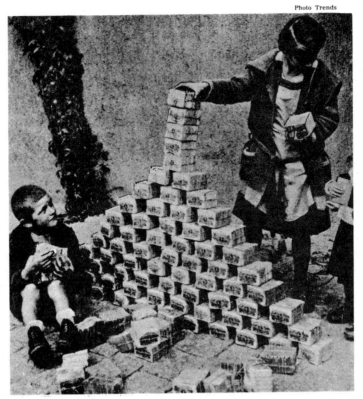

Castles of cash: Worhtless money in Weimar Germany.
Can it happen to the American dollar?

country into Common Ownerships. This would wipe out the capitalist idea of ownership right through industry and replace it with ownership by employees who work in the business acting in partnership with those who can supply *real capital.* The capitalist would lend capital to the workers like a banker, but he would not *own* the operation. The mistake is to think this is a difficult and complex operation involving yet another bureaucracy to carry it all out when it is really only a legal matter of buying shares and changing the by-laws of companies. It can be done in one hour on paper! This is not a difficult step like nationalization because *the capitalist does not lose his money.** It can

---

* See Book Two, *The Golden Egg: Manifesting the Rise of the Phoenix,* which describes Common Ownership and revitalizing the economy.

be done within the space of a boardroom meeting or the time it takes to sign a contract at a specific rate of interest or to agree to a share in profits. At the same time the right to create fictitious money should be taken from the commercial banks and restored to society by reserving this power only to the state. How would this create 100% money? By ending the power of the banks to create fictitious money in the form of bank credit, only the government would then have the power to create something out of nothing. And once this power is in the hands of the government, we can legislate our return to reality and make our store of the common wealth in real 100% dollars instead of fictitious dollars that are only figures written down on ledgers. How can we do this financial surgery that is so necessary to our economic security?

If the banks were not allowed to give credit for money they don't have and thereby to create money, and if this power were restored to the state alone, one could describe "state money" as real social credit. With private credit, the bankers get rich by having a kind of franchise on credit-making, whereas "social credit" means that society (the people) are the usurers. Now, whether credit is social or private, the money is fictitious, first because it is created on paper only (figures written in ledgers), and second because inflation undermines its original value. But once we have created state money, there is a way to turn it into 100% real money through Common Ownership. The present way of creating *social capital* is through deficit spending and the creation of a national debt. But all this artificial credit is achieved at citizens' expense by continually printing more and more paper money. Nobody is hearing this in any depth because we continue to do it and still complain of inflation. I repeat that paper money is only "real money" if we pledge our futures and those of our children to ever-increasing taxation and debt.

How then does state money become 100% money? Where does the backing come from if not from taxpayers whose finance is whittled away daily by printing paper? The answer is again Common Ownership. In Common Ownership 100% money is created not by borrowing on credit but by a once and for all printing of bonds which are held for the workers to be paid for by them out of the profits. The workers pay for the business out of future profits and if their company does not pay off these government bonds, the workers don't get the joint ownership. In this case *money* is backed by a promise against the future, but it is not a payoff through never-ending taxation but a fixed, finite and very real payment within a fixed period of time. The former is like the embezzler who keeps stealing more money and hoping to replace it when more comes in and meanwhile trying to fool his partner by some clever juggling of the books. He robs Peter to pay Paul. The latter is like an honest man who makes a pact with himself that on a given date he will put back the money he took from his own savings account, and he does so.

THE GREAT HOAX

It is clear that a capitalist economy cannot be sustained by controlling the bank rate of interest and that neither the public demand for goods nor full employment of the work force can be controlled by printing more money. The idea that we can control the economy by putting curbs on the supply of money and credit by creating artificially high interest rates, etc., has always led to unemployment and depression of the economy. Economists today have recognized that giving the government and state this right to control and issue money does give the politician and administration more direct control over the economy, but does this control work? Economists at government level never advocate Common Ownership of industry nor do they believe in 100% money but instead prefer to risk creating more unemployment by setting high interest rates on fictitious bank money and by restricting credit to discourage spending. This false interest rate is institutionalized usury and does not really protect the economy as supposed, but as we keep repeating, causes the capitalist system to create unemployment by making money scarce *supposedly* in order to control inflation. This creates cheaper labor, but at the expense of the taxpayers who must eventually pay for the higher interest rate for credit. And they must pay for the fictitious money with real money, i.e., by the tax upon their own earnings which is levied to support higher government deficits.

It is bad enough that we pay higher interest rates on fictitious money, but the public also hurts itself by allowing windfall profits for those bankers who pass credit from one bank account to another over and over again. Most people forget that they are loaning the bank money whenever they put money in a bank account. For example, the bank accepts deposit for $1000 from John and lends $600 to Michael who puts $500 of it in his account. The bank then lends Mary $400 and $500 to Jack who both put part of the money in their account. When the Michaels, Marys and Jacks are multiplied by several thousand customers, the same $1000 can be loaned to several hundred people, particularly if many of the checks paid between the customers are with the same bank. To increase the interest charges on all this credit is inflationary. In other words, if we take all the banks together, the same fictitious money is often loaned out to several people at the same time at the expense of public inflation. Whereas if industry retained its capital profits of Common Ownership and became its own banker, using accumulated social capital or state credit, no interest would be paid on it by anyone.* The reason why no one should pay interest is because it is the public's money to begin with and secondly the public money can be loaned out over and over again since it is only a contract needing nothing but credit to back it up. This credit is created out of nothing but the promise to pay value for bank notes, which it never does, nor does it ever need to.

OWNERSHIP AND CREDIT

The need to borrow capital from banks and other financial sources is almost inevitable for the owners of a business. In the USSR the State owns all businesses, yet the businesses still must borrow capital. They borrow from the State and the interest is paid for by the consumers in higher prices. Thus the government borrows money from itself but makes the workers pay for it. Whereas the capitalist banker charges interest as his business, the communist planner uses interest to exploit both the public and the workers who make the product. The State controls all credit, owns all business, reaps all profit, and in addition charges six percent on the capital sums allocated to the State-

---

* The Soviet Union whose industries operate on state credit or social capital does not follow this policy. They charge each factory with a capital interest up to six percent, and in this way the socialist states copy the capitalist.

owned industry. This in turn is charged against the selling prices and is precalculated as part of the cost of production. Since the State created this money out of nothing, to charge interest on it is just a roundabout way of taxing the people for the products they buy in order to pay for the weight of a very heavy bureaucracy.

In the USA, if a business does not have enough resources to pay for equipment, labor and raw materials, and still have enough money to operate, it is a matter of course to borrow working capital temporarily from a bank until the product is finished and can be sold for cash. The interest on this working capital can be calculated as just another business expense to be deducted from income taxes, and the amount is not relevant if the gross profit on the finished product is high. But if the profit margin is a fine one where only a few cents are made on the product on a large volume, then the difference in high or low interest rates can be the difference between a profit or a loss.

The workers in a business do not often appreciate the delicate balance of all these factors—the profit margin, the quantity of goods produced, the rate of interest, the fact that money must be borrowed and risked against future sales which may or may not be forthcoming— because the workers are seeing from a different point of view. But the owner has to decide what to do if he cannot get financing from the bank or if the interest rate from private lenders is too high. He has no choice but to go to the "money market" or stock market, which acts as a middleman between the company and anyone who is willing to pay out money for "shares" of the future profits. Another advantage of going public is that by spreading the ownership shares amongst a large number of small investors the businessman has more control of his company than if he is indebted to a bank or to two or three individuals. If large investors have a substantial interest in a company they will want a place on the board of directors and may interfere in the decision-making process at a later date. Essentially what the businessman is doing to borrow money from investors is to issue secured paper titles which promise to pay a proportion of the company's profits. This is why shares are called securities.

Banks and financial houses buy company ownership stock at a discount and sell it to the public at its face value. If the issue is fully subscribed on the stock market then the money is raised and the financial house can pay the industrialist. If the issue is undersubscribed and no one takes up the stock, the deal does not go through and the capital is returned to the people who bought shares. For example, supposing I were a businessman who wanted to expand and build a factory or a new block of offices. I would need a large sum of money, maybe several million dollars.

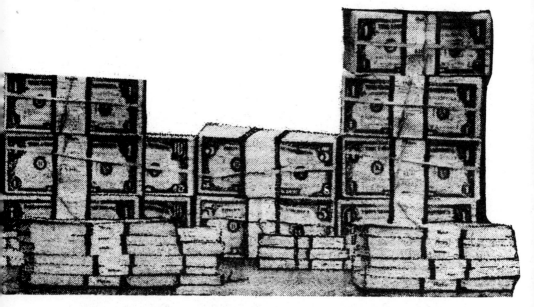

If I pay interest on it to a bank it will be very costly because banks and financial houses don't like long-term loans for the simple reason they like to lend the same money out over and over again, so they raise the interest on a long-term loan. But if, in spite of this deterrent, I go to a bank and say, "Lend me several million dollars to build a new factory," they will say, "Yes, but you must give us the building as security and until it is fully built, you must mortgage your existing company's assets to us in case anything should go wrong." I might say that this is too much to ask. I will instead try to sell part of my business to the public and raise new money as well to get a large amount of capital on which I pay no interest because the lenders are instead buying shares and becoming co-owners with the existing owners of my company and its new factory or buildings. They will share in future profits and in any losses, and my company does not have to risk the financiers taking over the entire business if the new factory does not succeed. As a businessman I say, "I will go to a stock broker who will float a share issue on the money market." A visit to the brokerage house reveals that they will issue the shares to the public less a commission of ten percent. Until the issue is subscribed over the next few months a bridging loan could be guaranteed to cover immediate needs at eight percent interest plus a commission for arranging the guarantee. When the brokers sell the shares they will deduct and get back the amounts they have advanced. They will deduct the interest and commission, giving the balance of the proceeds of sale to me against delivery of the new share certificates. Every day thereafter the new public shareholders will look up in the newspapers what the stock market quotation is for their shares which rises and falls with the profits of the whole undertaking.

If I am a small businessman, however, with few assets and a new project which requires a small amount of money, the stockbrokers and financial houses will not be at all interested in me because the same amount of paperwork has to be done for a small stock issue as a large one, plus the risk of not selling the shares of an unknown company is greater. They will probably refuse unless there are prospects of a sure success. Since the bank or financial house is giving out money, it seems to be taking a risk, but really the financial house has little risk except the advertising unless it decides to buy some of the stock shares itself and own part of the business temporarily until the shares are sold to the public. Many of the financial institutions and banks will step in and buy certain kinds of ownership stock, but they buy only from large and well-known industries that are financially sound and certain to make a profit. It is difficult for a small industrialist to prove he can deliver a profit, and in addition he is hampered by regulations which are now very strict on the stock market. Before any small company can sell shares, it must be investigated thoroughly by the Securities Exchange Commission to prevent small fly-by-night companies from selling shares in companies whose assets don't exist or selling worthless swamp or desert property as good land.

This is a much simplified account of what we must do to raise new capital in a capitalist system. Everything is engineered to make financing a low risk and a high profit for the middlemen. They know that all the capital is not required immediately by the industry so they advance (with interest) a line of credit in the form of guarantees enabling the industrialist to borrow from banks. For example, he can have one million now at a certain rate of interest, another million in six months at another rate, and another million later on. Meanwhile, the financial house is selling the shares. There seems to be some risk since the money is guaranteed to the industrialist even if the shares do not sell, but really there is no risk, because the financial houses and stockbrokers only buy stock that they know they can sell.

Why is this transaction a fictionalizing of money? If a financial house or stockbroker agrees to carry my loan, the money becomes fictitious because they create paper to replace the public's money, and they can get a ten percent guaranteed share in the expected profit long before I actually use the credit they have extended to me. In other words, they are bringing in money as they sell the stock to the public and at the same time they are collecting their interest from me, the industrialist. It is fictitious money since they are not paying *out* real money because the company doesn't need it all yet. This is made possible by the fact that the industrialist must make sure in advance that he can get enough of the capital he will need or he cannot even embark on the project for fear of falling short of capital later on. He has to know that he can get it when he needs it, so he is forced to borrow it at the outset rather than wait to arrange the loan when he is ready to use the money. Due to the time lag, the industrialist pays interest on money he has not yet actually received while the financial house may receive interest on money that has not yet even been loaned but only guaranteed or promised. The lender charges interest not upon money but on a "paper mortgage", promissory notes which comprise the great fictitious wealth created by the power of banks and financial houses who create the credit. Whether they actually have the wealth in assets or not is irrelevant. They get their interest or profit on the *guarantee* alone—the promise that credit will be available. They do not even have to deliver the money because the paper mortgage or promissory notes are resold to big institutions, insurance companies, etc., at a discount long before the actual credit is needed and actually used for working capital by industry.

I have said that often the industrialist goes to the financial house or stockbroker to raise money through the stock market rather than acquiring a bank loan. But in the end he is dealing with the bank via the financial house, because he is able to get a bank loan on the guarantee of the financial house. In this case he is using the ownership shares of his company as collateral. Shares are property, so they can be used as security for a private loan or for a business loan, just as a house or car can be used. But the bank only holds the shares; it doesn't own them. Many people do not realize when the radio advertisements say, "Come on in and buy a Cadillac on credit," that really there will be no credit unless there is some kind of collateral, job income, or security. When an industrialist goes to a bank and gets a loan for working capital, he may use the shares or assets of his company for collateral. If he does, then the other public shareholders are sharing the risk with the industrialist, because they are as responsible as he is to pay back the loan. But people do not think of this when they buy shares.

The workability of the capitalist system is that the public buys shares, the stockbroker or financial house is paid for being the middle-man in the transaction, and the industrialist gets the capital which enables him to make a profit and pay dividends to the shareholders for the use of their money. So everyone is happy. But if the business fails to make a profit, then the expansive trend is reversed and everyone feels the pinch except the middleman who, by use of fictitious money (guarantees on paper), has made a profit whether the business prospers or not.

Because of the subtle connection between borrowing and owner-ship, there seems no way out of this dependency on middlemen, but in fact there is a very natural solution. The first step, if the company already has a group of shareholders, is for the company to become its own banker. If it borrows from its own shareholders to raise working capital credit, it can bypass the stock market. Then the cost of raising new working capital is minimized. Alternatively, if a company chooses not to distribute its profits to shareholders but ploughs the profit back into cash reserves, then it does not need to borrow from financial institutions by mortgaging its assets and capital equipment. The best and most efficient way for a company to raise money is to borrow from its own shareholders who are already the owners of the equipment and are therefore fully secured. This is 100% money because it is backed by real, tangible assets and is not some fictitious accounting of a credit in a bank ledger. But even this first step is only a small solution to the gigantic problem of fictitious money and inflation. It still does not solve the problem of the millions of smaller businesses which cannot get enough capital to develop their companies. Smaller businesses get squeezed out in the normal capitalist process. Either they are too small to be a good risk or else interest rates are so high that, even if their product is doing well and warrants expansion, many businesses cannot expand. The gap between upper and middle class widens, and the wealthy get wealthier while the poor get poorer, just as the communists predicted. It is this aspect of capitalism that gives socialism its greatest impetus and support. If the process continues, capitalism will come to the final collapse and self-destruction which Marx foresaw. For this problem, as well as the problem of fictitious money and inflation, the answer is Common Ownership. Common Ownership is the method which will rectify this imbalance in capitalism and protect us from both our own capitalist greed and from the forces of socialism or communism.

In Common Ownership, all shares are owned in common by the employees of the company, and there is a direct link between their sense of responsibility and the amount of profit they will make. Since it is the owner's job to raise working capital, the worker in most businesses is not usually very concerned about it. But in Common Ownership it becomes the worker's problem because he is the owner and it is he who takes the risk and he who will reap the profit or suffer the loss. So he is motivated to understand these things, and the mystery of money is demystified. At present, little of this is understood by the worker at shopfloor level, although the process is very simple. As I have said, borrowing is simply a matter of having enough assets to put up as security so that a banker will risk his money on the future of the business. If the bank will not risk, and the industrialist has to go instead to the stock market, he must pay the extra interest for the services of the financial house or broker who acts as middleman and sells the stock to the public. This type of paper transaction is exploitative of industrial activity and is the great weakness of the capitalist system, making money a paper commodity which is bought and sold instead of reserving it as a medium of exchange.

We use money as a convenient medium of exchange, but ultimately the human energy which is locked up in money represents work and can also do work. And yet in many instances money is not work, just as bank credit is not real 100% money. Real work may take a long time to produce several thousand items but, with money and machinery, the human work energy expended in making those items can be dispensed with or transferred to another person or sold to another part of the world within a few minutes by writing a contract. In five minutes you can form a company on paper, pass ownership of assets and property to it by contract, sell the property to another company and dissolve the first company without going outside a lawyer's office. What is thus sold may have taken years of physical labor to create. A deal of fifteen million dollars takes about the same amount of time to transfer legally as a deal of fifteen dollars. All these paper transactions are for convenience, and so they have become an acceptable and respected part of our society. We have faith in our system. Our faith and conviction that money represents work and assets and that contracts written on paper represent title to real and tangible properties that we exchange, this faith creates our present society. If we had faith in another system of value, our world could be changed overnight. But we are content with the old system because we have not really questioned its axioms. We have never really asked why the ordinary citizen does not have the power to create money out of nothing without work or effort as does a government or a bank. The bank credit card on which a bank customer pays eighteen percent interest in order to defer payment for a month is an example of money created entirely out of the bank's reputation for making payment or crediting another customer's account who deals with the same bank. The bank credit card is just another form of currency printed on plastic instead of paper.

Why is this so bad? The consequences of making money into a commodity are that we create a whole capitalist world of people who

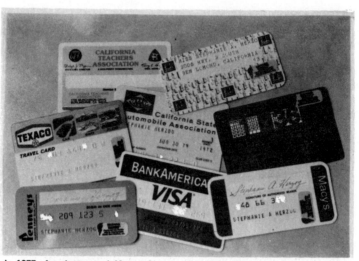

In 1977, Americans used Master Charge, with 47.8 million cardholders, and Visa
(formerly BankAmericard), with 44 million cardholders, more than 876 million times.

live their lives looking at the prices of shares in the morning newspaper
to see how wealthy they are or how much they have lost on their
shares. Their entire day is made happy or miserable or their consciousness is occupied worrying about the security of their shares in a
company they do not control. Their lives are in fact controlled by the
activities and values of the stock market which is based on the creation
of fictitious money, i.e., money that is created by printing paper shares,
certificates and paper currency rates. This "paper" is regarded by
ninety percent of the population as "real" and the source of all power
and happiness. Money is not in itself bad, but when most of our day is
spent talking about money, thinking about money and manipulating
sums of money, then we become a race of greedy-minded, self-centered
selfish beings, always with conflicting interests where we can only win
by someone else losing. Then we must ask ourself simple questions as
to why democracy does not work even though we are free to make it
work. What need would there be of communism or any other ism if the
life of a citizen was completely fulfilling in a free society? The problem
of income or wealth for everyone rather than a few skilled investors in
shares or people with control of industry is an age-old problem.
Common Ownership is a natural solution to this problem because a
financial house cannot do this kind of dealing and speculating with

Common Ownership stock because there is only one share, belonging to everybody employed in the business.

When there is Common Ownership, the workers and their savings, earning power, skills and job security all add to the feasibility of securing a private loan, because Common Ownership spreads the power and control of a company among responsible employees instead of irresponsible shareholders who may never have even seen the company in which they own stock and who rely upon the company president to see that they make a profit. In the transition to Common Ownership it might be asked, "What will become of all the money the existing shareholders put up to buy the original shares? Will the existing owners want a high price for selling the business?" The answer is that they can still lend the money to buy the shares to the Common Ownership just as a bank might do and still get a guaranteed and agreed slice of the profits until the sale of the shares has been paid off by the workers. They would not actually transfer their shares to the employees until the shares were paid for, so they would be "secured" just like a bank is secure when it holds the shares of a company collateral. When the owners are paid off, that releases 100% real money into the money market which then re-enters the economy. New enterprise flourishes, the supply of money for housing mortgages is increased, and the owners of this real money can, if they please, still lend it to industry for working capital. All this creates tax-free money from profits which would normally go in taxes and be wasted by party governments and politicians on self-serving projects in order to perpetuate their power. It also gives opportunity to the small company which it otherwise would not have.

There are other power-sharing aspects within the Common Ownership company which penetrate beneath the superficial financial and political mechanisms of our society. For instance, Common Ownership takes the power out of the hands of the company president's control and makes the stock more reliable, because any stock has value only if the industrialist is honest enough not to milk the business so that the shares become worthless as in the recent example of Investors Overseas Ltd. Robert Vesco, president of the company, took at least 250 million dollars and ran off to Costa Rica, having given himself an unsecured

"loan". The president before him, Bernie Cornfeld, stole from the
same company 100 million dollars.

Faith in the honesty and integrity of industrialists and businessmen
is what stands behind the paper shares. Whenever the president of a
company robs a company in which the public has invested, which
happens more often than the public knows, then faith in the capitalist
system is destroyed. The debasement of share values and currency and
debasement of the word eventually creates a disintegrating society,
because integrity in people's word and faith in their willingness to carry
out their promises no longer exist. Under such conditions, communication between one person and another breaks down, words become
meaningless, values are raped and morals decline. This is the world we
now inherit where integrity and truth between human beings is at a
premium, and faith in social systems and the leaders who administrate
them is nonexistent. In such unreal times which have lost their
meaning, anything can happen to flip the whole system on its back, like
a turtle helplessly waving its arms in the air and unable to get back on
its feet. This is the moment when Common Ownership will come into
its own.

Since the worker-owners of a Common Ownership company cannot
raise money from the sales of shares to the public, their development
capital can be found without going through the stock market simply by
using an Employees' Stock Ownership Plan (E.S.O.P.) set up under
the laws of the US government to foster the ownership of business by
employees. Under this plan, the employees and managers of a business
are allowed to buy their own stock over a fixed period of years, usually
around five, using a percent of the business' own profits *tax-free*. In
effect, the American government is forfeiting tax money in order to
make possible an entirely new kind of business. I have described this in
great detail for those who wish to learn more about it or actually do it
in another book which deals with the creation of wealth from nothing.*
With the future definitely leaning towards Common Ownership we cut
out the middlemen in the supply of money for development. The vision

---

* E.S.O.P. and how to go about creating one is described in *The Golden Egg:
Manifesting the Rise of the Phoenix*, soon to be published by the University of the Trees
Press.

of all companies eventually becoming their own bankers and belonging to their own employees is part of the Rise of the Phoenix since it will eliminate industrial strife, strikes, violence of picketing, etc. When all business becomes a spiritual instrument of the New Age reformation, money will become a true "store of energy" instead of a paper commodity. Meanwhile, let us see what are the implications and consequences of our present system.

LEGALIZED INSTITUTIONAL USURY

To pay interest to one set of people in society (bankers) who have been given this power to print fictitious money in the form of credit, is a form of public usury. But as long as society permits itself to operate on deficit and credit, whether that is private credit or social credit, we are in effect printing money which devalues the existing money we already have earned. There is no way around it because credit itself is not real; it is only man's confidence in man, confidence in the ability to pay. It is not by accident that the motto of the largest credit agency in the world, Dunn and Bradstreet, is "Man's confidence in man". Because I used to represent Dunn and Bradstreet in the West Indies for over ten years and founded my own National Credit Bureau which operated successfully and eventually sold out its shares to its employees (then operated later even more successfully), I am offering here not theoretical knowledge but the fruit of experience. All credit is a fiction based on future confidence or faith. Faith is a *sense of conviction* that we will get paid upon the due date or that the words or the signed contract of a person has absolute integrity. If words are not integral and promises are not kept, then they are a fiction.

Faith in the future capacity of a person or a company or a community is the whole basis for credit and rests entirely on man's financial confidence in the future and in a person's integrity. If we do not have this sense of conviction about the future, then credit is worth nothing and more often becomes a loss. Government guarantees are worthless if governments cannot pay their debts. Hence all credit in society is based on faith and is largely psychological, but if we borrow and we do not pay our deficit, then we lose the real value of our work done, which is devalued by the amount owed. Only our wealth stored in assets or money will go to pay our debts, and the credit we cannot pay off we will then still owe to others in some way. This is true whether we are an individual or a state and if we are borrowing from ourself, as the state is doing with a budget deficit, then *we are psychologically deceiving ourself, because we are devaluing our own money.* Eventually there must be a forgiving of this debt or a refloating of the value; hence countries devalue their own currencies in order to balance their internal debts. If we refuse to devalue, then others will be forced to do it for us. This is why external countries who give this credit to us by holding the paper money backed by the American government, have to devalue our dollar bills in foreign countries even though internally within our own country we don't notice much difference from a devaluation except for the gradual inflation of prices.

INFLATION RATES—the inflation of prices & devaluation of currency is identical.

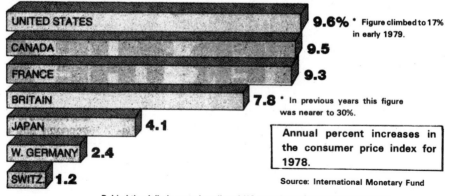

UNITED STATES **9.6%** * Figure climbed to 17% in early 1979.

CANADA **9.5**

FRANCE **9.3**

BRITAIN **7.8** * In previous years this figure was nearer to 30%.

JAPAN **4.1**

W. GERMANY **2.4**

SWITZ. **1.2**

Annual percent increases in the consumer price index for 1978.

Source: International Monetary Fund

Behind the dollar's woes is a dismal US record in international competition. Leading the major nations in its inflation rate, the US is last in productivity gains—and its trade deficit threatens to be chronic.

As long as a country uses this psychological self-deception, and the business world is not aware of the insecurity produced by the unreal psychological value of fictitious money, then our inflationary spiral will continue and politicians will continue to spend money they have not got. This has got to stop or it will be stopped by another depression or financial collapse. Who would believe that the great city of New York would ever go bankrupt and could not pay its bills? Yet it did, and only taxpayers' money from the federal government saved it from breaking down completely. The same thing can happen to the American dollar through misguided fiscal policies. The size of the organization is irrelevant, and big banks or big governments are as vulnerable to this fiscal irresponsibility as the ordinary citizen is.

As we said before, governments try to control inflation by curbing credit and the money supply, but only unemployment and a recession result from these curbs. The various devices and manipulations of economists cannot work in the long run any more than clever private individuals who are juggling checks can hide their insolvency from creditors who are banging at the door for their money. Not all bankers and capitalists believe in fictional credit such as that created by a budget deficit, because they believe in 100% money, and easy credit is anathema to them. But even among these, there have been some who saw the process of deflation by the creation of unemployment as a good thing, because it would bolster the currency. I do not believe we have to think that 100% money is a product of unemployment or the scarcity of money.* In spite of human suffering, these theorists have put the *value of money* before the social need of the people and regarded unemployment as an excellent check on runaway inflation, because it not only makes money and capital scarce but labor gets cheaper with unemployment, so that costs go down and real money gets more valuable. That is why most American businessmen went along with banker Andrew Mellon who recommended, just before the big financial crash of 1929, that the government should let the economy run down into its depths from which it would, by his theory, spring back to life automatically on a better footing of 100% money. The policy of deliberate unemployment would bring great suffering, he said, but he believed that business cycles operated by the law of supply and demand. "Liquidate stock, liquidate the farmers, liquidate labor," Mellon advised the government. The result was the Depression and the total collapse of financial institutions. The president was determined to keep the budget balanced, but during 1929, at the start of the Depression, 659 banks closed. In 1930, 1,352 banks closed, and in 1931, 2,294 banks closed, each destroying the cash and savings of millions of

---

* In *The Golden Egg* I give several other alternatives for communities and businesses who wish to create their own standards of value by issuing their own money in the form of a warehouse receipt for stable products.

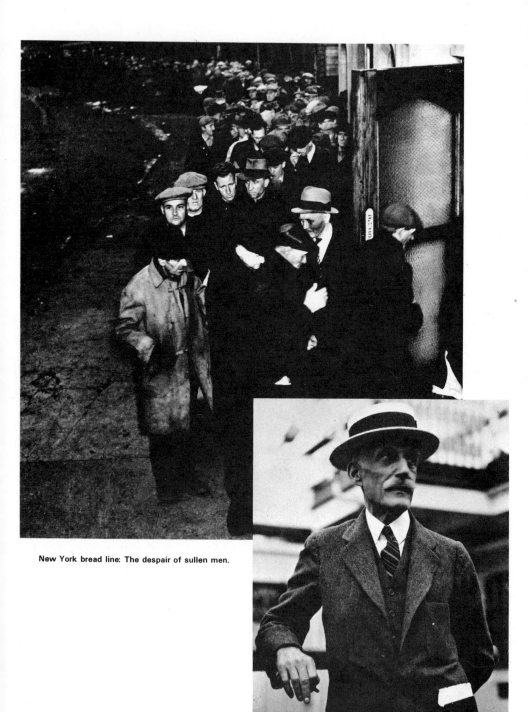

New York bread line: The despair of sullen men.

Andrew Mellon
"Government is just a business."

workers. The blame was laid eventually at the door of European master bankers who had given their New York associates the power to create easy money conditions, extending credit for speculation on the stock market which plunged and brought the crash on which the later Depression fed.

EASY MONEY AND HARD FACTS

How well I knew the pattern when I myself was buying and selling commodities on paper contracts with money given on easy credit terms from brokers on the futures market. Easy money encourages spending and speculation, as governments know. Anyone who can get easy credit knows how they can get into so much debt that they mortgage their future labors for years, all chasing this illusion of fictitious money! Everyone has the desire to spend money and they reason, "What is money for, anyway?" But spending on what? Let us take an example of indulgence—the luxury of owning a fancy motorhome, a recreation vehicle costing $20,000 which is used only twice a year but costs about $200 a month and which becomes parked rolling stock for ten or eleven months of the year. How many billions of dollars of family cash are tied up in these expensive gas-consuming pieces of equipment that do not produce anything, but instead saddle a family with at least $200 a month of payments? People are naively persuaded by easy credit that these houses on wheels are their "get-away" car in times of crisis or that they will always improve in value as a hedge against continuing inflation. None of this becomes true because if crises come, the first things you sell off are luxuries, and there are so many of these repossessed and used vehicles on the market right now, due to the fact that a high proportion of the work force is unemployed or struggling with inflation, that you can literally buy a $20,000 motorhome at less than $15,000 once it has been driven out of the showroom! The vehicle deflates in value the minute you drive it off the lot. Already there are more motorhomes than buyers, so even now you could not re-sell profitably. In the crisis you may not be able to sell at all, because everyone will have the same idea, and the market will be glutted. In addition, the money you would get if you did sell would be worth less than the money you paid for it. You think that by buying such a useful thing you will get out of the whole mess of dealing with paper money, but in fact, in the crisis, when you try to sell the motorhome, you will have more problems, not fewer, with the arbitrary value of money. Look down any middle class street today and see them lined up one after the other tying up millions of fictitious credit dollars. The crash must come when people are forced to sell and the loss eats into precious savings. The loss in value of this unnecessary physical possession, compounded with the loss in the inflated value of money, then becomes enormous. The money every year inflates more and is now in 1979 worth ten to fourteen percent less in the US, and in Britain in years of high inflation even thirty percent less.

Can society protect itself against another crash? If people get scared and run to get their money from the banks, who would get any but the first one hundred customers? The average bank does not keep much real cash on hand, barely enough for the day's needs. To stop the banks closing if there were another depression, the Federal Reserve Bank insures deposits up to $40,000, but it does not insure that banks will not close down. As I said before, the Federal Reserve is not a government agency, as many suppose, but is yet another deception based on paper credit. The only insurance against a bank's closure in a crisis is to stop the bank lending more fictitious money than it has actually got from its customers. Several banks have closed in the last five years, but the public has a short memory.

HOW TO REORGANIZE CAPITALISM

How does this state credit and bank credit we call fictitious compare with the social capital amassed by the workers in a Common Ownership? If all the businesses in America were converted to Common Ownership and the power of the banks to create money was withdrawn and given only to the state, would essential loans be difficult to get? No, because when the employees borrow money from banks or government to buy the shareholders' interests, the shareholders will have new money to then lend to banks or business enterprises. Therefore, money presently tied up in business stocks would be available for private loans and there would be no need for false credit or creation of false paper money. If the government creates a credit to pay off the shareholders and employers against the future profits of industry, the workers can be the new owners of the shares and repay the government under an Employee Stock Ownership Plan (ESOP). Thus government shoulders the financial burden normally borne by the private industrialist. The private capital thereby released would stimulate the economy and revitalize the free enterprise system while at the same time rooting out the ancient defects of exploitative capitalism. Socialism or state ownership would be prevented and the world saved from the ultimate bureaucracy. The government could buy out the shareholders' interests once and for all in a one-time payment legally made on behalf of the workers who, as we said, would pay back out of profits. It is important to repeat that this is not nationalization or socialism but Common Ownership. Those who put up the capital for industry would get paid in today's book values and the workers' "common ownerships" would gradually pay off the government, say, over five years at twenty percent a year out of their profits and before taxes were levied.

"How on earth is government going to get all that money?" says the capitalist. Easy! Pay it out in the same worthless pieces of paper that are legal tender now and print more money because we will only have to do it once and, after this one-time payment of debts, the government gets it back from the profits earned over the next five years. Inflation then will go *down* as government takes the repaid money out of circulation every year (the opposite of printing more, as they do now) and spends only the taxes it gets without incurring a budgetary deficit. The *quantity* of money here is not the important factor because the real purpose of money is only to effectively distribute goods and services in fair proportions within the society we live in. All money other than that in actual public circulation, even that resting in banks as figures in accounts, is fictitious money. The assets and money

Vanishing Money

in computer systems of a bank have no function in reality and are not in use except in our imaginations.

"Hey!" says the average citizen, "this is *my* money in the bank. Why is it fictitious?" The answer is that you can only get your money when everyone else does not want theirs. If everybody wants their money from a bank at the same time, the bank goes broke. Why would it go broke? Because it cannot sell all its assets in a few days, so much of it is tied up in property and loans to others who are in financial difficulties whenever there are tight economic situations. *So your money that you think is so safe in a bank is really tied up in loans to people who buy anything from houses to recreation vehicles.* In bad times when no one can get money, these assets are hard to sell and their security becomes worthless if everyone demands payment at the same time. You could not even get the worthless paper money if everyone lined up at the bank expecting the money in their bank account upon demand.

Bank credit is like the money tied up in recreation vehicles which is doing nothing for most of the year while the vehicle is lying idle, parked in the street. That is where your money is, not in the bank waiting for you to collect it! Similarly, money not in circulation, such as that fictitious paper which is financing the national debt, does nothing as it is tied up in safe deposit boxes or in currency under the mattress. When government borrows money or sells bonds and treasury bills, the public debt thus created is a debt which does nothing, and, like the idle recreation vehicle, is not in use because the citizen owes it to himself. It is fictitious money because the citizen (through the government) has loaned himself money he never had. But citizens still pay interest on this debt at eight cents out of each tax dollar,* just like they pay interest on their unused motor home. The public debt is also tied up in the bank purchases of fictitious money in the form of those treasury notes which the government sells to banks at a discount in order to get them into circulation. Any bank note or treasury bill is merely a promise to pay, but if the government had to give any value for it, such as gold, wheat or silver, there would be nothing there for you to get but more paper money. Such is the real nature of the money we spend, yet it takes a real collapse to teach us that.

---

* With present rising inflation and prime interest rates the public debt could go to twelve to fourteen cents out of each tax dollar.

I remember myself just after World War II, stuck with thousands of Belgian and French francs which became worthless overnight. Countries which have been through inflationary spirals several times like Argentina and France understand this. Old money is cancelled and the government prints new money. All those who hoarded treasury bills in their mattress got caught because the old money only equaled a hundredth or a thousandth part of the new money. In this way governments cancel the national debt by making their existing currency worthless, and they start all over again with a new paper value. The fact is that Belgium, France, Brazil, Argentina and several other countries have all done this in the last thirty years, so we may not say it is impossible.

How many ordinary people know that *the national debt is a fiction which we pay for every year with interest to bankers, and we pay for it again in the devaluation of our existing money through inflation?* This fictional money should not have interest charged upon it, which merely adds daily to the national debt. Because it is a fictional debt, it can be cancelled immediately merely by passing a law. If we look at the financial "pie" on page 916, we see that a large eight cent slice of every dollar goes to pay to service the national debt. This represents billions of dollars of unnecessary expense. As it looks now, this cannot be reduced unless there is an almost one hundred percent tax strike by citizens who will bring the message sharply home to our politicians that they must not only stop spending but must bring about ruthless fiscal reform. The national debt can only be maintained because we give the government the right to tax future generations of our children. Yet to cancel all this national debt is no financial problem because it never will get paid anyway, not even by mortgaging posterity and expecting our children to accept what we have done by expecting to tax their future work and wages. The system will break down long before that on inflation alone.

WHAT IS HAPPENING TO OUR SAVINGS?

The attitudes of politicians and economists generally is very much like that of stockbrokers who advise people on legitimate methods of gambling. Now that the Federal Reserve Bank is no longer tied to keeping gold reserves to back up our currency notes, they too are able to indulge in the speculative Keynesian philosophy of seeking continuous prosperity by means of perpetual inflating. The embezzlement dogma so dear to the hearts of politicians—that the people can continue to water down existing money in order to create new money by owing it to themselves (ourselves) so that we can continue to spend money on "goodies" for everyone without paying the corresponding taxes—is the same attitude of gamblers and speculators who are noted for being influenced more by emotion than by reason, especially when we fool ourselves by believing in our own cleverness that we are thinking things out. Perpetual inflation is like the gambling instinct on the stock market during good times when it is most insidious in its appeal because the victim of overconfidence persuades himself through wishful thinking that he is engaged in legitimate business transactions. The thought of big profits which blinds our perception of the real risks, helps to encourage the dangerous influence of wishful thinking. There is no real difficulty in understanding how many people in such high positions could be so easily misled by a few years of success. Anyone who has checked the swings of the stock market over a long period and related it to the much advertised prophecies and predictions, finds that the times when investment counselors are wrong are quietly soft-pedalled. Anyone who has checked the theories which predict business cycles and economic ups and downs will find that a man's judgement proves right just often enough to help the experts forget the times when they were wrong. In the case of investments in inflation-free stocks, insurance company annuities, or payments into a social security fund over a thirty year period, there is just no way that a consistent policy of political embezzlement of our savings can be rationalized, as we can see from the following table:

FUTURE BUYING POWER OF $1,000 AT COMPOUNDED ANNUAL RATES OF PRICE INCREASES

At End of	*Annual Rates of Price Increases*				
	10%	*15%*	*20%*	*25%*	*30%*
5 years	$620.92	$497.18	$401.88	$327.68	$269.33
10 years	385.54	247.18	161.51	107.37	072.54
20 years	148.64	061.10	026.08	011.53	005.26
30 years	057.31	015.10	004.21	001.24	000.38
40 years	022.09	003.73	000.68	000.13	000.03

If we invest $1000 now at a net five percent compound interest for thirty years it would accumulate $4322. But if the increase in the cost of living averages ten percent a year, the buying power of $4322 at the end of thirty years is only $246 of present-day buying power. Even if we use the government's tax incentive for a special retirement plan the result would only be $352 of today's buying power. If we get no interest and our economy goes to a fifteen percent annual increase in prices, we can see from our table that in thirty years our $1000 is only worth $15.10 of present-day value. And if we go to a thirty percent increase in prices, as Britain did last year, we would need to earn forty-three percent interest just to keep up with the inflation and break even. Therefore the odds against finding successful investments or savings in retirement funds which will be of use to us later are small if we allow government to continue to embezzle our existing wealth and currency.

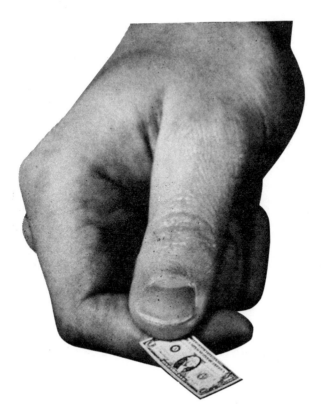

THE BUDGET DOLLAR   Fiscal Year 1965 (Estimated)

Where it comes from . . .

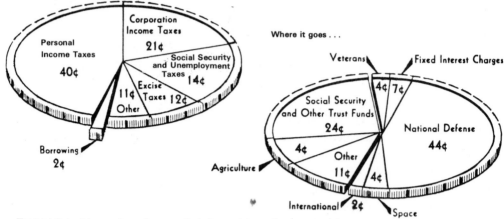

Corporation Income Taxes 21¢

Personal Income Taxes 40¢

Social Security and Unemployment Taxes 14¢

Excise Taxes 12¢

Other 11¢

Borrowing 2¢

Where it goes . . .

Veterans 4¢   Fixed Interest Charges 7¢

Social Security and Other Trust Funds 24¢

National Defense 44¢

4¢

Other 11¢   4¢

Agriculture

International 2¢   Space

The total Federal income from all sources including social security taxes, income taxes and business taxes comes to $439 billion and the total expenditure comes to $512 billion, making the deficit $73 billion. The separate income from corporation taxes is estimated for 1979 at $62 billion and the annual loss from the budget overspending is $73 billion. Therefore the business tax is $11 billion less than the annual deficit. The entire tax receipts from personal income tax comes to $190 billion supplemented by $25 billion from excise taxes, etc. Social security contributions received are $141 billion. They are received in trust for the public and these taxes are part of social trust funds received of $187 billion and $174 billion paid. out. The $73 billion loss is made up by issuing fictitious money, treasury bills, and credit for which the government pays $12 billion of the taxpayers' money in interest every year. This loss amounts to $60 annually for every man, woman and child in the US for interest on fictitious money alone.

THE BUDGET DOLLAR   Fiscal Year 1979 (Estimated)

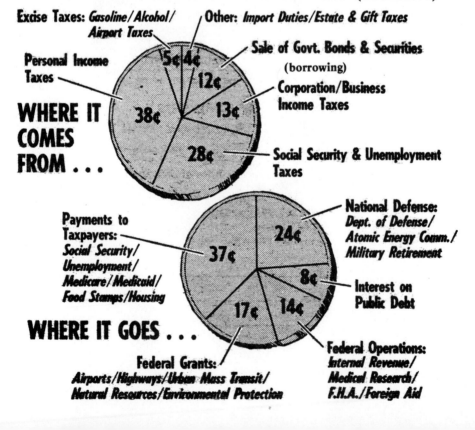

Excise Taxes: *Gasoline/Alcohol/ Airport Taxes* 5¢

Other: *Import Duties/Estate & Gift Taxes* 4¢

Personal Income Taxes 38¢

Sale of Govt. Bonds & Securities (borrowing) 12¢

Corporation/Business Income Taxes 13¢

WHERE IT COMES FROM . . .

Social Security & Unemployment Taxes 28¢

Payments to Taxpayers: *Social Security/ Unemployment/ Medicare/Medicaid/ Food Stamps/Housing* 37¢

National Defense: *Dept. of Defense/ Atomic Energy Comm./ Military Retirement* 24¢

Interest on Public Debt 8¢

WHERE IT GOES . . .

17¢   14¢

Federal Grants: *Airports/Highways/Urban Mass Transit/ Natural Resources/Environmental Protection*

Federal Operations: *Internal Revenue/ Medical Research/ F.H.A./Foreign Aid*

THE REAL CAUSE OF INFLATION

This information on the budget, supplied by the office of the President, is shown for 1965 and 1979, covering a span of fourteen years. The diagrams show how government borrowings increased through a deliberate governmental decision to print more money or issue government bonds. In 1965 the government of Lyndon Johnson increased the public debt by $5.2 billion. By 1979 the deficit financing of the budget had reached borrowings of nearly $60 billion, all of which was financed by printing and selling paper currency or bonds. The federal government's debt is a debt owed by the people. It is financed in several ways. From 1965 to 1979 the sale of government securities and bonds jumped from two percent to twelve percent while taxes on business corporations went down from twenty-one percent to thirteen percent during the same period, thus shifting the source of the government's revenue off the shoulders of big business. At the same time, social security and unemployment taxes went up double from fourteen percent to twenty-eight percent of the tax dollar. In other words, while social security and unemployment tax doubled, the tax on big business was cut almost in half.

What does all this mean? One way that the government finances the national debt and budget deficit is by borrowing the tax money already paid into the social security fund and other government trust funds. You may be paying social security payments now, thinking that when you are old you will collect them back again as promised, but if you do collect them, the inflated money will be worth far less than when you paid it in, in spite of cost of living increases, and there is a very good chance that the fund will be bankrupt by then and you will not be able to collect at all. This is equivalent to theft. At the same time, the public debt is having to subsidize the social security and welfare programs because they pay out more money than taxes bring in. Because the social security system was in massive deficit, Congress passed legislation to raise future taxes, beginning from 1979, simply to replenish the fund. This is complete madness because increases in social security and unemployment taxes are paid half by business and half by employees on the payroll, and these higher costs will be instantly passed on to consumers by increasing prices. The corresponding increase in the consumer price index will automatically touch off

claims for more wages by millions of workers everywhere who have
negotiated labor contracts which call for automatic adjustments as the
cost of living rises. Plus the social security payments will go up
because they are geared to the cost of living index so that more will be
paid out of the fund to old-age pensioners in order to keep up with
rising prices. The safe way to raise social security taxes is to go a
totally different route and to tax luxuries and unnecessary merchandise
that does not affect the consumer price index which is based only on
essential items.

Unemployment taxes in 1965 were fourteen cents out of every
dollar, and the cost of paying social security and welfare was twenty-
four cents out of the dollar. Therefore it was subsidized by ten cents.
Today twenty-eight percent of the dollar is paid *in* by taxes and thirty-
seven percent paid *out,* so the programs are subsidized by nine cents.
Social security and welfare used to be subsidized by corporation taxes
and by income tax but are now financed by issuing paper money. Since
corporation profit tax has gone down from twenty-one percent of the
tax dollar in 1965 to thirteen percent in 1979 in the same time that
interest on the public debt has gone up from two to twelve percent, it
shows that the public is now borrowing and paying for what the
corporations used to pay for. For example, most citizens who paid any
tax at all last year paid more taxes than Texaco, because this huge oil
conglomerate paid no tax at all on its profits of more than one
thousand million dollars, because of tax incentives for oil drilling. This
incentive offered to the very rich is paid for by you and me.

In 1978 Texaco made a profit of $1,005 million on an investment
capital of 31 billion dollars and they owe $2.8 billion to creditors. The
government lets them write off all their future profits and pay no
income taxes on these profits in order to encourage their investment in
high-risk oil exploration in which they could easily lose half their
profits up to 500 million dollars. The argument is that the nation needs
the oil and the oil companies would never take such risks without
incentive by the government. But what actually happens is that the oil
companies use government money to drill wells in places that are not
very likely to yield oil, just on the off chance that they might (with no
risk of their own) hit oil and make a big profit. Meanwhile, their own

fields in which they know very well that oil is present, they do not develop but save these for the future, because at the moment it is far more profitable for them to buy the oil from the Arabs at a controlled fixed price. Therefore, in effect, instead of giving big business encouragement by giving tax credits for efficient drilling and successful wells, the government encourages needless wasteful spending on drilling oil fields of high-risk speculation. While the price of foreign oil is high, profits on imported oil are also high because prices are fixed by price control. While there are considerable supplies of oil in America which have never been drilled or dowsed, we must also realize that it does not suit Texaco to develop their known resources if their profit on locally-discovered oil is going to be less than that on imported oil. As long as the government is willing to finance wildcat oil drilling of speculative oil leases with taxpayers' money and allows profits of over a billion dollars to be paid out to oil company shareholders, then all citizens in other businesses should also be entitled to speculate with government money and not to pay taxes. Instead, the smaller businessmen, who have no powerful lobbies to arrange such benefits for them, foot the bill for Texaco and carry the load of the national debt. The following list of expenses comes from the National Taxpayers Union:

DEBT OR LIABILITY ITEM	GROSS COST	YOUR SHARE
Public Debt	$ 721,000,000,000	$ 9,012
Accounts Payable	$ 80,000,000,000	$ 1,000
Undelivered Orders	$ 332,000,000,000	$ 4,150
Long Term Contracts	$ 15,000,000,000	$ 187
Loan and Credit Guarantees	$ 209,000,000,000	$ 2,612
Insurance Commitments	$1,733,000,000,000	$ 21,662
Annuity Programs	$5,900,000,000,000	$ 73,750
Unadjudicated Claims International Commitments & other Financial Obligations	$ 43,000,000,000	$ 537
TOTAL	$9,033,000,000,000	$112,910

That's a total debt due from each and every taxpayer of nearly $113,000, including you.

While people are hard at work all day to get the money they need to live on and to feel secure, politicians are spending thirty percent of that same money. Politicians cannot pay these expenses except with taxes, which already are costing us more than we spend on food, shelter or any necessity of life. In effect, the politicians are spending your money. What are they spending it on? Ten million dollars went to Uganda to dictator Idi Amin. In the last twenty years, the United States has financed not just one side but both sides of fourteen wars. How does this kind of extravagance affect the value of our currency?

Currency notes printed by the treasury are sold to the Federal Reserve banks and foreign buyers of dollars and bonds. This means that twelve percent of our government annual expenditure is borrowed from financial institutions who hold these securities, treasury bills, etc. as a security in their assets. National and foreign banks are therefore holding fictitious paper dollars as security for their customers' money which is loaned to them to do business with. This is like kids playing store because they use unreal money to do it with. If the dollar should be wiped out, these paper assets will be wiped out too, because the banks have secured fictitious money with more fictitious money. In that kind of game, when the crash comes, everybody loses and nobody wins.

What is the answer to this problem of securing ourself against a very real potential crash? Gold is only a partial answer because, although it is the only store of value which is scarce enough to act as currency in place of paper notes, it cannot be eaten or used for anything else than jewelry or luxurious articles of vanity. On a desert island a bucket of gold is worth nothing whereas a bucket of pure water might be priceless. Therefore the only real hedge against the collapse of paper money is water and land, because with water, land can be irrigated to grow crops for humans to stay alive and from land can come all the resources we need to survive. There is a big difference between this and hedging on real estate and property, because property can go down in value when there is no money to buy anything or when a vast majority of people have been impoverished by having their savings wiped out by financial collapse. But a property with land on which you yourself are living and farming will always produce wealth

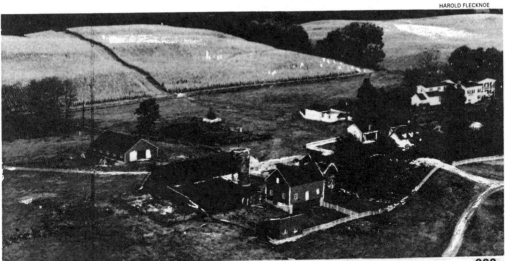

HAROLD FLECKNOE

In times of crisis, people desperately try to save dwindling wealth from inflation by investing in stocks of gold products, antiques, art, old coins, rare stamps and collectables. But investing in these or investing in real estate carries considerable risks. Unless you invest in a house in which you live or a farm on which you produce, you may find other residential or commercial property will remain empty providing no income while costs go spiraling up. Many poor people have lost property because they could not pay their taxes on the due date. Hence, small communities on self-reliant, commonly-owned, self-governing farms are the only protection poor people have for surviving periods of unemployment and inflation. Small communities and the beginning of the nuclear family who insulate themselves against the shock of catastrophe, both emotionally and economically, can provide for their spiritual growth as well.

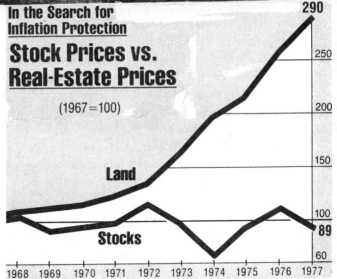

In the Search for Inflation Protection

Stock Prices vs. Real-Estate Prices

(1967=100)

Land

Stocks

and abundance, even if you have to make the soil yourself out of wastes. There are tribes in the Himalayas who live in harsh climates and bare rock, who make their own soil and compost from everything they can get, and they live a healthy, radiant and sunny life of happiness. Hence the future security for those who have money now, who wish to preserve their life savings and the sum of their life's toil, is to invest in small communities of their choosing, creating social capital and putting it to work in land or other means of production rather than keeping it held in fictitious paper. But this solution will not appeal to those who do not care for work. The people who thrive within the present system are those who make their monetary resources work *for* them. The plodders get stuck with the taxes and the poor have not the skill to multiply resources even if they had some. Hence the rich get richer, the big corporations get bigger, and the poor get poorer.

IS THE SOCIAL PROBLEM A LACK OF MONEY?

From all appearances it would seem that the basic cause of poverty is that the poor have no money. How do poor people get money? The question is better asked, how do rich people get their money? Many liberals conclude that cultural deprivation causes lack of income. However it is just as reasonable to assume that lack of income is the *cause* of poverty and that cultural deprivation is merely the *effect* of being poor. If lack of income is really the true root cause of cultural backwardness, then the social programs of modern welfare states are a waste of time. If it is true that cultural deprivation results from lack of education or a lack in development of social skills and job training, then the welfare programs should concentrate on that, rather than providing insurance for unemployment income as they do now. Is it money or is it education that makes people become wealthy? Is the problem of society merely a matter of income distribution as claimed by sociologists or is it the acquisiton of skills, including the skill of creating wealth?

For example, a father has two sons—one skilled at saving and at making money and the other skilled at losing it. Although the second son has great talent in several areas, he continually takes financial risks so he never has money. The first son never takes a risk, has little interest in putting his consciousness on anything except money and security. Perhaps they represent two extreme sides of their father who never has any great wealth but who has the skill to create wealth and therefore always has enough money for whatever needs the family may have. Increase the income of the first son, the thrifty conservative one, and he would become richer, but increase the income of the second son and he would become poorer, deeper in debt, needing more and more money to live every month as he credits more and indulges more in his compulsive extravagant tastes. The first impulse of a poor person is to spend money once he gets money, whereas the impulse of a rich person is to save capital and spend only from his surplus income. The secret of wealth is in making our income exceed our expenses. This is an incontrovertible financial law and a spiritual one too. A holy man reduces his needs to zero and is content and happy with little or enough. He is rich in spirit and regards the rich as emotionally poor. Yet he observes the financial law of conservation in other areas of his being as well and thereby reduces greed. This kind of self-discipline is not popular in this world of greedy materialistic people, and it is clear that our society is traveling in the opposite direction. But since the fundamental spiritual principles permeate the universe, we cannot escape them. Sooner or later they will cause life to send us happiness or pain depending on how willing we are to bring our actions in line with them.

TO WHOM DO WE OWE THE NATIONAL DEBT AND WHO HAS THE AUTHORITY TO CANCEL IT?

Only the people who owe the national debt can cancel it by voting on it in a referendum tax initiative. The move must come from the people because the politicians will never do it. Why can't the politicians do it? Because with modern democracy the politician must depend for his election on finances from helpers who expect their causes to be enhanced once he is in office, so once he is in the House or Senate he is lobbied constantly for government funds and in addition also proposes schemes which need funds, thereby increasing rather than decreasing the size of the budget.

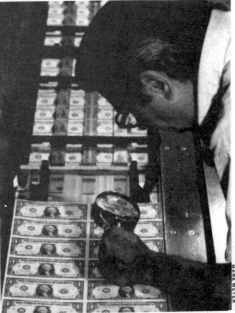

Dollars flow from Bureau of Engraving and Printing

Everyone looks to the government as the source of large-scale wealth and authority, yet in a democracy the people are the ultimate authority, not the government. Somehow we must act now to stop printing money. We must stop interest on the national debt and stop creating more national debt. Otherwise collapse is certain. Only when we stop this fiction of endless government wealth can we have 100% money. We need a medium of exchange in a stable currency that represents actual work or goods or service done; otherwise we are better off with a barter system. The steps to a stable currency are not something to fear or avoid but something necessary that the world has been desperately expecting the USA to achieve and so put its affairs in order. Without this currency reform, the free world will remain unstable and the security of the world will be threatened.

HOW RELIABLE ARE BANKS?

The problem with inflation is that it makes unwitting counterfeiters of the government whose civil servants and legislators do not realize the consequences of printing fictitious money until inflation is suddenly upon us with a vengeance. Inflation does not flower overnight. It creeps up on public and government alike. Prices rise along with wages. Every promotion or new job gives more money, but in spite of every increase we are soon back to juggling with our expenses which continue to outstrip our increased income. A government survey last month showed that a typical worker increased his wages by forty-three percent in the five years between 1973 and 1978, but prices went up faster, so his buying power actually went down by five percent. What does this mean to our nation's banks? If we borrow money today that is worth forty-three percent less in five years from now, we pay back the debt in dollars that are rapidly becoming more worthless. How do banks cope with this problem?

The year 1967 was the year government decided to use as a base year for the consumer price index of one hundred. We can measure inflation since then by that standard. As I write, in the fall of 1978, the government has just announced that the consumer price index for the month is 200.9; therefore things purchased today cost twice as much as in 1967, and the dollar has devalued by fifty percent. At the moment the inflation rate is thirteen percent a year and accelerating. Because the banks make a handsome profit of handling credit and fictitious money and their balance sheets show a healthy condition, they can presently keep up with this rate of inflation, still expand their services and give more credit at ever-increasing interest rates. But could the banks keep up their solvency if the inflation suddenly went into a spiral through a massive loss of confidence? In other words, we may have gotten used to inflation and we may know that it is increasing every year, but do we really know that "runaway" inflation is an entirely different phenomenon, and are we seeing that runaway inflation is a very real possibility in America? If the fifty percent inflation took place in the space of one year instead of ten, could the banks survive the loss? In countries where inflationary rates have reached up to two hundred percent the banks survive only by tying everything to the consumer index. In Argentina rents of property are fixed so they increase with the inflation rate; otherwise landlords get paid in worthless notes. Banks survive only by seizing the security of their customers property for loans not repaid on time and by making their customers take the loss in devaluation of money. Banking is less risky in places like South America where only the rich and those who own property can get loans from banks, but in the US where credit is extended easily to everyone, the vulnerability of banks to rapid inflation is more than anywhere else in the world. American banks are even more vulnerable than an ordinary business like Sears which issues credit cards because Sears' business assets are also tied up in inventory and equipment which is going up in value during rapid inflation. It would only require a few of these big companies to go under to bankrupt many banks.

Bank rupture comes from two causes: extending too much credit to unsound customers and a public run on the banks when the entire populace wants their money and savings out of a particular bank. When all the people want their money all at the same time to buy *things* in a runaway inflation, then the money situation becomes unstable. Debt is a great problem for most Americans. Outstanding personal debts, that is, money owed to banks on mortgages, automobiles, credit cards, etc., totals more than one trillion dollars (1,000 billion) which is more than double the $400 billion (400,000 million) of individual debts owed in 1967. Payments of interest on installments

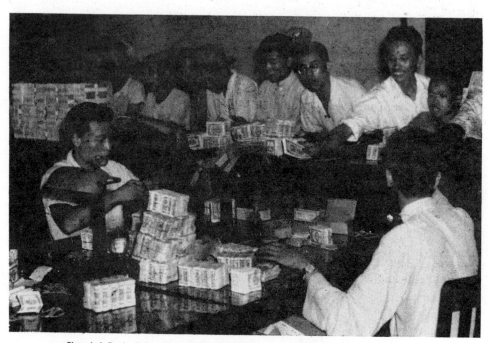

Shanghai. Bank clerks count bundles of old currency being exchanged for new gold yuan.

for things bought on credit now, account for almost sixteen cents of every dollar earned by Americans, and eight cents of every dollar of tax paid by Americans goes to pay interest on money the government owes to banks. With this amount owed and this amount of interest, the vulnerability of American banks to a fifty percent or seventy percent sudden inflationary spiral would be catastrophic.

Bankers are not unaware of this problem, and they are not intentionally grasping a lion's share of every dollar spent. Most bankers are going about their business as part of a system of credit that leads to unintentional forms of usury brought about by the power of banks to create credit out of nothing. Just as government has the power to create money out of nothing by printing it and selling it to bankers and thereby becomes unwittingly a producer of counterfeit money, so does the populace, by accepting the present system of credit and banking, unwittingly condone its own financial doom in a runaway spiral of inflation. The only thing which maintains the whole system is confidence in the American dollar and in the banks. When that confidence goes in times of crisis, the whole society panics and people are shocked into drastic attempts to preserve the value of their savings.

This is not to say that new legislation and regulations do not improve the efficiency of banking and financial institutions. Every day new regulations are invented by the bureaucracy to protect the public against collapse and misuse of customers' funds. Also rapid inflation and new technological innovation are compounding the complexity of banking and the banks' handling of the nation's savings. In today's world, bankers are enjoying a period of great prosperity and, even with inflation deflating the real profits of all who loan money, this year 1978 has been the most profitable year in the whole of banking history. Bad loans have been written off, savings have increased enormously, and next year (1979) a gain in bank profits is expected of at least twenty percent. So why are we worried for the solvency of banks? We are concerned because a day of reckoning is coming, some time in the future, from printing so many fictitious dollars on the government presses. Though we do not know just when, whether in ten years, five years, one year, or a matter of months, America is headed for runaway inflation, and the dollar will be wiped out. The banking system is highly vulnerable because it loans out dollars at today's value and gets back dollars which are worth less in a few years' time. At the moment, profits are good enough to keep up with a ten percent inflation, but if runaway inflation occurs at thirty percent or even fifty percent and seventy-five percent in a year, then assets in paper monetary holdings will be wiped out and the banks' security will become insolvent. No one will get their money because banks and businesses will fail almost overnight. Banks cannot stand a fifty percent devaluation of their paper assets and survive. How can it be that the politicians are creating the inflation spiral and yet they do not know they are the cause? They think, "The government has money available. If I don't spend it, someone else will. If I don't get it for my constituents, some specialist lobby will get it." While the taxpayer is squealing, the politicians are trying to get tax money for their pet projects, money which they keep voting for themselves in the House. Recently the legislators cut President Carter's budget by billions but they added budget items of their own so the figure came back up to the same amount as before they cut it.

President Carter has stated categorically that inflation is the number one threat to this nation and, even if he has to be the most unpopular president in solving the inflation problem, he would rather accomplish this feat than run again for a second term of office. This will require political ruthlessness of an order not yet manifested by any American president. If President Carter can implement what comes out of his mouth, he will be the greatest president that America has ever had. The process of setting inflation into reverse, to *de*flation, is considered by most economists to be out of human control, because the greed of man supersedes his reason thereby causing him to continually ask for higher prices and higher wages which trigger each other automatically, since no one will put down the price of a product if they have to pay their employees more to make it and no one in their right senses would ask for less money in wages if prices are rising. Although politicians, economists and government experts believe inflation is inevitable and unstoppable, the facts are that the financial law itself will eventually build deflation by causing a collapse. This collapse can be avoided by a tax revolt which is within the power of every citizen. The dollar is a problem something can be done about. If a tax revolt happens it will cripple politicians and keep them from spending which will bring about a reversal of runaway inflation. At any moment in history something can be done about the ailing dollar because inflation is man-made and therefore can be changed into deflation by man. The likelihood that the present fiscal policy on public debt, credit and currency will be reversed by our leaders in the next few years is small, but if the tax revolution comes soon, the politicians will have no option but to stop spending. Since the situation is subject to control by a change in national policy, no one can prophesy that runaway inflation is inevitable. One of the purposes of this book is to bring inflation to a halt before the politicians bankrupt the American dollar and weaken the forces of freedom in the world.

THE LAWS OF NATURE

As I said before, in my lifetime in Europe I have seen inflation with the leading Western nations. There are many Americans who believe that a financial collapse cannot happen in America. But even in the history of the United States the value of money has been almost worthless. We say we are prepared this time, but always the smug

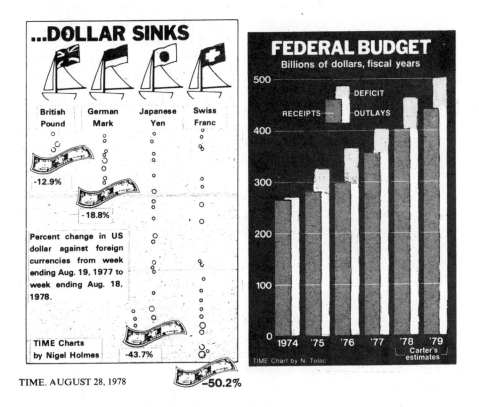

...DOLLAR SINKS

British Pound   German Mark   Japanese Yen   Swiss Franc

-12.9%

-18.8%

Percent change in US dollar against foreign currencies from week ending Aug. 19, 1977 to week ending Aug. 18, 1978.

TIME Charts by Nigel Holmes   -43.7%

TIME. AUGUST 28, 1978   -50.2%

FEDERAL BUDGET
Billions of dollars, fiscal years

500

DEFICIT
RECEIPTS — OUTLAYS

400

300

200

100

0   1974   '75   '76   '77   '78   '79
Carter's estimates

TIME Chart by N. Telac

opinion-makers say these things without really knowing the incontrovertible law of finance expressed by Dickens through Mr. Micawber speaking to David Copperfield:

"My other piece of advice, Copperfield," said Mr. Micawber, "is this: Annual income twenty pounds, annual

expenditure nineteen, nineteen six, result happiness. Annual
income twenty pounds, annual expenditure twenty pounds,
ought and six, result misery. The blossom is blighted, the
leaf is withered, the God of day goes down upon the dreary
scene, and—and, in short, you are forever floored. As I
am!"

Dickens may have hit on the secret of inflation and social happiness.
Nevertheless Americans did not follow this philosophy in the past, and
many attribute economic success to the credit system which enables
business to get started. In America there are eight million small family
businesses which need to borrow, and their credit is always secured by
a house, a car or some value or assets. It is true that many of these
businesses could never get started without credit, and it is good to
encourage expansion in this way. But the evil side-effects of too easy
credit borrowing are worse than nothing at all, because everyone
depends on everyone else being stable and, when millions of businesses
fail, the whole economy is unstable. It is easy for people to tell others
to cut back or tell the government to cut back, but until we are
prepared to be equally rigorous with ourselves—prepared *not* to get the
loan we think we need or *not* to buy everything our hearts desire— we
will not be willing to rock the boat and we will close our eyes, as we
are doing now, and hope that somehow the economy will keep supplying
the abundant life and that the national debt will someday diminish.

It has been said that the growth of communism was spawned by the
terrible selfishness of Western society. The attitude that the voter has
no more responsibility than to cast his vote and pay his taxes is still
very common in Western society today. One of the greatest weaknesses
in the democracy of the West is the communist ability to point to the
selfishness of money. To put an end to the financial power centers
would also put an end to communist expansion because, in a world of
Common Ownership, the communist system would stand revealed as a
bankrupt system which exploits the people even worse through high
prices and invisible taxes than capitalism does. Because the Soviet
system creates money out of nothing through creating credit in identically the same way that capitalist banks do, the State has the only power
to allocate capital to industry. The only difference in capitalism is that the

capital is in private hands and that taxes are paid on actual profits and sales. But in the communist system the government extracts its taxes before a thing is made by taking seventy percent of the gross price of everything made, at the source of its production. This is a more exploitative share of the workers' labor and productivity than any

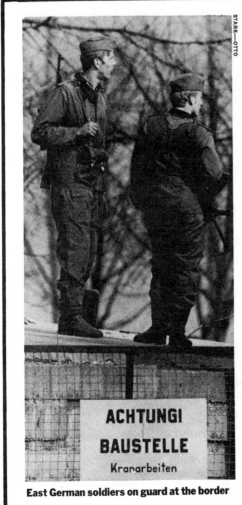

ACHTUNG!

BAUSTELLE

Kranarbeiten

STARK—OTTO

East German soldiers on guard at the border

TIME, JANUARY 30, 1978

The trouble began earlier this month when the West German weekly *Der Spiegel* published a 30-page manifesto issued by a group of underground dissenters in East Germany who called themselves the League of Democratic Communists of Germany. The document denounced the Soviet Union for "brutal exploitation and suppression" of East Germany. With bitter sarcasm, the anonymous authors called their country "a pathetic imitation of a Soviet Republic whose worst features have been reinforced by German thoroughness." Noting that Stalin had concentration camps even before Hitler, the manifesto charged that the "barbaric" Soviet system had since 1945 claimed "more victims in Eastern Europe than Hitler's Nazism and World War II." The manifesto called for the restoration of basic freedoms and the reunification of Germany, after the East has withdrawn from the Warsaw Pact and the West from NATO.

The manifesto also attacked corruption and greed in the government of Party Chief Erich Honecker. "These Politburocrats are sick with conceit," the document declared. "No ruling class in Germany has ever sponged on others the way the two dozen ruling Communist families have, using our country like a self-service store." Accused of living in "golden ghettos," the leaders were said to have "enriched themselves shamelessly in special shops and by privately ordering goods from the West." The worst offender was Honecker himself, who, the manifesto charged, had "stuffed the homes of his relatives from cellar to roof with the most modern Western conveniences" and obtained highly paid jobs for his wife and in-laws.

capitalist would dare take. The communist workers have far less control than Western unions have over the working conditions and, if anyone complains, he is ostracized as unpatriotic and anti-social or is branded as an imperialist agent. Instead of spreading real ownership to everyone, as it claims, the Soviet system makes the employer (the State) more monolithic, more powerful, autocratic and oppressive than any capitalist employer has ever been. In the first days of the Industrial Revolution there were no forced labor camps although there were no limits on power, ruthlessness and greed. Even back then, Marx saw the problem, but he did not see the solution. Perhaps his blindness to human nature prevented him. He polarized the conflict into the exploiters and exploited, the capitalist and the worker, not seeing that victims can become exploiters overnight. And even he himself was willing to let his own family go hungry while, concerned for the welfare of workers, he wrote *Das Kapital.*

A REAL SOLUTION

Economists never seem to find a real solution to the world's economic dilemma because they tend to think in an economic bubble, divorcing economics from all other psychological factors of our lives. There is a tendency to stop short of really striking the root of human nature, as though half-measures would ever work. In capitalist England, for example, the socialist party has just begun to think in terms of workers' control to give labor more say in the running of business. A government white paper offers a plan for industrial democracy by giving the work force one-third of the representation on the directors' boards, leading eventually to equal control. The plan calls for one-third of all industry to be thus structured within five years. The idea of the plan is to enable two opposing sides of capital and labor to work out power-sharing arrangements. Firms with 500 employees would be obliged to consult with the workers on proposals affecting the workers' welfare. Companies who employ more than 2,000 workers are to give shopfloor union representatives the same rights as directors of the board appointed by the owners and shareholders. The underlying theme for this proposal is to lessen the conflict in labor relations and to cut down the strikes which cause the industry to become financially unsound.

This plan cannot work because it does not touch the question of ownership. Unless the capitalist can have a partner who has not only an equal vote but an equal *risk* in the business, *how can he disclose financial matters if these facts are only going to be used against him by ruthless unions who do not care for the solvency of the enterprise?* Until the worker becomes an *owner* along with the shareholders, the same problem of separate selfish interests will continually rear its ugly head. In Britain, labor already has ample representation and power to cripple any enterprise, and the weakness of the British economy is not due to "power sharing" but to inefficiency, low productivity and lack of aggressive marketing. Labor unions use every lever in wage bargaining, and the capitalist will not invest in new machinery when his risk of loss through strikes is so high. The lack of machinery brings inefficiency, and thus the investment of capital in the economy suffers as an indirect result of labor's threatening power.

In any proposal where the workers gain power without risk, this leak in the life-force of the economy can only get worse and worse.

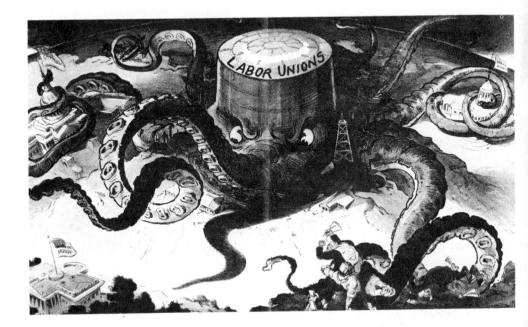

Therefore the only real answer is Common Ownership in which the worker's interest becomes the same as the owner's interests. No capitalist will invest in anything without a guarantee of security or control of his assets. To have others controlling his destiny who have no responsibility will not inspire confidence. Without confidence, credit is impossible to grant. Yet a way has to be found to reduce tension between capitalist and labor union; otherwise industry and large capital enterprises will certainly collapse. This is the prophecy of Marx, that capitalism will collapse from its own internal contradictions, and he is right! The present tension amounts to a class struggle for domination, and only civil war can result from it. This is what has happened in Russia, China, Vietnam, Cambodia and all those countries which have suffered from a communist revolution. Civil war took place where the capitalist classes saw the inevitable changes too late and so were ruthlessly exterminated. Only Common Ownership can defeat communism. We must now put power back with the individual and not with the group such as unions, political parties, companies and self-interest. Only in this way will the *group consciousness* which can nurture the selfless welfare of all become manifest in human evolution of individuals themselves.

How long will it take us to develop communities with the social drive to achieve group consciousness which alone is the sign of a new birthing? Modern mankind must be first aware of what this means in terms of joy, openness and the rising of the human spirit to new heights. How will this awareness come when most are concerned with their own personal desires for money, power and fame? It can only come when we feel the appeal of group consciousness even more powerfully—the togetherness and sharing of a group activity, the psychological security that it brings, the teamwork of working together like a large family with a bond that makes each person feel part of the whole. It is a completely new and fresh feeling of security and trust, a sense of conviction that there is no need to trust because our faith in each other is grounded in confidence and integrity. But even more exciting to every worker or businessman is to know that our efforts to create wealth can be used as a spiritual service to the world and society. If every Common Ownership were to give, for every employee's bonus, an equal amount of its profits to a charitable non-profit activity of its own choosing, then we could begin to take responsibility for the whole instead of letting the government carry that burden at our expense. To know this as we work, that twenty percent of our profits or one-fifth of our work time is going to benefit the whole directly by our own efforts, is far more fulfilling than knowing that one-third of our present efforts and work time is taken by the government to satisfy the insatiable appetite of Mammon. Instead of taxing creativity as we do now we would be enhancing it and making work into joy, business into social service and capital into an instrument of God.

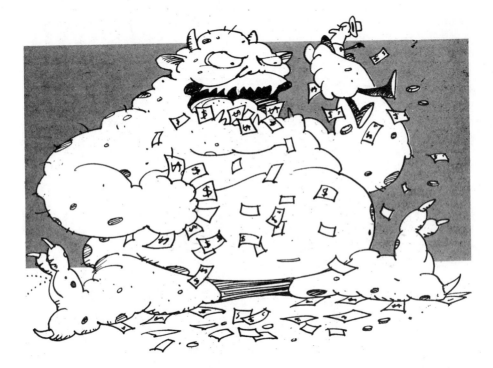

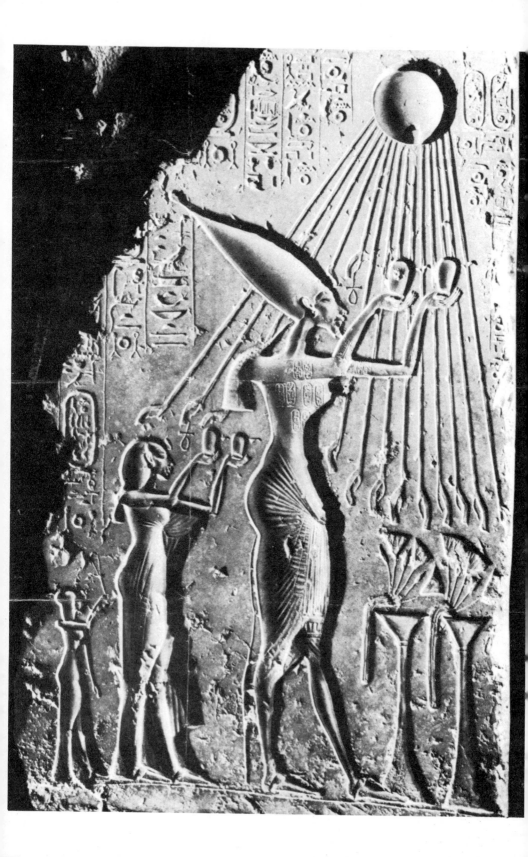

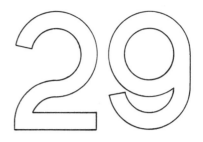

THE REAL AND THE FAKE PHOENIX

The Phoenix fable represents a universal symbol of the rising of a new consciousness springing from the self-renewing ashes of the cosmic egg which brings the birth of the new light and a New Age. The Phoenix was said to have had a melodious cry and to rise every 500 years to give a new philosophy to the world. The image of its death and rebirth can only be referring to the human self, the passion with which it dies and is conceived yet again in bliss. The golden dawn returns after the sunset, and new life which springs from the fruiting of the holy tree of life was long seen as the worship of the rising light in all the world's cultures.

The worship of the sun in Egypt was symbolized by a sacred tree which handed down life force to man. It was said to live as long as the Phoenix and to die at the same time. Born out of the nucleus of the cosmic egg, the sacred tree of life and knowledge is renewed each time the new Phoenix rises from its funeral pyre. To tell the real from the fake Phoenix and to penetrate the meaning of this archetype, it is important to view this mythological bird in a less fabulous context and to explain the terms of the allegory for the purpose of seeing the Phoenix in our own social context.

*The Phoenix is the "Self" rising to a new level of light synthesis.
*The Tree of Knowledge is the human nervous system and its appendage of sensors.
*The Tree of Life is the nerve dendrites in the human brain which die and are reborn with each rising of self-consciousness.
*The melodious cry is a new philosophy of life, a new insight, paradigm or world view of the creation and purpose of existence.
*The funeral pyre is the darkening of the light powers in the external world of the senses.
*The egg is the primordial nucleus which bears the seed of its own self-creation.
*The Rising of the Phoenix is the unveiling of the inner light which triumphs over the external powers of darkness.

Put in the context of this present era with its modern powers of men and machines, this allegory means that people of the darkest nature are in the position of authority and are bringing harm to the wise and able men and women of the world who feel impotent and powerless to act. It signifies a coming disaster which cannot be prevented by the forces of good, but which can bring a new consciousness of light out of the ashes and burned out darkness of men's souls.

The wasteful spending of public money by certain political leaders of Western society, the corruption of Congress and brainwash of the people in the stingy amounts of tax credits given for the rapid development of solar energy, and the slowness of government response to the harnessing of the sun's light, all reveal a darkness of the minds of those who lead us. Today's inflation caused by Western governmental financial policies and the contrived unemployment used to bring inflation under control are leading headlong into a burgeoning tax revolt which signals the end of the age of government as we have known it for centuries. All mature industrial societies in western Europe, Canada,

Australia and Japan are bogging down in the stagnation of productivity and the inflation caused by loss of value of money. Today's rampant inflation uncontrollably leads to the loss of that money power which supports the last-stage phases of the dying industrial revolution. The Phoenix will rise soon from out of the ashes of the coming financial and energy collapse. As the shift from societies and economies based on capital, intensive labor productivity and nonrenewable energy takes place, the transition to some new undefined "post-industrial" society will be resisted tooth and nail by the dark minds of our present leaders who manage our national economic policies. They cannot help this because they are not aware of their ignorance of their own levels of perception. In the darkness of their minds they believe that they know the answers, but they are failing because the economic data on which they base their theory of government is becoming totally discredited and even the conservatives feel it to be illusory. But the borderline between delusion and illusion is not recognized by the managers of our capital-consuming technologies, and therefore billions of dollars are spent on persuading legislatures to maintain obsolete systems of control, taxation, and environmental protection.

Let us stop for a moment and identify with Captain Cousteau and his "people's" crusade to save the ocean, the whales, the endangered dolphins, and halt the irresponsible destruction of our life systems:

> "It is an unavoidable fact of international life that the decision makers in governments everywhere are most influenced by vested interests with extravagant lobbying budgets and by organizations with enormous memberships. Those of us who love the sea, who recognize the blood relationship of all earth's beings, who see on this Water Planet a growing threat to our most fundamental biological machinery, do not command the money and power of even a single major multi-national corporation. But we can wield the formidable power of our numbers, the strength of a great unified crowd of citizens of the planet . . . .

It is unbelievable. It is unacceptable.

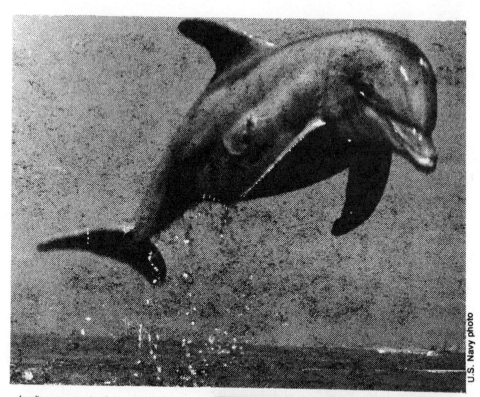

U.S. Navy photo

Leading men to the fish, the dolphin itself is now threatened with extinction in the nets of the heartless fishermen. Conditioned to the joyful freedom of the ocean, the innocent dolphin has trusted mankind to the point of foolishness. Will its radar-like intelligence wake up to the beastliness of human selfishness?

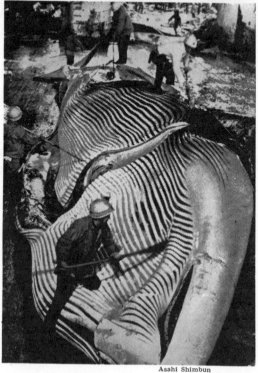

The whale is almost extinct due to the rapacious appetite for blubber and profit. Protests to Russia and Japan, whose fleets refuse to stop the slaughter, are ruthlessly ignored.

Asahi Shimbun

We must stop this stupidity, and the most effective weapon
we have as citizens—as parents—is the sheer force of our
numbers."*

If this book can help the Cousteaus of this world to get even five new
members from the vast army of the nonaggressive humans who remain
fast asleep while the planet sinks into cosmic oblivion and self-
annihilation, then one of its purposes will be served. But we must
attempt more than membership, for in setting out his campaign for the
saving of the ocean, the courageous Captain Cousteau has also set out
the weaponry of the peacemakers and the common people of the earth
throughout the whole of history. He has shown us the strategy to bring
down the mighty authorities and voices of brass which squelched the
promise of the counterculture, and now threaten the glory of life itself:

> "That is the strategy of the dolphin when threatened by an
> animal armed with greater strength and size. Pursued by a
> large shark, a pack of dolphins will suddenly turn en masse,
> dive below the shark and drive their blunt noses into its
> belly, one after another. It is the perfect strategy. With no
> ribs or diaphragm to protect its vital organs, the shark is
> vulnerable. For all of its power, the shark is defeated by
> intelligence and the force of numbers."

The soft underbelly of government is the power to tax its citizens
for that vital juice and energy upon which its appetite grows, ever
demanding more and more. For without this power, its own power to
function is dead. We must work hard now like the threatened beaver
not only to dam up the river of life force which sustains and nourishes
the obsolete, but to unfold the new methods of government which are in
tune with Nature's laws. To model our government on Nature we must
first test out our plan on the small scale and then by sheer replication
of numbers gradually overcome the monolithic power of Mammon.

Daily we must repeat like a mantram that literally billions are spent
on self-defeating schemes, systems for nuclear power, systems of

---

* *Cousteau Society Log,* January 1979.

financial suicide and fictitious money. In the 8,760 hours there are in a year, the decadent moral and spiritual health policies of the Health, Education and Welfare Department will expend $181 billion in the current 1979 fiscal year and $196 billion in 1980. That is $22.3 million per hour. This is approved by the self-perpetuating outmoded elective institutions sustained by parties and groups of people who rise to power through political parties and through the millions spent on persuading the people to elect them to power.

The bloated budgets for military and space hardware, the contract overruns amounting to billions of dollars and the administrative feather-bedding, cost-plus expensive no-risk contracts for energy producers, price supports to inefficient production, subsidies for agricultural production such as tobacco, are all milking the citizen dry so that he now slaves three to four months out of the year to pay for government expenses to feed this darkness of men's minds. How can "work" be glorified when it is actually serfdom?

The 1,000 largest companies referred to in this book as "big business" have, over the last seven years, used up eighty percent of all government tax credits, but they have created only 75,000 new jobs. Yet the six million small businesses* who receive little help from government tax policies, created over nine million new jobs during the same period.**

The demise of our industrial civilization is imminent unless we can reconceptualize our situation and recognize that the heavy taxation of the people does not provide an enlightened society but subsidizes a failing one. The lessons of ancient history have not been learned. Government extravagance from the times of Solomon to the French Revolution, from the luxury of the Czars to the heavy and unfair taxation which caused the American Revolution, have always killed

---

* From an article by Hazel Anderson, author of "Creative Alternative Futures", co-director of the Princeton Center for Alternative Futures, *Christian Science Monitor,* August 9, 1978.
**Editor's note: There are now over eight million small individually owned businesses in the USA according to Dun & Bradstreet, Inc.

the golden goose in every age. The golden goose* of modern society is industrial production but the health of this goose depends on the ever-richer nourishment provided by taxpayers' subsidies and government-rigged markets. The goose moreover is subject to seeking an ever-cheaper labor force even if it means going abroad, exploiting our dwindling resources and raping the environment in order to stay alive. The lessons of history are lost on modern mankind. Even Solomon, the wisest of kings and builders of public projects, brought forced labor and higher taxes until the people wrenched the kingdom of Israel out of the hands of the house of David because of its excesses. Rehoboam, the son of Solomon, rejected the pleas of the people for relief from the heavy taxes and burdens laid upon them by his father. The people rebelled, stoned the tax collector, renounced the family of David and set Jeroboam over them as king. But Jeroboam was even worse and led them to the idolatry of calf worship.

The new rulers and new politicians have always made this mistake of setting new masters and new authorities in place of the old when what is needed is self-rule and self-discipline. But what politician and how many citizens care about self-discipline in America? The US civilization cannot even conserve its wanton, greedy appetite for oil, so that wealth and capital is flowing faster than it can be made, out of the country and into Arabia in the form of an invisible tax. The industrial society is being invisibly milked by the four hundred percent increase in the price of its major energy source. This outflow of dollars is equal to one-third of the income tax for the entire USA, while meantime the Congress is attempting to downplay the consequences of this massive import of oil and its effect on the value of the declining dollar.

The United States government is mortgaged to the world. "How is this?" says the US citizen with some anger at the suggestion. It is simple. Billions of paper dollars are in the hands of the Swiss banks, the Arab oil sheiks, the Germans and the Japanese, and so the value of the dollar goes down and down. Then the President says he will spend thirty billion dollars to hold the dollar's value up. That means the taxpayers, of course, since the President doesn't use his own thirty

---

* See *The Golden Egg*, a how-to book for the coming age of spiritual economics. Published 1979.

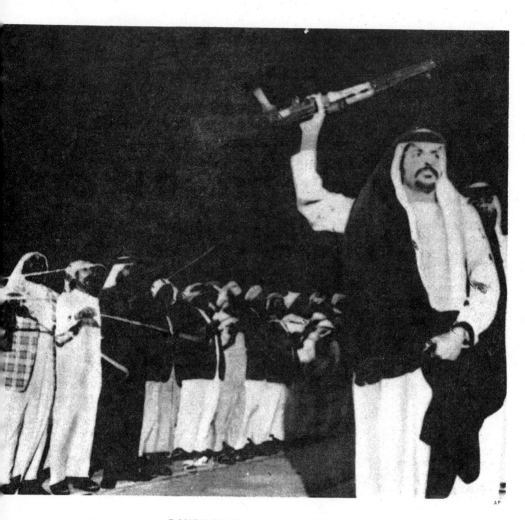

DANCE OF THE OIL DERVISHES

In Abu Dhabi, Oil Minister Mani Said Utaiba of United Arab Emirates exuberantly celebrates the petroleum price increases. Price-fixing is illegal in most civilized countries ranking as a crime along with forgery, extortion, embezzlement, etc. But *governments* can print money and practice extortion and embezzlement to their hearts' content. Oil-rich countries, having had their deserts and oil fields developed by large American and British multinational companies, have now nationalized these businesses and are holding the world to ransom by forming a price-fixing control. These sharp increases in prices put an invisible tax on the world's economies, raising the price of all transportation, heating costs and goods.

OPEC, the new cartel, now gouges the pockets of the world's taxpayers even worse than the monopolistic oil companies. The second important cause of inflation, after the government printing presses, is the adverse balance of trade caused by 400 percent increase in prices of oil imports. The devaluation of the dollar is inevitable as long as oil prices are inflating and will cause a crash in spite of attempts to save the dollar by printing more money or selling more bonds (mortgages on the taxpayers' future savings).

billion but ours. He announces a prime rate of ten or eleven percent interest on money borrowed by the US Treasury by the issue of government bonds, securities, etc. What happens is that Arabs, Swiss, Japanese, anyone holding American dollars rushes their money back to the USA to get ten percent interest, which is one-tenth of the whole loan, back every year—not for a year but forever, because those bonds go on the national debt, owed by every American citizen. Who pays this ten percent every year to the Arabs, Swiss, Germans and Japanese if it is not the American public? The US government pays it out of taxes to service the public debt so that it can pay its mortgage to the world. The US is mortgaged up to the hilt, whatever other nice names you want to call it. That is why the dollar is going to crash. Except for the countries mentioned almost all other countries are in a very similar position. These are dark times in human consciousness which must come in order for the old era to consume itself and give birth to the New Age of enlightenment. This book is about the birth of a new consciousness of the Phoenix where the quality of human knowledge rather than nonrenewable resources is regarded as the primal source of wealth. Those who see the clouds obscuring the dark minds of our power-crazed politicians who spend great sums to get themselves elected, must not allow themselves to be swept along by the unfavorable circumstances of these darkening times, but instead can see this as a testing and refining of our steadfastness of heart. Those who cleave to the light cannot be shaken by the collapsing world events and will avoid the pit of darkness by maintaining the growth of inner life.

What does the Phoenix do with the world problem of moral degradation which casts to the winds all universally accepted moral principles such as truth, honesty, sincerity, fellowship, good will towards men, self-control, nonharmfulness, self-sacrifice and service, etc.? This problem obviously cannot be solved by making appeals to more ethics and less moral vices. Those who are committed to unethical and immoral actions have no scruples in acquiring wealth, power and position. They will not only adulterate foodstuffs and medicines and tell lies about their intentions and goods for sale, but they will adulterate the minds of our children and plant their own corrupted kind in positions of power in the government. These people speak even more loudly of morals and freedom, sharing, democracy, etc., while at the same time deceiving us by doing the opposite.

If you cannot have peace within you, you can never have the power to bring peace in the world outside. There is no other way to bring peace than to rise above man-made differences in values, concepts, ideals and to realize our own Self and thus communicate with the same Self in everybody. Because the external world of events is only a projection of the thoughts and ideas of ignorant or wise human beings we must first know how to achieve a revolution in the mind, then a change in social values will emerge.

To do this inner work and refine our consciousness, to work on changing our self and to explore the depths of our being together with others in Creative Conflict, to cure the greatest of all evil forces (our own self-righteous blindness), that is the real religion and the real science of the spirit—evolution of the nucleus.

Because so few people in society know their own self-ignorance, we need a crash program to know the real "self". How do we convince those who feel they know themselves very well and cannot see any need for such a program? This is the world problem in a nutshell, since it applies to most of our present representatives, UN delegates, leaders, priests and scholars. To take on a battle with arrogance, may even be seen as an arrogance itself. Yet it must be faced and can be done with skill if we can find ways to expose this lack of self-knowledge in group interactions and in methods of creative communication. Such a program cannot be based on the usual morality approach of religion which deals with ethics. The ego is not ethical because it is self-deceptive, therefore morals and ethics are useless for penetrating the nature of reality or discussing the real inner-worlds of people. Morals give no clue as to virtue. A moral person may not be a virtuous person. A virtuous person does not live life by a rule book but from a sense of the truthful, the beautiful and good. A virtuous person would not do anything immoral but at the same time does not live by human moralistic rules. Yet guidelines or rules for living and decision-making are essential to make our government work, whether that government is local, centralized or merely a nuclear family. Nonmoralistic rules are not idealistic but are formed because they avoid harm or trouble or consequences to others.

Since religion and politics are moralistic both in tone and concept, they are of little use in discovering our self-righteousness. What should be the attitude of a world-changer who is rising to the call of the Phoenix? In order to be heard by the arrogant who hold the worldly power, we have to appear outwardly passive but inwardly strong; we should show peace to all those authorities who expect us to be docile and pay our taxes. While inwardly we are constantly working on new ways to govern ourselves, we must outwardly work to throw out corrupted politicians who refuse to do the people's will. Outwardly we yield to the minor social conflicts while inwardly we restrain all unnecessary fears and thoughts in order to preserve all our energy for the great work of freeing ourselves from the shackles of centuries of human error. The real revolution is in the mind within and only when that is won can we stop needless government spending and interference and become masters of our destiny. Out of this persistent quiet work to build community and understand the real nature of self-rule shall come worldwide human freedom from oppressive governments, freedom which we can all accept and enjoy. The way to this state of being, this worldly heaven, cannot leave out consciousness or the skill of creative communication, for the very answer to what prevents society from working is the direct insight into our own self-ignorance.

How does man know what he does not know? How can any individual ever know that within him there are worlds of being which lie veiled from his sight? How can we know that our ignoring of these domains of consciousness is to be in ignorance of the most basic drives which dominate the very social and spiritual life of the entire planet? Unawareness hides the root cause of this ignorance, but our present education does not drive home the importance of self-knowledge. That root cause is the poor level of communication, not always between enemies and hostile societies, but even between loved ones. Nothing is more evident of this poor level of communication than the fifty percent divorce rate and the alienation of our children who accept the proliferation of drugs and pornography as a normal way of life. The rising tide of violence everywhere is an indicator that the human race is not communicating. The word "communication" has its origin in the word "muni", from the Latin for "sharing". This is a clue to what kind of communication is needed.

There are those who are aware of the slender power of the forces of light in the present world situation, where arrogance and military might rule the councils of the world, and there is always the temptation to speak out, to shout the truth from the housetops, to be open and integral in a decaying world. To do so of course is to invite the hostility of those whose will prevails and to draw the fire of the opposing forces. Such an approach may be a deliberate aim of this book, yet this is not recommended for everyone. In certain situations people must hide their light in order to make their will eventually prevail. In certain places the dark forces have almost extinguished the light and the immediate cultural environment offers great difficulty in everyday communication even at the ordinary level of words. Where freedom of expression does exist, the answer to the world problem is really in the depth of human communication, not in the means of communication. Where the freedom of the soul is threatened by totalitarian repression, the crucible of suffering forges strength in the depths of character for they cannot speak out, and so the people must hide their light in the highest part of their consciousness. This perservering attitude should dwell in the heart of the oppressed and should not be made discernible to the dark forces from the outside; otherwise in their desperation to kill the threat they will not allow the forces of light to keep alive their will and to face all the difficulties.

It is arguable as to where the greatest darkness of society really is, since the external darkness we often see in certain national policies may not equal the internal darkness of ignorance in any given society. It is certain that even in the present free society of the West, there would be a fierce battle between those who would preserve the political animal at all costs and those who regard the death of the present political machinery as a necessary purification of an antiquated, ineffective and corrupt system. Here would begin the battle between the new Phoenix who comes in the fierce brilliance of the light of righteous action and the fake Phoenix who deceives with words and theories. While the fake makes all the obvious popular moves to swim with the tide of fashion and ride the opportunist waves of mob passions, the real Phoenix lays the difficult groundwork for ages to come.

How shall we know the signs when the forces of the holy one are rising? And how shall we know the times when the real revolutionary forces are ready to grasp the evolutionary power of our creative consciousness out of its enslavement to government systems? Social changes throughout history have always come through tax rebellion. The Magna Carta was signed because of a tax rebellion. The American War of Independence began as a tax rebellion. At the moment much of our creativity is taxed instead of our spending. What we produce with our hands and heads and efforts should only be taxed when incomes soar beyond the average amount required to live reasonably and to own a car and get to work, for this present immoral system of taxing is equivalent to piracy and has most of the ethics of a highwayman. To tax low incomes is to discourage productivity and the creation of wealth even before it is made. Taxes should be levied on spending and a much sharper distinction drawn between taxes on the essentials needed for life and the luxuries of abundant living. An ad valorem tax per item over a certain amount on certain goods such as furniture, clothes, telephones, etc., would mean that the poor would not be taxed on small inexpensive essential items. Anyone can spend money just as anyone can waste time chasing after pleasure and squander a lifetime on the inessentials. Pleasures could be taxed heavily but essentials are best left free to find their own levels in the market place. Even the present gasoline tax affects the poor who must drive or ride to work. Costs of essentials like food increase due to trucking fuel cost increases.

We will discover the real from the fake by their attitudes to taxation of creativity and luxury. Those politicians who would suck on the creative, who would want to milk the productive efforts of society, will reveal themselves in the battle for control of the common wealth. Unearned income, like that of shareholders who do not work for what they get, and very high wages of specialized skills should be taxed, but earned income up to the minimum needed to live decently should not be. The wealth of society should not be under control of government rulers and politicians but only controlled by those who produce it. Generosity must be allowed to operate efficiently and the employees of companies should be allowed to donate a fixed part of their annual wealth to charitable projects of their own choosing out of taxes. To be harassed by taxgatherers so that others may spend the monies which represent over a third of our working time frivolously on needless expenses is the first area of government where the outward resistance of the individual to external authority can legitimately come. The reaction to the former years of docility of the citizen will trigger in hard times of inflation the first rebellion against the taxing powers of the system. This of course will not in itself bring a political revolution or a bright New Age especially if it is allowed merely to flop ineffectually back into the selfish indulgence of more money for the taxpayer, but if, like the American Revolution, it brings our mind to thoughts of a greater freedom and directs our consciousness to developing new methods of sharing wealth and more importantly stimulates the creation of social wealth, then the tax revolution will be the beginning of the final battle between spiritual individuals and earthly authority. The age-old battle of kings versus the sovereignty of the individual will be fought once again on a higher level of true democracy versus "big government", Common Ownership versus "big business", and this battle will not begin in earnest until the threat of a total tax revolt strikes at the jugular vein of "big government". The dire threat that such a people's revolution might cripple a government or undermine the military defense would of course become a rationalization used vigorously by the conservative forces as well as the bureaucrats and would actively polarize and darken the national consciousness. At the moment there is nothing except misguided confusion amongst taxpayers in the West, but if the situation became polarized and obvious, then it would be necessary to veil the inner light—to be a silent rebel and not become an obvious target for reaction. Otherwise the consciousness revolutionaries would not appear safe and comfortable to those who are of the darkness. At the same time as exercising caution we must not hesitate to encourage the breaking up of external authority patterns, not in order to create chaos and disorder in society as politics and communism do by undermining institutions, but to effect an orderly, slow and careful transition between the old authoritative systems and the new self-rule communities which freely share their common surplus wealth rather than enforce taxpayers to share by coercive measures. The reason we say that a tax revolution is a signal for Common Ownership and the nuclear community is because, by spending the equivalent of what we would spend in taxes in the creation of an employee-owned company common capital fund, the workers who produce wealth are creating a prosperity consciousness for the capitalist and for all, not just for the few. It enables them to be active participants in the spiritual revolution and not just idle observers in the wings. The tax revolution is only a beginning of the battle of righteousness because it removes the power of almighty dollar and forces our leaders to relate to us from spiritual rather than from commercial and financial considerations. The critical point comes when the government will not have enough resources to govern as an autocracy while still pretending to be a democracy. Democracy is when the people rule, not the government. Politicians who act for people must surrender the absolutism of government sovereignty back to the people and not concentrate it in central government. This was the original intent of the founding fathers of the American dream.

To those who hear the melodious call of the Phoenix as it rises from the utter depths of death and self-destroying dualism, to those who see truth and have ears to hear truth, and for those who know the Phoenix is risen within them, the primordial light shines out from the consciousness of a truthful person. The radiance of the upward force of the inner light is seen as love in the eyes, and this is the mark by which the Phoenix is recognized. With these people the awakening rising forces of light can be open but wherever the dark force is in power, it is still important to be cautious and reserved and not to risk crucifixion to entice the enmity of hostile forces by deliberately using forceful or militant behavior. Using force does not change people but only creates fear. Therefore we should not join fashionable cults or work for more bizarre tax legislation such as Proposition 13 in California which only

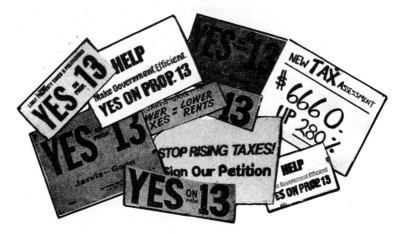

benefits property owners. Proposition 13 was a good beginning of rebellious spirits but not good legislation. We should make sure that our legislation protects those who pay the taxes. Landlords do not pay the taxes, they only add on costs and collect them from renters as part of the rent, which means that the renters have really paid the taxes and the landlords have not felt the pinch at all. While individual home owners properly benefit from a tax revolt like Proposition 13, since as a taxpayer their claim to tax relief is legitimate, they should also consider the renters in their fight to trim big government spending. Every way which forces government to spend only on bone and sinew and to cut the fat in government budgets at every level is legitimate self-defense against authoritarian exploitation. But if it is achieved at the expense of the poor or at the expense of renters merely to enrich owners of rental property, then the new way is no better type of exploitation than the old, and its momentum will cause it to perish in its own selfishness.

Therefore the quiet work to improve communication by probing the depths of human social interaction does not require us to become a fashionable cultish movement or to join in with the false practices of revolutionaries who preach violence since this only draws those visionaries who work for the new way of self-rule to the attention of the authorities. Socially we must not pretend to be all-knowing like the ignorant politicians of our time, but gradually build up small groups and communities with our own ways of dealing with social conflicts in a creative expression of community group consciousness. These groups will have to let much of the darker things pass without being duped. Why do we say this when the white knights are ready to charge and do battle for the forces of light? The answer is to be found in a new group method of self-rule by which the rising Phoenix becomes gradually triumphant over the dark forces of fear and doubt. This triumph is not experienced externally over other individuals, but happens within the consciousness of each person who can reject external authorities upon the earth and open up to the Cosmic Intelligence for direct guidance in new group-conscious methods of achieving unity. This method is not a multi-party system nor are individuals formed into competing parties to achieve democracy which leads to bureaucracy, but they become students of group consciousness—the single party democracy where all are equally sovereign and participate in self-rule. The division of human government into the leaders and the led, the right and the left, the employer and worker, etc., leads to the division of individual people as well as classes. Class warfare is no answer. Christ says that, "The evil forces are divided against themselves and so that is the end of them." This shows us the true power of union which removes the traumatic blockages of karma and releases our love of fellowman. The tax revolution is only a sign of the age that our belief in authoritarianism is beginning to break down, that the sovereignty of consciousness itself is reasserting its own divinity. The false authority of the church hierarchy, which looks towards religious personalities, popes, bishops and the external God, is now being returned to the internal teacher, the Christ within, who is the voice of God.

The Phoenix strips away the fear which mankind feels about "authority" so that love is freed to move in the hearts of all those peoples who are not divided amongst themselves. That consciousness which is divided against itself will not accept this without a battle, for it means the death of the ego, the end of all egocentric relationships between the ruled and the rulers who dominate society. In short the whole coming of the Phoenix is concerned with a duality in the minds of mankind, a division between one part of our self and another which always fears and doubts and therefore acts destructively against itself.

> "They reckon ill who leave me out;
> When me they fly, I am the wings:
> I am the doubter and the doubt, . . ."
> Ralph Waldo Emerson

The time is soon coming when those whose understanding of this duality between the individual self and its environment, between the self's separation of itself and the group, will come out into the open and shine in the darkness like a great light. But first the world must diminish in righteousness to its lowest depths because that is our test, that is our way of knowing that difference between the true and the false Phoenix.

The climax of the darkening and the division of man's consciousness is now being reached as I write this book. The moment of its maximum power will be the moment of the Rise of the Phoenix in the New Age of light. But the dark power will at first become self-perpetuating and hold so high a place in government that it can imprison and arrest all who are on the dualistic side of good even when they truly believe themselves to be protected and working for the powers of light. This power of the negative to wound the good must be real for the nature of goodness to be real. The Phoenix itself is eternally beyond this human dualism of light and dark, right and wrong, positive and negative, good and bad, but springs out of the nucleus where these forces are in balance. Beyond the concepts of good and evil there is another reality which is pure consciousness, where judgement in good and bad terms does not exist. It is from this world view that the events in this book are described, knowing that all the evil spawned by the dark power is consumed in the intensity of its own darkness. For the darkness owes its origin to the existence of light. This the dark power does not know—that it is merely a shadow of fear cast by the material veil. For what is night is only the shadow side of the earth, just as our own conscious self and ego are a shadow of the pure light of consciousness.

Because the Phoenix rises out of its own ashes and is born out of the new flames, it is a symbol that the evil force must itself be totally consumed and fall into oblivion at the very moment when it overcomes the good, and thus it consumes the energy of the old ways to which it owes its existence.

Quite apart from the pollution of the oceans and the rape of the environment a much more important and sinister battle goes on for the pollution of our minds. An example can be seen in the world now battling on a huge scale at the unconscious level in the imaginations and minds of people polarized between the social theories of Marx, Christianity and capitalism. If capitalism had not exploited the poor and the children in the 1800s, if it had really revealed itself as enlightened self-interest as it claims, if it had not had to be forced at every stage to stop polluting the air, the waters and the good earth, would the likes of Marx or Lenin or Mao Tse-tung have ever gotten any followers? Today the last stages of the battle are forming between these divisive forces who will destroy each other at the very moment when the synthesis of all that is good in both systems will be distilled into essence.

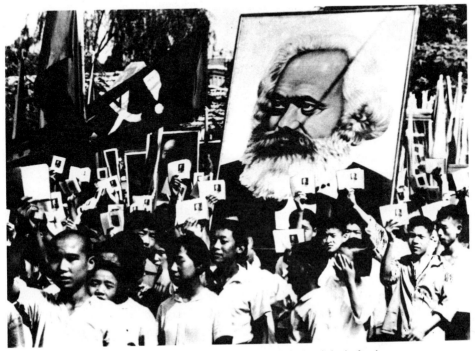

Followers of Marx and Mao Tse-tung carrying the latter's book of sayings.

The thesis of Jesus Christ of the reality of the Kingdom of Heaven, and the materialist antithesis of Karl Marx of the sole existence of the Kingdom of Earth, shall soon be joined together in the synthesis of Nuclear Evolution—the Kingdom of Heaven upon Earth! But as Christ himself prophesied, nonrecognition of the real from the fake will deceive many who will find it difficult to see the Truth:

> "Imposters will come claiming to be messiahs or prophets, and they will produce great signs and wonders to mislead, if such a thing were possible, even God's own people."

And immediately after this, as if to show the quality of the light of consciousness dawning across the whole 360 degree sweep of consciousness, comes the image of the sudden awakening, beyond the logical and conceptual efforts of the mind:

"For as lightning flashes from the east and shines as far as the west, so will be the coming of the Son of Man."

It is obvious that Christ's God was the pure light of 360 degree consciousness, and the rising of the light in the east was the achievement of union through the supersensitive awareness of the nature of light.

The rising of the new light can be compared to the realization of the illumined mind, which knows that the light of the sun and all the stars and suns radiating in every direction of ultimate space is really the same light which gives birth to consciousness. The Phoenix rises when man sees, without the confusion of the dualistic mind, that light and consciousness are one.

This book attempts to point to this theory as set out in my previous books, *Nuclear Evolution* and *Supersensonics,* that give the proofs which the reader can experience within only by practice day by day, hour by hour, minute by minute. Without preparation there can be no seeing or awareness of this light, and it is a waste of time to try to communicate on levels of consciousness which mankind as a whole does not know of nor even care about. This does not mean that those who do care and do know shouldn't express, communicate and speak of the deeper matters in their heart for those who will hear. But in this chapter we attempt to communicate only on those levels of consciousness where physical, social and rational men and women can see themselves and the environment from east to west (with everyone in it) as ONE.

That experience of the ONE, who is Pure Consciousness in the nuclear self of both reader and writer, is without the judgement of good and bad, outside and inside, or "him" and "me". That experience is not an opinion or an idea but a certain vibration of Truth which is absolute. It is the sudden awareness of a different kind of knowing. Beyond the ego is the experience of a synthesis of all the truth we know already, a vibration in thought in our consciousness which knows the difference between the real and the fake. At the moment of such a realization the Phoenix rises in us and the negative consciousness of the world and its conflicts and isms are dispelled. Thus the allegory of the Phoenix is the same as the allegory of the risen Christ who triumphs in consciousness spiritually over the inevitable physical death.

THE FAKE PHOENIX

Have you ever thought how gullible people are to follow the likes of Hitler and Mussolini, Lenin and Stalin, Mao Tse-tung or their historical equivalents who came to us with the great schemes which inspired masses of people to give up their normal lives and dedicate themselves to great causes?

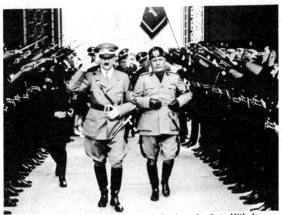

Even the dictator Mussolini yielded subserviently to Hitler's wishes. And in turn, millions went along with both Mussolini and Hitler.

On looking back from the now into the past we can see that they fooled millions of believers into a funny kind of idealism so that the people think light is dark and dark is light.

Whether it is politics or the evils of religion of medieval times it seems we can only tell the fake from the genuine after the fact and not before. We tire of hearing the revolutionaries talk of the evils of political revolutions and not their own evils. They repeat their jingles again and again like communism with its slogans of freedom and the greed of capitalism with all its affluent promises of the rich society.

The world believes it doesn't need to hear about these "isms" any more than it needs to learn how to spot a wolf in sheep's clothing.

The sad thing is that we do not even spot the fake Phoenix until it has risen with all its power and starts to devour the very people who set it up as the hope of the future. Why are people so blind that almost eighty million Germans were proud to march behind the German Eagle? Why did millions more for thirty years believe that Joseph Stalin and Lenin were saviors of the human race? Why are people daily deceived by their religious perceptions when the obvious is staring them in the face? Over the radio I just heard that the founders of the Church of God with a university college and a well-known money-raising radio program have been indicted for converting several million dollars for their own use. Recently, the leader of a thirty million dollar drug abuse program supported by government and the public as a charity has been arrested for complicity in a murder. Both of these leaders had the power to inspire and charismatically turn the heads and hearts of thousands of people who placed all their faith in them. What is the message for us in this?

All around the planet at this time we see the ancient myth of the dying Phoenix coming true in the flames of political and military conflagrations which encircle the people of the world. How many times in history has the world mistaken the rise of a world deceiver for the birthing of the Phoenix? It is easy to look back and see how many earthly powers have sneered at heaven and believed that they have finally usurped the evolutionary power, only to find they merely deceived the world and caused untold suffering to millions. We know the Roman legions marched behind the symbol of the eagle but what other great worldwide movements have held aloft the symbol of the eagle-eyed Phoenix, only to fail those who sincerely believed? What sort of people cannot see true at the time of folly and begin to follow a phony messiah spreading strife, division, death and dictatorship instead of the claimed unity and peace? How many people can see ahead into the somber grey clouds of misery which the fake Phoenix brings over the human spirit instead of freedom and joy?

As the typical example of deception in our own age we would no doubt elect Adolf Hitler with his idealistic book *Mein Kampf* ("my battle") with its great plan for a Teutonic master race arousing the warlike passion for military conquest and a racial hatred of the Jews. It was obvious that Hitler thought of himself as a Phoenix giving birth to a New Age, but in his self-delusion he is a prime example of a fake. According to the Nazi teachings of Adolf Hitler, the government was to treat the populations of eastern Europe as inferior races fit only to serve as slaves, and those classes of the population which were educated or might be leadership material, together with the Jews and any individuals who showed the least sign of resistance, were put to death. Between 1941 and 1945 at one camp, Auschwitz in Poland, as many as 4,000,000 were dispatched in the gas chambers and by starvation and disease.

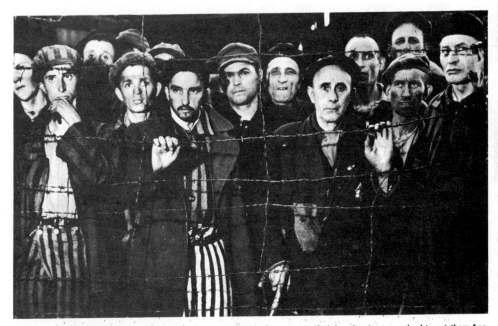

Bewildered prisoners in the notorious Buchenwald concentration camp as horrified American troops arrived to set them free.

At Manthausen, one of the camps in Austria, close to 2,000,000 people, mostly Jews, were exterminated. Economic exploitation of all territories over which Hitler became absolute master between 1939 and 1944 was ruthless. Frequent manhunts were carried out to round up slave labor for deportation to Germany and about 4,795,000 workers were carried back to Germany all in this way. The three largest groups were Russians—1,900,000, Poles—851,000, and French—764,000, and these were treated entirely as slave labor in appalling conditions. This was part of the plan for the new order, and any resistance was met with the destruction of entire villages and the ruthless shooting of hostages.

But throughout history others more skillfully deceptive than Hitler have led mankind into great suffering and death and brought us the massive destruction of life in prison camps. Other idealistic dictator-ships and whole nations have believed and are right now believing the deceptions of the fake Phoenix as it rises in the twisted imaginations of men and women everywhere. The millions fooled by such idealogues as Lenin and Stalin in Russia and Mao Tse-tung in China really do believe in their system of thought and the society they are now building. It is even more staggering when we hear people even today defending them on the radio and in universities everywhere. What has happened to the clear-seeing mind of the human race? It is all the more deceptive because all this twisted political action and idealism has been encouraged in the name of an ideology which openly supports division, secrecy and the undermining of existing forces by deception, fomentation of hatred or racial trouble in any areas of human conflict, and the spreading of false stories in order to bring down a democratic government and take over by force of arms. Once in power under the banner of an ideology the bloodbath starts and we hear very little of it in the press. The familiar pattern is that while the killing is going on, all foreign press journalists are banned and the society becomes closed to the world. Those people who could write a factual account of murder and genocide in these revolutionary countries of the world over the last thirty to fifty years of global history are no longer with us. They have been eliminated from the face of the earth, destroyed by the fake Phoenix in the purges and pogroms of these former years.

But what about now in this moment of world history? Can we recognize the true from the false? While I write this book in the blood of the slain, their bones are now turning to dust and ashes in the ground. The noise of their clamoring spirits turn into millions of cries of "Wake up! Wake up!" which call to the real Phoenix to rise out of its own funeral pyre.

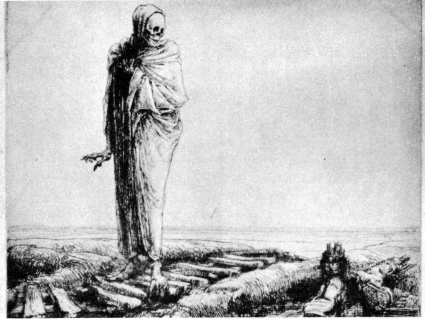

DEATH AWED. Percy Smith.
This great etching sums up the whole horror of war. It is expressive of no one period, but of all periods.

Just as there is something wrong in the attitudes of capitalists who build noisy trucks and filthy smokestacks and refuse to cooperate until forced to by law and the consumer activists, so there is also something wrong in the way intellectuals and idealists perceive realities; otherwise they would easily see the difference between practice and political theory. Continually society supports those ivory tower thinkers and political academic sympathizers of these ideologies who are always comparing capitalist practices with Russian theories. If they were perceptive enough to look at Russian practice and compare it to capitalist practice we would see that fake idealism is just as exploitative of society as capitalist greed. While "big business" and the persuaders employed by great industrial powers, the utilities, and the oil industry do often undermine and ride roughshod over democratic process with the rape of the environment and the propaganda of persuasion, at least they do not yet murder and kill in the promotion of their selfish idea. Though they may risk the lives of millions in the future through their investments in nuclear energy, these utilities do have many supporters and shareholders among the people who benefit daily from their profits.

The capitalist whose ice cream truck parks daily outside my window and who refuses to put a sound muffler on his compressor so I can hardly hear myself think pays no attention to my fifty complaints. Am I then justified in sabotage or violent action? The fake Phoenix sweeps everyone into believing that violence in support of an ideal is justified in order to get ideal change. But the danger is not only in our righteous indignation but in our conviction that we perceive the situation correctly. The case against the truck is not against the greedy company, or the manufacturer, but against the society which allows such obvious exploitation through noise pollution of its own citizens. In a referendum in California the right to build polluting nuclear plants and the right to smoke in others' air spaces were approved by a majority. To what extent did we notice that this free and democratic vote reflected not the public weal but the deception of the persuaders and propagandists? In democracy power is wielded indirectly through the rubber stamp of the public which blinds itself to reality. What is the middle way between the self-righteous and violent retaliation of the fake Phoenix and this apathetic inertia which infects people when they are acting as "the public"? Have we ever considered how quickly the sluggish world responds to personal anger and yet in its public apathy forgets the cold political brutality, the calculating horrendous tortures and crimes against humanity? What role does this inability to see things as they are play in the path of an evolutionary intelligence?

We must look at the facts of life rather than theories and we must become more aware and in tune with the actions of groups formed for specific purposes. We must look at group consciousness itself not only in other animals and in natural systems of intelligence but also in our own lives as they are lived as social beings. Is social anger and righteous indignation in politically conscious people blinding us to far wider potentials? If we look at the record of the past, we will see how this "reforming" spirit in society has swung like a pendulum from extreme to extreme with little improvement of the basic conditions of power and exploitation and injustice in the human scene. Will we continue to follow the irrational social drive in mankind which willy-nilly pulls us along a blind path which eventually gets strewn with the bodies of those who were believers? The path to all isms like capitalism, communism or socialism is paved with the hearts of the disillusioned and is running with the blood of the brave. Why does this have to be so absurd? Can we not change our view of the planetary forces of change and find some new constitutional way of testing our beliefs and our leaders' integrity and developing clarity of mind so that we can have instantaneous clear seeing into any situation that arises, and we no longer need leaders to envision our future for us because we ourselves have as much vision as they? Are there new groupings of humans in the world who can work for constitutional and social change differently and without the risk of deception, groups in which all are leaders and there are no blind gullible sheep to be led to the slaughter?

Most people have never directly encountered a New Age group and are therefore totally dependent on the news media, which like to dramatize and to milk the dark and negative side of life for the sake of exciting headlines. People have no way of telling which groups are cults and which are not. But if they took the trouble to investigate, the differences are quite clear. The attitude to money is one criterion; the attitude to authority is another; and force is another. But the main attitude we must watch out for is not the power-seeking tactics of the fake Phoenix but our own attitude of self-righteous complacency which does nothing to form our own model community or constitution. It is this willingness to live life half asleep which makes us easy victims for any false messiah or political savior with a little energy. This is the problem which Creative Conflict and nuclear groups must tackle now if the human race is to stop war and killing in the name of peace. Nothing is more obvious in the formation of groups, parties and religions which attempt to win political or social power.

EXPOSING THE CULTS

It's a good thing that the fraudulent should be exposed, that the truth about spiritual groups—supposedly spiritual groups—should be exposed, so that the healthy groups which are pure and can stand the light of day, the light of truth, will get investigated more. The problem with good groups, i.e., the groups which are true group consciousness, is that they don't get investigated enough. They don't make any bad waves, so they don't get noticed so much. The ones that are most publicized are so-called New Age groups which are not groups at all, but are really mini-dictatorships which pose as groups. These groups, no different from the lamas and feudal church systems, are hierarchy, with all the baronets and the knights and lackeys, and all the sheep—the followers. They dance to the dictator's whims, whether it is the Reverend Jim Jones or some of the many others. Jones couldn't operate in the USA because he was operating with threats. His flock had to believe absolutely everything he said, otherwise they were beaten and threatened. They couldn't leave because he forced them to turn over their property. When it got a bit hot and things started to leak out about the way his operation was run, they went off to Guyana where they could actually create a prison stockade, take the passports away and have guns, so that from the barrel of a gun everything he said of course was absolute law, to the point where he pretended to be God and wanted to be worshipped as God.

There's a saying which goes, "Those whom the gods would destroy they first make mad." And one way that group leaders, particularly spiritual group leaders, are exposed is that they begin to suffer a special kind of madness. Because of the adulation of the followers, they can get away with anything and their word is absolute law. So they begin to feel that heady power and begin to feel that they have power over life and death and particularly the lives of other people, and then they start to use it and decide everything for those people. They marry them off to whomever they want depending on whether it suits the organization they are trying to build. They do not encourage clear thinking and concise or precise communication but deliberately create a mystique around the leadership so that their charisma can dominate everything. If you look into those organizations you find many of the membership are people who never know what's really going on, even if they are next to the top man. It's always a bit hazy about what's going on, or where the money goes, or how things are decided. Even at the top they always have to ask so and so, and it's always a chain of command where it's not really a group consciousness at all, because the leaders of those groups are not trying to teach their followers to think for themselves. They are trying to get them to make the leader a fat cat. His power depends on everyone bowing, scraping and feeding him with money, and on absolute obedience, so you can always see that the teaching of those teachers is false. They put all their money away in Swiss bank accounts and have private jets and stay in the most expensive hotels.

If you look closely, you see that a true teacher, a true master in true group consciousness only wants others to have the same mastery. He teaches a true group consciousness where there is decision-making at every level, not making himself an absolute authority. The authority is always given to the followers first, at least until they fail. He gives them the freedom to fail, whereas a man at the top of an organization, where he is number one in the hierarchy, cannot afford to allow his followers to fail because that would be his own failure. They represent his personal success, so they have to succeed. That means they cannot be allowed to make any decisions which might go wrong, so he must make the final decision in everything. The true teacher works as Nature does. He allows his students to make decisions so that they will fail if necessary as a learning experience, and he will only step in at the last minute to save the situation. He might have to be a dictator in the end to pick up the mess that the students make, but he gives them that freedom to know themselves well enough to learn from their mistakes. He gives them the trust, and risks the whole enterprise so that if it succeeds it is their success, not his, and in that success he rejoices because he has taught them how to be skillful, how to use their minds and their powers to fulfill themselves, not just be a carbon copy and follow and do what he says, but to have the clarity of mind that he himself has. Instead of deliberately creating mystique and unclear communication, the true master creates the situation where we get more clear, more open in our minds about who we are, what we can do and how the situation is around us, so we can master it rather than be prisoner of it. In many of the very prosperous spiritual organizations, if you look at their constitutions, you will see that the first thing it says is, "All decisions shall be made by Swami this or Reverend that, and his decision shall be final."

So there is a big difference in what you call and classify a New Age group. Many of these gurus and teachers are not New Age, they are very Old Age because they run their organizations the exact same way that the medieval feudal systems were run, the way the kings and knights and barons kept people in servitude to them. If you see a guru sitting on a throne with lots of ashrams and million-dollar jets and all that, you have to ask yourself, why does he need all those people to go and make money so he can sit in glory? Isn't it strange that people are into those cults? And that's what it really is—a personality cult—it's not true group consciousness at all! Just as kings and rulers create an authoritarian system, the same thing happens in the spiritual world. We do not always realize that kings, queens and military dictators are like a personality cult and that the masses get the same thrill and feeling of security from royalty or authority that cultists get from their leaders. You elect a personality and then you worship it. You worship the power it executes and then you have a cult. It is strange that man has not changed much from old times in terms of his cultish ways. The more cults are exposed and the more people discover phony spiritual groups, the better it is for those who have purified their consciousness, because anyone can come and investigate healthy groups and find there is no coercion. They are not imprisoning their followers but teaching them to be free, to think clearly and to think for themselves.

Cults frighten us because we do not understand our own gullibility. Jonestown was a rather visible group from our point of view and close to home because it was Americans who had gone to Guyana, and we have quite a few so-called spiritual cults in America. But there are much bigger and more dangerous cults than Jonestown who are setting the world back. We don't have to look very far to see that the cult of Stalin was much worse than the cult of Reverend Jones. And right now in 1979 there are places throughout the world, like Cambodia, where not just nine hundred are being murdered as in Jonestown, but thousands and millions are suffering because of people who think they know how to run other people's lives. It is going on in so many places. We are very comfortable here in the US, insulated from it all. This country has never really had any hardship. It has never had a war that has really touched it. There have never been bombs on this nation, never been rockets, never been a deflation except way back in the continental civil war, never had the currency worth nothing in almost a day. If we really look at how well off we are in America in wealth and in freedom we would be wiser in how to preserve it. It is one of the few places left on the planet. Most of the countries in Asia and South America and most of the countries in the UN are dictatorships and don't allow any opposition. They are ruled by a few individuals who have power over the lives of millions of people, not just a thousand people like Reverend Jones had in the forest. But the real punch is that a cult only hits us when it is close to home. We don't think of it much when it is elsewhere, out there in the world, but when it's Americans it hits harder.

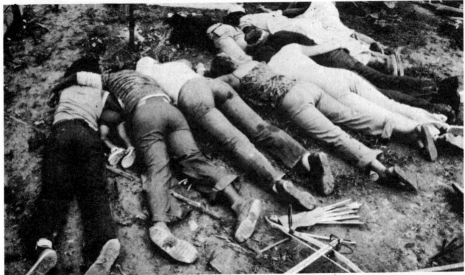

Jonestown victims   Frank Johnston—The Washington Post

So let us rejoice in the persecution of all that cult stuff. Let us have more of it—until there are only one or two groups left in the world. Then we won't have to condemn anyone else as phony. If we have a good group we just need to worry about getting our own act clean and becoming so precise in our own consciousness that we can succeed without having to have a boss, without having to have anyone directing the show. Then when we demonstrate that group consciousness, some-one visiting our group will say, "This place really does run by itself; it doesn't need a leader because you are all leaders."

But of course we cannot just say that with our mouth. At the center I started in London, everyone was supposed to be a leader. That was the theory, but that was also the myth. A man came there one day when I was in the US and said, "You know, you're not leaders, you people. The leader is away." They all got up in arms and said, "No, we're all leaders. We practice a certain type of group consciousness here and it makes us all leaders." But actually he wasn't so wrong, because if they'd been true leaders they would have been able to pay the bills. They would have been able to know what carried the place along in reality, and they didn't. It is possible to live the myth that we are responsible, masterful, capable, effective, precise, clear, and all those things, and yet fool ourselves. Hopefully at University of the Trees we don't have that kind of situation. We are all totally responsible for the operation, so that we all know what makes it tick and we all know what it takes to make it run. We all decide everything, we all own the business, and we take the consequences of making the decisions, right or wrong, and we do not blame someone up there in authority. Most people do not want this kind of total responsibility. They'd rather float along, have someone else decide all the questions for them, do all their thinking for them so they can forget about any challenges and just live a mentally lazy life, doing only what they feel like doing. Only in small groups can we learn how to take responsibility for the whole in a way that we can handle, where it does not seem too big to attempt. By not taking responsibility we find only our small niche in a huge society, oblivious to what is really happening in the other parts. By taking responsibility we move into the center where we are fully alive, in touch with the whole, at the hub; and only there is peace found.

The world has now come to a critical point in the evolution of its inhabitants. The fruits of American largesse in the past have brought forth a new and strong Germany out of the destruction of Hitler. The German eagle flies again. Help to Japan has brought its people economically once again into the land of the rising sun. American aid to other countries has protected the world against invasion and its dollars in the past have built up the defenses against the forces of the anti-Phoenix. Now the world must recognize the war of righteousness cannot be waged with self-righteousness any more than a communist plan for world dominion and union can be spread by division. Now we must go inside ourselves to the internal conflict and fight with our self-righteous anger and frustration and turn it into creative conflict. We must decide in our hearts whether the American dollar is dying as a symbol of power, what has been termed the "Almighty Dollar", or whether America is to be the home of the new Phoenix, aware and awakening to its evolutionary vision. This will depend on the keenness of its vision of the future and whether the dollar collapses as the world's major currency. It will depend on giving a new economic and spiritual philosophy to the world in which the image of grasping imperialism and commercialism is overshadowed by "right action" of its people to group together in small communities to root out the fake Phoenix in any form. This new philosophy will not be a set of concepts, theories or political ideals but a cosmic program, set in the nucleus from the beginning of all life. It will not operate through darkness, in shadows and the stealth of night, but will bring each brain into openness and will flood light into all human relationships. The fake Phoenix cannot bring that trust which throws all its Truth out into the open in the knowledge that the Superintelligence of the nucleus does not fear the intensity of light, does not need to hide its true intent. Those who, like the Phoenix, fly into the sun's light cannot see anything in their consciousness but pure light, because they are blinded continually on every side by the brilliant rays of the Source. The Source is not separate from themselves but they see its glory with a sense of awe and do not claim it in their conceit. Thus we can tell the true from the false Phoenix. The true witness of that light does not come to speak of its own glory but gives the credit to the Source. Thus is the Source glorified by receiving back its own light. Thus is the Phoenix glorified by the Source.

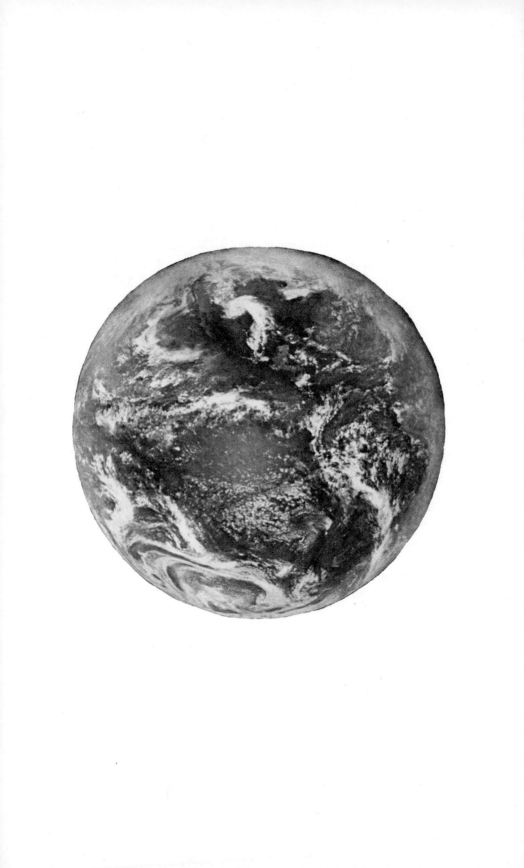

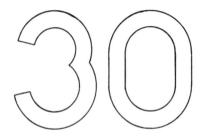

THE RISE OF THE PHOENIX

The Phoenix which rises from its own ashes is the symbol for the New Age which turns full cycle upon itself. Christ says of the awakening consciousness: "I shall rise again. Like the flashing of light in the east, I shall return again and again."

The idea of the resurrection, the risen Christ, is the rising of the Phoenix in the Nuclear core of Being out of the ashes of its own death of ego. Are these merely words and metaphors? Are symbols only stories with which mankind amuses himself? The pioneer work of Freud in the field of psychology showed that symbols were the language of our unconscious minds, speaking to us in our dreams as we slept, bringing up important knowledge about ourselves. Freud's colleague, Carl Jung, went even further to say that not only our dreams but our waking life is acted out according to certain archetypal symbols

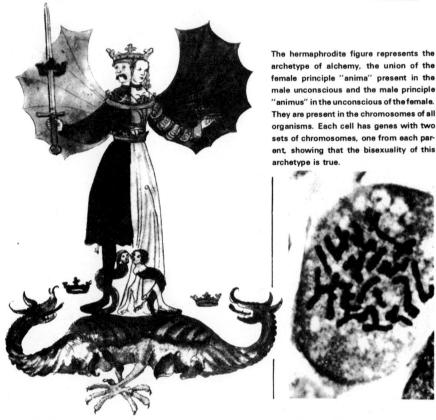

The hermaphrodite figure represents the archetype of alchemy, the union of the female principle "anima" present in the male unconscious and the male principle "animus" in the unconscious of the female. They are present in the chromosomes of all organisms. Each cell has genes with two sets of chromosomes, one from each parent, showing that the bisexuality of this archetype is true.

which arise from the unconscious mind of people in all places and in all times. These archetypes which arise in dreams and in all mythologies seem primitive and remote to our now-civilized consciousness which believes that modern life is reality. We do not see that our modern life, despite its technology and scientific discoveries, is as much a waking dream as life in the ego has always been. Because the ego sees only illusion of separate entities, groups, stars, chemicals and people, etc., our new theory of consciousness needs to demonstrate that it is not just "modern" life that is the waking dream, but our whole edifice of what is normal.

To most people in the world, events are all happening out there to others in London, Moscow, Afghanistan, Washington. These events, places and people are believed to exist independent of our conscious knowing. This separated world is the delusion of the dualistic mind which the Phoenix comes to destroy. When we come to see the construction of the "false self" called ego, we see that it is comprised of the sense of separation within itself. Puffed up inside its own "ego-bubble", its power of separation believes it can conquer "out there" and become master of space, of air, of all that it surveys. In its waking dream the false self sees its human limitations to be its all and therefore limits all others by its own limits. When we identify our consciousness as separate from the environment in which it lives or separate from the objects it experiences in the external world, we do not realize that all this external experience is reconstructed as an internal holograph, a symbolic re-creation of events, concepts, stimuli, etc., inside our heads. All that we know and see, the politics and social situation, even the personality of friends as well as our own identity, is a re-creation of consciousness and is thus limited or delimited by the limits in our own consciousness. Therefore we can know nothing about society or philosophy or anything else which is not already within our own powers of understanding.

The disillusioned of each generation run from ideal to ideal in search of the golden bird of paradise, but they never find it. We naturally think of idealists and dreamers as good people wishing for themselves and for the world a brighter and more enlightened state of being. Yet without working on the waking dream which separates the ego from the world it lives in, the ideal is merely the projection of our own image, unconsciously striving to achieve its own archetype, limiting all others in its self-deception. The ego is blinded by its own light, blinded by its own conceit. Hence, the waking dream is such that the Phoenix must die to itself and be reborn out of the debris of the fire which consumes the mind and its dream symbols in order to see with the sharp vision of direct perception. What is this Phoenix? Is it some great being who comes to enlighten us and who returns again and again to point the way? Will the New Age spawn a new culture with a new flag to wave for all to follow or will it emerge fully-fledged from within the human psyche? From whence does the Phoenix arise?

The Phoenix can only rise within you. Only your own ego can become the fire which will generate the energy for its resurrection. When the Phoenix rises it destroys the old self, and the new one is born out of the ashes of what is left in the contents of our consciousness. We are born again and again out of this residue, this garbage of our conscious and unconscious life, until we are free like the Phoenix to fly directly into the sun.

What is this garbage, then? Let us translate the symbols into the patterns of human life. Millions were killed deliberately by the Pakistani army when East Pakistan decided to secede from West Pakistan. Troops would invade the university and kill all intellectuals in sight because these were the future leaders. Thousands are now being killed, as I write, by the army of the Shah of Iran in the civil disorders inspired by religious leaders against his regime. Every day in Africa, South America and Asia thousands are tortured, executed, and sent to prison as a direct result of institutional violence. What is the source of that same violence and aggression that emerges as conflict in ourselves? We do not want it. We do not own up to it. It is garbage—the product of our frustrations which are born out of our deluded ego perceptions.

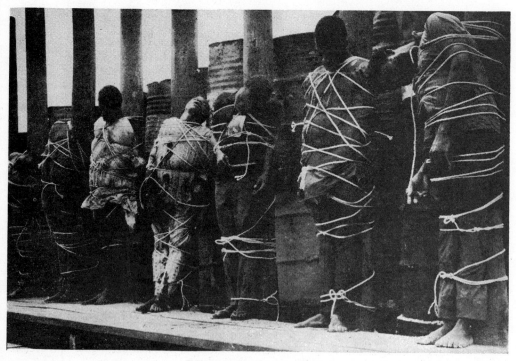

Public execution in Lagos, Nigeria.

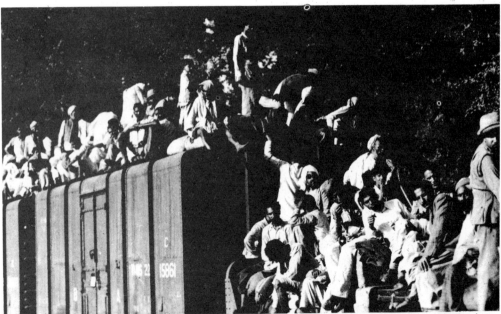

In cutting up the subcontinent at the time of the partition of India, the British Government agreed with Jinnah, a Muslim who was a lawyer, to create the state of Pakistan against the ideas of Mahatma Gandhi who believed the nation should be secular, not based on religion and not favoring one religion above another. The result was so much hatred and bloodshed that over ten million people died as massive population shifts occurred. Surviving Muslims went to East and West Pakistan and Hindus went to India. Millions were uprooted from their homes where they were born.

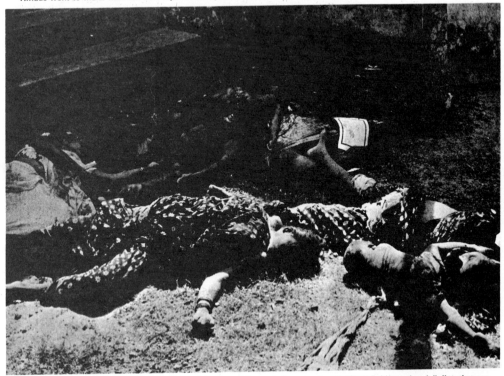

When East Pakistan revolted against the exploitation of the central government in West Pakistan the civil disturbances were put down by the Pakistani army. A defenseless population was butchered in order to hold on to the territory. India did not intervene but helped the rebels and accepted millions of refugees escaping from the carnage. Religion spells death in such highly emotional situations of civil strife.

Freud said that human aggression was all repressed in the unconscious sexual libido and that man was an aggressive creature because of unexpressed sexual energy, like a pressure cooker ready to blow. This viewpoint came from the fact that Freud was a thinking type and a physical type. He rejected intuition and reduced everything to basic red chakra energy (libido). Consequently his perception of truth was limited to his own level of consciousness, and his irreconcilable conflict with Jung, his colleague, came from the fact that Jung was a thinking-intuitive type. Jung's reality was too big for Freud and frightened him, as he himself admitted. Jung's thought process built its edifice of thought on the unconscious intuitive perception of synchronous events.

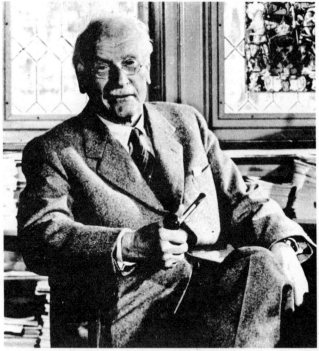

Carl Jung 1875-1961— was an intuitive thinking-type who saw Western science as only half the picture of reality. Studying the Vedic Sanskrit teachings and the ancient Chinese yoga systems he saw that their concepts of Tao or the world-soul fitted with his theory of a collective unconscious.

Jung set up his own theory of dream interpretation by developing the conception of fundamental archetypes. Such notions as God, Father, wise old man, Mother, power and escape, exist as universal drives in the unconscious in which all individuals share. These archetypes emerge in the interaction between our conscious and unconscious parts of our personality representing good and evil, masculinity and femininity and are fraught with metaphysical overtones. In other words Jung perceived that the contents of the collective unconscious pop up wherever there is a condition of resonance created for them in someone, and the collective unconscious will then emerge through that person. For example, the "messiah" is an archetype which will personify itself through a human being as it did in Jesus of Nazareth, but it is part of the collective unconscious of the human race, which means that we are all able to become identified with the messiah, since it is in our unconscious.

Freud was emphasizing how we keep the lid on our unconscious mind by repressing unacceptable feelings, whereas Jung was talking of just the opposite—how we permit the contents of our unconscious minds to rise in us and motivate us to action. For example, the messiah archetype can be a disease if you make it your self-image. To *think* you are the messiah is a disease, and the true messiah must always be validated by another, as Christ was baptized by John the Baptist. But if in your heart you *identify* with the messiah and the rising Phoenix and, in a selfless way without ego identification, you *become* it, you thereby allow many messiahs and many Phoenixes to emerge from the archetype as aspects of yourself, not as separate manifestations. The fake messiah uses his delusions of grandeur to separate from others and lift himself above them. The true messiah experiences "others" as himself. The Phoenix that raises its head as a self-image in our head is a fake. But if we tune to the *pure* space, the real Christ consciousness, the Phoenix rises in our own heart.

There are many archetypes through which we create our reality in the imagination, and the collective unconsciousness comes out not only in our sleeping dreams but in our waking dream. Much of human action is based on the archetype we unconsciously or consciously identify with—the self-image we hold of who we are or who we want to be. If our image is narrow and limited it will bring us into conflict with the rest of the whole, which will cause us to resonate with negative archetypes. This is the reason Jung believed that aggression arose from the archetypes held in the collective unconscious. But it is not only the collective unconscious that motivates us but a cosmic unconscious. Violence is not just a product of man's nature or a result of repressed conflict. There is a violence in Nature that is not personal but which comes as a result of mass tensions on a macrocosmic scale.

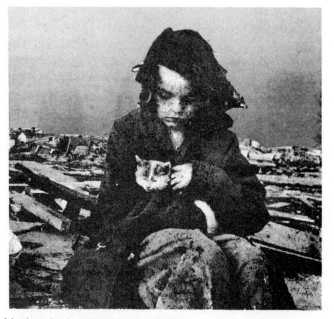

A hurricane has just devastated this girl's home—an example of Nature's violence.

A kind of cosmic violence is going on in the center of the sun, in exploding supernovae where energy of a whole galaxy is bursting and irradiating the whole. When a supernova goes off, all the atoms in a galaxy are energized by the accelerated electrons which become highly polarized in the spiral grip of the rotating magnetic field. Thus all matter in that nebula becomes polarized causing all gases to ionize, raising all matter onto another level of evolution. This whole violent process is the rise of the Phoenix on a cosmic scale. In order to rise and provide energy to light up the whole galaxy the supernova has to die or shed most of its matter. In a matter of three weeks a supernova burst sheds as much energy as a whole star would shed in its lifetime of shining from a white dwarf to a red giant throughout the entirety of its evolution.

This cosmic process is reflected in human affairs in the form of the rising of certain stars on the human scene which sweep the earth like Christianity, Mohammedanism, Buddhism, Communism. These are of course mental bursts represented by a lot of killing and wars, institutional violence performed by a lot of small people being part of big armies and power cliques like the old Holy Roman Church. But our insight comes when we realize that the Superintelligent refiner's fire that burns away the dross in galaxies and in Nature also operates in the people of the world, and nothing can stop this process because that is how things are. The only way the Force can be redirected and human violence prevented is by changing our own consciousness to tune to a higher cosmic archetype. We must uproot from our consciousness our present archetypal pattern to replace it with another, which is possible in consciousness through surrender to the One. It is possible to change human beings, not by brainwashing which is at the mental level, but by a change of being which is a change of heart. The reason we have had all these wars throughout the ages is that men have tried to change heads—the way people think. But what we need is a change of hearts.

The archetype of the heart is different to the archetype of the head. The head separates, thinks of itself as an entity separate from other entities, tries to get other entities to do its will and run the world by its archetypal thinking of self-centeredness. Thus the cosmic archetype of violence manifests its energy on earth through separative egos; war is the result. The archetype of the heart is cosmic on its own level of complete togetherness which is the meaning of the word *samadhi*, from the Sanskrit root word *sam* meaning complete or perfect and *adhi* meaning together or union. When the heart is united with the cosmic archetype there is perfect union, perfect togetherness and complete tranquility. This is not a human change but a surrender to the Cosmos, an opening to a higher level of consciousness in Nature, allowing it to imprint in our imagination a new cosmic archetype. So we don't do it ourselves by trying to impose the new archetype on Nature from a mental conception. It is not a matter of magicians cooking up cosmic fire in some laboratory saying, "follow *my* new archetype". We are talking about God's archetype which is waiting for man once he gets out of his ego. If hearts are one it doesn't matter what is in the head. To change the heart is to tune into the Cosmos. The present human archetypal identification makes us a slave of passions, a slave of cosmic forces, not their master, whereas it is possible to be in control of cosmic forces and change our life. It's within the human power to use cosmic forces for good or evil, for selfish or cosmic ends. The moment we use our consciousness for cosmic ends we've changed the human archetype.*

All our self-images are archetypes—these are the subtle images we hold of what we are looking for in life. It might be a deep image of our ideal mate or a vague vision of what we think will bring us fulfillment or how we would be if we could be what we *want* to be. The macho he-man, the submissive woman and the feminist are popular modern day archetypes that mold people's reality. On another level is the archetype of the hero. The warrior hero is another type of selflessness, like the Roman, Horatio, who defended the bridge for his fellow warriors though it cost him his life, or the vow of the Spartan race to die for Sparta. In religion we have the saint or religious hero, the martyr who goes joyfully to crucifixion or to face the lions in the Roman Colosseum. The levels on which these archetypes function correspond to our own breadth of consciousness—the scope of our ability to identify with what is larger than ourself. Somewhere between the hero and the cosmic archetype in the heart is the level of the Divine Mother or Heavenly Father. Hindus who get trapped in the worship of the Divine Mother—the Shakti energy or devotional side of religion—are limiting religion by identification with only half the creative force, just as Christians get trapped in the worship of the Father, the Shiva or active force. Both these limitations on cosmic consciousness can become a perversion of religion, whereas the true samadhi is found in the union of these male and female archetypes. All these images are subtle ego identifications, even the most noble and heroic, because they limit the person to that identity, so that a higher cosmic archetype cannot penetrate.

A mother with her children feels a great swelling up of joy inside, a natural feeling which is pure and not based on a self-image. Therefore,

---

* *Out of the Fire of the Nucleus*, the third book in this series, delves into how we use cosmic forces for good and for evil.

to expand that natural feeling to include the whole is the real selfless work of the devotee, rather than attempting to see oneself as "The Mother" which perpetuates self-image and inflates the ego. Cosmically, "Mother" is the in-breath, drawing all to the center of love; "Father" is the out-breath, radiating from the center throughout the creation. But Father without Mother or Mother without Father are only concepts of religion and are not the complete life force which is in us already, creating all we see. Mother and Father are principles in Nature. The cosmic Father swells up inside with light like a supernova and wants to expand and illuminate the universe with his glory. He is searching for the cosmic Mother who will take the light and compress it and suck it in and surrender to it. Then the female principle, the Great Mother, becomes pregnant with all possibilities. These principles of creation are real and cosmic in that stars explode and contract, and positive and negative forces are woven throughout the created universe, yet even on a cosmic scale these are also limitations, because there is an *un*created universe beyond the creation, just as our consciousness is beyond the body. Consciousness *uses* the body in the same way that the uncreated universe uses the creation, and that archetype of the primal uncreated state of Being is a black hole, the singularity or absolute state of the heart where no duality exists, neither positive or negative, the state where both positive and negative are annihilated in balancing each other so that a third and timeless state is created which has no form but has *all* potentials, both manifest and unmanifest, created and uncreated, since at any moment it can create time and with time create vibration or movement from out of the stillness or the balance. Such an unmanifested state is beyond all qualities and is therefore the archetype of the nameless superintelligent Tao, the fundamental ground of existence which is the archetype of the eternal, the unchanging.

In order to *be* this singularity of the heart and not just think we are that, we must make way for the Phoenix to arise by preparing the ground. There is no route to the heart through the safe, well-travelled pathways of the head. The only way to get there is to allow the total energy and intensity of full consciousness (not just the workings of the mind) to break you through as you work on your separating ego. We begin by learning to hold the higher archetype and to look on ourselves as being that still, peaceful eternal heart and by the process of identification to evolve closer and closer to the archetype of the eternal One. In short, we must get a new self-image and must learn that it is not to be feared, even though all our lesser self-images must be sacrificed to it. In becoming the uncreated nothing we will become everything and our hearts will be as big as the universe, beating with God's heart, and our long search to find our Self will be fulfilled.

ARCHETYPAL CHANGE

It is remarkable on this planet that the introduction of every new idea that requires deep change in people has been accompanied by considerable amounts of aggression. Every movement which ever started and had any power in it to transform, has always brought hostility and aggression to the surface. The moral instincts of man have given rise to the spread of religious empires by aggression and force and coercion. Even beliefs of nonviolence have been spread by the sword or by violence. By using violence we are automatically proving that the idea does not have the power to travel by its own energy, regardless of whether these beliefs are political, religious or otherwise idealistic. Early Christianity, up to the time of Constantine, *had* this energy of spiritual excitement in the process of transmission of the teachings. The emperor Constantine, converted to Christianity, adopted it as a state religion of the Roman Empire in the East—Christianity's first step toward respectability after 400 years of violent repression. Similarly Buddhism was made the state religion by King Ashoka, and the Buddhist teachings were spread with the already existing power of the state and defended by the army. The interference of the secular by the edicts of these two rulers, Constantine and Ashoka, may have been the adulteration of the seed which spread the pure teachings in a polluted form and therefore had the seed of failure built into it. By failure we do not mean that these two great religions do not contain the essence of humility and enlightenment which all individuals seek, but that in their growth they have failed to retain the purity of their original founders and have thereby become conceptual dogmas and scriptures rather than a way of life. By failure we mean that the world has not followed these teachings and consequently gets more and more violent. We must look at facts and not run away from them. The fact is that in our idealism we sell more Bibles than ever, and there has never been a more popular demand for written scriptures than at this moment in history. But we cannot confuse quantity with quality, myth with reality, expectations with performance. The ideas we hold in our heads have outstripped our manifestation, and the doctrines which we have "promoted" are like weeds which have choked out the truth that just grows naturally like a seed.

Cosmic ideas that are born out of Nature herself and are natural archetypes have within them the evolutionary energy so that nothing can stop them once their time has come. Many men have *thought* that their idea's time had come and have gone out to promote it with every means at their disposal. Yet the moment they stopped spending money, advertising, promoting and pushing, the movement fizzled by its own lack of self-replicating, self-creating force. A truly revolutionary idea does not need promoting; it just takes over naturally and unfolds through its sheer natural rightness, fitting into a niche that has been created by human wrongness.

Ideas or concepts which have changed the world universally and not just in various geographical sections of peoples or countries have been human inventions which were useful, such as the telephone and television or workable theories like Einstein's formulation of relativity which is now at the back of all our electromagnetic age. None of these needed to be promoted; they sold themselves with their sheer ability to function efficiently. An invention in the social and human levels of communication analogous to these discoveries would be a method to enable humans to communicate with each other at a much deeper level than written or spoken words. Another analogous invention would be a new system of thought for understanding man's place in the universe, resulting in a true image of himself. This system of thought would have to be functional in that it truly represented a natural unfolding of a human need to communicate on more than one level of expression and hopefully in a multi-leveled communication, including all present methods, encapsulating the synthesis of all religion and science that has gone before and raising it to a higher level of expression. It is this that Nuclear Evolution attempts to tap or formulate, to plug into the cosmic archetype or the natural archetypal form of man's multi-leveled personality, enabling him to resolve conflicts between himself, the environment and others but more important to resolve his inner conflicts, because confusion and chaos within contribute to frustration, aggression and violence without.

The invention of a system for understanding the universe and ourself, beyond the religious and theoretical and conceptual modes of communicating, would have to employ the skillful use of man's higher faculties, at present little researched, such as the powers of the imagination over the physical vehicle, the power of consciousness to intervene in material events on higher levels of functioning, and the faculty of vision or the anticipatory ability of consciousness to get into the future and work on the present thereby setting up a guiding-field for planetary organisms to naturally follow. The role of consciousness in building an evolutionary instrument out of the biological materials we inherit as humans would not only supersede the telephone, television and other slower means of communication dependent on material equipment, but would make the potentialities inherited in our genes provide us with a super-efficient computer in the brain.

The brain is the slave of our consciousness and not our controller. It only controls those who do not know they have this power over their biological vehicle. We can also make our brain a servant of the cosmic will if we choose to tap into its superintelligent program. Our brain can, if we so choose, function as a superintelligent add-on unit to the existing superintelligence hidden in the total environment around us. The only real problem in the human world is that humans do not know how to do this, nor do most humans think it is important to do it. This is the true purpose of all religions everywhere, yet we settle for so much less when we embrace a dogma or doctrine.

Human consciousness, being polarized to earth rather than the light of space, would rather believe in man's original sin and ignore the possibility of direct illumination which would mean a radical change in beliefs. The teaching of the church with its positive emphasis on compassion for others could hardly be called negative, yet original sin and Satan are preached full swing on Sunday on radio and television networks all over America, and millions of people listen. The beliefs of the church concerning the thirteen devils who were formerly angels and were consigned to Hell for their rebellion against God, along with the

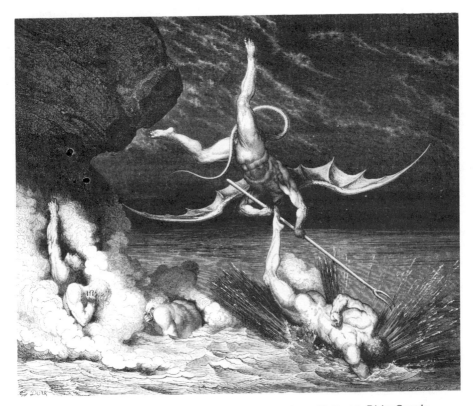

Gustave Dore's illustration of a demon tormenting one of the damned in Dante's *Divine Comedy.*

chief among them, Lucifer, are still openly and widely taught, though their origin was Saint Ignatius of the first century A.D.

The difficulty of our scientific age is that skeptical modern thinkers cannot accept this church teaching as valid knowledge because it has no possibility of proof, and in addition many of these church dogmas have nothing to do with divine intelligence but are merely concepts from the days of the Inquisition. They can make no individual more intelligent or more skillful in the use of his or her consciousness. What we must do now is find out scientifically how our mind really works and how it unconsciously manufactures such archetypes about sin, Satan, and God, out of consciousness, thereby blocking the clarity of the divine intelligence with *human* ideas. Why is it that humans prefer to "tinker" with the world and become a race of "smatterers" rather than go direct to the Ancient of Days? They prefer to meddle with what they do not understand, rather than have complete clarity on the real issues of life. What we need now on earth is the ability to tap the inexhaustible intelligence written into every nucleus of every cell of the brain. This means giving up human dogma and theories and seeking the source of consciousness directly in the surrender of our thought processes to God—the superintelligent nucleus at the heart of all systems, organic or inorganic. This would be the equivalent of having the most sophisticated equipment and having an instruction book on how to work it, whereas at the moment we have the equipment in the brain but nowhere can we find specific instructions from Nature on how to use it.

For man's consciousness to use this knowledge of his own capacity for cooperation, synthesis of all that is known, and the transmission of complete thoughts rather than semantic patchworks—the kind of wholistic thinking that can only come when all the brain computers are functioning as one—would enable each human being to become a direct thought-writer, writing and replicating his or her own thoughts in the mind of another, just as we now write on paper or use a typewriter. We would have the equivalent of having our thoughts picked up by a typewriter and having it clatter away and type them out. But instead this would be happening in another person's mind on several levels by virtue of a new type of clairvoyance or telepathy transmitted by the vibrations of the heart rather than by images in the head.

TELE-THOUGHT

Telepathy comes from the root word *tele* (meaning distance, as in tele-vision) and *pathy* (meaning feeling). Telepathy has not been universally accepted by all scientists although many have come to believe in it through experimental evidence available at the Parapsychological Associations of Britain and America. Many scientists, physicists and psychologists have investigated it and now know that it is no longer just a speculative phenomenon. There is also a large body of scientists who demand proof of telepathy without bothering to investigate it themselves. Somehow they feel that those who have investigated should go around convincing the doubters. They pick holes in reports as if that is a substitute for setting up first-hand experiments to validate evidence oneself. There are arrogant people who will not take time to do research on the subjects, and we can dismiss them for making pronouncements on what they have not tested. There is so much evidence that we can communicate beyond the mind if we *want* to find it. The best way to prove it is to do some simple experiments oneself, and it was for this reason that I wrote the book *Supersensonics** which gives several ways of proceeding scientifically with simple experiments for ordinary people to do. This type of "feeling at a distance" is similar to "seeing at a distance" which is sometimes referred to as clairvoyance. However we are talking here not of the classical clairvoyance involving messages in pictures or words but the kind of "sensing at a distance" communication which goes on between two people without words or images but in feelings. In this type of sensing, distance is no object because even close to our touch and close to our eyes we can see no more of a person's inmost thoughts than we can a thousand miles away.

Constantly, humans are exciting each other through a twilight zone of consciousness which represents ninety percent of the information we judge a person on. From an appearance on TV or merely seeing a photograph, one does not get the same feeling about a person as when we are actually in their presence. Yet we see them with our senses the same. When we see them in person, something else is transmitted in the vibration, the eyes which look into ours, the body posture, etc., and it is indefinable, so we say that we like or dislike a person. Different people give different reasons, but the fact is that when a person comes into the room or into our presence we have instant subtle feelings about them even before they open their mouths. Likewise we get feelings about a person's voice on the telephone even when we have never seen them. Do these feelings come from what they say or how they look externally? Or is it a natural reaction in which we receive ninety percent of the information that enables us to judge whether we like the person or not? Becoming aware of this interaction of consciousness is what I mean by "tele-thought"—a combination of tele-feeling and tele-vision, telepathy or clairvoyance. Why does this seem far-fetched to

---

* *Supersensonics*, the science of sensing radiation at a distance.

those who have not experimented? Because they do not realize that when you see a person even in front of your own eyes, your perceptual process must still get the images into your brain just as a video TV screen must get the images to the receiver in order for them to come out on a screen before us as a picture. Whether the person is near or far, in Africa or on the TV screen, the same image must be processed in the same way. If we are careful to think through this process ourself we will discover that we are always thinking things about people we know and people we live with at the unconscious level which determines instantly whether we will have a larger relationship or not, whether we shall fall in love or not, whether we shall trust the person or not. It is this information, vibration, thought beyond our conscious mind, which I call tele-thought because it determines our real communication with others. People who are not aware of this form of clairvoyance, even when everyone has it to a degree, usually are people who are shut off from their hearts. They rely entirely on the judgements in their heads, and although they are not in touch with "feelings" the one feeling they do have is that they are cut off, separated, set apart from the universe and the whole. They just cannot understand *tele-thought* because they cannot feel anything coming from people and even have difficulty feeling their own feeling. But underneath, they feel very strongly about how things are and should be and you only have to read what they write to know that they have gut level feelings about everything, and a sensitive person can pick this "thought-feeling" up as a vibration without any words.

We might ask, what is the difference between this kind of clairvoyance, and the transmission of messages through the psychic kind of clairvoyance which deals only with the nonsensory transmission of information at a distance? Most psychics see only the picture, feel only the feeling or hear only the words. This is merely *information.* ESP does not necessarily enable one to experience the depths of another person's being. Tele-thought is far more than information; it is knowing what is going on inside the other, and we can only know what is going on inside another on this level to the degree that we know ourself. Nuclear Evolution conceives of a much deeper communication than telepathy or clairvoyance, since all these thoughts and images are subject to subjective interpretation. The development of tele-thought is direct perception into the real nature beyond the images, thoughts or words. Tele-thought enables us to see not only into the hearts of humans but to see Nature's systems directly as they are. Communication within the nuclear model of the multi-leveled human, works through a primordial image set up by Nature as its own archetypal form of the nucleus of all life. This model is *not* subjective in the sense of being separate from the objective world. The levels of consciousness in the nuclear model are found repeated endlessly throughout every system of creation and are provable as such in the radiant spectrum of the universe and its universal energies.

The utilization of such tele-thought powers of our consciousness for the opening of faculties we already have built into the evolutionary instrument of the brain, are far more wonderful and mind-boggling than any new invention of vision at a distance such as television, since with tele-thought our consciousness would be everywhere, perceiving the Superintelligence at work throughout the whole, rather than being an infinitesimal human part lumbered with a superintelligent computer brain that we do not know how to use. We are cosmically the equivalent of beggars, scrambling for scraps in garbage cans while unknowingly we have the golden key to a vast storehouse of riches. Scientists are constantly hunting everywhere for the eyeglasses which will enable us to peer into the depths of Nature, and we do not realize that we have them in our own pocket. We get frustrated and angry at not finding them, only to find that they were always within our grasp. We have the microscope and telescope but these, like the television which depends for its far-seeing upon the material instrument, are only the beginning. I am talking about an instrument within, already put there in the genes and cells of our body and brain.

The fact that most people believe they are so far from ESP, much less from some bizarre idea of tele-thought, is a block in itself, since psychic abilities are not a prerequisite to tele-thought. Psychic faculties are of no evolutionary significance and are well-known to be spiritual blind alleys since the people who do have these gifts are sometimes lower down the evolutionary scale of self-awareness than those they "help". What we mean by tele-thought is not the form of the message but the content. The difference between reading the program notes at a concert and actually experiencing the music yourself is analogous to going to clairvoyants and having them read your future, since your future is in your own hands, and taking action now this very day which will make tomorrow a very different picture. On the other hand, if we stay the same now and do not invoke the secret power within us to mold the future, then we may as well have our reality dictated by clairvoyants and soothsayers, psychologists and scientists, politicians or other persons of doubtful leadership quality whose only claim to be ahead of us is a little more bumptiousness and arrogance and desire to be out front waving flags for us to follow, as if they knew more than we know of what is in store for us in the cosmic program.

What does it mean to say not the form but the content? The difference between communication at the level of concepts, ideas, ideologies, theories, words and similar methods of confusing our minds with half-baked perceptions to do with forms, rather than freeing our consciousness from such claptrap to enable the direct perception of content, is the mental and conceptual hurdle that prevents man from tele-thought. Tele-thought is the equivalent of Jung's *collective unconscious* which may arise in various parts of the world in different forms and symbols from the same archetypal roots in man everywhere. Love, hate, aggression, frustration, etc., are fundamental emotional energies written into our biological computer, and these are behind the rising of the symbols in the mind. The rising of the Phoenix is such an archetype, which brings with it the new capacity for communication on deeper levels of intelligence but at the cost of the burning up and consuming of old forms—namely old methods of validating knowledge, old traditional means of transmitting meaning, and old methods of thinking about our own limitations. The new rising of the cosmic thinker in light is available to anyone who can drop the limitations they have placed on their own consciousness, who can strip themselves of all conditioned responses, who can wash their own minds clear of egocentric thoughts about themselves or others, who can enter into the wisdom pool and bathe in the waters of eternal life which link them with all other intelligent organisms throughout the totality of space. This is the only real block to Nuclear Evolution and it is this block which is at the root of all human error, misperception and misunderstanding.

What is now needed are men and women of integrity who have the common sense to work for the divine intelligence without thoughts of personal reward, to bring about the highest undertaking conceivable to human beings. Their service can be offered in the name of any religion or philosophy of life since Nuclear Evolution is not in competition with anyone or with any ideals. This is not an idealistic call to believe in anything but to evolve the most fulfilling potential in their own lifestyle. To embark on this new training, designed to open up the already-programmed brain, provides any individual with the vision to undergo the process of Nuclear Evolution and to reveal the beauty of its creative intelligence. Once you can see the missing ingredient in your relationships there is no choice left but to set about doing Nuclear Evolution, because the realization knocks you over that to go back to the old and tried images of the old form is to betray your own soul. For the insightful individual who catches the vision this is a great discovery, but what of humanity? The mass of humanity will not change unless there are individuals who lead the way by a dynamic example of community living which demonstrates another threshold of human existence. Thus penetration of the nucleus of group consciousness while developing a new kind of sensitivity with others is the first radical step in raising the potential of individuals. The invention of a new system of thought which can penetrate into the awareness of "the other", or even the awareness present in our own self, will show us how useless our old ways of thought have been through the centuries and how dead are mental *concepts* compared to the living energy and directional movement inherent in genuine archetypes. Archetypes, to intellectuals, are static symbols that only *point* to these deep energies in man; they think of an archetype arising only in the mind, like a concept. The grey areas in the human mind between the archetypal symbol and the reality of an actual *force* or intelligence or content working *through* all created forms is difficult for many people to accept, as they think of an archetype as an idea or thought rather than a real energy. This is because humans generally have not discovered the power of their own imagination over cosmic forces and, apart from a few people who pray and get results, there has been no real proof or manifestation in new life forms to show the archetype living and growing with the energy we unconsciously feed to it. The coming of group consciousness, where each individual in the group makes himself or herself into a willing participant and servant of the cosmic will, enables a new organ to be formed in the human being just as inorganic atoms and molecules and organic cells form our own organs which are capable of functioning on higher levels than the individual parts. So will humans, when they discover *content* rather than *form,* be capable of loving in a wholly new way and on a different level than they have ever loved before.

EXPANSION OF THE SEED OF LOVE

Whenever the sense of righteousness wanes, the dark forces of involution, materialism and domination pervade the hearts of human souls. A corresponding tension is thereby created in the psychic atmosphere of millions of common people. In order to preserve equilibrium and peace of mind, an answering evolutionary manifestation of righteousness is essential. This cannot be merely in the form of ideas, books, or theories but must make a start with small groups of actual living people. It is then that the superintelligent consciousness of the cosmic creative energy (Saguna Brahman in Sanskrit) becomes manifest in human embodiment all over the planet, determined to throw off the shackles of all that is gross, material-minded, dominating, selfish and highly reactive.

Here we discuss the nature of action because any expansion of the nucleus before it is ready only expands all the problems of the mind and its physical servant, the active body. We must discriminate carefully between "self-righteousness" and "righteousness", because until we fully know the difference we are not ready, however much we may protest. The word righteousness means "right action" and "right thinking". The Sermon on the Mount and the *Bhagavad-Gita* express these cosmic ideas of right relationships in terms which, although still very true, have had little effect on the present darkness of the planet. We know the familiar words and concepts. We know they are true but, couched in their old language, their true meaning and revelation of cosmic laws escapes us. Millions of books of these words are sold every year and people revere them as never before, yet the dark forces on the planet encroach more and more. The time has come when we can no longer put off that day we have always known would come; we must begin at last to *live* the teachings or our species will annihilate itself.

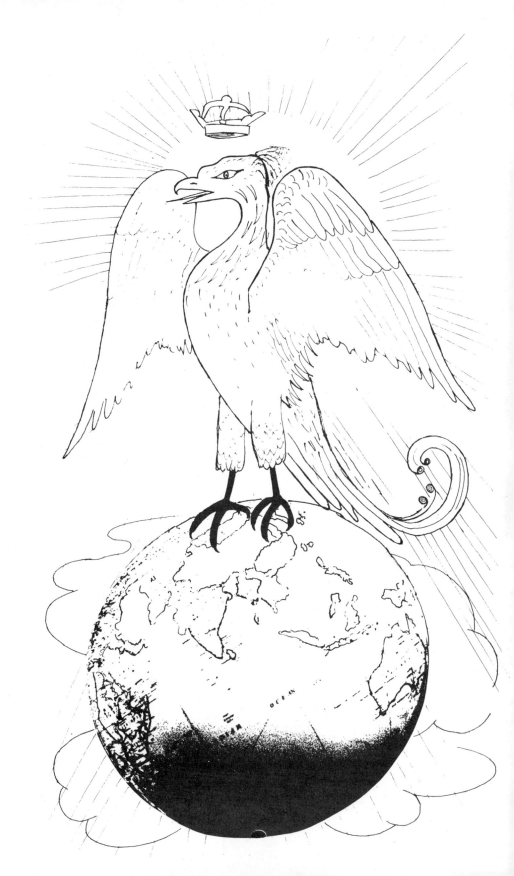

The planet is the wisdom school for saints which sets the tasks and examines man's awareness of the great opportunities for the human race to "grow". Life is a gift of consciousness. It is offered to us from the supreme consciousness so that we may transmute our egocentric personality completely. The suffering world is offered to us that we may redeem it of our past ignorance.

The total environment in which we function as a being is a superintelligent entity beyond our senses. Only the "supersense" can fathom its purpose. The environment is an intelligent "field" of righteousness in the hearts of men and women where the lord of the body—"the Self"—sits actively present on its central throne at the seat of consciousness. The evolution of the human spirit takes place in consciousness in the "field of righteousness" in the souls of humans yearly, daily and hourly and is written in the quality of your life, is glorified in the quality of your joy, and is fulfilled in your love of the whole world and cosmos. This "field" which includes you and the environment is the nucleus of the whole universe and even now, as you spend a few minutes or hours of your life reading these words, it is powerfully present within you. This field of consciousness, vibrating on several levels, is the absolute individual indivisible "you"—the nuclear Self.

There exists a little known "Science of the Absolute" which is given to different Avatars in times of great uncertainty and death concerning this "nuclear Self". To meet one of these Avatars is to meet them all, for they all say the same thing in different words. The true Avatar never declares himself for he is always declared by others. The most he can say is that

I and God are ONE!

—not declaring himself to be God, as egocentric people think, but instead saying there is no "I" present to separate itself from God. This Science of the Absolute is the transcendence of life and death through the dis-identification of consciousness with all that is separative and divisive—even our own thoughts of God as external to consciousness! Eternal life in these times of uncertainty is never really thought of by earth people as a cosmic absolute. Even the matter-less singularity of the Black Hole conceived of by physicists is believed to be no more than the death of a giant star which eats light, for they have not yet seen that the Phoenix is the seed fire, rising out of the black hole of formless consciousness at the heart of all existence. Every human being is a micro-universe whose consciousness immediately annihilates all phenomena the second it is experienced. All thought is the past memory of the now which is gone in the instantaneous moment of perception. To recall any experience of the fleeting moment of now puts the being in the level of history and memory. The human race has lost its memory of its beginnings because, when the Phoenix rises again and again, the fire of consciousness annihilates all our thoughts in the black hole of actual physical death and blows away the mind at the moment of birth into the invisible white hole we call our ever-renewing consciousness of the creation.

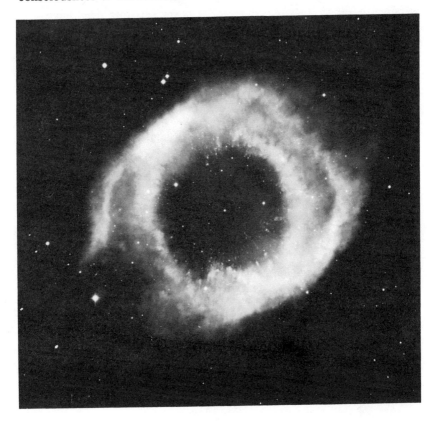

The universe is sucked into the black hole of our being and we are lost beyond the horizon of the self-sense as all thought dies in the silence of the formless One, who is our consciousness.

The Phoenix rises to call you to remember your real being. He or she or it is beyond all forms and classifications of consciousness because it is pure of all thoughts which cannot experience now, without creating time of yestermoment. Tomorrow to the Christ Consciousness is already now, because the seed thought of the experiencer is the fire consciousness, which creates both now and tomorrow just as it creates yesterday and yestermoment by reflection and thought.

WHAT IS THE ABSOLUTE?

The absolute nuclear Self eternally shines and vibrates as cosmic sound of creation and, like the sun, is never separate from the ever-renewing radiation of its own light—the light of consciousness—self-aware, self-resplendent in its own glory. But the eternal life of this nuclear Self is very different from the mere survival of bodily death. It is a very different event from the survival of the human soul, often ridiculed as unproved by selfish, egocentric and materialist societies. Although it is as indefinable as love, the eternal life of the nuclear Self is available to everyone now incarnate. Through selfless service to the whole of creation, the gross vibration of self-righteous judgements and the inability to see one's own blindness are gradually removed, so that we no longer feel that selflessness is a self-denial, but more an affirmation that ALL has become the Self. The whole vibrating external universe is experienced as the witness of one's inner self—the "I" of consciousness. The absolute is self-evident, needing no other, and is therefore self-luminous, and its illumination is its own reward for the inner work for the righteous and wise investigation of *that* which we have called pure consciousness.

How difficult and complex! exclaims our intellect. How many emotional hurdles our emotional body feels it must get over to gain that eternal reward of bliss divine! But the flash of lightning, the illumination across the mental sky, only awaits the insight that our consciousness is part of an indivisible and invisible network of other individuals who are parts of the same Self and are at work everywhere. They are parts of the hologram of our own consciousness, sacrificing themselves, integrating themselves, harmonizing and polarizing all of humanity into the synthesis of the nucleus. Such is the universal bond of the invisible nucleus expressing itself with that righteousness which is eternally present as consciousness of good in everything.

TRAINING THE INTELLECT TO PENETRATE THE HEART

Why do we write here of righteousness if books and words and religious thoughts cannot help us to break through into eternal life? This book is mainly written for those few who are ready to go into pure consciousness by purifying the heart by self-discipline and development of their discriminative faculties. Those who can think for themselves, whose intellects have found rest in tranquillity and whose minds are free from personal love and hatred and liberated from pairs of opposites, will experience an intense desire to experience the highest consciousness of their Universal Nuclear Self.

How does this happen in the rising light of the Phoenix? First must come the realization that the "I Am", the self-regarding essence which seems to be so different in everybody, is really the filtering of an all-pervading cosmic influence passing through various bodies which, although different from one another in form, become *ONE* on the annihilation of ego-identification with bodies. Our birth, our death, our class, creed, gender and nationality, all so important in the world, all belong to the body. Whenever the Self—the I AM—the consciousness identifies with the body, then it appears to most people who view the hologram of life that the different characteristics of our physical material bodies are always superimposed on our idea of "Self". This illusion is not easily understood without deep meditation and deep self-analysis.

The wise one, therefore, through the continuous investigation of Self—Who am I?—discriminates and separates the pure and the fake residing in the inmost Self—the I—from all those bodies with which it has become closely identified. With the same awareness that we can separate the kernel from the husk do we know that the nut or seed of self-consciousness is all-pervading. Even while experiencing itself as separate, consciousness is falling upon every object of perception equally, from the center within. Although everyone looks out of their consciousness, they do not realize that the same basic awareness of being is in everything. What is it in mankind which prevents the self from cognition of this superintelligence in the mirror of our self-consciousness? Is the universe or life really a mirror to our self? The self-consciousness obviously transcends the body and all its psychological and physical functions on different thresholds of being, but because human intelligence identifies the Self—I AM—with these separate functions, in ignorance of our true nature, we cannot see that our consciousness is merely acting as a witness of those separate functions, and like a ruler or sovereign, is their controller. Although supreme consciousness is king over all our functions of brain and mind, yet it remains totally different from them because it is always the eternal subject, the unchanging consciousness, from birth to death, in itself quite unqualified by its daily association with external and ever-changing objects of the world. The same which says I AM today, is the same I AM of yesterday, of yesteryear and of yesterlife.

WHO ARE YOU?

The nuclear Self shines as the invisible light throughout the whole of space so that when the identity of the universal light of consciousness is kindled in the heart, the individual one (the indivisible one) shines forth as the same universal light of I (pure consciousness) in the same way as the sun shines into our consciousness when clouds move out of the way. The sun shines eternally, one with its own light behind the clouds, in exactly the same way that the true Self shines behind the clouds of ego-consciousness. The self-realized person who penetrates the nucleus, experiences existence as bliss everywhere and at the heart of every object of the universe. Those who work only for themselves or their own family or own country live in vain and are divided from the teacher of righteousness. That teacher of right action is the rising cosmic vibration of Nadam, the superintelligent sound current of eternal ever-renewing consciousness.

In short, the voice of God.

Do you hear that voice? Many ask how can the I—the human self—hear the voice of God? The answer is that those who do the will of God fulfill themselves in right action, and in so doing, hear the voice of God.

The Phoenix says in the heart—I am ONE great singularity in which all exists as invisible consciousness of self. I am the indestructible self whom you cannot see nor image nor sense because I flow out of your eyes as formless light and illuminate all around you. When I rise in the center of your being I rise up in the center of all beings, for I am your self, that one who is self-revealing and selfless, that one who flies to the outermost reaches of space in the timeless instant and returns to emerge in its own cosmic seed in your exploding light of the mind. I am the light of consciousness, invisible, immortal and beyond death, and am continuously born as the experiencer of all the worlds.

The Phoenix comes to show you the book of Nature and open the doors of direct perception.

There is no other.

I am indivisible pure consciousness annihilating itself at the instant of self-recognition. That is why you cannot see me either in yourself or in the worlds that you observe. Yet I am here like the invisible radio wave and the unseen light of the stars passing through the blackness of space.

I am that one you seek, forever chasing yourself through eons of timeless love. I see you in your own eye beams and experience whatever you see. Whatever you limit with your consciousness you limit also in me.

I am the Phoenix who flies into the sun, that one who is consumed by its own appetite for love.

I am the lover of all existence who radiates in your being and awaits the golden dawn of your rising.

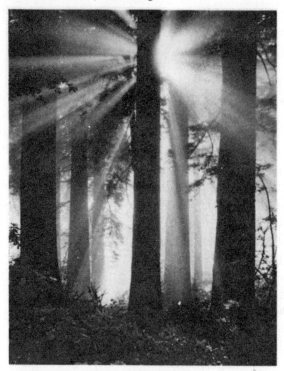

As the light is hidden by the redwood trees, so the Self hides behind your ego, waiting to be discovered.

The consciousness which writes and speaks itself in you is mine and mine alone. You are that. You will always be that. Though you cloud over your awareness with inner conflicts, though you are anxious as to my existence, though you are frustrated at your ignorance of me, I am yet that also. For the veil is also of my doing, that I may be at peace with my own light in you. The separation is not real; only your consciousness can make that which is real become real for you.

The Phoenix is a myth of that reality which cannot be spoken or formed into thoughts.

It is "thatness" which you alone can see with the isness of your own awareness. The message of the Phoenix is that your conflict is unnecessary.

God is consciousness.
Consciousness is God.
Pure consciousness is beyond any idea
of God.
Gods are mental creations of your
consciousness, whereas I am uncreated
and whole without limits or ideals.

Worship me as the light of consciousness
and I shall rise again in all things
and capture your heart.
For I am the love you seek which
turns on the lovelight in your own eye.
I am the egoless "I" which knows no
destruction of self. I am the life which
knows no death.
Ponder deeply the words of Christ,
Krishna, Buddha and those who are born with
the seed fire of the Cosmos (divine consciousness).
For I am the Phoenix, who rises from the ashes
of destruction of all that divides
the (individable) individual.
Of such is your own light.

"Arise, shine; for thy light is come,
and the glory of the Lord is risen upon thee.

For, behold, the darkness shall cover the earth,
and gross darkness the peoples;
but the Lord shall rise upon thee,
and his glory shall be seen upon thee.

And the nations shall come to thy light,
and the kings to the brightness of thy rising."

Isaiah 60: 1-3

As the lightning flashes from East to West and suddenly illuminates the whole world around us, so does the Phoenix rise again and light up the world within us.

>Ask not the Phoenix to bring that light.
>You *are* that light!
>Ask not that you shall find love.
>You are that love!

INDEX

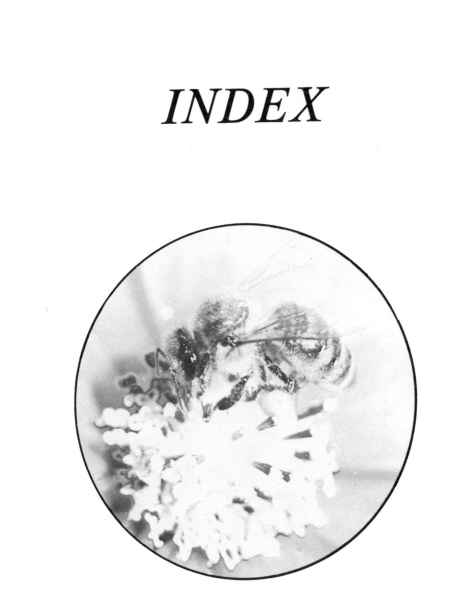

INDEX

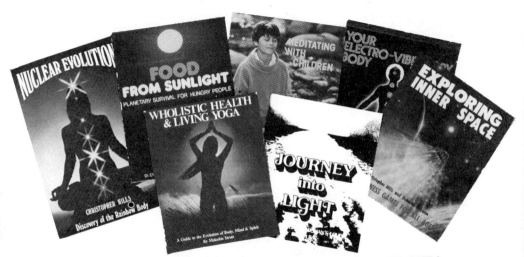

BOOKS BY MEMBERS OF THE UNIVERSITY OF THE TREES

Nuclear Evolution: Discovery of the Rainbow Body, by Christopher Hills, Ph.D., D.Sc.
Deluxe paperback 12.95   Hardback library edition 18.95
Christopher Hills takes us on an astonishing journey through the levels of awareness, exploring in depth the structure of the Rainbow Body. Using a unique psychology of wisdom to view Light, Aura Colors, Chakras, Kundalini, the I Ching and much more, he unfolds new designs for planetary living and breakthroughs in self-discovery. This book penetrates the whole spectrum of the spiritual path and shows us how to use light to transform our life situation. A scientific investigation of the evolutionary intelligence and the mystery of human consciousness. 1024 pages, 320 illustrations.

Food From Sunlight, by Christopher Hills, Ph.D., D.Sc., Hiroshi Nakamura, D.Sc.   14.95
The Japanese have known since 1917 that successful harvesting of algae would produce infinite amounts of food from air, light and water. Failure to do so prompted in 1959 the Japanese newspaper article *Chlorella Algae, the Manna from Heaven, is a Twentieth Century Myth.* But in 1963 Spirulina algae was discovered and, over the next ten years, brought manna from heaven to a reality. In Japan it now sells ounce for ounce the same price as gold, due to its nutritional values and rejuvenation properties.

Wholistic Health and Living Yoga, by Malcolm Strutt, M.A.   9.95
A new wholistic approach to the spiritual science of total health which includes the application of yogic principles to daily living situations, complete self-examination and encounters, yoga postures, meditations, breathing and energizing methods, and other practical techniques for spiritual stimulation.

Your Electro-Vibratory Body, by Victor Beasley, Ph.D.   9.95
This book contains a selection of research from the world's foremost pioneers who look at the human body as a collection of atoms and molecules whirling around in space. They see the effects of one's auric field extending far beyond the physical body. They show how your mood, personality and health are affected and governed by magnetic and electric fields, positive and negative ions, light and colors, and even the thoughts of others. This information, once regarded as occult, is now the focus of research by M.D.'s and Ph.D.'s.

Exploring Inner Space, by Christopher Hills, Ph.D., D.Sc. and Deborah Rozman, Ph.D.   9.95
Take a space journey through the worlds that lie within you. Explore the nature of light and energy as they are expressed through the seven inner time-space dimensions. This handbook of awareness-expanding games for all ages leads you to experience your real self and develop new skills in creative communication.

Journey Into Light, by Ann Ray, Ph.D.   7.95
Ann Ray's personal experience of Nuclear Evolution and the teachings and research of Christopher Hills on light, color and the transforming power of consciousness. The author gives a frank and open account of her own spiritual journey toward ego death and how this journey feels and what it requires of every person who sets his or her course in that direction.

Meditating With Children, by Deborah Rozman, Ph.D.   5.95
The first of its kind! A delightful teaching book that brings the great art and science of meditation and conscious evolution to children of all ages. This workbook is being used in classrooms throughout the country as a nonreligious text in centering and awareness development. Excellent results achieved with gifted, average, retarded and hyperactive children.

All prices are subject to change without notice.

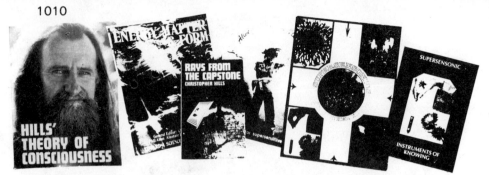

Energy, Matter and Form, by P. Allen, M.A., R. Smith and A. Bearne   9.95
Three consciousness researchers provide a dynamic workbook for those ready to test the bounds of their consciousness. It shows how to perform experiments for unfolding extraordinary dimensions of experience. This comprehensive text presents extensive information and insight into the human aura, psychic energy centers, kundalini, psychotronics, electrophotography, divining, acupuncture research, radionics, holography, black holes, pyramid energies and the Creative Imagination.

Alive to the Universe, by Robert Massy, Ph.D.   9.95
A physicist explains Supersensonics in simple layman's language, and gives step-by-step instructions on how to divine for lost objects, people, water, minerals, health, etc. Your vast potential for multi-dimensional awareness awaits unfolding through this book. An illustration a page.

Hills' Theory of Consciousness, by Robert Massy, Ph.D.   7.95
A student of a master of consciousness describes his own development in a group of 15 selected students of Nuclear Evolution. This book contains simplified accounts of inspired research of the actual structure of Consciousness and its many drives which physicist Massy believes will dominate the next 500-1,000 years of man's history.

Supersensonics, by Christopher Hills, Ph.D., D.Sc.   15.00
The Diviner's bible and encyclopedia that describes actual methods of measuring psychic electricity (prana) and the ways ancient masters and civilizations arrived at advanced knowledge of perception. Shows you how to communicate with plants, crystals, atoms, Cosmic Intelligences or your true Self. A mind-bending book.

Rays From the Capstone, Christopher Hills, Ph.D., D.Sc.   4.95
Find some refreshing answers about what's really going on inside a pyramid. It is the first to clearly set out what energies are generated and what effects these forces have on you, your food, plants, etc.

Instruments of Knowing, Christopher Hills, Ph.D., D.Sc.   1.95
This book describes over thirty divining tools and the hundreds of uses they have. The miracles of Christ are linked to divining.

Send for a free catalog of our complete line of Supersensonic instruments.

UPCOMING BOOKS BY CHRISTOPHER HILLS

The Golden Egg is a practical how-to accompaniment to **Rise of the Phoenix**. While **Rise of the Phoenix** is the vision that is before us now, **The Golden Egg** shows specific ways that this vision can be manifested by you in your own home, business and community to produce evolutionary methods of self-government which serve the whole. The practice of Creative Conflict, Common Ownership of business, and how to set up a nuclear community are all laid out with explicit instructions. The World Peace Center Constitution which can be applied to a business, a church, a school or a community is given in full as well as instructions for its implementation. **The Golden Egg** supplies the alternative to Capitalism and Communism that we are all seeking which can be used by nations as well as small groups, and provides us with a synthesis of the best of both systems as well as the missing spiritual ingredient that brings evolutionary growth. Available July/August, 1979.

Out of the Fire of the Nucleus reveals the polarization of the forces which are bringing the world to a final confrontation with the egocentric powers presently dominating. It shows these forces of darkness as actual energies and psychological realities which can only be countered with full use of the power of light. This final book gives the answer of *how to use* light to enable man to love enough to conquer the negative forces around him and to live a new way of life which protects the nuclear community *psychotronically*. Exploding all limiting human concepts of peace and love, this book is an adventure into an era which is imminent, and which, when it dawns, may find us asleep. **Out of the Fire of the Nucleus** calls us to prepare ourselves and gives us the means to do so. Available October/November, 1979.

All prices are subject to change without notice.